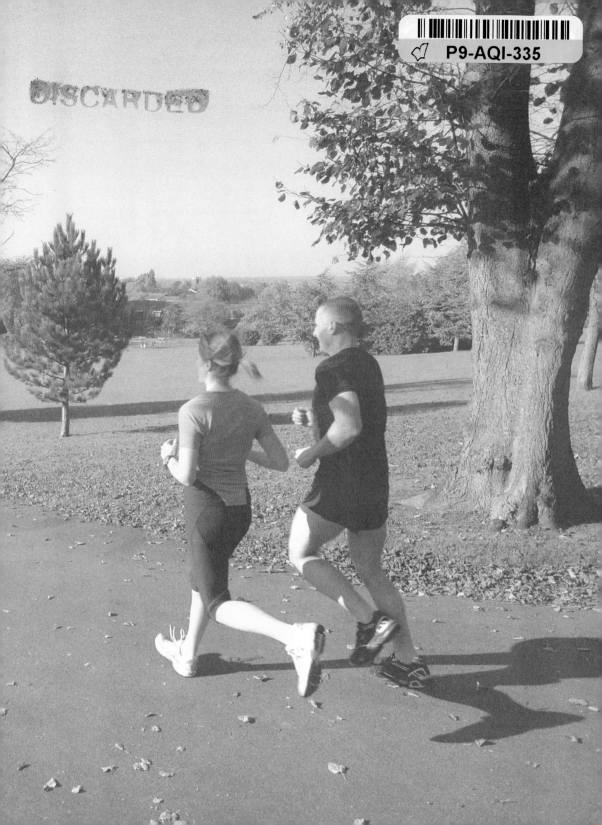

THE COMPLETE PRACTICAL ENCYCLOPEDIA OF
RUNNING, CYCLING
& FITNESS TRAINING

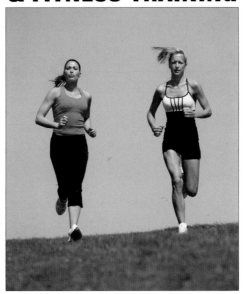

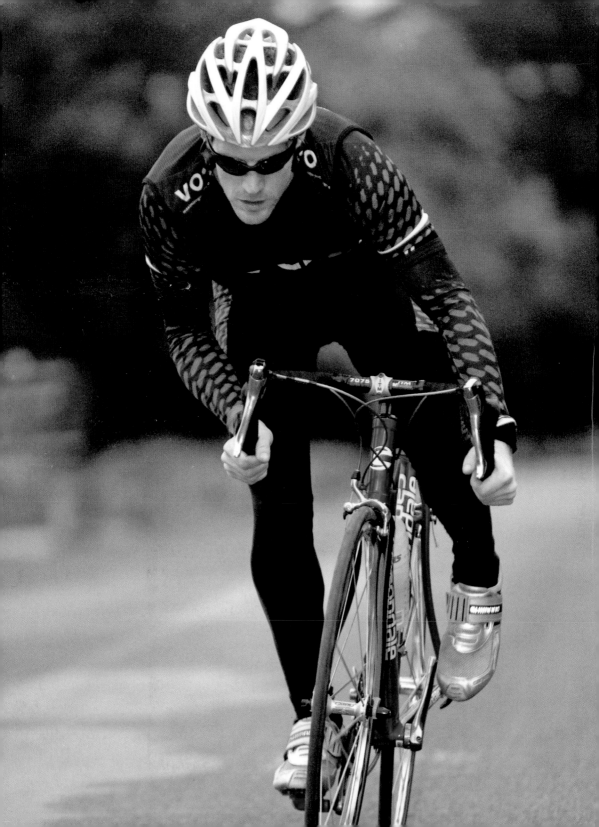

THE COMPLETE PRACTICAL ENCYCLOPEDIA OF

RUNNING, CYCLING & FITNESS TRAINING

THE ULTIMATE COMPENDIUM FOR STAYING ACTIVE, GETTING FIT AND IMPROVING YOUR SKILLS, WHETHER YOU RUN AND CYCLE FOR LEISURE OR FOR COMPETITIONS AND RACES

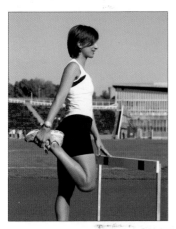 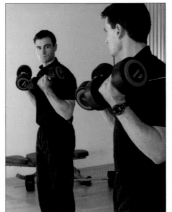 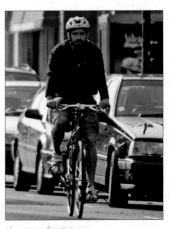

STEP-BY-STEP INSTRUCTIONS, TRAINING PLANS, NUTRITIONAL INFORMATION AND EXPERT ADVICE, ALL SHOWN IN MORE THAN 1350 FANTASTIC PHOTOGRAPHS AND ILLUSTRATIONS

ELIZABETH HUFTON • EDWARD PICKERING • ANDY WADSWORTH

LORENZ BOOKS

This edition is published by Lorenz Books, an imprint of Anness Publishing Ltd, Blaby Road, Wigston, Leicestershire LE18 4SE

Email: info@anness.com

Web: www.lorenzbooks.com; www.annesspublishing.com

Anness Publishing has a new picture agency outlet for images for publishing, promotions or advertising. Please visit our website www.practicalpictures.com for more information.

ETHICAL TRADING POLICY
At Anness Publishing we believe that business should be conducted in an ethical and ecologically sustainable way, with respect for the environment and a proper regard to the replacement of the natural resources we employ.
As a publisher, we use a lot of wood pulp in high-quality paper for printing, and that wood commonly comes from spruce trees. We are therefore currently growing more than 750,000 trees in three Scottish forest plantations: Berrymoss (130 hectares/320 acres), West Touxhill (125 hectares/305 acres) and Deveron Forest (75 hectares/185 acres). The forests we manage contain more than 3.5 times the number of trees employed each year in making paper for the books we manufacture.
Because of this ongoing ecological investment programme, you, as our customer, can have the pleasure and reassurance of knowing that a tree is being cultivated on your behalf to naturally replace the materials used to make the book you are holding. For further information about this scheme, go to www.annesspublishing.com/trees

© Anness Publishing Ltd 2011

Parts of this book have previously been published in three separate volumes:
The Illustrated Practical Encyclopedia of Running, The Illustrated Practical Encyclopedia of Cycling and The Illustrated Practical Encyclopedia of Fitness Training.

Publisher: Joanna Lorenz
Project Editors: Amy Christian, Anne Hildyard, Brian Burns and Hannah Consterdine
Photographers: Phil O'Connor, Mike King and Geoff Waugh
Designers: Nigel Partridge and Steve West
Illustrator: Peter Bull
Production Controller: Mai-Ling Collyer

PUBLISHER'S NOTE:
Although the advice and information in this book are believed to be accurate and true at the time of going to press, neither the authors nor the publisher can accept any legal responsibility or liability for any errors or omissions that may have been made nor for any inaccuracies nor for any loss, harm or injury that comes about from following instructions or advice in this book. You are advised to consult your doctor before commencing a new exercise programme.

CONTENTS

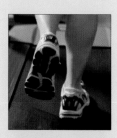
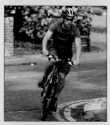
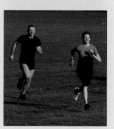
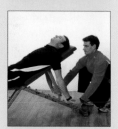
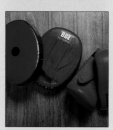

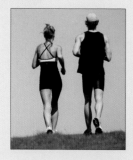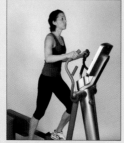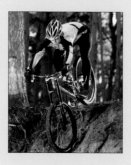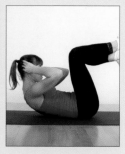

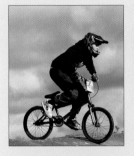 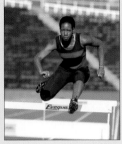 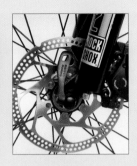 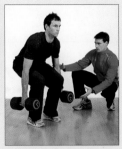

Introduction

With the wealth of running clubs, cycle paths and gyms around today, there has never been a better time to get involved. However and wherever you like to exercise, this book will show you how to start running, take up cycling, or improve your personal fitness.

This comprehensive compendium is an inspirational guide to two of the best known and most popular leisure activities, running and cycling, teamed together with an informed and practical general section dedicated to fitness training and achieving a healthy lifestyle.

The book covers everything you need to know to get started, improve, and then excel in both disciplines, whether you are a casual runner or cyclist for leisure, or looking to compete in local or national competitions. A complementary and essential section on fitness training shows you how to build up your stamina, strength and muscle, and also how to eat more healthily.

Below: Cycling is not only a practical way to get around but is fun and a great way to keep fit.

Part 1: Running

The running section begins with Getting Started, covering basics such as pre-run health checks, clothing, warming-up and stretching. In the opening chapters we will show you how to create a programme that works for you, and also how you can safely and effectively build up your miles and fitness, while staying healthy and injury-free.

Starting Events explains how to get involved in organized runs, with advice on which to choose, whether it's a 5K fun-run for charity or a 26-mile marathon. Detailed training plans take you right up to race day, all set at different levels so that you can train at a pace that is right for your fitness and experience.

Sprint and Middle-Distance Racing guides you through the different short- and middle-distance track events, with

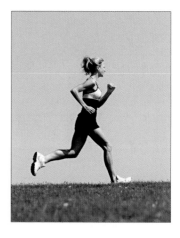

Above: One of the appeals of running is how little you need to get started – just find a pair of trainers and a nearby park.

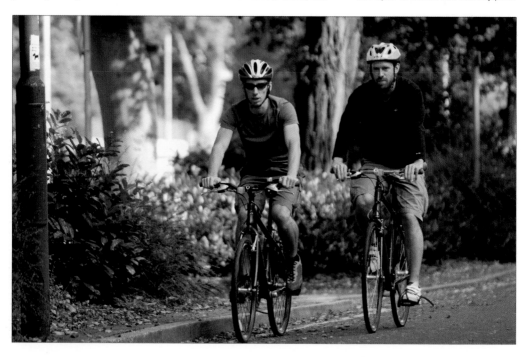

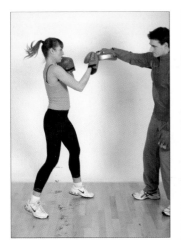

Above: Sparring with a partner helps to strengthen and tone your upper body – especially the arms and abdominals.

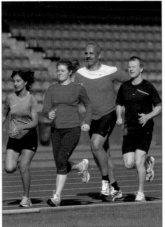

Above: Running with friends helps you to stay motivated in your training and can even be an enjoyable social activity.

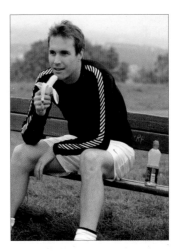

Above: It is important to eat and drink the right things to complement your training and exercise regime.

comprehensive exercise plans for drills, strength training, working with weights and building up speed endurance.

Advanced Long-Distance Running picks up where this chapter leaves off, providing dietary advice and training schedules for those with more experience, who may wish to race competitively or take part in more strenuous runs.

Part 2: Cycling

This section will explain everything you need to know to make the most of your cycling experience, whether you are a beginner or an expert, a road rider or a mountain biker.

If you are riding for pleasure, we will explain the basic skills you need to get started. We'll describe leisure cycling, commuting, cycling for the family and how to get your children involved. For the more adventurous, we will look at the ultimate in leisure cycling – touring. We'll explain how you can make your bike part of your holiday, and advise you on what to take and where to go.

The second chapter, Fast Riding, shows you how to use your bike to get fitter, or to take part in semi-competitive events. The section on sportives will guide you through the preparation, training and tactics for a

middle or long-distance sportive event. Then the action moves off road, to take you through the different disciplines of mountain biking. We'll look at cross-country trail riding and freeriding, and give advice on where in the world you can enjoy mountain biking.

The last chapter is about fully competitive cycling – racing on- and off-road, with explanations of tactics, strategies and skills. We'll also take a look at the world's greatest bike races, from the Tour de France to the Giro d'Italia.

Part 3: Fitness Training

This third section of the book covers everything you could need to implement a new exercise regime and improve your general fitness.

The opening chapters explain how to plan your training and the tests that you can do to judge your current level of fitness. It then introduces Cardiovascular Training; outlining the benefits and techniques, showing you how the most common equipment works, and looking at more unusual activities such as boxercise.

We move on to Resistance Training, with detailed step-by-step instructions for how to exercise specific muscles and parts of the body with specialized machines, dumbbells or free-weights.

There is also a key chapter on how to improve your flexibility and core stability, with a number of training plans designed for different levels of ability.

A final chapter on Nutrition explains how important healthy eating is to an active lifestyle. We'll show you how to adapt your diet to your personal needs, dietary requirements and fitness regime, with detailed notes on the benefits of certain foods, vitamins and minerals.

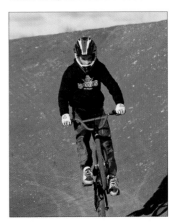

Above: Many children's first experience of cycling comes through BMXing, which enables them to develop riding skills, confidence and agility.

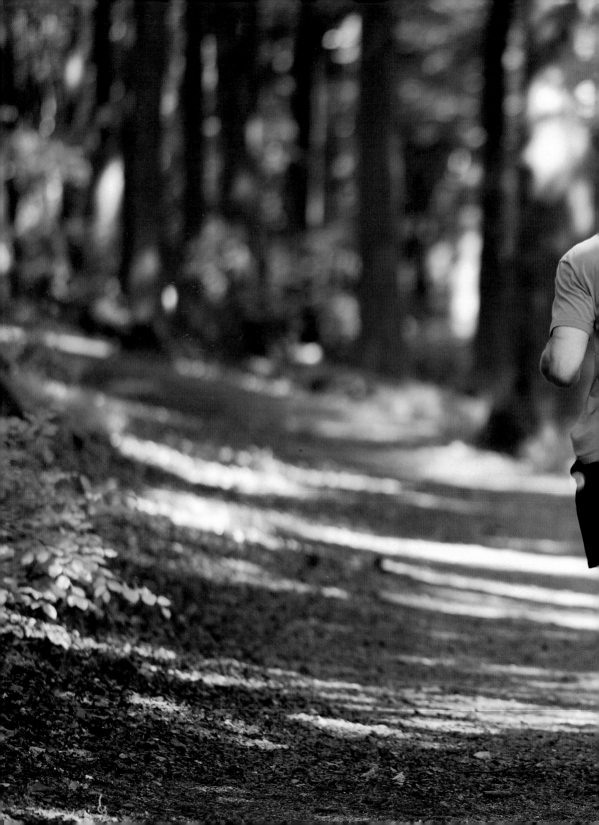

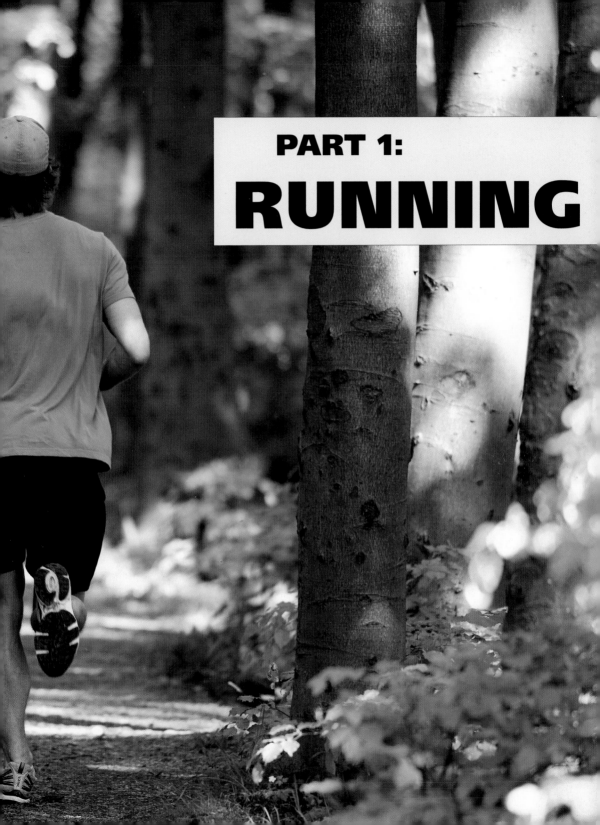

PART 1:
RUNNING

Introduction
to Running

Running is a natural activity. Almost as soon as a child can walk, he or she will try to run. Thousands of years ago, this natural instinct was born out of a need to run to survive, but these days many people have no need to run and, once we reach adulthood, often no desire to. Perhaps it is because of this, and the complications of modern life, that the last 50 years have seen a gradual growth in the number of people choosing to run; the simplicity and naturalness of the action appeals to people with otherwise cluttered lives.

Ironically the surge in participation and interest has made running more complicated; an entire industry has grown up around it, with fierce competition to develop more technical running shoes, clothes, and computers to analyse running data. At the same time, for all the millions of people running today, there are countless different reasons for doing so, and someone who starts with one goal in mind soon finds their motivation has changed. A recreational runner who starts out to lose weight becomes faster; he wants to race, then to race well, then perhaps to try to win. At the competitive end of the spectrum, the days of the have-a-go amateur athlete are gone, and training, nutrition, racing and recovery have become finely tuned scientific processes.

This is not bad news. As the runner becomes more involved in the finer details of the sport, he finds he has a better understanding of, and connection with, his own body. As a sport, running is perhaps the purest means of pushing the body to its very limit and finding out what you can do, since the basic technical ability is in all of us. This is as true for the elite athlete, pushing to find out whether the marathon can be run closer to the two-hour mark, as it is for the everyday runner curious to see if he can break three hours for a marathon or just make it to the end of his first 10K race.

No matter what your running origins or future, this section aims to help you make the most of the sport you love, from beginners to advanced runners, children to veterans, sprinters to marathon runners and beyond. It contains all the information you will need to fine-tune your running, and, hopefully, the inspiration you will need to enjoy running for pleasure, whichever direction you choose to take.

Right: Running is the perfect sport for connecting with your body and with the world around you. You don't need any special equipment to get going.

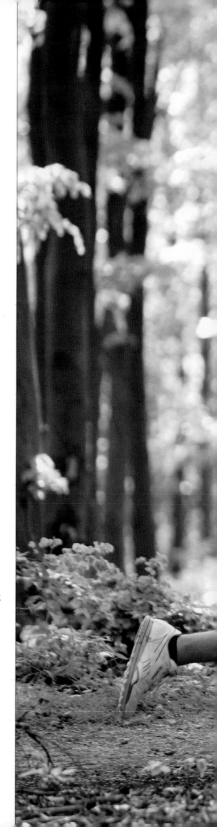

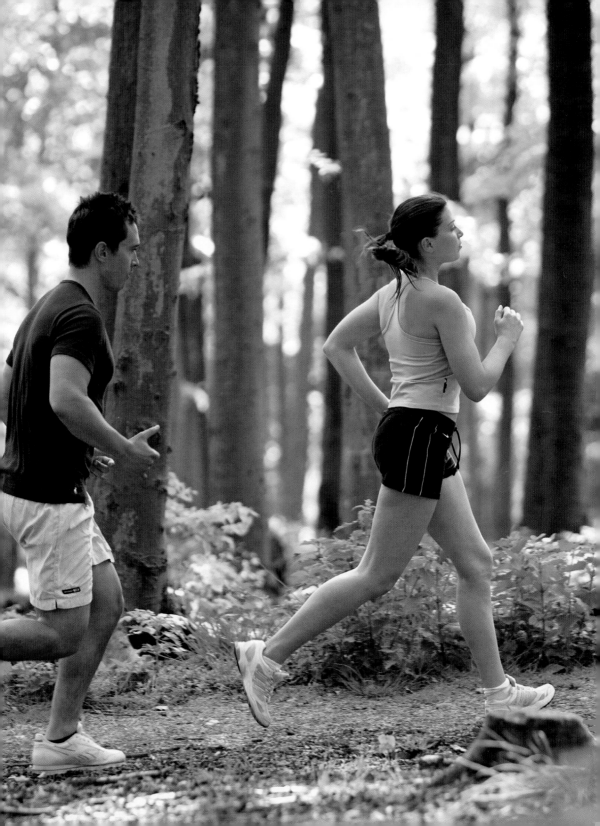

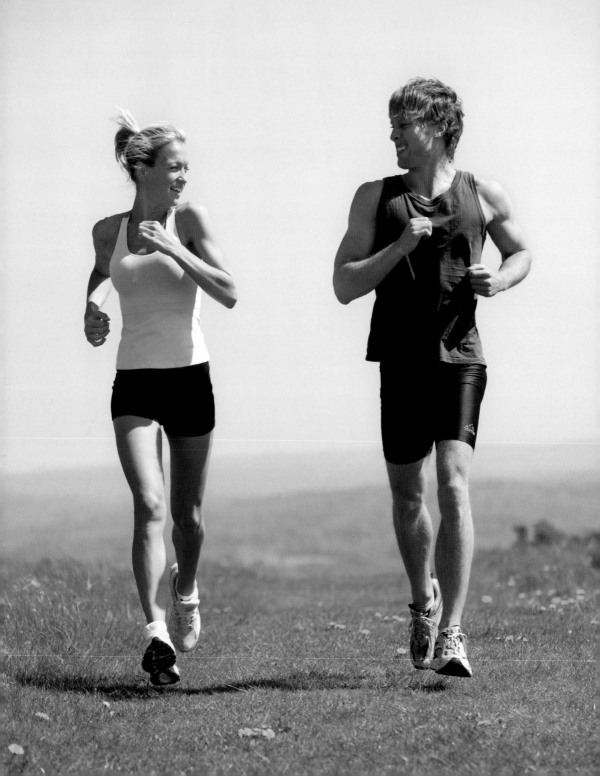

GETTING STARTED

Despite its simplicity, running is a misunderstood
form of exercise. Start out on the wrong foot, and
you could be turned off immediately. This chapter
looks at how thousands of people have found
the right way to run over the last few decades,
and how and why you can and should join them.
It provides all the information you need to get
from no exercise at all to being able to run for
30 minutes, five times a week, and to build the
foundation for more advanced running later on.

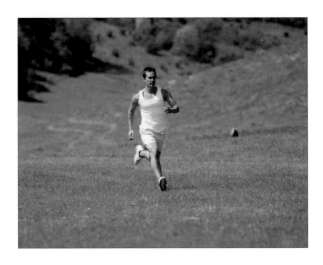

Above: Your first runs should be fun and energizing, so keep them easy.
Left: It's hard to take your first steps as a runner – starting out with a friend will
keep you motivated.

Running Today

From the streets of New York and London, running has now reached a peak in the USA, Europe and around the Western world. In a movement described as the second running boom, the sport has reached a wider base of participants with varying reasons for getting involved.

It is impossible to give an accurate figure for the number of runners worldwide – or even in any one country – because the very simplicity of running that draws so many people is such that there is no need to register or tell anyone that you run; in fact, many who do so may not consider themselves to be 'runners' at all. Nevertheless, it is safe to say that the second running boom is even bigger, more encompassing and more prolonged than the first.

Running the numbers

The only thing that can be said for certain about the typical runner today is that he or she could be anyone. However, there is no doubt that the face of marathon running has changed.

	1980	1995	2006
Women as % of runners	10.5%	26%	40%
Men as % of runners	89.5%	74%	60%
Masters (over 40)	26%	44%	46%
Average marathon times: Men	3:32:17	3:54:00	4:15:34
Average marathon times: Women	4:03:39	4:15:00	4:46:40

(Figures for USA, source: Running USA Road Running Information Center annual marathon report)

Keeping pace with change

While the first running boom was inspired (at first) by the performances of elite athletes such as Frank Shorter,

Below: The Paris Marathon is the second biggest in Europe, attracting runners with its wide streets and flat course.

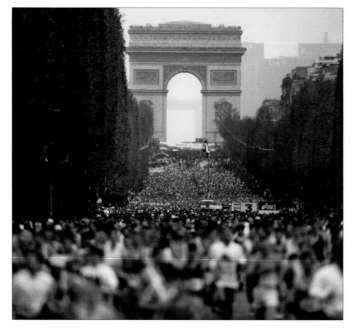

and focused on the challenge of running a marathon as quickly as possible, the second surge has a different focus – or lack of focus. Runners in the 70s and early 80s were usually male, under 40 years of age, and ran to compete, but there is

now a roughly 50:50 gender split, with more masters (or veterans) running, and reasons for running range from a means of losing weight, to raising money for charity, or a way to beat stress.

The second running boom has been driven by a number of factors. The most noticeable has been the increased involvement of large charities setting up their own running events, with an emphasis on taking part rather than fierce competition. This change in atmosphere has drawn more women to the sport. In particular, women-only charity races such as Race for the Cure in the USA and the Race for Life series in the UK have created a new type of event, encouraging participants to run to improve their health and fitness while raising vast sums of money for charity. Over 3.4 million women have taken part in the Race for Life, raising over £200 million for Cancer Research UK – an event which began with a single race with just 680 runners in 1994.

A sport for everyone

This 'taking part' ethos has flowed through to more established events, such as the big city marathons that started the first running boom. Where runners may once have given

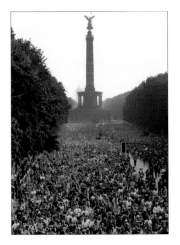

Above: The Real Berlin Marathon was the setting for the men's world marathon record in 2008, 2:03:59.

up at the age of 40, frustrated that they could no longer compete at the front of the field, many of them now continue, choosing to compete against their age-group peers, creating the phenomenon of Masters (or Vets) competitions. Running has also benefited from increasing concern about public health: with rates of obesity, diabetes and lifestyle-related conditions increasing, exercise is seen as part of the solution. Running is cheap, accessible and perhaps the most time-efficient form of exercise available, and public health bodies recognize its importance particularly for those whose socio-economic backgrounds put them most at risk of lifestyle-related health problems.

At the same time, a running industry that helps to support newcomers has grown with the second running boom. Never has so much specialist running equipment, information and so many resources been available to people thinking of taking up running. Where once athletics clubs only catered for those willing to train extremely hard for top-three race places, clubs now cater for all ages and abilities, and a new type of informal running network has sprung up.

Professional race organizers stage huge events in countries all over the world, creating 'destination' events, to which people are willing to travel great distances for the experience of visiting a place rather than a fast finishing time.

Now the process has gone full circle. With participation at an all-time high, more people are discovering a talent for running and hunger for competition that they didn't know they had, so the traditional athletics clubs are benefiting from a new influx of fast runners.

Below: The Chicago Marathon, part of the World Marathon majors series, is home to the women's World Marathon record.

World's largest marathons: 2007 (finishers)	
ING New York City Marathon	38,557
Flora London Marathon	35,667
Real Berlin Marathon	32,638
Paris Marathon (2006)	30,739
LaSalle Bank Chicago Marathon	28,815
Honolulu Marathon (2006)	24,573
Marine Corps Marathon	20,622
Boston Marathon	20,348
City of Los Angeles Marathon	20,120
Conenergy Hamburg Marathon (2006)	16,375

How many runners are there?

The only country to carry out a census of runners is the USA where, in 2005, 37.8 million people reported running at least three times a week. Elsewhere, a reasonable estimate of the numbers of regular runners can be made from the circulations of different countries' specialist running magazines (figures shown here are from 2006):

UK	1,670,000
Germany	1,200,000
France	1,040,000
Netherlands and Belgium	760,000
Sweden	100,000
South Africa	360,000
Spain	560,000
Japan	2,400,000
Australia and New Zealand	160,000

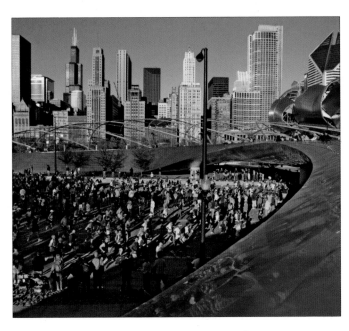

Why Run?

Running often comes under attack as being more damaging than other forms of exercise, but the truth is that just about every aspect of a person's physical and mental health will benefit from moderate running.

Apart from the sheer enjoyment and satisfaction you will gain from running, here are just some of the proven benefits that you can acquire by running three or four times a week for 20 to 30 minutes each time.

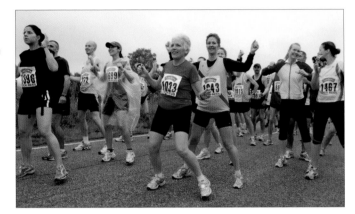

Healthy heart and lungs
Running reduces your risk of heart disease, lowering blood pressure and levels of 'bad', artery-clogging LDL (low density lipoprotein) cholesterol, while raising levels of 'good' HDL (high density lipoprotein) cholesterol, which helps keep blood vessels clear. Your heart is a muscle, so working it harder at safe levels will build its strength and size; as you become fitter, your heart rate will gradually drop slightly, showing that the heart has

Below: You don't need to run particularly far or fast to start feeling the benefits of regular running.

become more efficient. Meanwhile your body's ability to transport oxygen improves as capillaries (tiny blood vessels) develop in working muscles. Not only will running become easier, but everyday activities will seem to take less effort.

Above: No matter what your age, you can use running to become fitter and, more importantly, happier!

Below: Moderate exercise – such as a track session – helps to use your body's 'fight or flight' hormones.

Reduced body fat
Of course, running helps people lose weight and maintain a healthy body weight, decreasing the risk of obesity-related conditions. Even if you are a healthy weight to begin with, you will benefit: research has shown that excess body fat around internal organs is a risk to your long-term health no matter what your overall size. Regular exercise is the best way to reduce your body fat levels.

Reduced stress levels
Going out for a run may be the last thing you want to do at the end of a hard day, but it will help you to relax. When we become stressed, whatever the reason, our bodies react as though faced with danger and produce what is known as the 'fight or flight' response, developed in early man to fend off or escape from

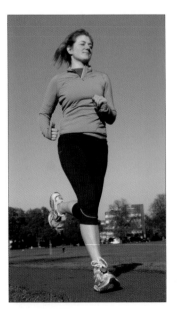

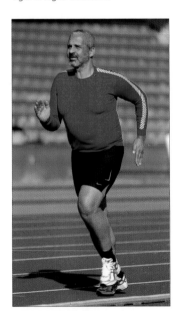

predators or other humans. Stress hormones called catecholamines are released in to the bloodstream, raising the heart rate and blood pressure and speeding up breathing, to prepare the body for physical activity. Running provides a release for these chemicals, thus reducing the more unpleasant symptoms of stress such as anxiety, shaking and wakefulness.

Better bones and joints

Many people avoid running, believing the impact to be bad for their joints and bones. However, running improves bone density, helping to fend off osteoporosis (brittle bones). While often cited as a cause of osteoarthritis, particularly in the knee, there is no evidence to suggest regular runners are more at risk than anyone else. In fact, regularly activity can help to maintain joint mobility as you get older.

Improved mental health

Once you have been running a few times, you will understand why people become runners for life. Moderate

Below: Women are more prone to osteoporosis, but running can help to decrease the risk.

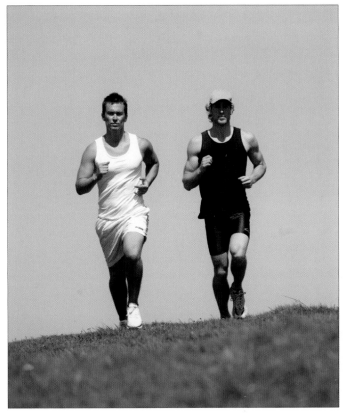

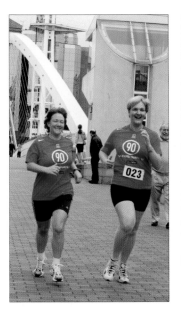

exercise produces a 'high' feeling that can last for hours afterward. Scientists are unsure why, but exercise has been linked to the release of endorphins, natural painkilling chemicals that are released during prolonged and intense activity. More recent research has shown an increase in levels of another substance, anandamide, in the bloodstream of runners and cyclists after exercise, which makes them feel relaxed and 'high'. There are longer-term effects, too. Anecdotal evidence shows that running improves the symptoms of depression, and many doctors now recommend exercise to help depressed patients.

Better gut health

It may not be an obvious benefit, but running also helps to keep your bowel movements regular. It is thought

Above: Over time, your body fat will reduce through running, so you'll look good as well as feel great.

that increased levels of stomach acid, improved blood circulation and muscle tone, and the repeated impact of running could all contribute to this effect.

Improved muscle tone

As well as these largely unseen health benefits, one of the main reasons people run is simply to look good. Running increases muscle mass and improves tone, and not just in the obvious areas (your legs). If you maintain good form, running will help improve your posture, tone up your stomach and back muscles and, as a consequence of reducing your level of body fat, your new-found muscle tone will be all the more visible.

Before you Run: Basic Health Checks

We have seen that running has many health benefits, but only if it is done properly. Before you head out on your first run, it is important to consider some of the risks – though usually small – involved in taking up exercise.

Being aware of the impact exercise can have on the different parts of the body is particularly important if you generally lead a sedentary lifestyle. Rushing into a demanding exercise regime is inadvisable – you could do yourself some real damage. Before you start running, visit your doctor for a thorough health check and to discuss with them whether more in-depth tests may be necessary to ensure you get the most from your running.

Below: Start training very gradually to avoid over-stressing your body, even if you feel perfectly healthy.

Pregnant pause

If you think that you may be pregnant, you should take a test before you start any intense exercise programme. Running is no longer considered unsafe during pregnancy and can be beneficial for women who already exercise regularly, but pregnancy is not a good time to start running (or any other form of strenuous exercise) from scratch as your body will be unused to the extra strain of the activity.

Right: If you are new to running, wait until after your baby is born to start; try gentle walking instead.

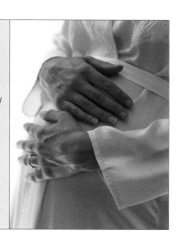

Family history

Talk to older relatives about any conditions that run in your family. These may be anything from heart problems, high blood pressure and cholesterol, to early osteoarthritis. Some allergic conditions may affect your sport – for example, asthma can be triggered by exercise and often runs in the family. The information you uncover about your family's health history will enable your doctor to test for particular conditions.

Blood pressure

All exercise helps to lower blood pressure, but if your blood pressure is very high to start off with, you may require regular check-ups and medication to control it.

Blood pressure measurements show systolic pressure (the maximum pressure in your blood vessels as the heart pumps blood around the body) and diastolic pressure (the minimum pressure, between beats). Normal values may be anything from 100/70 to 130/90. Some people suffer from white-coat syndrome, where the

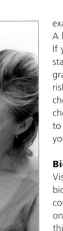

example 68/(1.74 squared) = BMI 22.5. A healthy BMI is between 20 and 25. If your BMI is high, you may need to start your exercise programme more gradually; you will have an increased risk of high blood pressure and cholesterol so should have these checked. If it is low, you will need to ensure you eat more to fuel your exercise.

Biomechanics

Visiting a specialist podiatrist or biomechanist before you start running could save you painful injuries later on. While obviously there is no such thing as a 'perfect' gait, if you have any particular problem such as a leg-length discrepancy, it could have a serious knock-on effect once you start running.

A podiatrist or biomechanist can perform a full gait analysis by examining your standing posture, walking and running gait; using slowed down video footage or electronic pressure plates to show the finer points of your running cycle. If potential problems are spotted, they can be dealt with using exercises or special insoles for your running shoes (orthoses).

Above: Regular exercise will keep your blood pressure down, but check it before you start.

doctor's surgery setting causes stress and raised blood pressure. In this case an electronic home blood pressure gauge can give a more typical reading.

Exercise ECG

An ECG or EKG (electrocardiogram) measures the electrical activity of heart muscles, which can show irregularities and help to diagnose any heart problems. This test involves exercising on a treadmill or stationary bike with electrodes attached to your chest. The electrodes pass information to the ECG machine, which produces a printed representation of your heart's activity. It is arranged through your doctor and would usually only be carried out if you had experienced chest pains or had a genetic risk of heart problems.

Current level of fitness

There are many ways to test your fitness, but many health centres use heart rate during and after exercise as a simple starting point.

Wearing a heart-rate monitor – a chest strap with an electric transmitter that sends signals to a computer – you will be asked to exercise at increasing

intensity for a few minutes. After you stop, the time taken for your heart rate to return to normal helps a fitness instructor, or your doctor, to determine your starting level of fitness and advise you on how to progress your training.

Body Mass Index (BMI)

A standard measure of whether you are a healthy weight for your height, BMI is worked out as your weight in kilograms divided by your height in metres squared, for

Below: An exercise ECG makes sure that your heart is as ready to run as you are.

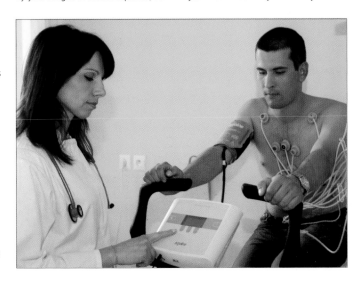

Starting a Walk/Run Programme

It will take time for your body to adapt to the unique stresses of running, so you need to ease in gently, build your fitness gradually, and learn to walk before you can run. This six-week plan will help you adjust to new levels of exercise.

Your first jogging sessions should be exhilarating, but for many the experience of taking up exercise is marred by trying to do too much, too soon.

If you are completely new to exercise, or coming back from a long break, build up time on your feet by walking at first. Slowly introduce periods of running, which can become longer as you become fitter, until you can run comfortably for 15 minutes. Some people choose to continue using walk breaks and never switch to continuous running; this can be a particularly effective strategy for longer sessions as the walk breaks allow you to recover. In fact, some athletes have been known to complete sub-three hour marathons using this technique.

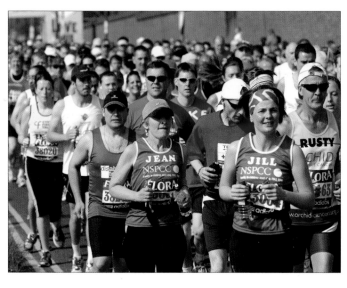

Below: Follow a walk/run programme to help you build your fitness steadily and enjoy making progress with your running.

Below: Walk confidently and briskly in between run segments to stretch out your body and freshen up.

Above: Using a walk/run method could one day help you to conquer a race; maybe even a marathon.

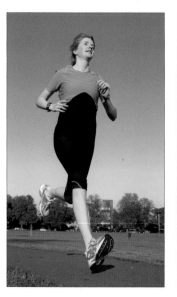

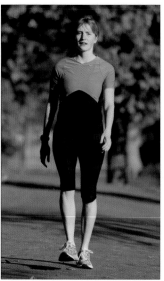

Walking tall

In a walk/run programme, your walk breaks should provide recovery time from running, but do not be tempted to relax so much that you begin to slouch. You will find the transition from walking to running much easier if you walk 'tall'; this will also help to stretch out your muscles as you go and to encourage good posture as you speed up. Imagine a string attached to your head, drawing you up tall. Keep your shoulders back, dropped but relaxed, and your neck relaxed. Make sure you look forward, not up. Take long, fast but relaxed strides and swing your arms from the shoulder, breathing deeply. Keep your spine neutral, so that your pelvis is neither tucked right under, nor tilting back.

How to use this plan

Treat the sessions as a guide and choose days on which you know you will be able to exercise. Decide in advance which days you will do your walk/run sessions, write these sessions in your diary and treat them as 'unmissable' appointments. If possible, try to fit your session in early on in the day – before work or any other commitments – to prevent anything getting in the way. Don't be tempted to push yourself too early by running for longer periods than stated in the plan, as you will run the risk of injury. It's also important to remember that the sessions described should be in addition to any activity you already do. You may feel more tired than usual at first, especially when you're adding run intervals to your walks, but by the end of the six weeks this should wear off and you'll find you have more energy, rather than less.

Below: In just six weeks you can build up to a daily 30-minute walk/run, a precious half-hour to yourself in a busy day.

Six-week walk/run programme

Week one
Session one: Walk for 15 minutes
Session two: Walk for 15 minutes
Session three: Walk for 15 minutes

Week two
Session one: Walk 20 minutes
Session two: Walk 10 minutes; run 1; walk 10, run 1
Session three: Walk 10 minutes, run 2; walk 8, run 2

Week three
Session one: Walk 8 minutes, run 2; walk 8, run 2
Session two: Walk 8 minutes, run 2; walk 5, run 2; walk 3, run 1
Session three: Walk 8 minutes, run 3; walk 4, run 2, twice

Week four
Session one: Walk 5 minutes, run 2; x 4
Session two: Walk 5 minutes, run 2; walk 5, run 3; walk 5, run 2
Session three: Walk 5 minutes, run 3; walk 5, run 4; walk 5, run 3

Week five
Session one: Walk 5 minutes, run 4; x 3
Session two: Walk 5 minutes, run 5; x 3
Session three: Walk 5 minutes, run 5; x 3

Week six
Session one: Walk 4 minutes, run 6; x 3
Session two: Walk 4 minutes, run 6; walk 3, run 7, twice
Session three: Walk 4 minutes, run 10; walk 3, run 5

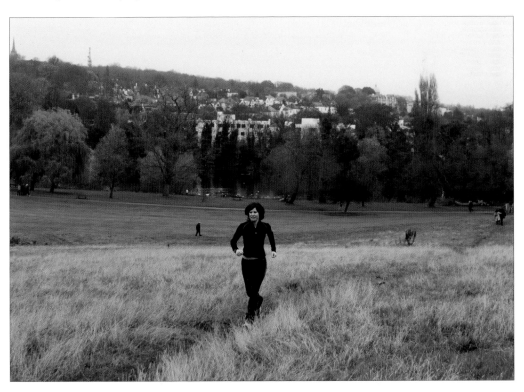

Running for Fitness: Six-week Plan

You will be amazed at what you can achieve in six short weeks. Even if you don't see yourself as a 'sporty person', a little application and a structured plan will take you from just a few walk/run sessions per week to becoming a real runner.

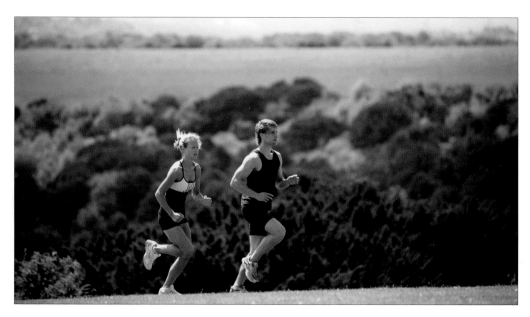

Once you have become used to regular exercise, you will be surprised how fast you can progress. This plan aims to bring you from walking and running three times a week to the recommended minimum of 30 minutes of moderate exercise, five times a week.

While any physical activity improves your health, building up to and then maintaining this level will keep you at a good level of fitness. Research has shown it will reduce your risk of developing heart disease by 50 per cent, as well as reducing your risk of obesity and several forms of cancer. It is also a good basis for moving your running up to the next level, should you choose to do so.

Building up slowly

When you have come from no activity at all to regularly managing three sessions per week, you can feel as though you're ready to tackle anything, but try to hold

something back. It is right that you should feel stronger and stronger as your sessions build up, but the way to maintain this feeling is not to let it fool you into doing more than you intended. Keep to the planned sessions, leaving your walk breaks in as scheduled, to make sure your body becomes fitter and

Above: Follow the plan and by the third week you will be ready to try some harder run-only sessions.

doesn't breakdown due to early overuse. Similarly, while it's useful to get in to a routine, don't be tempted to exercise every day. Even at the early stages of

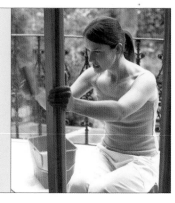

Making the most of fitness

You should think of 30 minutes of exercise as a bare minimum. Research shows that it doesn't matter if your total exercise time is broken up, so take every opportunity to boost your fitness. Walk up stairs, give yourself lunchtime errands that require a ten-minute walk; even ten minutes of housework counts toward your total.

Right: The more active you are generally, the more energy you'll have – even housework helps!

Six-week plan				
	Day one	Day two	Day three	Day four	Day five
Week one	Walk 5, run 10 x 2	Rest	Walk 3, run 12 x 2	Rest	Walk 5, run 10 x 2
Week two	Walk 3, run 12 x 2	Walk 3, run 12, walk 5	Walk 3, run 12 x 2	Rest	Walk 5, run 10 x 2
Week three	Run 5, walk 2 x 4	Run 7, walk 3 x 3	Run 12, walk 3 x 2	Run 7, walk 3 x 3	Run 13, walk 2 x 2
Week four	Run 5, walk 1 x 5	Run 8, walk 2 x 3	Run 13, walk 2 x 2	Run 5, walk 1 x 5	Run 13, walk 2 x 2
Week five	Run 5, walk 1 x 5	Run 20	Run 15, walk 2, run 10	Run 5, walk 1 x 5	Run 20
Week six	Run 5, walk 1 x 5	Run 25	Run 5, walk 1 x 5	Run 10, walk 1 x 3	Run 30

your fitness-building regime, your body needs rest days to adapt to the training you've done. Watch your speed as well – getting fitter makes you feel more energetic but throwing that extra energy into bursts of fast running before you're ready could jeopardize the work you've done, leaving you injured.

How to use this plan
If it seems daunting, think of this six-week plan as having three two-week phases. In the first phase, you are gradually building up the total amount of running you do each day. In the second phase, you are becoming used to exercising five times a week. Finally, in the third phase, you will introduce some more difficult run-only sessions.

In weeks one and two, focus on your posture as you run, carrying your tall walking frame into your running and keeping your strides long and relaxed. As you run for longer periods, it can be easy to allow yourself to slouch, but this can lead to injuries.

In weeks three and four, you should start to feel fitter. At this stage it is really important to keep your running pace even, as you may feel ready to speed up; make sure you are able to chat or sing as you go.

In your continuous run sessions in the final two weeks, maintain the steady pace you have learned through most of your run, but as you near your finishing point – say when you are 100m (330ft) from your front door – imagine you are racing someone and give yourself a sprint finish.

Below: After a few weeks of building up your training, you'll be able to speed up to run home.

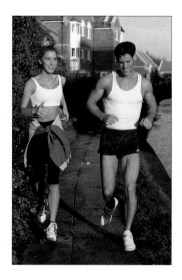

Above: Take a friend with you so you can talk as you run, a great way to keep your pace steady.

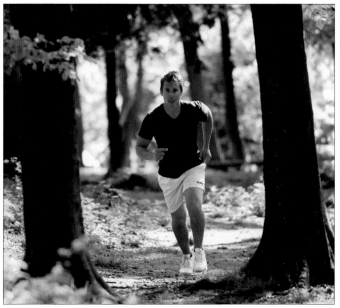

Running and the Human Body

One of the joys of running is that it increases your appreciation of the human body.
Although your legs may appear to do all the work, almost every part of the body is
involved in or affected by the act of running.

Learning about the basic processes
involved will not only give you a better
understanding of what happens when
you run, but will also help you to
develop your training over the months
and years to come.

Heart
The resting heart rate of an average
man is around 70 beats per minute
(bpm), and slightly faster for a woman.
When you run, the rate increases to
pump blood to the working muscles.
Your resting heart rate will go down
with months of training, and your heart
rate will not go up as much during runs;
your maximum heart rate (calculated
using the formula 214 – [0.8 x age] for
men, and 209 – [0.9 x age] for women)
will also stay level as you age if you
continue to train, where it would
usually drop for people with a more
sedentary lifestyle.

Lungs
You will become more aware of your
breathing as soon as you start to run
and, like your heart rate, your lungs
respond to training over time. Your lung
capacity (the volume of air you are able
to breathe out in one breath) will
increase. The oxygen you take in is
essential for powering your running, as
it reacts with sugars, fats and proteins
from food to create energy that enables
your muscles to contract. Efficient
expulsion of carbon dioxide is also key
to running well.

Blood and blood vessels
It is blood which transports the oxygen
and fuel your muscles require to run
well, and the waste products that need
to be removed to keep running for
long periods of time and to recover
afterward. Your blood volume increases
with regular exercise, as does the number
of oxygen-carrying red blood cells.

Immune system
Any moderate exercise increases
the body's resistance to minor
ailments, though intense training
such as marathon running blocks the
action of some types of white blood
cells, lowering immunity. You can
counteract this by consuming higher
levels of carbohydrate before and
during running.

Digestive system
Your body requires higher levels of
most nutrients once you start training
regularly, from carbohydrates, proteins
and fats for fuel to vitamins and
minerals that help keep your muscles
and nerves functioning well, and help
metabolize the food you take in.

Brain
Since the brain controls all movement, it
is the starting point for all your running,
but you can train your mind to help
improve your performance in less
obvious ways. Elite athletes use a
technique known as neuro-linguistic
programming (NLP) to prepare for
events, and ordinary runners can use
exercises such as visualization – seeing
a successful outcome – to build
confidence. The more intense your
training becomes, the more important
the power of your mind will be.

Muscles
Your working muscles respond to training
and will develop differently depending on
the kind of running and cross-training
you do. There are two broad types of
muscle fibre: fast-twitch and slow-twitch.
Good sprinters have a higher percentage
of fast-twitch muscle fibres, while
endurance athletes have more slow-
twitch fibres (the average person has
roughly a 50:50 split). Whether you are
better at fast or long running depends
on your natural starting level of fast or
slow-twitch muscle fibres, though specific
training can have some effect on the size
and action of the fibres. Most recreational
and fitness running uses slow-twitch
muscle fibres. Your muscles are able to
store a small amount of energy as
glycogen (a type of glucose), which is the
first and most accessible source of fuel
for exercise. More glycogen is stored in
your liver; around 2,000 calories in total,
enough to fuel around 32km (20 miles),
or three hours of running.

The human body: main systems

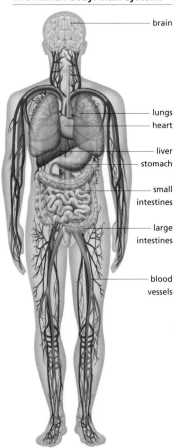

brain

lungs

heart

liver

stomach

small
intestines

large
intestines

blood
vessels

Main muscle groups: front and back

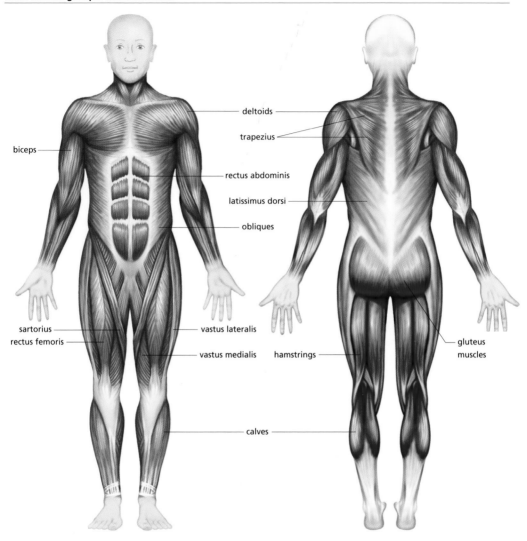

deltoids

trapezius

biceps

rectus abdominis

latissimus dorsi

obliques

sartorius

rectus femoris

vastus lateralis

vastus medialis

hamstrings

gluteus
muscles

calves

Muscle groups

Throughout this book, and as you train more, you will learn more about how different muscle groups work to create a smooth, strong running action. Some of the muscles you might strengthen are:

Gluteus muscles and hamstrings: the 'glutes' run around the pelvis, and the tops of the thighs; the hamstrings run down the backs of your upper legs. They provide forward propulsion when you run.

Quadriceps: the muscles down the front of the thigh, which extend the legs and stabilize you when running downhill.

Calves: the muscles at the back of your lower leg, which help with forward propulsion while running.

Back and shoulder muscles: the latissmus dorsi (lats) and rhomboid muscles in your mid and upper back, and the trapezius and posterior deltoid muscles in your

shoulders, help you to stay upright and maintain good form, especially when running longer distances.

Abdominal muscles: these work with the muscles in your back to stabilize your trunk, allowing for more efficient driving movements with your legs. The deep stomach muscles, together with some deep muscles in the lower back, are sometimes called your core.

Basic Stretching for Runners

Stretching is a vital part of any runner's training routine. It helps get the muscles moving easily and eliminates the risk of injury during a run. Running and stretching go hand in hand, but still many runners neglect flexibility, particularly at the start of their career.

Even though you may not feel like it after a run, it is important to spend a few minutes stretching. You will feel the difference if you don't. Stretching is attributed with reducing muscle soreness after running, decreasing the risk of injury, and improving performance by enhancing the range of motion in joints. Complete these eight basic stretches wherever you finish your run – you don't need any special equipment. Hold each stretch for 20 seconds before swapping to the opposite side and repeating.

Gluteals

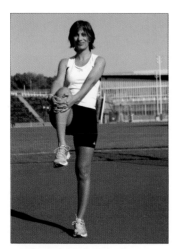

Raise one leg and bend the knee, drawing it in toward your chest. Wrap your arms around your raised leg and pull it in to your body; hold for 20 seconds. Draw the leg toward the opposite side of your body to stretch the smaller, deeper gluteals muscles.
Watch point: *make sure you bring your leg up to your chest, not the other way around; keep your back straight or the stretch will be less effective.*

Hamstrings

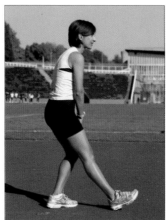

Stand with your feet hip-width apart. Step forward, place the heel of your front foot on the ground and bend your back leg, with the front leg straight. Lean forward from the hips, with your back straight, holding your front leg. Feel the stretch along the back of the straight leg.
Watch point: *you may find the hip on your supporting side will swing out as you lean forward, but keep your hips level to focus the stretch on your hamstring.*

Iliotibial bands

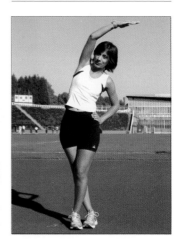

Cross one leg in front of the other, with the outsides of your feet together. Raise the arm on the side of your back leg and lean from the hips in the opposite direction. Feel a stretch along the outside of your back leg, from hip to knee.
Watch point: *the iliotibial band is difficult to stretch, but do not be tempted to overcompensate if you are unable to feel it by twisting your back. Make sure your torso faces forward.*

Stretching rules
- As a beginner, save your stretching for after exercise. You only really need to stretch beforehand if you are going to run very fast
- Before each stretch, take a deep breath, and perform the movement of the stretch as you exhale
- Try to relax when you are in each stretch; it should pull, but not hurt
- Do not bounce or jerk. Go in to each stretch slowly, then stay still

Right: Stretch well after exercise.

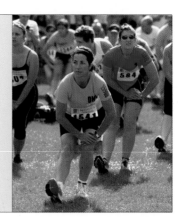

Quadriceps

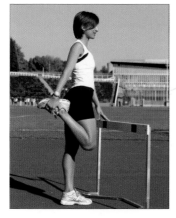

Stand with your legs together, holding on to a chair or wall for support. Bend one knee and bring the heel of the foot toward your bottom. Use your free hand to pull the foot farther in, keeping your hips level and facing forward.
Watch point: *point your knee down toward the floor against the action of your hand pulling the foot back, rather than pulling your entire leg backward.*

Calves

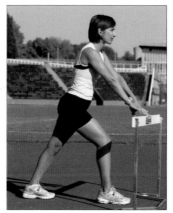

Stand with your feet together and take a step forward. Lean forward keeping your back straight, so that your front leg is bent while your back leg remains straight (you may need to hold on to a support for balance).
Watch point: *make sure your back heel stays on the ground throughout; push it into the floor to feel the stretch more.*

Lower calves

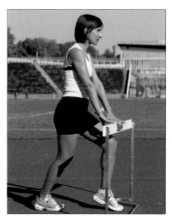

After stretching the upper calves, bring your back leg in slightly. Again, bend your front leg, but allow your back leg to bend, which will bring the heel off the floor. Push the heel down to feel the stretch in the bottom part of your calf.
Watch point: *this may not feel as intense as the main calf stretch, but resist the urge to put all your weight on the back leg.*

Lower back

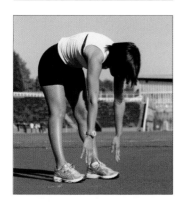

Stand with your feet hip-width apart. Stretch up, lengthening your spine, then bend forward from the hips, gradually allowing your back to relax down as though trying to touch your toes (don't worry if you are unable to do this!).
Watch point: *do not force this stretch, as you may damage your back; it should be relaxing.*

Hip flexors

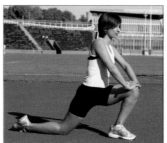

Kneel on the floor and bring one leg in front, so that your foot is flat on the ground and your knee is at a right angle. Stretch your other leg behind you, and point your toes so the upper side of your foot is on the floor. Lean forward, feeling the stretch at the front of the opposite hip.
Watch point: *if you cannot find any soft ground, don't flatten your back foot, instead keep your toes tucked under. The stretch will be less intense.*

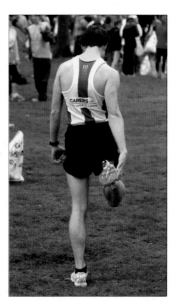

Above: You will often see more experienced runners stretching; it is a good habit to form early on.

Basic Strength Training

All-over body conditioning is not just about looking good. Strengthening the major muscle groups with these eight simple exercises will soon help you to become a more comfortable, efficient and faster runner. No special equipment is needed; they can be done anywhere.

There is no need to join a gym or buy any equipment to begin with, as your own body weight will provide all the resistance you need for a simple but effective workout. Between runs, perform these basic exercises in the order given here, and as you become stronger, and the exercises begin to feel easier, run through the same sequence twice in a row.

1 Wall Squat

Works: Gluteals, calves, hamstrings, quadriceps
Watch point: keep your knees pointing forward.

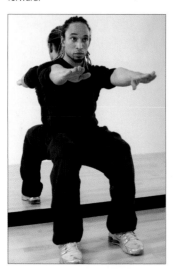

Stand against a wall with your feet hip-width apart and about a foot in front of you. Keeping your back straight against the wall and looking ahead, bend your knees to lower yourself toward the floor until your thighs are parallel to the ground, so that you are 'sitting' as if in a chair. Hold for a count of 10, then slowly push back up. Repeat 5 times.

2 Push-up

Works: Arms, shoulders, pectoral muscles, back muscles, core abdominal muscles
Watch point: keep your abdominal muscles tensed throughout to protect your back.

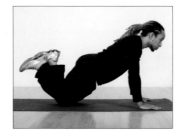 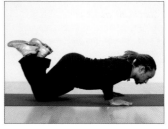

1 *Start on your hands and knees. Raise your feet and cross them over, and slowly walk your hands forward so they are level with your shoulders.*

2 *With your weight forward over your hands, lower your body until your elbows form right angles, then slowly push back up. Aim for 10 to 15 repetitions.*

3 Lunge

Works: Quads, hamstrings, gluteals, calves, hip adductors and abductors
Watch point: keep the movement controlled; do not jump forward or back up. If necessary, use your arms to balance.

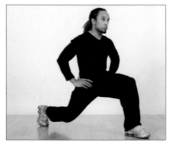

Start with your feet hip-width apart and your hands on your hips. Step forward so that one leg is in front, then lower yourself toward the floor until both knees form roughly a right angle; keep your back straight and look forward. Push your front heel into the floor and push back up again. Repeat with the other leg and do 10 on each side.

4 Chair squeeze

Works: Hip abductors and adductors
Watch point: keep the rest of your body relaxed through the exercise; it can be tempting to twist your back, but avoid this.

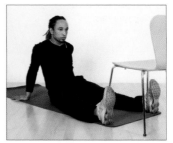

Sit on the floor facing a sturdy chair (not a folding chair) or small table. With your legs straight, squeeze the legs of the chair together using the inside edges of your feet; hold for five seconds and repeat 10 to 15 times. Then switch so that the outsides of your feet are pressing the chair legs outward.

5 Bicycle

Works: Abdominal muscles, obliques
Watch point: avoid rocking from side to side during the exercise. Your back and pelvis should stay still throughout.

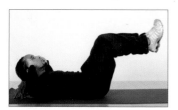 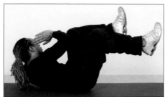 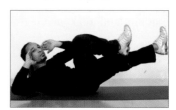

1 *Start in the crunch position. Lift your legs off the floor, keeping your feet side-by-side and your knees bent at right angles.*

2 *Tense your stomach muscles to pull your shoulders off the floor, then pull your right shoulder up toward your left knee, bringing the knee in to meet it.*

3 *Then repeat the exercise on the other side. Do 15 to 20 repetitions on both sides. Do this without resting in between repetitions if possible.*

6 Standard crunch

Works: Abdominal muscles
Watch point: do not tense your neck or use jerking movements to pull yourself up. Breathe out as you pull up to keep your neck soft.

7 Lower-back raise

Works: Erector spinae, gluteals
Watch point: do not jerk. If you feel pain, stop – you are overarching your back.

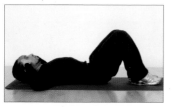 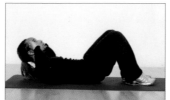 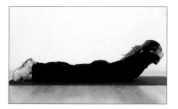

1 *Lie down on the floor with your knees bent and feet together, flat on the floor. Bend your arms at the elbow so that your hands are lightly touching your ears.*

2 *Tense your stomach muscles, keeping your pelvis in a neutral position, and draw your shoulders up, pulling your ribs toward your hips and with your stomach flat. Slowly lower. Repeat 20 to 30 times.*

Lie on the floor on your stomach, with your hands touching your ears. Slowly raise your shoulders and upper back so that you are looking up and ahead, then lower the body to the floor again.

8 Tricep dip

Works: Triceps, abdominal muscles
Watch point: keep your legs straight and steady throughout; if you are wobbling, practise with your legs and bottom on the floor.

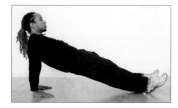 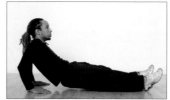 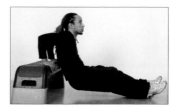

1 *Sit with your legs straight out and your hands on the floor behind you. Draw your abdominal muscles in, pushing up. Your body should be in a straight line, with your arms supporting your weight.*

2 *Bend your elbows to slightly lower your torso toward the floor, then push back up. Repeat 10 to 15 times at first, increasing the repetitions as your arms become stronger.*

3 *To make the exercise harder, use a step to raise your hands off the ground. Lower your torso toward the ground in the same way, then push back up, repeating 10 to 15 times.*

Tracking Your Progress

Running brings fitness gains quicker than any other recreational sport. There are no technical skills to master, at least in the first few months of training; all you have to do is go out and run and you will see the results fast.

Get in to the good habit of keeping checks on your overall fitness early on in your running career and it will serve you well in future. You don't need any special equipment to carry out a quick check on how you are doing, although if you have access to a gym or personal trainer it makes sense to ask for a full fitness assessment to be carried out every six to ten weeks.

Your training diary

To see how well your fitness is progressing, you will need to keep some kind of record of your running. Even without specific fitness tests, writing a training diary and reviewing it from time to time will tell you a great deal about what you are doing right and, when problems arise, what has gone wrong.

How much detail you record in your training diary is up to you, but a basic diary should show how far you ran

Below: Keeping a training diary can help you analyze why your runs go well – or not so well.

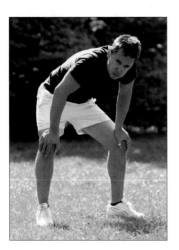

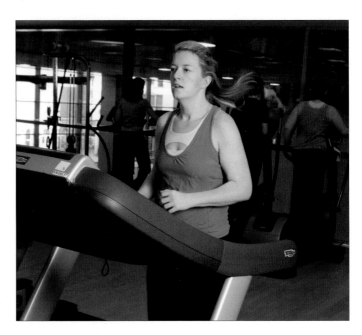

that day, how long it took you, and how you felt during the run. You might also want to record your resting heart rate, your weight before and after the run, what you ate and drank before and during exercise, and the route you took and who ran with you. All of these details can have a bearing on your performance that day and may help you to spot useful patterns in successful or unsuccessful training periods.

Your training diary should not be just a list of numbers. Some general guidelines to help are:

Go into detail. At first it may seem obsessive, but try to be as precise as possible with your measurements: time your runs with a watch, and measure your routes on a map or using a speed and distance monitor. When describing your feelings about

Above: Your gym instructors should be able to give you full fitness checks every six to ten weeks.

the run, make notes of how you felt: physically strong, fast, sluggish, heavy footed, any aches or pains, and emotions. If you think anything may have affected your run, make a note of it.

Take measurements at the same time each day. Always record your resting heart rate as soon as you wake up and before you get out of bed, which is when it will be slowest. If you track your weight, do it first thing in the morning before eating or drinking, and ideally unclothed.

Be honest. You may not have been able to run quite as far or as fast as you had planned to, but make sure your diary entries reflect this and include any reasons why that might have happened, even if you simply did not feel up to it. This is bound to happen from time to time. If you are not completely honest with yourself then the diary stops being useful.

Simple fitness tests

The following tables contain very simple fitness tests. These four tests are all measures which can help you to track your improvements over time. These tests will only provide very rough guidelines to

your overall fitness but after just a few short weeks of training you should start to see a real improvement in all of these different areas. Take the tests regularly to keep track of how you are progressing.
(Source: American Council on Exercise)

Cooper test

This test was designed by Kenneth H. Cooper in 1968 for US military use. Run as far as you can in 12 minutes, and measure how far you have run.

Sex/age	Very poor	Poor	Fair	Good	Excellent
M20–29:	1,600m	1,600–2,199	2,200–2,399	2,400–2,800	2,800+
F20–29:	1,500m	1,500–1,799	1,800–2,199	2,200–2,700	2,700+
M30–39:	1,500m	1,500–1,899	1,900–2,299	2,300–2,700	2,700+
F30–39:	1,400m	1,400–1,699	1,700–1,999	2,000–2,500	2,500
M40–49:	1,400m	1,400–1,699	1,700–2,099	2,100–2,500	2,500
F40–49:	1,200m	1,200–1,499	1,500–1,899	1,900–2,300	2,300
M50+:	1,300m	1,300–1,599	1,600–1,999	2,000–2,400	2,400
F50+:	1,100m	1,100–1,399	1,400–1,699	1,700–2,200	2,200

Heart-rate recovery

On a treadmill in the gym, begin running at a comfortable speed. Increase the gradient by 1 per cent every minute, until you reach your maximum effort. Record your heart rate (ideally using a heart-rate monitor, otherwise take your pulse). Stop exercising, and record your heart rate after two minutes rest. Note the difference between the two numbers.

Very Poor	Fair	Good	Excellent
Drop of less than 12 beats per minute	Drop of 15–25 beats per minute	Drop of more than 25 beats per minute	Almost complete recovery (within 10bpm of standing heart rate)

Body mass index

Weigh yourself, then divide your weight in kilograms by your height in metres squared. The best time to weigh yourself is first thing in the morning.

Very poor	Poor	Fair	Good
Below 18.5 (underweight) or above 30 (obese)	25–29.9 (overweight)	18.5–20 (slightly overweight)	20–24.9 (within a healthy weight range)

Body fat

Have a personal trainer measure you with callipers to work out your body fat percentage, or use a pair of body fat scales, which you should be able to find at your gym. Alternatively, you can buy a pair of scales for home use.

Very poor	Fair	Good	Excellent
25%+ (men)	18–25% (men)	14–17% (men)	6–13% (male athletes)
32%+ (women)	25–31% (women)	21–24% (women)	14–20% (female athletes)

Troubleshooting Early Problems

The best laid plans go awry, and your training schedule is no exception. Don't be disillusioned if you suffer setbacks after a few weeks' running, as a few simple measures will get you back on track in no time at all.

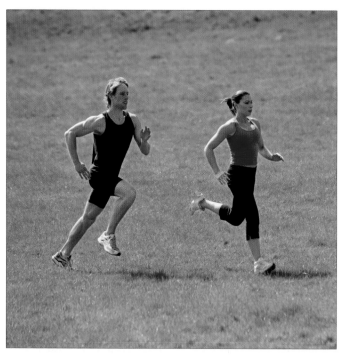

Upper back and shoulder pain. This is probably a result of poor posture. Pull your shoulders back while running and make sure you are looking straight in front of you, not down at the ground.

Calf pain. This is also a very common problem for new runners, particularly for women who wear shoes with high heels most of the day. Loosen your calf muscles by stretching them after every run and strengthen them with calf raises: stand on a low step with your heels hanging off the edge. Slowly lower yourself down then push up until you are up on your tiptoes. Repeat 10 times.

Left: You'll be full of energy as your fitness grows, but listen to your body to make sure you keep running strongly.

Below: Calf pain can be a problem for women who wear high heels, so stretch your calves regularly.

For the first few weeks of your running life, every run will be a pleasure as you find you can run farther and faster than you ever thought possible. Then one day you pull up with a calf pain, it happens again the next day and then you feel like giving up.

Teething problems are likely in any new exercise regime and can leave you feeling disheartened and demotivated after all the hard work you have put in. Thankfully these niggles are usually very simple to fix, leaving you free to continue on your journey toward becoming a runner.

Aches and pains

Generalized aching is an accepted part of taking up exercise and is a good sign that you are working your muscles hard enough. However,

localized pains should not be ignored as they could be early signs of long-term injuries. Some common problems for new runners include:

Shin splints. This is a general term for pain in the shins, often caused by running on very hard surfaces. Make sure you are wearing well-cushioned shoes and switch some of your running to softer surfaces such as grass; stretching your calves will also help. For instant relief, kneel on a carpet and sit right back on your heels.

Foot pain. This is usually the result of poor footwear. If you are wearing old trainers (sneakers), these can cause pain underneath the foot, while over-tight lacing can cause sharp pain over the top of your foot.

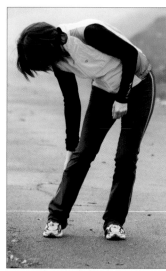

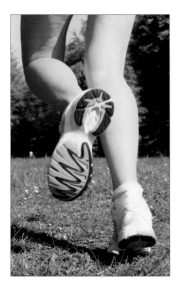

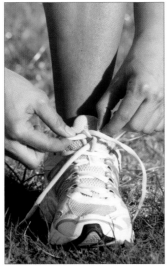

may have hit a fitness 'plateau'. If you are running three to five times a week for an hour or less, and have been doing so for some time, then it is time to pick up the intensity of your running with one or two faster sessions per week. If you are not ready for that, simply changing your route or finding a new running partner could provide the lift you need.

If you have been training particularly hard – for more than an hour each day – then your plateau could be the result of overtraining. Other symptoms include fatigue, lack of motivation and mood swings. In this case have a few weeks of easy running and build back up slowly.

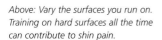

Above: Vary the surfaces you run on. Training on hard surfaces all the time can contribute to shin pain.

Above: Sometimes the cause of pain can be as simple as the way you tie up your shoelaces.

Finding time
The more you train, the more you will want to train, but fitting it in can become a problem. Set your alarm half an hour earlier and run first thing in the morning, or arrange for a long lunch hour two or three days a week in which you can run. Try running all or part of the way to work – a great timesaver, which means you beat the rush-hour traffic, too. In time you will find that running makes time for itself.

Restlessness
Though regular exercise generally promotes good sleep, some people find they become wakeful the more they run. Try to avoid running within three or four hours of bedtime – switch your run to lunchtime or early morning – and develop a relaxing bedtime routine, such as having a warm bath then stretching. If you run in the afternoon or evening and are hungry afterward, avoid foods that contain a lot of sugar or caffeine, as these may keep you awake.

Digestion
Most runners are affected at some point by 'runner's trots' – stomach cramps and diarrhoea brought on by running. If it has become such a regular problem for you that you are afraid to run, try experimenting with your food. Avoid eating for two to three hours before you run and cut down on high-fibre foods. Caffeine can exacerbate the problem, so stick to water or sports drinks. If this fails, you should investigate whether you have a food intolerance – many people find that gluten and dairy products can cause diarrhoea, so speak to your doctor if you think this may be the case.

Fitness plateau
If you have stopped seeing big improvements in your fitness – perhaps you are slowing down, or your breathing is more laboured – then you

Below: Shin splints are painful enough to stop you running, but this stretch gives instant relief.

Below: Running to work saves time and money, and is a great way to avoid rush-hour stress in the morning.

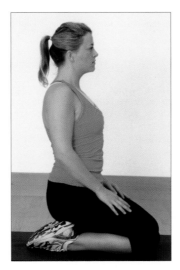

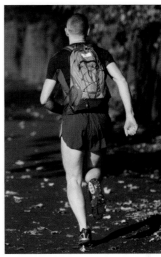

Staying Motivated

No matter how much you grow to love running, there will be times when it's hard to keep your momentum going. Learning to overcome the barriers between you and your favourite activity will make the difference between a passing phase and a lifetime of fitness.

Even the most committed runners will suffer from dips in their motivation. During your first few months of running it can be especially hard to keep going, as you readjust to your new routine. As you continue running, though, you will find that it is as much a mental exercise as a physical one, and consciously working on your drive to run is one of the keys to a long, successful running career.

There are many reasons for loss of motivation. Perhaps you are frustrated at your slow progress, or are not seeing the radical changes you had hoped for. Maybe you feel that running means making too many sacrifices in other areas of your life. Even a spell of bad weather can sap your will to go out and run.

Below: Arrange to meet up with friends so you don't skip a run.

The first thing to remember is that missing one or two runs is not necessarily a problem. It is good to allow your body to recover from all the hard work you have put it through. At the same time, it is important to stop yourself from drifting into a habit of making excuses. A good place to start is revisiting the reasons you took up running in the first place, whether that was losing weight, getting fit or relieving stress. If running is not helping you meet those targets, ask yourself why – for example, if you wanted to lose weight but are failing to do so, perhaps you are eating more to make up for training without realizing it. Think about the other, less tangible benefits of running, such as its effects on your long-term health (if you are short of inspiration, re-read 'Why Run?').

> **Instant motivation**
> • Run with others
> • Set an immediate goal – for example, beating yesterday's time
> • Give yourself a reward – maybe your favourite dessert, or a long bath
> • Buy new kit – you will want to try it out straight away
> • Run with music
> • Go for a short run – the chances are that you will keep going once you are out

Finding solutions

If external factors are giving rise to excuses for not running, think about solutions that will deal with these problems permanently. For example, if your family or partner is resentful of the time you spend running, try to get them

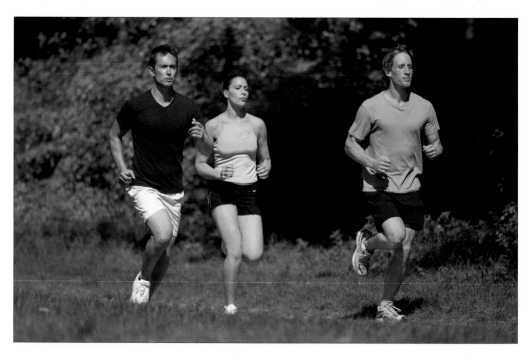

you get up or get home from work; make the rule that once you are wearing the kit, you have to run. Have an answer ready for every excuse, and tell yourself that you are only allowed certain treats on the days that you run.

Managing expectations

Often people lose motivation to run because it fails to live up to the expectations they had when they started out. In most cases there is a reason that running has not fixed a particular problem or given you a desired outcome, and in some cases the problem is just that your expectations were too high. Common reasons for disillusionment are:

Failing to lose weight. If you took up running to shift a few pounds and it's not working, first of all ask yourself if you're doing enough. Remember that to lose 450g (1lb) per week you need to burn an extra 3,500kcal (14,700kJ) – that's equivalent to running for 50 minutes, every single day! Try being more active in other ways (such as walking more or cycling to work), and keep a food diary to make sure you're not eating extra to 'make up for' running.

Not feeling fitter. Though you should feel some benefits after just a couple of runs (mainly because of the feel-good chemicals released in to your bloodstream when you exercise), it will take six to eight weeks of regular running before you find it more comfortable, as your heart, lungs and muscles need time to adapt.

Being 'bad' at running. Perhaps you were a great runner at school, or maybe you thought you were naturally athletic – either way, being slower than you hoped is disappointing. Again, you need to give your body time to adapt to training before it can run fast – even the best athletes take years to reach their peak, so be patient.

Feeling stressed out. Aside from the physical benefits of running, you may have heard that it's good for stress relief, only to find that it's another thing on your 'to do' list, leaving you feeling even more

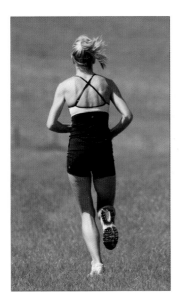

Above: Remind yourself why you started running, whether it was to get in shape or to reduce your stress levels.

involved by having them cycle with you along the route; if they don't want to be involved, plan to spend quality time doing something they enjoy. You could also encourage work colleagues to run with you; set up a lunchtime running club and show your boss how running can make the team more productive.

At the same time you may find that applying some of the techniques you use at work to your running will help your motivation. Review your running goals at regular intervals as you would those at work. If you find that they have gone stale – or were unrealistic in the first place – set new goals. For example, if an original goal was to lose 5kg (11lb) and that has been achieved, look at setting a goal to improve your running instead. If your goal was to lose 10kg (22lb) and you have only lost 2kg (4½lb), find a more achievable target. Make sure your running goals are SMART: specific, measurable, achievable, realistic and timely.

Forge good running habits by setting yourself golden rules that will last all of your running life, so that lack of motivation never stops you. For example, change into your running kit as soon as

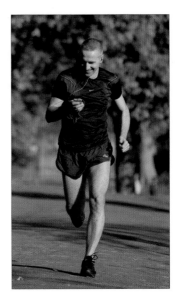

Above: Music can be a powerful motivator – use your favourite songs to inspire you to run again.

strung out. Reorganize your timetable before you commit to running regularly, so you can always fit it in easily. For most people the simplest way to do this is to run early in the morning – then it should help to relieve stress about the day ahead and it's one thing off that 'to do' list before you've even reached the office.

Group support

The best way to tackle lack of motivation is to run with other people – often the idea of letting someone else down is more powerful than the thought of letting yourself down. If this is impossible, you can still share your training with others: try setting up a blog, or visiting forums on running websites for support. Showing your training diary to a friend regularly can also help, as you will be embarrassed by any skipped sessions. Try being your own coach, too. Remind yourself how much you have achieved since you started, and give yourself pep talks – if you find yourself thinking 'I can't face a run this evening,' tell yourself 'I always feel better after running. I've done this in the past and know I can do it again.'

Gear Basics: Shoes

One of the best things about running is that it doesn't require lots of equipment, but the one essential piece of kit is a good pair of running-specific shoes. Learn a little bit about them, and you won't need to spend a fortune.

The one piece of running equipment you need to invest in before even taking your first step, is a good pair of running shoes. These will help to correct problems in your gait, in turn helping you to avoid any injuries and to run faster and more comfortably.

The key factor that determines which type of running shoe you need is the degree to which your feet pronate – that is, roll inward – when

Below: Shoes help prevent gait problems such as overpronation (where your feet roll too far in) as seen here.

your foot hits the ground during a run. Pronation is your natural shock absorption. In a normal runner, the heel hits the ground first, then your weight rolls through the foot and the foot falls inward slightly, so that you finish each step with the inside of the front of your foot to push off again.

When buying your first pair of running shoes, it is best to have your gait analysed by a podiatrist or by experienced staff in a running store. Tests you could have might include the following:

Video gait analysis. You are filmed running on a treadmill, then the film is reviewed in slow motion to analyse the movement of your foot.

Pressure plate analysis. You are asked to run over a mat which is fitted with pressure sensors. Readings from these sensors are used to produce an accurate diagram showing where your foot places most pressure through each stride.

Running outside. At specialist running stores, you will often be asked to run up and down outside the store while the

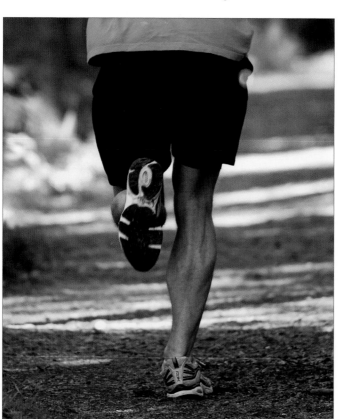

Buying the right shoes
The best place to buy your running shoes is from a specialist running store (rather than a general sports store). If at all possible, ask experienced runners in your area where they buy their shoes from. When you find a good shop, take the time to talk to the staff; the best advisors will be experienced, enthusiastic runners themselves. Avoid buying very cheap shoes, but do look at shoes in the sales: these are usually just last season's models and will be just as effective as the newer, more fashionable versions.

Below: Take your time choosing trainers and make sure you get expert help in the store.

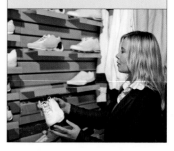

assistant watches your gait. You may feel self-conscious doing this, but this test has the advantage that your run will be more natural on the pavement than on a treadmill or over a pressure plate.

Static examination. Podiatrists may examine the range of movement and natural stance of your feet, ankles and legs while sitting and standing.

Following any type of gait assessment apart from a static examination, if you're then trying on shoes, the store assistant should ask you to repeat the test in different pairs of trainers to look at the effect they have on your gait. They should be able to demonstrate how the shoes are correcting any problems – remember, if you are not convinced by what you're told, you should always try to get a second opinion.

The wet foot test

The wet foot test is a quick and easy way to find out about your degree of pronation. Wet your feet and walk over a piece of cardboard, then look at the shape of your footprint.

1 Neutral/normal foot. The heel and forefoot are clear and even; the outside of the foot will have made a wide band connecting the front and back of the foot. Runners with a normal degree of pronation usually need stability shoes.

2 Flat/overpronating foot. Almost the entire foot makes contact with the ground, so the band between the front and back of the foot will be much wider and straighter. Runners with this type of footprint will need a motion-control shoe, which is usually heavier and firmer.

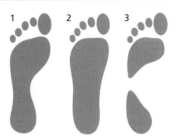

Above: Your degree of pronation will affect the way you run; it is easily detected by looking at a wet footprint.

3 Supinating foot. Runners who supinate have high arches, so there will only be a thin line, if any, between the rear and front of the foot. Neutral or cushioned shoes are best for these runners.

Running shoes inside out

Different brands have their own technologies, but there are some features which most shoes have in common.

Upper: the fabric part of the shoe, usually designed to be as light and breathable as possible, though in motion control shoes this may be firmer or more fitted to help provide support.

Midsole: the cushioned interior of the sole, between the outsole and insole, containing most of the shoe's motion control and comfort features.

Insole: the removable sole inside the shoe, which may be shaped to support the arch and help prevent pronation. If you need orthoses, these will go in place of your insole.

Forefoot: the wider front part of the shoe. Generally, the wider the forefoot, the more stable the shoe.

Heel counter: a hard cup in the heel of the shoe used to provide stability and prevent pronation from the rear foot.

Midfoot shank/arch bridge: plastic supports built in to the midsole to support the arch in flat-footed runners.

Medial post/rollbar: a firmer piece of foam in the midsole of the shoe used to force the foot upright, and prevent excessive pronation.

Outsole: the tough outside of the underneath of your shoe, with lugs of varying depth for different terrain (the bigger the lugs, the more grip the shoe has).

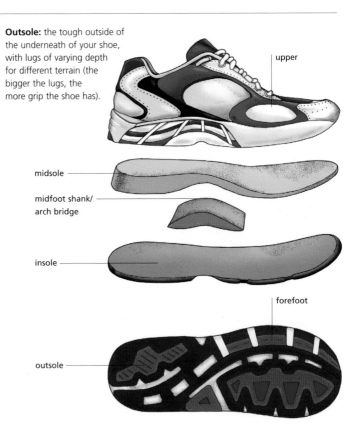

upper

midsole

midfoot shank/
arch bridge

insole

forefoot

outsole

Gear Basics: Apparel

Running kit may look simple, but behind the humble-looking shorts and T-shirt is a host of technologies designed to keep you cool, comfortable and confident while you're exercising. It may not make you run faster, but it will help you enjoy the experience a lot more.

For many people the bold step of a first run is a spontaneous decision, so an old cotton T-shirt and basketball shorts might stand in for technical running kit. After returning home weighed down in a cold, clammy top and rubbed raw from chafing shorts, you will realize why it is worth treating yourself to some proper apparel.

Spring and summer kit

T-shirts. A summer running T-shirt should control moisture, wicking sweat away from your skin and drying quickly, to help keep you cool. The cut of the top is also important: it should be fitted to allow ease of movement, and may even feel odd when you are standing still, as some tops are cut for a running motion. Other features to look for are flat or welded seams, to avoid chafing, and venting down the back and under the arms to keep you cool.

Below: Traditional split-leg shorts.

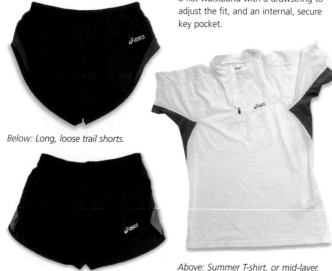

Below: Long, loose trail shorts.

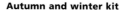
Smart kit

Running apparel is becoming more technical and might include:
Odour control: Silver yarn (X-Static) woven into the fabric helps reduce odour; sometimes material is treated with antibacterial chemicals to prevent odours developing. The best T-shirts might include self-refreshing odour technology, which uses sugar molecules to catch sweat as it forms.

Temperature regulation: Increasingly, manufacturers are using fabrics that react to moisture and heat. The weave of the fabric changes shape to change the flow of air around the body.
Sun protection: Most summer kit has a loose weave, which means you can get sunburnt through it, but some manufacturers now make kit that offers protection up to factor 50.

Singlets may keep you cooler but can chafe under your arms, so be sure to try them on first.
Shorts. Again, these should ideally be made from wicking material. Traditional running shorts are cut very short with a split up each side, so your legs are able to move as freely as possible, and have a supportive inner mesh. If these make you feel too self-conscious, go for trail shorts instead, which are slightly longer and looser. Look for features like a flat waistband with a drawstring to adjust the fit, and an internal, secure key pocket.

Autumn and winter kit

Tights. The best and most effective winter tights will incorporate several panels of different materials: water resistant areas on the thighs and shins, thermal material down the calves, and cooler mesh panels in the inner thigh and back of the knee. Calf zips help to give a better fit, but make sure that the leggings are the right length, or the zip will chafe on your leg. If you expect to be running at night-time, in the dark, look for reflective flashes winding diagonally around the calf, as these will be much more visible than stripes or flashes on the upper leg.
Tops. In sub-zero temperatures, you may need three thin layers: a wicking layer against your skin, a light insulating layer in the middle, and a windproof and waterproof layer on the outside. If the weather is slightly warmer, leave out the middle layer. Remember that even when it seems incredibly cold outside, you inevitably warm up when running, so don't wear bulky layers.

Accessories

Hats. These are useful in winter, though really only necessary in sub-zero temperatures. Go for a hat made from wicking material with a brushed

Above: Summer T-shirt, or mid-layer.

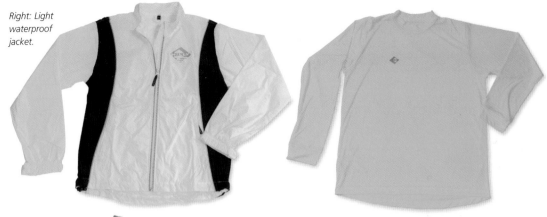

Right: Light waterproof jacket.

Above: Long-sleeved winter base layer.

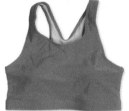

Above: Crop-top style sports bra.

Below: Shock-absorbing sock.

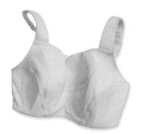

Above: Moulded, underwired sports bra.

Above: Wicking winter hat.

Right: Long, warm winter tights.

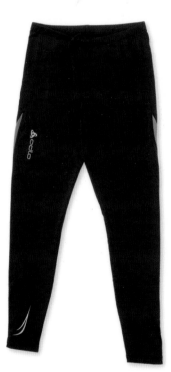

Supporting acts

Sports bras are as essential a piece of kit for women as running shoes. Breasts are naturally supported by the Coopers ligament which, once stretched, cannot regain its original shape. Research has shown that during running, breasts move in a figure-of-eight motion, but a good sports bra can reduce this movement by up to 80 per cent. Crop tops are fine for A to B cups, while larger-sized women should look for high-fronted, moulded bras with thicker, non-elastic straps.

interior that will not irritate your forehead. In the summer months, wearing a cap can be a good idea to keep the sun off your head and shade your eyes; try to find one with a folding peak so you can carry it easily in your pocket if you want to take it off.

Sports socks. These are becoming increasingly complex and can add extra shock absorption. Some manufacturers even claim that they can add support for your feet by using different weaves and thicker pads in key areas of pressure. Double-layered running socks can help to prevent blisters forming on long runs.

Gloves. These are another useful item in very cold weather. Avoid wool and go for light, wicking gloves. Useful features are rubber pads on the fingers, so you won't need to remove them to undo zips or use keys, and towelling on the outside of the thumb for mopping your face.

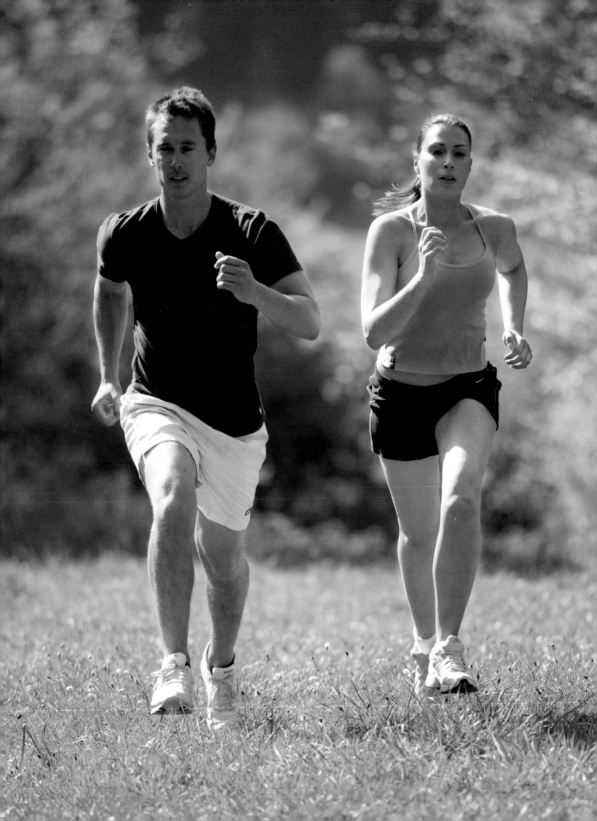

BUILDING FITNESS

Regular running transforms your health, but
once you are running a few times each week you
will find you want to know and do more.
This chapter will help you to make the step up
from running for health to improving your running
for the extra fitness gains this will bring. Your
running will become more technical, but more fun, too.
This means not only running faster, but also adding
strength training, reviewing your diet, and bringing
other forms of exercise into your life.

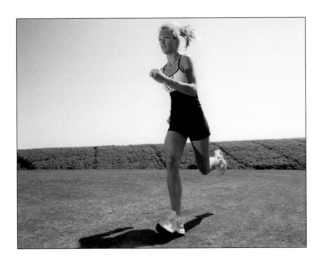

Above: Push yourself with faster sessions and you'll reap the benefits.
Left: Building up the distance you run is the first step to increasing your fitness.

Building Up Miles

A solid base of mileage is the foundation on which all good running is built, but be careful: try to take a shortcut to extra miles and the cracks will start to show. This simple guide shows how to increase your training volume the right way.

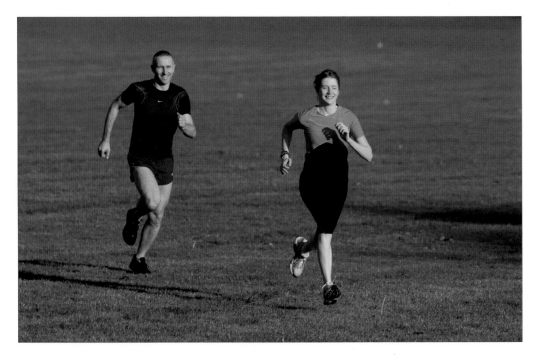

In an easy week, the British marathon world record holder Paula Radcliffe runs 160–190km (100–120 miles) – ten times as much as someone running for fitness. Unless you are training to challenge her in a marathon, your weekly mileage is unlikely to reach three figures, but gradually building up your distance will improve your fitness and give you an invaluable base should you decide to start training for events. For beginners, building up running volume is the simplest way to keep enjoying fitness gains. It helps your body to become used to the action of running. You will develop more capillaries (tiny bloody vessels) in your working muscles, helping your body to deliver oxygen to power your running. Once you have built

your base, adapting to more intensive training will be easier, with a lower risk of injury or overtraining.

Building frequency
A good rule of thumb when increasing your training is to do so by no more than 10 per cent a week, so if you run for 30 minutes four times a week, add only 10 to 15 minutes the next week, then 20 minutes the next, and so on. Running more often should be your goal before increasing mileage, as this helps to build the habit of regular running (which makes it easier mentally) and gives your metabolism a boost every day. This may mean shortening your route temporarily for example, you might go from three half-hour sessions to five 20-minute sessions. After that, try adding

Above: At first, just add short loops on to your regular runs to increase your mileage gradually.

5 minutes to your run every week until you are running 40 to 45 minutes, five or six times per week.

Running for longer and more often can initially prove difficult to fit in, and you may struggle with motivation as inevitably you forgo half an hour in bed, or lunch with a friend to run. Find strategies to trick yourself into running: run as part of your commute or, on weekends, add running to regular activities such as visiting relatives or buying a morning newspaper. Add an extra 5-minute loop at the start of your regular route (rather than at the end when you will be more tempted to stop from tiredness). Allow yourself

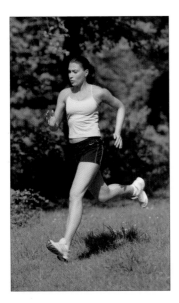

Above: Running farther makes your body more efficient and powerful, so you can run faster.

to slow down slightly and enjoy the scenery, so that running is a relaxing time to look forward to rather than something to cram in.

Building distance

As well as running more often and for slightly longer each time, you should plan one long run per week, aiming to build up to between 90 minutes and 2 hours. This long run will teach your body to be more efficient at using fat for fuel, which means your body fat levels will drop and you will be able to run farther comfortably, without 'hitting the wall' – running out of carbohydrates to fuel your muscles, resulting in sudden tiredness and jelly legs.

When building up your long runs, as with regular training sessions, think in terms of time rather than distance to begin with. That way you will soon discover your natural pace, which will help you work out how far you are running. Remember the 10 per cent rule – don't build up your long run on the same weeks that you increase your other runs.

The idea of running for 16–19km (10–12 miles) at a time can be quite daunting, so try running three or four loops near your home or base so that you feel safe and are able to stop if you need to. On the other

hand, if you feel you might be too tempted to stop early, an out and back route should encourage you to keep going to reach home quicker. Start your long run early in the day so it doesn't interfere with your other plans, and take a sports drink so that you don't run out of energy or become dehydrated.

Below: Keep your pace easy on your longest run of the week and then take it easy the day after.

> **Rules for long runs**
> • Increase your total weekly mileage by no more than 10 per cent each week
> • Don't try to run faster at the same time – build your foundation first
> • Drink and eat more as your body uses more fuel
> • Record your mileage and make sure you replace your shoes after about 800km (500 miles)
> • Keep your pace easy, so you are able to chat or sing as you run
> • When you introduce a long run, make sure you take it easy (and short) the days before and after

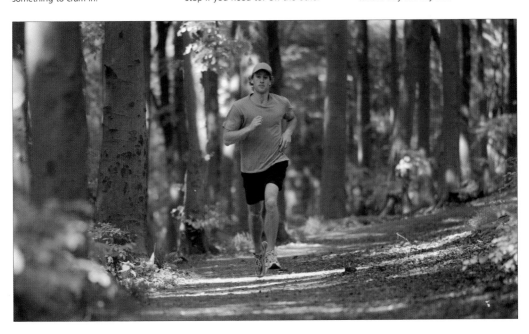

Learning Good Form

Becoming a runner is not just about getting into good habits. It's also about losing bad habits, and that includes many of the little quirks that make your running style unique – because those 'quirks' could prevent you from running to your best ability.

Running is as simple as putting one foot in front of the other. At least, that is the commonly held view. In fact, if you were to watch 100 runners, you would see 100 completely different ways of moving. There is no perfect running form, or even anything that could be truly described as normal. Instead individuals develop their own running style based on body shape, learned habits and, to an extent, the speed and distance they are running.

There is a limit to the extent to which you can change your running form, since most of your movements are made without conscious thought, but there is also a limit to how much you would want to change – after all, your body has developed a running style to deal with its own particular quirks, and even a style that looks unnatural and uncomfortable is not

a problem unless it causes injuries. However, thinking about your form can help you run more efficiently.

Legs

Your leading knee should drive up high so that your thigh is parallel to the ground (or perhaps slightly higher). The lower part of the lead leg should stay tucked neatly under until your knee is high, then push down quickly to the floor. Your foot should not land too far ahead of you, but should be close to being underneath your body as you run,

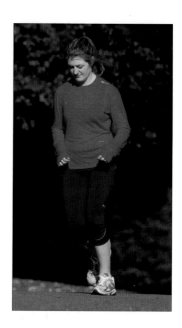

Right: A self-conscious, shuffling gait is not uncommon, but straighten up and you'll find that your running becomes a lot easier.

Below: Use your upper body as well as your legs to help you move forward.

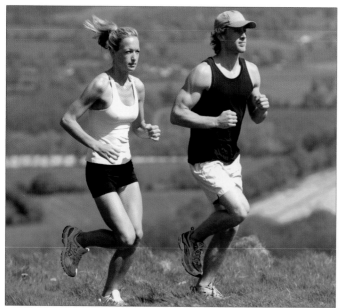

Exceptional elites

Elite runners are always exceptional, and they can also be exceptions to the rule that better running style leads to better running.

The British long-distance runner Paula Radcliffe has a very distinctive twisting nod of the head as she runs, which often becomes more pronounced as her races go on, yet she still holds four of the world's five fastest women's marathon times.

Sprinters are usually encouraged to run leaning forward with a relaxed, smooth style, but the American athlete Michael Johnson was the exception to this rule. He ran with a stiff-looking, upright style and quick, short steps, but even so he managed to win no less than five Olympic gold medals and in fact still holds the world record for the 400m.

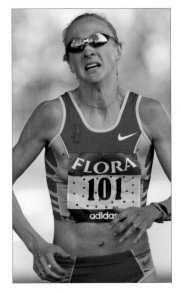

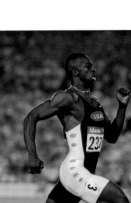

Above: Marathon runner Paula Radcliffe's style looks tense, with a famous 'nodding head', but it certainly works for her.

Above: Michael Johnson says that his strange, upright sprinting style made him the successful athlete that he is.

and you should be able to claw the ground underneath you with this foot then push off strongly into the next stride.

Pelvis
Your pelvis should be in a neutral position; that is, neither tilting forward nor sticking out backward. It should remain fairly still during running, without moving up and down or

twisting from side to side. Lack of stability in the pelvis is the root of many running injuries, as muscles around the pelvis and in the legs can easily be overworked when trying to keep your hips still.

Torso
The middle of your body, the torso, should always be strong and static as you run. Your abdominal muscles

should naturally tense up to stabilize your body, but try not to squeeze these muscles. There should be no twisting from the waist.

Arms and shoulders
The action of your upper body, and in particular of your arms and shoulders, has a surprisingly high impact on your overall running efficiency. Your shoulders should always be relaxed, positioned down and back so that your chest is open and you can breathe easily. Your elbows should be bent to about 90 degrees, and your arms should swing back and forth (rather than across your body) in time with the movement of your legs; this can help keep your leg speed and rhythm up.

Head and neck
Your neck should be long and relaxed, and you should be facing forward, looking straight ahead. Your face should also be relaxed; scowling, grimacing or grinding your jaw may seem inevitable during a hard run, but any movement, however small, wastes energy and has a knock-on effect, making your neck and shoulders tense, too.

Quick form fixers	
Problem	**Solution**
Poor knee drive	Get in to the habit of driving your knee by adding sets of four or five 100m sprints into your runs; running faster naturally encourages you to pick your legs up, and the habit will filter into your slower running.
Slouching and hunched shoulders	If you catch yourself slouching, try taking as deep a breath as you can, and imagine you have just seen the finish line of a race. This should encourage you to straighten up and open your chest.
Lazy arms	Run with very light weights in your hands (not more than about 500g/1¼lb each) or around your wrists. Carrying weights will make you more conscious of your arm action and help you to build momentum.

Simple Speedwork

There are many different ways to train your body faster, and all of them involve pushing yourself out of your natural comfort zone. But don't let that put you off – speedwork is time-efficient, satisfying and even enjoyable.

Introducing speedwork to your training can be a daunting prospect. Traditional speed sessions look, on paper, complicated and technical and you may think that running very fast is the sole preserve of experienced athletes. But introducing speedwork, which is any session that involves running faster than you have been, after just a few months of running is straightforward and has huge benefits.

Just one faster run per week will gradually extend your comfort zone, so that your relaxed running pace becomes faster naturally. It improves your cardiovascular fitness, so your heart rate stays lower for longer and recovers more quickly; it recruits fast-twitch muscle fibres, which you will need if you plan to race in future; and it burns more calories overall than slower runs. Speedwork is also enjoyable, adding an element of variety to your training.

Below: The track may be intimidating at first, but it's a forgiving surface which makes speed sessions easier.

Technical terms

There is really nothing complicated about speedwork in its purest forms, so try not to be put off by technical-sounding terms often seen in running schedules:

Reps: simply means 'repetitions' or 'repeats' and refers to the faster-paced parts of your speed session (for example, 4 x 400m reps indicates running 400m fast, four times).

Recoveries: in the context of a speed session, a 'recovery' is a period of easy jogging, walking or sometimes stopping altogether, in between faster reps.

Strides: a technique of fast but relaxed running, often used to inject some speed in to longer, easier runs.

Intervals: the term interval training actually covers all speedwork (and is used in other sports, too). It simply means interspersing intervals of hard and easy effort, though often in running it is used to refer to longer periods of fast running (that is, reps more than one minute long).

Fartlek: a Swedish word meaning 'speedplay', this is an unstructured form of speedwork.

Speedwork rules

For all its benefits, speedwork places extra stress on your body, so take care when you start out by following a few simple rules. Firstly, add speed slowly. Just as you need to increase mileage gradually to avoid injury, so you need to introduce speedwork gently. Start with just one session per week, and try not to sprint all-out; you will need practice to find out how to pace your faster runs.

Secondly, as you build more speedwork into your training, it is important that you make sure that you plan easy runs in between hard sessions. Your body needs time to recover to make fitness gains, so fit in a rest day or cross-training between long or fast runs.

Below: Speed sessions, especially on the track, add focus to your training and help you pace yourself.

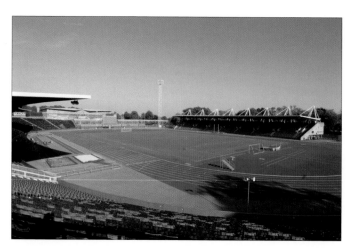

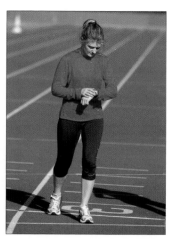

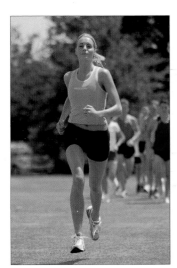

Above: You don't need a track to run fast, but it is best to choose a softer surface to run on – smooth, flat lawns are a good alternative, and give more space to train in a group.

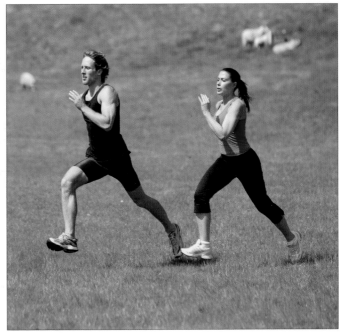

Above: Workouts with faster friends build your own speed and prevent speedwork becoming a chore.

You will also need to pay extra attention to your running style. You may find yourself striding out longer than usual, but it is more efficient to concentrate on increasing your leg speed, so you take more steps rather than longer steps. The more you push your body during a run, whether you are running farther or faster, the more your running style will count.

Making changes

Running tracks can be intimidating, but remember that hard runs need soft surfaces. Shin splints and joint pain are very common in runners who have just introduced or increased their speedwork sessions. The faster you run, the greater the impact will be on your body, so to counteract this, do faster sessions on grass or soft trails (or on a track if you can face it).

As well as changing venues, you may need to adjust your eating pattern on speedwork days. Pushing yourself harder can make you feel nauseous, so leave more time between your pre-run meal and the training

session. You have probably been avoiding caffeine before long runs to avoid dehydration, but research shows that a shot of caffeine before a fast session can help you run faster and may help to burn fat.

Finally, even if you usually prefer to run alone, speed sessions are much easier to do with other people, if only because you might need an extra push to get through the session. Training with faster friends can be a great motivator.

Below: It's a good idea to hire your local track with a group of friends for regular mixed ability sessions.

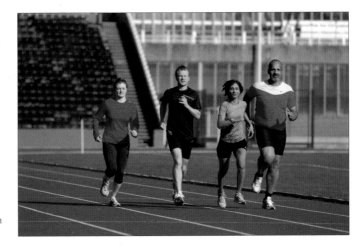

First Fast Runs

Speedwork takes many forms and for the fastest athletes it's finely tuned and technically perfect. For a beginner, though, your first fast workouts should concentrate more on variety and enjoyment so that you can push yourself without punishing yourself.

Although training faster will improve your overall speed, it would be a mistake to simply go out on your usual run and try to speed up from the outset – you'll almost certainly run too fast and won't be able to finish the session. Instead you need to practise running at different speeds for different lengths of time, from short, very fast sprints to longer sustained intervals of 10 minutes or more. It will take time to learn the different paces you'll need for speedwork but approach it as a bit of fun and you should become used to the way it feels to run faster. You don't need a track, a coach or set of complicated set of instructions

Below: Make use of the landscape for fartlek runs, changing pace as your surroundings change.

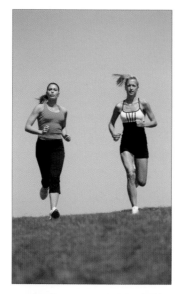

to speed up. Try these easy ways to speed up one of your regular runs, remembering to run easy for the first 10 minutes of every session.

Fartlek
From the Swedish word meaning 'speedplay', fartlek is the most enjoyable and easiest form of speedwork. It may sound difficult, but it just means including a few faster bursts into your run at random points; you could try using lampposts or street signs as start and finish points; changing speed when you change running surface; or, if you run with music, running faster during a particular song.

Left: Most runners enjoy the fast, relaxed feeling of a strides session, with short, intense bursts of speed.

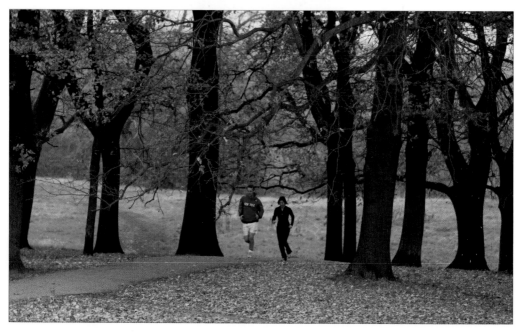

Right: Spiral sessions in your local park help you learn to run at varying paces.

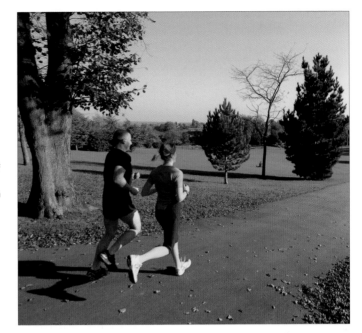

Race yourself

Just as you can build up running using a walk/run strategy, you can build up periods of faster running using slow then fast intervals. Pick a short route that usually takes 30 minutes to complete, and introduce five faster spurts of 200 to 300m (or 2 minutes). Gradually increase the length of the faster intervals and reduce the length of the slower sections, aiming to take five minutes off the whole route time over a period of a few months.

Strides

This involves using short, fast bursts used to pick up your overall pace and improve your form. During the last 10 minutes of a regular run, speed up for a 20-second burst, keeping your running action smooth and relaxed; you should feel as though you are floating. Slow down for

Below: Many people new to running find that their form naturally improves when they start to run faster.

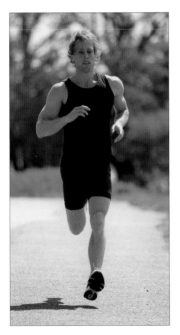

40 seconds, then repeat six to eight times. Increase the number of strides on your run as you become stronger.

Musical sprints

If you are unable to vary the terrain of your run easily, try varying the soundtrack. Use an MP3 player to create an interval session by making yourself a playlist with songs of different tempos, and run in time to the music. Alternatively, run fast during the chorus of songs and slower during the verse. Make things more interesting by asking a friend to make the playlist for you, so you don't know what is coming up (or run with a radio, which should have the same effect).

Spiral session

Go to a large park that you know well, and run four or five loops starting with a large, outer loop and gradually decrease the distance. For the first, longest loop, which should take you about 10 minutes, stay at an easy jog. For each successive smaller loop, speed up slightly, until you finish with a 1- or 2-minute, very fast circuit. After your fastest loop, run the circuits back out in reverse order, finishing with an easy 10 minutes.

Team efforts

You might usually prefer to run alone, but arranging to do harder sessions with a group of friends means you are less likely to duck out and do another easy run. Team sessions offer you more variety and help to keep your mind off your aching muscles, too. Here are a few to start with.

Hares and hounds: slower runners in the group head out first and choose the route; after an agreed time (say 3 minutes), the faster runners head out to try to catch them.

Mixed intervals: play cat and mouse with a friend by running the same route with different intervals: after a warm-up, one partner could run 2 minutes fast, 2 slow, 2 fast while the other continues to run easy; then the first runner has a 5-minute slow recovery while the second runs a continuous fast 5.

Team fartlek: head out with a group of friends and, after your warm-up, take it in turns to shout out the start and finish of fast periods, so the rest of the group don't know what is coming.

Hill Running

When planning running routes, most people choose to avoid hills. This seems to make sense – after all, running is about moving quickly, not trudging up steep slopes and stumbling down the other side. However, hill running has many benefits.

How you run hill sessions depends on your goal, but there are some benefits that are common to all hill running. The most important is that it builds your overall strength; research has shown that the muscles in your legs are forced to work harder for each step when running uphill, so they become more powerful, which translates to faster running and better endurance on flat surfaces. It is not just good for your legs; your upper body will become stronger as you need to use your arms to drive yourself up the hill, and your core strength and balance are improved by holding yourself steady on uneven downhill sections. Hills can be used as a threshold session, since your heart rate invariably rises on the climbs, and the mental strength you learn from repeatedly running a tough climb will

Below: Choose hills that level out at the bottom, giving you space to recover.

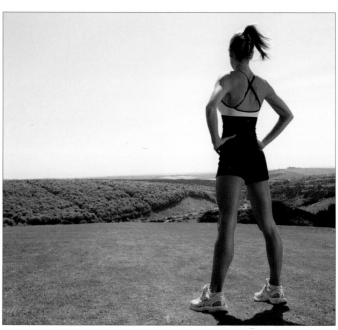

Above: Conquering tough climbs makes you stronger – and rewards you with great views at the top.

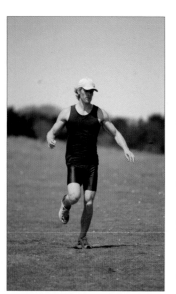

serve you well when you return to the road. Few race routes are completely flat, so learning to run up and down hills will always give you an edge over competitors if you choose to race.

How to run hills

First, choose your hill carefully. Look for a hill with about a 10 per cent gradient, ideally off-road as this will be more challenging for your muscles, but less damaging in terms of impact. You need at least 400m (¼ mile) of hill, with a fairly flat area at the bottom for recovery running. If you can, find a hill in a park or open countryside, so that you have good views to take your mind off the hard sessions.

Prepare yourself mentally before running a hill session. Running uphill can be demoralizing since you slow right down and struggle to find a

rhythm, so remind yourself of the goals behind your session, whether that is getting fitter, racing or just the satisfaction of a hard run (see box). Decide whether it will help you more to focus on the task in hand or look for distractions.

Form is important when running hills to avoid injury and becoming tired. Lean in to the hill slightly as you run up, but do not hunch over. Keep your back strong and pump your arms back and forth. Run on the front of your feet and keep your strides short. Look ahead of you rather than up toward the summit, otherwise you will strain your neck and could lose your footing. Try to

Hill sessions

Endurance (for fitness and long-distance running). Run uphill for 2 minutes, jog down and immediately start your next run up. Your effort should feel continuous even though you are not sprinting up the hill. Start with a 10-minute block, increasing each session by 2 minutes every week.

Threshold hills (for 5K and 10K running). Run uphill for 45 seconds to 1 minute, fast enough that you can utter only one or two words. Jog easily back down and repeat 10 to 12 times.

Power hills (for sprinting and middle-distance running, or to add speed in the final few weeks before a race). Find a steeper hill and power your way up for 30 seconds; jog or walk back down slowly, then repeat. Make this session harder by using soft ground – try it on sand dunes. Do 10 to 15 repetitions, rest for 5 minutes, then another 10 repetitions if you can.

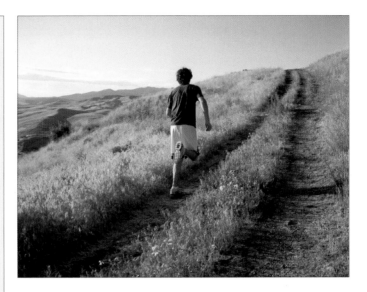

Above: As you climb hills make sure you keep your form strong and powerful to maximize the benefits.

keep your effort even when running uphill, even if that means slowing down. If you do have to walk, be purposeful and strong rather than trudging up.

Running downhill is, for many people, even more daunting than trying to run uphill. The trick is to be confident and allow gravity to carry you down, using quick, light steps and holding your arms out to the sides for balance. Keep your core muscles engaged to keep your balance and try to avoid leaning backward – you are more likely to injure yourself if you are constantly trying to put the brakes on. Watch the ground ahead of you and plan your route down as you go.

Below: Running down hills can be scary as you lose control, but it helps you to work on your balance.

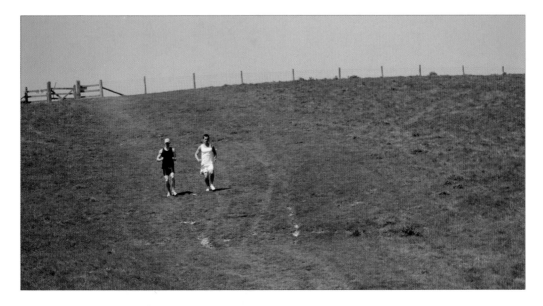

Threshold Training

Pain in the muscles after a hard run is caused by the breakdown of a substance called lactic acid, which is produced when you train. Deliberately training at or just below this 'burning legs' level is known as threshold, or tempo training.

When you have worked hard on a run your legs burn afterward, and the elevator looks more appealing than staggering up the stairs. The reason for this discomfort is the build-up of hydrogen ions in your muscles, which raise the level of acidity of your muscles.

Although threshold training is probably the most difficult kind of running, both in terms of learning how to do it correctly and in terms of physical and mental endurance, it is well worth including in your schedule once a week. At the most basic level it helps to improve your ability to run at a sustained, fast

Below: Threshold training sessions are perfect preparation for the pain of running fast races.

pace. It encourages you to run with good form, which carries through into the rest of your running, and teaches your body how to use fuel and oxygen more efficiently. Training at this level raises your lactate threshold, so you can run harder for longer. However, the real value of threshold training is seen when you race. During any race of more than a 1.5–3km (1–2 miles) you will be running at your lactate threshold for long periods of time, and learning to cope at this level is crucial to staying strong to the finish line.

How to run at your lactate threshold

Judging your threshold pace is almost as difficult as running at it. Lactate threshold can be measured using analysis

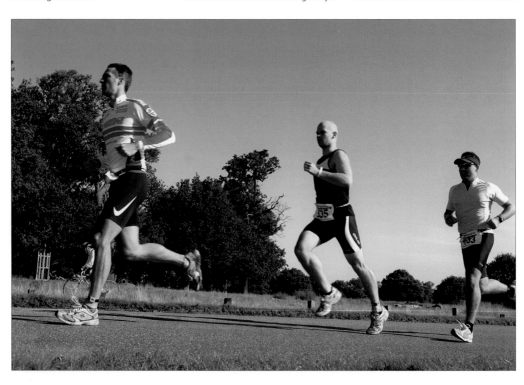

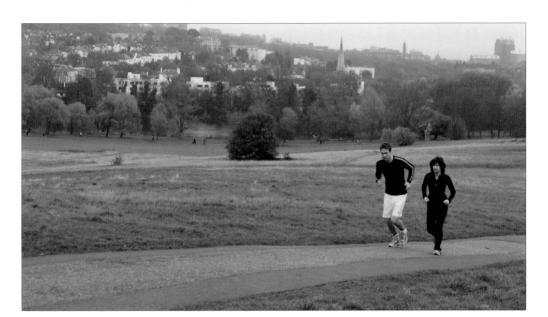

Above: Training with a faster runner will keep you at threshold pace when you're ready to stop.

of your blood (taken during exercise) or analysis of the gases you breathe out during exercise; this determines the heart rate at which you reach your threshold. However, these methods are expensive and, for the everyday runner, unnecessary.

In real terms it is better to think about running as fast as you can for a prolonged interval – say 20 minutes.

Lactic acid explained

This is a by-product of your energy producing system. When you run steadily, your body uses the aerobic system, in which oxygen is used with carbohydrates to produce energy. When you run harder, you cannot breathe in enough oxygen to continue this process, so your muscles switch to anaerobic energy production. The different system for breaking down carbohydrates results in the production of lactic acid. In fact, lactic acid is not what causes the burning, heavy-legs sensation. When you train hard, lactic acid breaks down in to lactate and hydrogen ions, and it is the ions that cause the problem.

Even this can be difficult to judge, as you should not feel as though you are running fast to begin with; the trick is to find a faster than usual running pace that you are able to sustain all the way through your threshold interval, but which leaves you feeling as though you could not have run any farther at that pace. A good guide is the talk test: after a minute or two of running at threshold pace, you should only be able to utter one or two words at a time. If you are alone, use the breathing test: if you usually take two steps for each breath, when you are at your threshold pace you will breathe harder, with two steps for the inhale and one sharp breath to exhale. You can use a heart-rate monitor if you have one: for most active people, the lactate threshold is reached at around 80 to 85 per cent of their maximum heart rate (estimate your maximum heart rate by subtracting your age from 220), so aim to stay at or just below that. However, the best way to ensure you are running at the right pace is to practice.

Different approaches

There are two ways to approach threshold training. First, you can run long intervals with short recoveries, for example you might run a distance of about 1.5km (1 mile) – or for 5 to 10 minutes – three or four times at threshold pace, with just 1 minute recovery between each interval. Secondly, you can run continuous threshold loops, building up each week, starting with 10 to 15 minutes and gradually building up to 30 to 40 minutes at threshold pace.

Below: Learn to tune into your own body and focus on the sensations of sustained fast running.

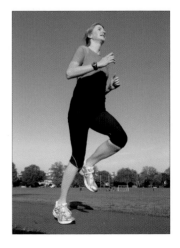

Running Surfaces

Conditions underfoot can make a huge difference to your running and generally speaking, the faster the surface, the more damage it will do in the long term. Choosing the right surface for the right sessions will help you to stay clear of injury.

The great thing about running is that you can do it wherever you are. If wherever you are happens to be in a city centre, however, you will soon find that your legs and joints take a pounding as you bash out thousands of steps on concrete. Here is a quick guide to some of the most common running surfaces, and which sessions they suit best.

Concrete

For many people, this is the surface they run on most often, as it is what you will frequently find outside your front door or office. However, the crushed rock that forms the basis of concrete paths makes it an incredibly solid surface to run on, with the added benefit of being faster than other surfaces. It is also usually a fairly smooth, even surface. However, this hardness also produces a bigger shock through your

Below: Synthetic tracks are a joy to run on and are perfect for measuring your speed intervals.

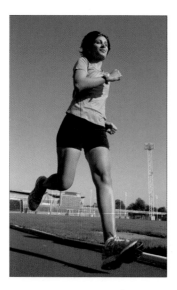

joints, and regular running on concrete can lead to impact injuries such as shin splints. If the pavement is poorly maintained you also run the risk of falling or twisting an ankle.
Best for: short, easy, convenient sessions that cannot be done elsewhere.

Asphalt

The vast majority of roads are made from asphalt and, as a result, most road races will use this surface too. It has slightly more 'give' than concrete, and usually provides a smooth, fast, even ground for running. However, like concrete, it offers little cushioning and should not be the base for most of your miles. Running in traffic also poses obvious risks, while drains and potholes could catch you unawares and cause accidents.
Best for: race practice or short runs.

Track

Although they can be intimidating for beginners, tracks are great fun to run on. They are usually made from synthetic materials to give a softer landing and some bounce, and because they are so flat and even, your running should feel much easier. They also provide the simplest way of measuring your run. The downside to track running is that the repeated bends can put a strain on your knees and ankles (alleviate this by changing direction often) and that it can become boring running in circles.
Best for: speed training and races.

Trail

Man-made woodchip trails, or natural forest trails, provide great running surfaces. As well as being soft underfoot and usually quite even, they are often in relaxing, traffic-free settings such as parks or woodlands. On the downside they can be badly affected by extreme weather – treacherously muddy when it

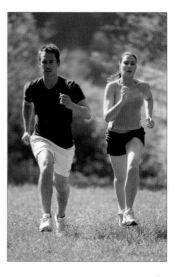

Above: Running on grass gives your legs a welcome break from harsh concrete surfaces.

rains, or baked hard when it is sunny – and sometimes hide hazards, such as tree roots or potholes.
Best for: long runs.

Grass

Short, well-kept grass is a pleasure to run on and has the best balance of soft cushioning and firm ground for fast running. Unfortunately some of the best grass for running may be in forbidden areas, such as golf courses or maintained parks, but even hopping on to grass verges for short sections of your normal routes will give your legs a break. The soft ground also makes your muscles work harder so you will be stronger when you race on the road. On the downside, like trails, grass can be slippy when wet and the surface is sometimes uneven.
Best for: longer speed sessions, long runs.

Alternative surfaces

Sometimes a trip away or desire for a change of scene will find you running on more unusual surfaces.

Sand: provides a great workout for your legs; wet sand is a good soft surface for longer runs if you can find enough of it. Running on the beach can place a strain on your Achilles tendon and calf, as your heel sinks down into the sand every time your foot hits the ground.

Moorland: a soft, springy and forgiving surface, this is great for longer off-road runs. Can be a trip hazard.

Rocky trails: if you are lucky enough to live near mountains, you might encounter scree and rock trails. These are very good for working on your balance and co-ordination, but you will need special trail shoes to protect your feet from bruising on the hard, sharp rock.

Treadmills: when the weather is bad, treadmills are a great alternative to running outdoors, and their soft, flat, even surface is good for runners returning from injury. However, they don't really replicate running outdoors, so should not be a base for all training.

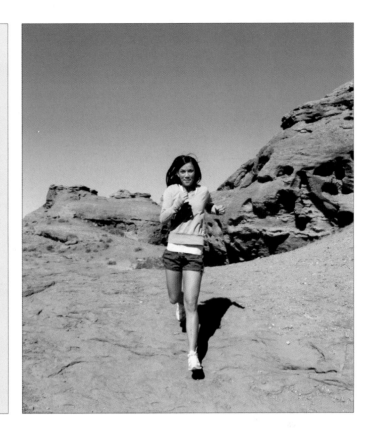

Below: Soft, smooth treadmills are perfect for returning to running after a period off due to injury.

Above: Off-road running can be glorious, but you'll need to watch your footing, especially on rough terrain.

Below: Training on sand is hard work – so many runners use it as a way to strengthen their legs.

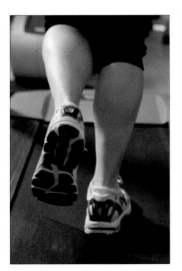

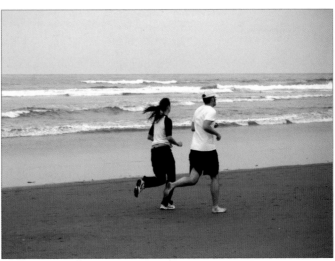

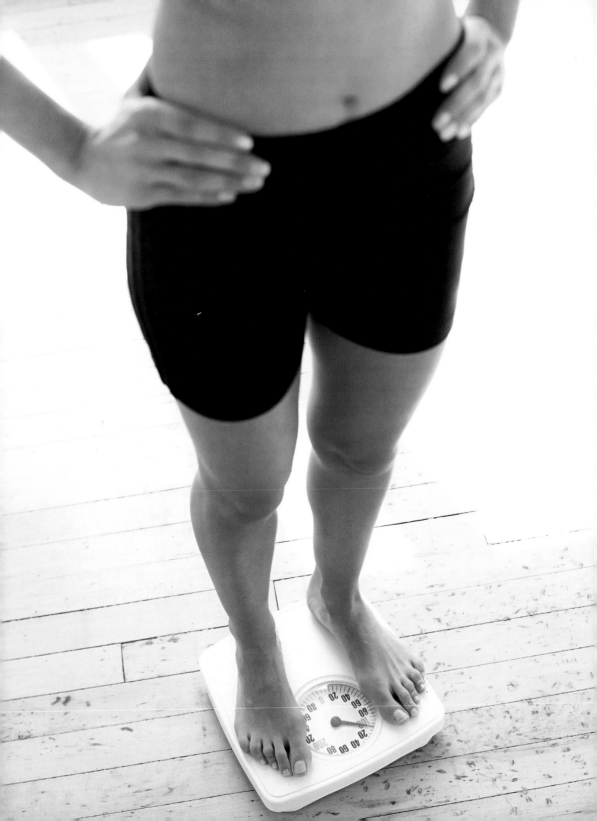

NUTRITION FOR RUNNING

For many people, starting to run is just the first step in a move toward a healthier lifestyle. Whatever your reason for running, good nutrition enables you to perform well, make the most of your sessions and avoid injury and fatigue. Traditional diets do not fit with the special requirements of runners, so even if weight loss is one of your goals, you will need to think carefully before cutting down what you eat and drink.

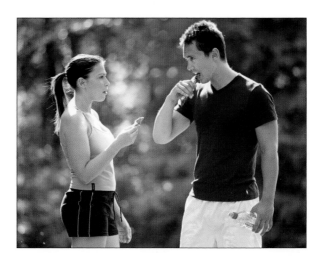

Above: Runners should think of food as fuel for their training.
Left: Running helps you lose weight, and losing weight helps you run.

Runners' Golden Food Rules

Becoming a runner means changing your attitude to food. Yes, you will be able to eat a bit more of what you fancy, but at the same time, eating a healthy diet is more important than ever to improve both your performance and your enjoyment in running.

There is nothing complicated about eating well – just follow these basic nutritional guidelines.

Never run on empty
Skipping meals is a bad habit for anyone, but for active people it can ruin an exercise session. Even if you run first thing in the morning, you should aim to eat a light snack an hour or two before you run. Good options include a banana and a small pot of yogurt, a handful of raisins, or if you find it impossible to stomach solids before running, try a sports drink.

Eat little and often
Using this strategy will keep your energy levels constant throughout the day, avoiding the surges and lethargy-inducing dips caused by eating large, heavy meals. By planning healthy snacks or light meals every two or three hours, you will be less tempted to give in to cravings for unhealthy foods, or skip a run because you are so hungry you choose to eat instead.

Below: Take healthy snacks, such as fruit, to give you an energy boost when you go out on long runs.

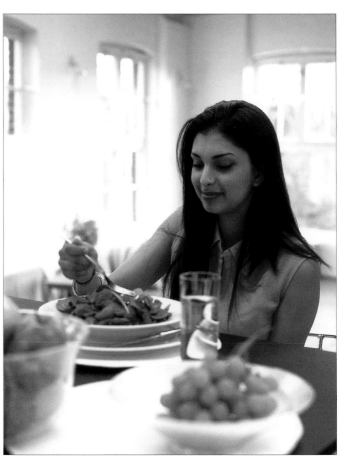

Above: As a runner you'll need to eat more so don't be tempted to skip meals.

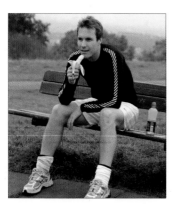

Eat the right carbohydrates
You will probably have heard that eating platefuls of carbohydrates (often abbreviated to carbs) is vital to fuel all exercise. While it is certainly true that the carbohydrates in your diet should give you most of your energy – around 60 per cent of the total calories you consume – all carbohydrates are not equal in terms of how quickly they are metabolized in the body. It is therefore important to plan exactly which carbohydrates you eat around your training sessions, making sure to use slow-release carbohydrates most of the time, with faster fixes for just before and after your training sessions.

(For a more detailed guide to the role that carbohydrates play in your diet, see pages 490–1.)

What are antioxidants?

Antioxidants are nutrients that help to combat the effects of free radicals – the molecules in the body that are linked to ageing, muscle soreness, heart disease and cancer. Intense exercise produces more free radicals in the body (as does smoking, ultraviolet light and pollution), so runners need to consume more antioxidants in their diets to counteract this effect. Antioxidants include vitamins A, C and E, carotenes (found in fruit and vegetables), the minerals selenium, copper, manganese and zinc (found in whole grains, cereals and meat), and flavanoids (found in tea, red wine, garlic and onions, and fruit and vegetables).

Below: Including a wide range of fruit and vegetables in your diet gives you plenty of antioxidants.

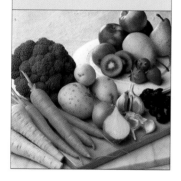

Inject some colour

As a runner, it is particularly important to make sure you have enough vitamins and minerals. The best way to do this is to accurately measure your food and work out how much of each nutrient you are eating – but no-one wants to plan their meals with a calculator. A simple route to getting enough vitamins, including essential antioxidants (see box), is to make sure you eat a variety of different-coloured fruit and vegetables.

Eat some fat

Forget the idea that all fat is your enemy. Between 15 per cent and 30 per cent of your daily calories should come from 'good' fats – that is, polyunsaturated and monounsaturated fats as found in foods like vegetable oils, eggs, nuts and avocados. These fats can help lower levels of 'bad' LDL (low density lipoprotein) cholesterol, keeping your heart and arteries healthy. They are also an excellent source of fat-soluble vitamins (A, D and E) and omega-3 fatty acids, which have been shown to improve athletic performance as well as keeping the heart healthy.

You should try to avoid foods containing too much 'bad' fat. Saturated fat, which is found in meat and full-fat dairy products, can raise your levels of LDL cholesterol, while trans fats (hydrogenated fats found in some ready-made products such as bread, cakes and margarine) are worse still.

Include protein at every meal

The more active you become, the more protein you will need. Your body uses it to repair tissue damage and to build muscle, and it can also be used as fuel for exercise. Protein also helps fill you up, so you are less likely to crave unhealthy snacks. Make sure you include some protein in every meal: sprinkle seeds on your breakfast cereal, snack on handfuls of nuts, and have some lean meat, fish or eggs in your lunch and main evening meal.

Below: Not all fats are bad; for example, eggs are a great source of fat-soluble vitamins.

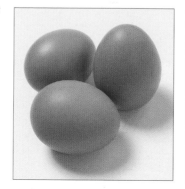

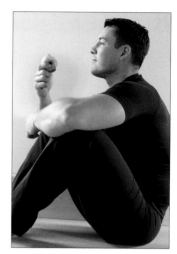

Above: Change the way you think about food – view it as fuel for your running, not 'excess calories'.

Do not diet

Most adults have been on a diet at some point in their lives. However, you will be a healthier, better runner if you can break out of the dieting mindset. Think about what you eat as fuel for your body's activities, and don't feel guilty about having the odd treat – your running can help you to burn it off. Look at building healthier eating and exercise habits long term, and you will be far more successful at keeping your weight down than you ever were with dieting.

Below: As well as healthy fats, nuts contain plenty of protein, so a handful makes a filling snack.

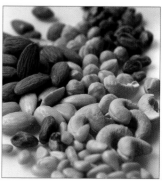

Runners' Golden Hydration Rules

One of the first pieces of advice given to novice runners is to drink more. But as most of us find, drinking gallons of water every time we run is neither practical nor effective. Here's how to solve your drink problems.

You have probably been told that you should always have a bottle of water on you at all times and should be sipping regularly when you exercise to avoid dehydration, which will not only damage your health but impede your performance. To an extent, this is sound advice. Getting hydration right is essential for comfortable, safe running.

The often-quoted fact that even a tiny drop in hydration – just one or two per cent of your body weight – leads to a much greater drop in performance is also true. However, drinking as much as you can, as often as you can is not necessarily the answer. During an hour of running

Below: You should be especially careful to monitor your hydration levels when training in hot conditions.

How much to drink

You will need to use trial and error to a certain extent to find a comfortable and beneficial amount of fluid for your training, but here are some good general hydration rules to follow:
• Drink 500ml (about 1 pint) of fluid during the two hours directly before your run
• Aim to drink 2–3 litres (3½–6 pints) each day (depending on your size and exercise level)
• Drink little and often rather than large volumes at once
• For every kilogram (2¼lb) of body weight which is lost during a run, drink approximately 1.5 litres (2½ pints) of water
• On short runs (up to one hour) there is no need to drink during exercise

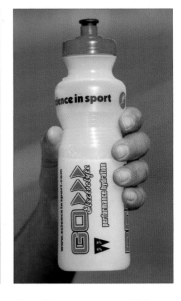
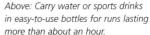

Above: Carry water or sports drinks in easy-to-use bottles for runs lasting more than about an hour.

you might lose up to 2 litres (3½ pints) of fluid, but your body is incapable of replacing that amount over the same time period.

Monitoring hydration

Instead of thinking about hydration in terms of filling up with liquid before and after a run, think about staying well hydrated generally. It is easy to monitor your hydration using one of these simple methods:

Weigh yourself (naked). Do this before and straight after a run. Every kilogram lost equates to one litre of fluid.

Monitor the colour of your urine. It should be very pale yellow (almost clear) most of the time. If it is very dark, you are dehydrated.

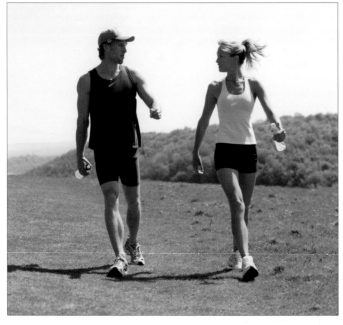

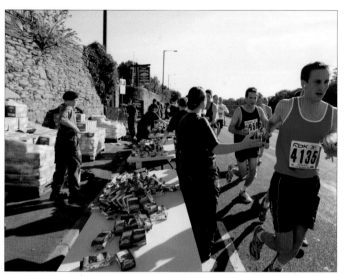

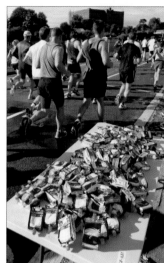

Above: Regular practice makes it easier to judge what and when you should drink during races.

Pay attention to your thirst. The old wisdom of drinking before you are thirsty is overly cautious, but it is certainly true that as soon as you feel thirsty your body is telling you to take in some fluid.

Although some level of dehydration is inevitable after a long run or race, it should not severely hamper your session. In fact, studies have shown that elite athletes regularly perform at modest levels of dehydration, and may even benefit from being slightly lighter as a result of carrying less water. However, it is important to be aware of the symptoms of severe dehydration, particularly if you are running in very hot or humid conditions, as in extreme cases this can be fatal. Signs to watch out for include: severe thirst, headache, lack of sweating, and confusion.

Drinking too much
While dehydration is still one of the biggest problems facing runners, particularly over longer distances, drinking too much water can be just as dangerous. Your body needs a certain level of sodium to function properly,

and filling up with plain water without losing it through sweat or urine can lead to a condition called hyponatremia, which means lack of sodium but is often known as water poisoning or over-hydration. This condition is increasingly common in larger mass races, where runners are slower and more likely to be overly conscientious about taking on water. The slower you run, the less fluid you lose through sweat, and the more opportunity there is to take a drink. Taking ibuprofen (an anti-inflammatory drug often used for joint and muscle pain) or aspirin will increase a runner's risk of developing hyponatremia. The symptoms are very similar to dehydration: headaches,

Above: Special sports drinks contain electrolytes which replace those that are lost through sweat.

nausea and confusion usually develop, along with bloating. Many runners are rightly very reluctant to reduce the volume of fluid they drink, as it can be difficult to judge how little is too little, so the simplest way to avoid hyponatremia is to drink sports drinks instead of water. These drinks contain electrolytes which replace those lost through sweat and they maintain your sodium levels. They also have the added benefit of containing carbohydrates, which will improve your running performance and fight off fatigue.

Good and bad drinks

Generally speaking, any fluid can be used to stay hydrated, but some are more beneficial than others, and some have side effects.

Good
Plain water: for runs up to one hour's duration, if required.
Sports drinks: for long runs over one hour.
Diluted fruit juice: for long runs.
Coffee or cola: just before hard or fast sessions, to increase alertness and speed.

Bad
Fizzy drinks: the gas in carbonated drinks makes them hard to take on the run, so many runners can't take on enough liquid to stay hydrated.
Thick drinks: some smoothies and shakes contain food that needs to be digested, so are absorbed slowly into the body.
Alcoholic drinks: any drink which contains more than 4 per cent alcohol speeds up the body's urine production, causing dehydration.

Pre-run Training Snacks

It is tempting to reward yourself for running by filling up on chocolate bars or chips, but what you eat before and after training can make a real difference to your performance and recovery. These snacks can all be made in less than ten minutes.

Think about planning your diet and you probably focus on the largest meal of your day. This is not a mistake – after all, your main meals account for most of your daily calorie intake and are your best chance to take in essential nutrients. However, a good diet can easily be undone by poor snacking and choices of light meals. The simple solution is to prepare your own easy snacks both to fuel your running and to help your body recover afterward.

Aim to eat two to three hours before running if you can, choosing slow-release carbohydrates to avoid peaks and troughs in energy as you run. Your body can only hold enough carbohydrate to fuel two to three hours of running, so during a long session (over one hour) you might want to take in some energy as you go, in which case special sports drinks and gels available from sports stores, may be the best choice.

Below: Drink diluted fruit juice before a run – it will be easier for your body to digest than solid food.

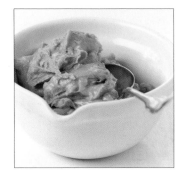

Banana and peanut toastie

1 small banana
1 slice wholemeal (whole-wheat) bread
15ml/1 tbsp smooth peanut butter

Mash the banana in a small bowl with a fork. Lightly toast the bread, then spread with peanut butter, adding the mashed banana on top. Fold in half to serve.

Nutritional information per portion:
Energy 392kcal/1646kJ; Protein 12g; Carbohydrate 56g; Fat 13g.

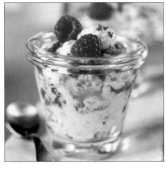

Breakfast pot

2 plain (unsalted) rice cakes
100g/4oz fresh raspberries
50g/2oz pomegranate (flesh and seeds)
150ml/¼ pint/⅔ cup low-fat fruit yogurt
15ml/1 tbsp clear honey

Break the rice cakes into pieces and place in a small bowl. Mix in the fruit and yogurt. Drizzle the honey on top.

Nutritional information per portion:
Energy 318kcal/1335k; Protein 9g; Carbohydrate 70g; Fat 1.8g.

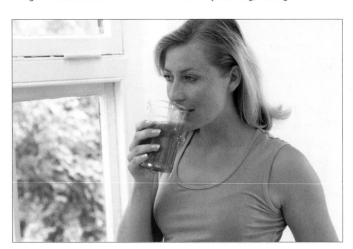

Digestive problems

Many people find it difficult to eat before running, particularly early in the morning. If your food sits in your stomach, at best you will suffer from a stitch or heavy legs, at worst you may feel sick or have diarrhoea. However, it is best to eat something before training, so try to eat a little before running. The more liquid a food, the easier it is to digest, so start with sports drinks or diluted fruit juice, then try soft fruit, such as a ripe banana. As you become used to running on that, try more solid foods. Two hours between eating and running is usually plenty of time for your pre-training snack or drink to leave your stomach.

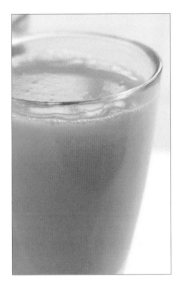
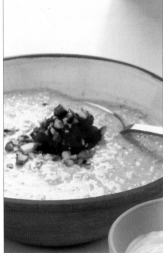
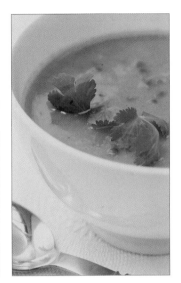

Energizing banana citrus shake

15ml/1 tbsp lemon juice
100ml/3½fl oz/scant ½ cup
  fresh orange juice
1 banana, mashed
150ml/¼ pint/⅔ cup low-fat
  natural (plain) yogurt
100ml/3½fl oz/scant ½ cup
  skimmed milk
5ml/1 tsp clear honey
5ml/1 tsp finely grated fresh root
  ginger or 10ml/2 tsp ground ginger

Place all the ingredients together in
a smoothie maker or blender, then
process on a low setting until the
mixture is smooth. Adjust the amount
of milk in the smoothie to change the
consistency. Serve immediately, or
keep chilled in the refrigerator for
up to 24 hours.

Nutritional information per portion:
Energy 296kcal/1243kJ; Protein 13g;
Carbohydrate 60g; Fat 2g.

COOK'S TIP
Investing in a juice extractor is
worthwhile if you want to be sure that
your fruit juice is fresh and pure. To
make orange juice, peel the fruit and
cut into large chunks before using the
juice extractor to juice.

Porridge with fruit and nuts

35g/1¼oz rolled oats
15ml/1 tbsp ground almonds
25g/1oz raisins, plus extra for topping
5ml/1 tsp cinnamon
100ml/3½fl oz/scant ½ cup skimmed
  milk, mixed with 100ml/3½fl oz/
  scant ½ cup water
15ml/1 tbsp clear honey
15ml/1 tbsp pistachio nuts, chopped

Place the rolled oats, ground almonds,
raisins, cinnamon, skimmed milk and
water in a large heavy pan over a low
heat and cook for about five minutes.
When the porridge is cooked, and
the milk has all been absorbed into the
oats, stir in the honey and leave to
stand for a minute. Sprinkle the nuts
and raisins on top of the porridge and
serve immediately.

Nutritional information per portion:
Energy 400kcal/1680kJ; Protein 13g;
Carbohydrate 59g; Fat 13g.

VARIATIONS
Add different toppings to your morning
porridge for variety. Try the following
combinations: chopped dried apricots
with pumpkin seeds, mixed berries and
natural (plain) yogurt, or sunflower
seeds, dates and sliced banana.

Quick tomato soup

5ml/1 tsp olive oil
1 small onion
1 clove garlic, crushed
400g/14oz can chopped tomatoes
400g/14oz can chickpeas, drained
  and rinsed
15ml/1 tbsp tomato purée (paste)
10ml/2 tsp mixed dried herbs
5ml/1 tsp chilli powder (optional)

Finely chop the onion. Heat the olive
oil in a large, heavy pan over a
medium heat. Fry the chopped onion
in the olive oil for about two minutes.
Add the crushed garlic, chopped
tomatoes, chickpeas, tomato purée,
mixed dried herbs and chilli powder,
if using, to the pan.
  Stir the ingredients together
thoroughly and simmer over a low
heat for about five minutes, or until
the soup is heated through thoroughly.
Serve immediately. You can also
make a larger quantity of soup by
doubling the ingredient amounts,
then freeze individual portions for up
to one month. This recipe makes
approximately two servings.

Nutritional information per portion:
Energy 253kcal/1062kJ; Protein 13g;
Carbohydrate 33g; Fat 9g.

Post-run Training Snacks

It is important to take on some food or drink as soon as possible after running.
A combination of carbohydrate and protein is best to restock your muscle glycogen
and help your muscles repair any damage done by hard training.

After training is a good time to eat fast-acting carbohydrates, so if you are a fan of white bread or sugary foods, this is a good opportunity to indulge, though as always you should be mindful of eating empty calories. Your immunity is lowered by fast or long running so whatever your post-training treat, you should try to include plenty of antioxidant vitamins in the hours and days after a hard session.

Eat as soon as you can after finishing your run. You may find that you don't feel like eating, particularly if it is a hot day or you have trained harder than usual, in which case try to drink some fruit juice or a glass of milk. Eat some solid food once you feel better. Think of your post-run refuelling strategy as your pre-run snacks in reverse: start with something small and easy to digest, then an hour or so later have a light snack, then when you are hungry again go for a heavier meal.

Below: Drinking milk after training is a good way of ensuring you get your protein if you don't feel like eating.

Antioxidant boosting smoothie

1 small banana
80g/3oz mixed berries, such as
* raspberries, strawberries, blueberries*
* or blackberries (fresh or frozen)*
250ml/8fl oz/1 cup skimmed milk
1–2 drops vanilla extract

Peel and roughly chop the banana. Put the chopped banana into a blender or smoothie maker and then add the fresh or frozen mixed berries, milk and vanilla extract.

Blend all the ingredients together until the mixture is a smooth consistency. For extra protein, add a scoop or two of protein shake mix. Serve immediately in a tall glass, or chill in the refrigerator for up to 24 hours.

Nutritional information per portion:
Energy 204kcal/856 kJ; Protein 10g;
Carbohydrate 42g; Fat 0.6g.

Below: Fruit juices and smoothies are a good way to take in antioxidant vitamins and are very easy to digest.

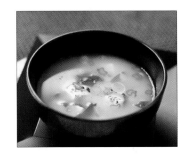

Miso soup

1 sachet miso soup or 15ml/1 tbsp
* miso paste*
400ml/14fl oz/1⅔ cups boiling water
100g/3¾oz/scant ½ cup beansprouts
100g/3¾oz firm tofu, cubed
100g/3¾oz spring greens (collards),
* roughly chopped*

Mix the miso and water together in a pan. Add the beansprouts, tofu and spring greens. Heat for 5 minutes.

Nutritional information per portion:
Energy 238kcal/ 1000kJ; Protein 20g;
Carbohydrate 20g; Fat 9g.

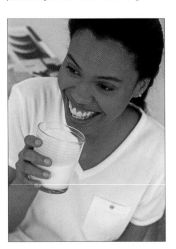

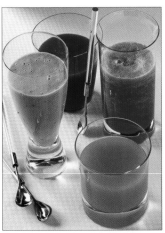

Quick protein fix

Eating enough protein is essential to enable your body to make a quick and full recovery from hard training sessions, but it can sometimes be a struggle to fulfil your daily requirements. A simple fix to this problem is to add protein shakes to your diet.

These come in powder form and are usually based around whey protein, providing about 15g (½oz) per serving. They often contain different vitamins and minerals as well as 200–300kcal (840–1,260kJ) of energy. If you don't like the taste of the shakes, you can always add a scoop or two of the powder to other foods such as porridge, desserts or fruit smoothies.

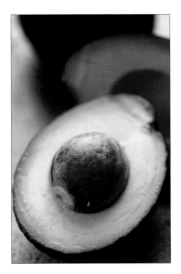

Above: Avocados have a high carbohydrate content and are full of the 'good' fats that your body needs.

Guacamole pasta

40g/1½oz wholemeal (whole-wheat)
  pasta
1 small avocado approx 50g/2oz
150g/5oz/⅔ cup low-fat natural
  (plain) yogurt
1 clove garlic, peeled and crushed
5ml/1 tsp lemon juice
1.5ml/¼ tsp chilli powder
2 tomatoes, chopped
15ml/1 tbsp pumpkin seeds

Fill a large pan with water and bring
to the boil. Cook the wholemeal
pasta for about six minutes (or
according to the packet instructions)
in the boiling water. Meanwhile,
mash the avocado in a large bowl
using a fork. Add the natural yogurt,
crushed garlic, lemon juice, chilli
powder and chopped tomatoes.
Mix together well. Strain the pasta,
put into a bowl and stir in the avocado
mixture. Sprinkle the pumpkin seeds
on top to serve.

Nutritional information per portion:
Energy 380kcal/1596kJ; Protein 17g;
Carbohydrate 41g; Fat 17g.

Sandwich fillings
A fresh sandwich makes the perfect
recovery food after a lunchtime run.

HUMMUS AND VEGETABLE
50g/2oz hummus
1 carrot, grated
50g/2oz chopped red (bell) pepper
15ml/1 tbsp fresh coriander (cilantro)

Nutritional information per portion:
Energy 138kcal/580kJ; Protein 5g;
Carbohydrate 15g; Fat 7g.

CHICKEN SALSA
100g/3¾oz roast chicken breast, sliced
30ml/2 tbsp salsa
1 handful spinach leaves

Nutritional information per portion:
Energy 231kcal/970kJ; Protein 28g;
Carbohydrate 3g; Fat 5g.

EGG AND PESTO
1 hard-boiled egg, sliced
15ml/1 tbsp red pesto
1 handful rocket (arugula)

Nutritional information per portion:
Energy: 200kcal/840kJ; Protein 13g;
Carbohydrate 1.5g; Fat 15g.

PRAWN AND SPINACH
5ml/1 tsp curry powder
Small pot of natural (plain) yogurt
100g/3¾oz prawns (shrimp), cooked
1 handful spinach leaves

Mix the curry powder and yogurt
together in a small bowl. Add the
prawns and spinach and mix.

Nutritional information per portion:
Energy 204kcal/856kJ; Protein 32g;
Carbohydrate 12g; Fat 3g.

Nutritional values for bread
When calculating nutritional values for sandwiches, remember to add the nutritional values of
the bread you choose (values per slice):

	Energy	Protein	Carbs	Fat
Seeded Wholemeal	234kcal/983kJ	9g	32g	8g
Wholemeal (whole-wheat)	172kcal/722kJ	7g	33g	2g
Rye	153kcal/642kJ	6g	32g	1g
White	160kcal/672kJ	6g	32g	1g
Plain bagel (1)	216kcal/907kJ	7.7g	42.8g	1.6g
Multigrain wrap	185kcal/777kJ	5.1g	32.2g	4g

Below: Rye bread contains the least
calories so is a good choice if one of
your running aims is losing weight.

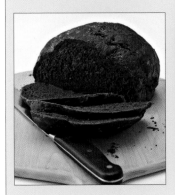

Below: White bread is full of fast-
acting carbohydrates so is best eaten
after training, if possible.

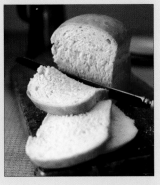

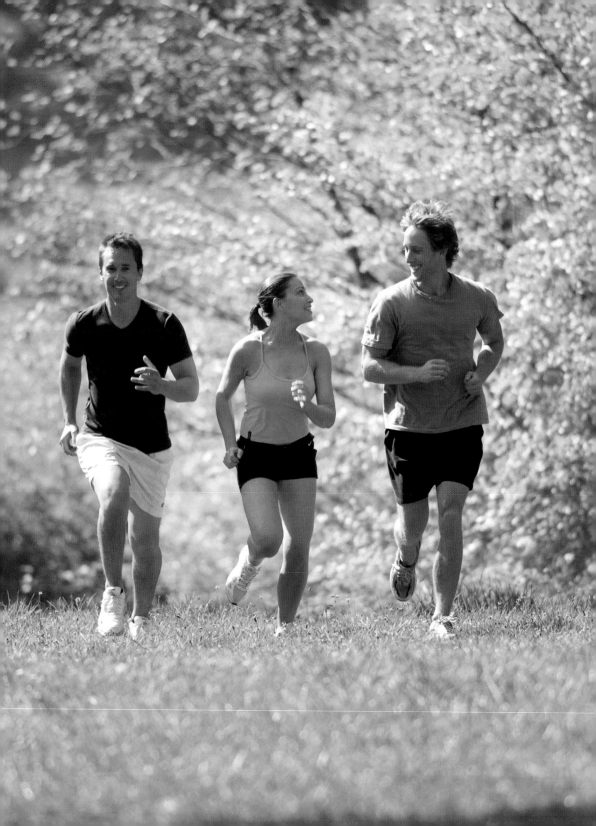

HEALTH AND INJURY

Runners tend to be more aware of their body than other people. This is a good thing, since it is rare to spend a lifetime running regularly without encountering injury. The good news is that running injuries can usually be cured within a few weeks, and most can be avoided altogether. This chapter will guide you through the symptoms and treatments of some common running injuries, and show you how best to run throughout your life, no matter what age or life stage you have reached.

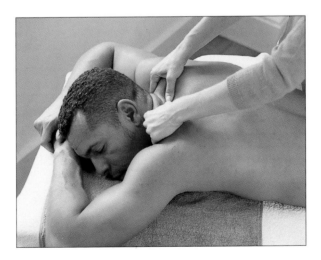

Above: Sports massage is a common treatment for running injuries – but it's not always this relaxing!
Left: Steady, sensible training increases are key to avoiding serious injury problems.

Common Injuries

Running has a reputation for causing more injuries than other sports. While this is not really fair, it is true that the repeated impact of thousands of steps places strains on your lower body. Here are some of the most common problems, their causes and how to deal with them.

Plantar fasciitis

The plantar fascia is a thick band of tissue under your foot running from front to back. Plantar fasciitis occurs when the tissue becomes inflamed, causing a dull pain under your foot. The pain may be worse on waking and, at first, feels better once you start walking or running, as the foot warms up.

Causes: High, stiff arches in your feet or low, flat arches can put a strain on the plantar fascia. A tight Achilles tendon or calf also puts more pressure through the foot, as does overpronating (your feet rolling too far inward on impact). Your shoes might also be the culprit: worn out shoes or too firm soles are another cause.

Treatment: This may require weeks of rest, during which stretching of the fascia itself is recommended: you can do this by rolling a golf ball under your foot, from big toe to little toe. Stretching your calf and Achilles may help. It is also worth seeing a podiatrist to check you are wearing the right shoes.

Instant relief: Freeze water in a paper cup, then peel off the cup and roll your foot over the ice. If you need a quick fix, use a cold drink can.

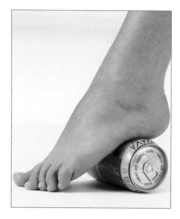

Above: Rolling the sole of your foot over something firm and cool alleviates plantar fasciitis pain.

Ankle sprain

A sprained ankle is the overstretching (or, in severe cases, breaking) of the ligaments around your ankle, usually on the outside.

Causes: This injury is always sudden, generally caused by stepping on a sharp camber or obstacle. Weakness in the ankle and fatigue are also factors, as you will be less able to correct your ankle position.

Treatment: RICE is always the best treatment (see box). You will usually need to take six to eight weeks off running. Once the initial swelling has died down, you can start balance exercises to rebuild strength and balance in your ankle.

Instant relief: Painkillers are effective – and often necessary – with this injury. Anti-inflammatory drugs may be taken to reduce swelling.

Achilles and calf pain

The Achilles tendon runs from your heel up to your calf muscle. Tightness in the Achilles often leads to problems in the calf, and vice versa. Achilles pain is usually sharp and felt just above the heel, while a calf strain is felt farther up.

Causes: Weak or inflexible calves cause both Achilles and calf problems. Running on hills and soft ground aggravates the problem. Speedwork

Achilles and calf pain

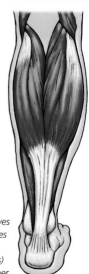

Right: Tight calves and tight Achilles tendons (under the calf muscles) often go together.

Plantar fasciitis

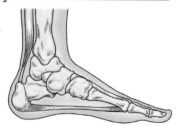

Above: The pain comes from inflammation of the plantar fascia, which runs under the foot.

Ankle sprain

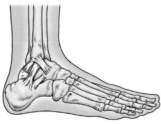

Above: The delicate, complex ligaments around the ankle become stretched in an ankle sprain.

Right: Calf pain can often be a result of tightness in the Achilles tendon at the back of the heel.

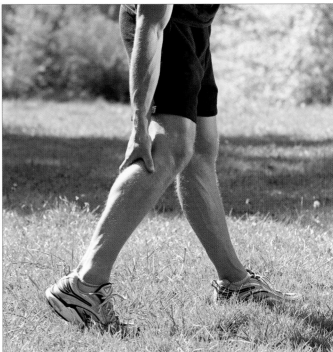

RICE

This is the first treatment for any acute injury that could become inflamed. It stands for rest, ice, compression and elevation. Stop running straight away, ice the injured area for 10 to 20 minutes, apply a compression bandage (ideally, have a sports professional apply the bandage so that it is not too tight), and if possible, raise the injured area above your heart.

Below: It is important to elevate and apply an ice pack to an ankle injury.

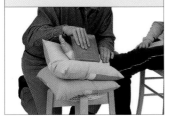

---

can contribute as it tightens up the calf muscles. Overpronation can sometimes be a factor.

Treatment: Stretching and strengthening of the calves should help. Try heel raises on a step, raising yourself up using your good leg and lowering with your weight through the injured leg. You may be able to run through a mild calf strain, but Achilles injuries usually require rest.

Instant relief: Wear shoes with a slight heel, or place heel lifts (no greater than 1cm/½in high) in your shoes to take the pressure off. (However, regularly wearing high heels can be a contributing factor to the injury.)

Shin splints

The term shin splints refers to any pain felt down the shins. Although worse during running, pain may be felt when walking.

Causes: Inflammation in the muscles, tendons or around the bones in your shins. Sometimes shin pain is caused by compartment syndrome, an inflammation of the thin fascia over the compartments of the muscles in your shins. Shin pain is often a result of sudden increases in mileage and running on hard surfaces. Worn out shoes and overpronation are also factors, and the pain may be linked to tight or weak calves.

Treatment: Stretching the calves and shins helps, as does deep tissue massage carried out by a physiotherapist. Self massage can help: place one thumb on top of the other on the inside of your shin, press hard and run up to the knee, repeating this right across the shin. It may be worth visiting a podiatrist to analyse your gait and recommend the correct shoes, or orthoses (special insoles to correct your gait). If you have severe compartment syndrome, surgery can be used to make a small incision in the fascia and release the pressure.

Instant relief: Simply kneeling with your feet flat on the floor (top down) provides some relief, and ice is very effective.

Shin splints

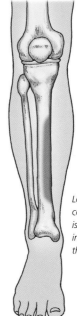

Left: Shin pain is very common in runners. It is often caused by inflammation around the bones in the shin.

Runner's knee

Otherwise known as patellafemoral pain syndrome, runner's knee is a sharp pain directly underneath the kneecap. As well as making running painful, it can be difficult for sufferers to use stairs or sit for long periods with their knees bent.

Causes: This condition was once thought to be the result of worn-down cartilage in the knee, but is now believed to be the result of the kneecap tracking to one side. This movement could be due to the wrong shoes (either too cushioned, allowing the kneecap to move too much, or not providing enough support for overpronation), weak quadriceps (particularly on the inside of the leg), tight hamstrings, or high-arched feet.

Treatment: Correcting the problems in the runner's gait that cause the kneecap to move is the best form of treatment. This could involve stretching the quads and hamstrings, or seeing a podiatrist for advice on shoes or orthoses. Performing slow, single-leg half squats (so you don't fully bend the knee) can help the kneecap to track properly.

Instant relief: Rest and ice, keeping the leg as straight as possible.

Runner's knee

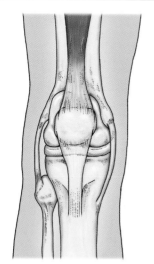

Above: The sharp pain of runner's knee is thought to be caused by the kneecap tracking to one side.

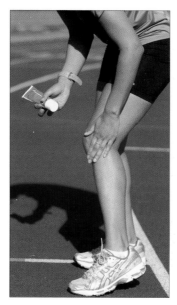

Above: Applying a freeze gel to the knee provides temporary relief, but don't ignore symptoms.

Other knee problems:

Anterior cruciate ligament (ACL) injury The ACL crosses underneath the kneecap, helping to keep the bones in the lower leg in place. It is most commonly damaged through twisting or sports involving a lot of lateral movement, such as football or hockey. This injury is too painful to run through and usually requires surgery.

Baker's cyst An inflammation of the bursa (fluid-filled sac) between the bone and muscle at the back of the knee, which becomes painful (the swelling is clearly visible). Anti-inflammatory drugs and RICE usually cure it in time.

Meniscal injuries There are two menisci (thin, fibrous cartilages) on the surfaces of the knee, one on the inside and one on the outside. The meniscus on the inside is more commonly damaged, and can be torn through twisting or bending the knee. Small tears may repair on their own but often keyhole surgery is required to remove the damaged part of the meniscus (recovery is very quick after surgery).

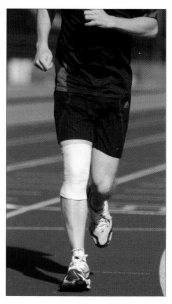

Above: Support bandages can help keep the knee in place and ease the pain of some injuries.

Iliotibial Band Syndrome (ITBS)

This condition has a very distinctive kind of pain, a dull ache on the outside of the knee, which can occur about ten minutes into a run. If you run through it, eventually any bending of the knee becomes very painful, especially walking downhill or down stairs. The ITB is a thick band of tissue running from the hip to just below the knee, and the pain is caused when the ITB becomes tight and rubs across the bones at the side of the knee with every step.

Causes: Running too far on a cambered surface or downhill can bring on this problem, though it may also come on through sharp increases in mileage. Overpronation and wearing the wrong running shoes can be factors. Lack of flexibility in the gluteus muscles and hamstrings can also cause the ITB to tighten.

Treatment: A notoriously difficult problem to cure, ITBS can be treated simply if caught early. Complete rest for a few days as soon as the symptoms appear can make a difference, after which stretching and deep tissue massage (performed by a physiotherapist) are the usual treatments. You can stretch the ITB by standing up straight with your legs crossed over (the painful leg should be behind the 'good' leg), then leaning sideways in the same direction as your back leg.

Instant relief: Straightening the leg and icing it as soon as symptoms appear should provide some relief and help recovery. It is best not to attempt to run through any symptoms of ITBS.

Hamstring injuries

A large tear in the hamstring usually happens mid-run and will be painful enough to stop you running. It may bruise and swell. Even a minor overuse strain in the hamstring can be very painful as the muscle is so large and so involved in running.

Causes: The hamstring helps propel you forward at speed, so sprinting and jumping are common causes of sudden tears. Introducing speedwork

and hillwork too quickly, or changing running surface or shoes are also common culprits.

Treatment: Massage can help with strains, though a severe muscle tear will take several weeks of rest to heal. Improving general flexibility right through your legs and hips should help the injury to clear up and stop it recurring.

Instant relief: For a tear, ice will provide pain relief, while if you are planning to run through a strain, try wearing compression kit to keep the muscle warm and flexible.

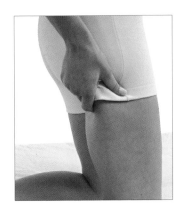

Below: Injuries to the hamstring muscle often occur quite suddenly in the middle of fast sessions.

Above: Regular massage, including self-massage, can help you to recover from muscular injuries.

Hamstring injuries

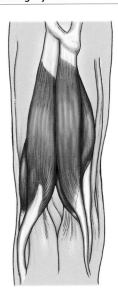

Above: The large hamstring muscle helps propel you forward and tears are very painful.

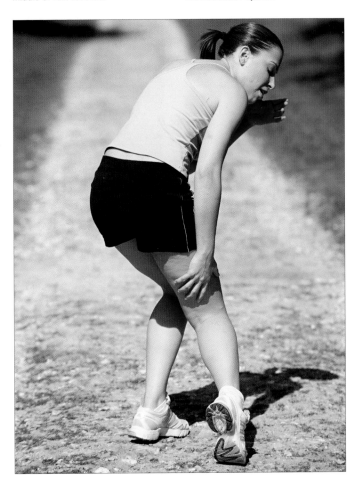

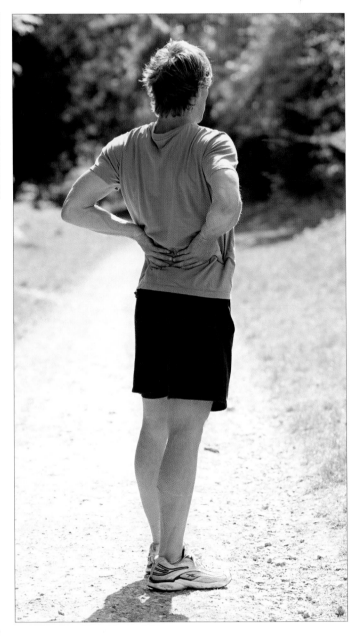

Right: Pain in the lower back is often a symptom of a problem elsewhere, such as around the pelvis.

Piriformis syndrome

The piriformis is a muscle deep in the buttock that helps rotate the leg outward and stabilizes the hip. If it becomes tight, you will feel a pain deep in the buttock when running, and if you try to run through it you might also have tightening and pain down the back and inside of your thigh, or in your lower back.

Causes: The piriformis usually becomes tight when it is forced to do the work of other, larger muscles, so weak gluteal muscles, abductors and core abdominal muscles can all contribute. Increasing speedwork or mileage too quickly are also factors, and lack of general flexibility makes the problem worse.

Treatment: Once the piriformis is tight enough to be painful, it usually requires deep tissue massage to release the muscle. Strengthening the core, glutes, hip abductors and adductors should help, and stretching all the major muscle groups is also essential.

The piriformis itself is hard to stretch, but try lying on your back with both knees bent; rotate the leg of the affected buttock outward and bring the ankle up to rest on the opposite knee in a figure 4 position, then reach around and grasp the back of your other leg, pulling both legs in toward your chest.

Instant relief: Give yourself an easy massage by lying down on the ground with a tennis ball under your buttock. Slowly roll the ball underneath you, putting as much of your weight as possible on the affected hip.

Osteoarthritis (hip)

This is much more common in older runners than younger ones. Osteoarthritis is a degenerative condition which produces a dull ache and stiffness in the hip joint and may reduce your range of movement.

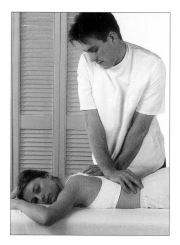

Above: Osteopaths can help make sure that your spine is aligned correctly, preventing injury.

Causes: Age and genetic factors are often behind osteoarthritis, and while running may aggravate it, it has not been shown to increase your likelihood of developing the condition (contrary to popular belief).

Treatment: Regular stretching should help to keep the joint mobile, and you should switch to soft but even running surfaces to reduce the impact through the joint. Glucosamine supplements

Pelvis

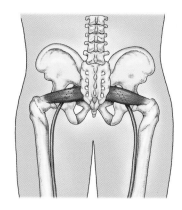

Above: The pelvis is a complex structure and problems with its alignment cause pain both above and below it.

can help. In severe cases, hip replacement surgery may be necessary.
Instant relief: Anti-inflammatory drugs should ease the pain.

Back pain

Most people will feel back pain at some point in their lives and, for runners, this tends to be in the lower back. Problems in the lower back may be hard to self-diagnose as you could feel the pain lower down – for example sciatic pain can be felt right down your leg.
Causes: If your back pain is chronic (rather than the result of a sudden, twisting or bending movement), then it could be the result of a number of problems. Weak abdominal muscles, resulting in poor posture, are a common cause. Gait problems, including leg length discrepancy, can lead to back pain. Problems in your gluteus or piriformis muscles can also be felt in the lower back.
Treatment: Though you may be able to run through mild back pain, you should look for the cause and correct it as soon as possible to avoid further problems. Strengthening your core and back muscles should help. You should have a gait analysis to rule out biomechanical problems,

A holistic approach

No matter how precisely you can pinpoint the painful area, no part of your body works in isolation. Running injuries, unless caused by a specific accident (such as an ankle sprain), are usually the result of chronic problems in more than one area of the body. Instability or weakness in your core can lead to a misaligned pelvis, which in turn stresses the muscles in your legs when you run.

If you have a recurring injury, or one which refuses to go away, visit a physiotherapist to work out the cause of your problems so you can correct it in the long term.

and it is worth visiting an osteopath to make sure that your spine is correctly aligned.
Instant relief: Alternating hot (using a hot water bottle) and cold (using ice) should help to relieve the pain temporarily. At night, try sleeping on your side with a pillow between your knees.

Below: Simple, regular stretches can help to alleviate back pain and prevent problems worsening.

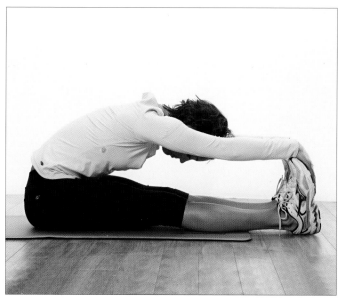

Avoiding Injury

There is nothing more frustrating for a runner than being incapacitated by an injury. That frustration is usually heightened by the knowledge that the problem could have been prevented, or at least its impact lessened.

Running injuries are almost always the result of a number of controllable factors. Here are some of the most common causes of injury and how to avoid them becoming a problem.

Too much, too soon
The list of sports injuries that can be caused by this basic error is almost comprehensive. In between sessions, your body becomes stronger by adapting to the stresses you place on it during training. By piling on miles or intensity, your body has little opportunity to adapt, and damage occurs. Never increase your mileage by more than 10 per cent a week. Don't increase more than one element at a time, be it speed, distance, or cross-training, and take into account other increases in activity, such as a new cycle commute to work, or even just an increased workload in the office.

Below: Stretching should be a relaxing part of your training, so use the time to reflect on your workout.

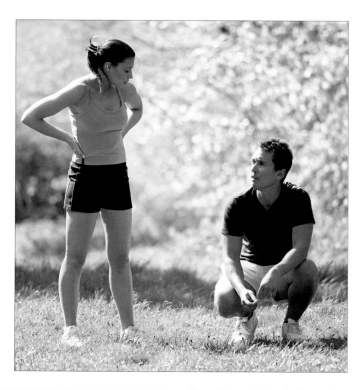

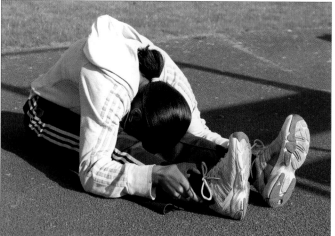

Above: Take regular breaks from training to avoid overtraining, which can lead to a decline in performance.

Overtraining syndrome
If you are training hard but not seeing a noticeable improvement, or carrying a chronic, low-level injury, you could be suffering from overtraining syndrome, which is brought on by long periods of intensive training. Symptoms can include extreme fatigue, depression, persistent colds and a decline in running performance. Fix the problem by taking a complete break from running for two weeks, which you can spend reviewing your goals.

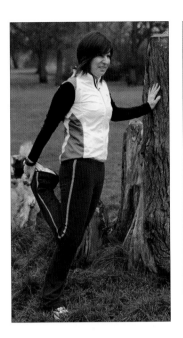

Above: The best athletes make stretching an essential part of their post-run routine to avoid injury.

Regular rest is important to help your body recover from training. Never train hard two days in a row. Schedule one rest day per week and have an easy training week every six to eight weeks.

Poor shoes

If you don't replace your shoes regularly, you can't expect them to provide enough cushioning and support for the thousands of footfalls that they will endure. They can be costly, but avoiding the expense of new shoes usually results in the much greater expense of sports injury treatment. As a general rule you should replace shoes every 800km (500 miles) or six months, but this will vary on different factors like your shoes, gait, weight and running surface. You should check your shoes for wear and tear at least once a month. If possible, buy two pairs of running shoes and alternate wearing them, so each pair has a chance to decompress and dry out after every use.

Yoga and Pilates

It may not necessarily be the first thing that springs to mind as a runner, but taking a few classes in yoga and Pilates is a very good way to improve your core strength, flexibility and body awareness, all of which can help you to avoid injury. It is always better to attend classes rather than attempt exercises on your own, as doing them incorrectly is at best useless and at worst potentially harmful. Before starting a new class, ensure it is at the right level for your experience, and in the case of yoga, that it is the right type: you should try to avoid overly strenuous forms such as power yoga or bikram yoga (where the room is kept very hot).

Right: Even learning the very basics of yoga and Pilates can help you be more in touch with your body.

Poor conditioning

Becoming a better runner is not just about running. The more you run, the more obvious your weak points will become, which is why good overall conditioning is essential. Start every run with a 10-minute warm-up jog, and spend 10 to 15 minutes afterward stretching all your major muscle groups. As you build up your training, you should also include strengthening work such as hill running or weight training, so that your body is stable and balanced when you take to the roads. Lack of flexibility combined with muscle imbalances (for example, if your quads are stronger than your hamstrings) is a recipe for injury.

Do not ignore biomechanical faults either, as these become exaggerated when you run. Give yourself a quick check standing straight in front of a mirror: you should be able to see, for example, whether one shoulder sits higher than the other, or if your hips are level. Do a single leg squat slowly and see whether your knee points forward all the way down. If you spot anything potentially troublesome, see a podiatrist or physiotherapist for a full assessment.

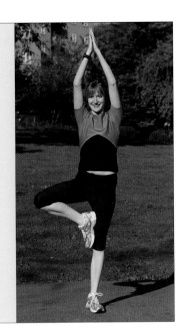

Running environment

Where and with whom you run can be a major factor in avoiding injury. If you run on very hard surfaces such as pavement or asphalt, you are at risk from impact injuries. On the other hand, if you always run on sand, you risk straining your Achilles tendon. Running the same route all the time is problematic, as you will be running on the same camber and potentially stressing one side of your body.

Below: Rest and relaxation are just as important for your development as hard training sessions.

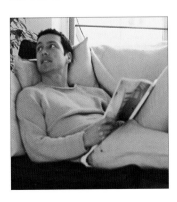

Injury Specialists

It is difficult to know who to turn to when you become injured through running. There are a range of health professionals who can help with sports injuries in different ways, but the most important thing is to find someone you trust and who cares about your sport.

Though running is undoubtedly good for your overall health, you'd be extremely lucky to go through a lifetime of the sport without becoming injured at some point. Unfortunately treating these injuries can be expensive, especially if you don't get the right diagnosis – and that depends on you finding the right health professional in the first place. Whichever route you take, if you have a persistent pain that doesn't respond to rest quickly, don't just hope it will go away. See one of these people who can speed your recovery and, perhaps more importantly, help you to find ways of preventing a relapse.

Your family doctor

As with any health problem, your family doctor is a useful first port of call for running-related trouble. Though he is unlikely to solve the problem himself, your doctor will be able to make a first diagnosis and refer you to a specialist for further treatment. For acute injuries, a doctor may be best placed to help, as he will be able to assess how serious the damage is and order X-rays or scans; he can even refer you to a surgeon if necessary.

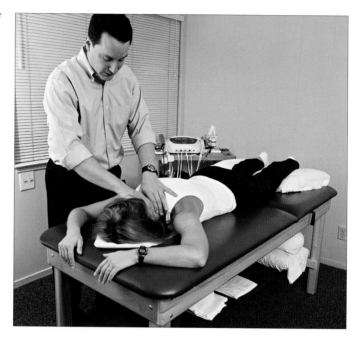

Physiotherapist

If you have a long-term or relatively minor injury, your doctor will often refer you to a physiotherapist, and

Above: Sports physiotherapists are trained to use different treatments for a range of injuries.

many runners go straight to the physio once an injury has set in. A physiotherapist can diagnose and treat almost all sports injuries, and will look at the injury in the context of your whole body, often examining your overall posture and gait to determine underlying causes. Physiotherapists usually treat injuries using massage, and by prescribing stretching and strengthening exercises. They are often trained in a wide range of disciplines including deep tissue massage, acupuncture, strapping and using ultrasound to break down scar tissue. Some physiotherapists will also refer you for for further examination in the form of scans and X-rays.

Finding Dr Right

Most sports-injury specialists operate privately, so check that they are fully qualified; most disciplines have regulatory boards so start with these organizations to find a trustworthy professional. Before you book an appointment, check that the person you have chosen has interest and experience in sports injuries. Don't be embarrassed to ask about their qualifications. If you know other runners, ask them for recommendations.

Right: Do not be embarrassed to ask your doctor about their qualifications.

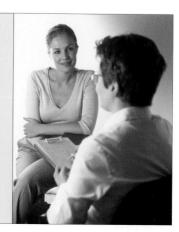

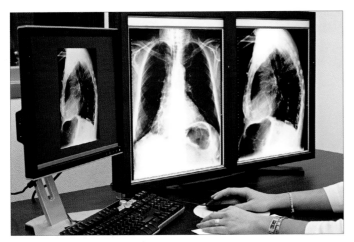

Left: Health professionals can refer you for tests, such as X-rays or MRI scans, to aid diagnosis.

and strengthening exercises, and may be trained in acupuncture and strapping (to support your muscles).

Sports masseur

While not usually able to help with serious injuries, sports masseurs can offer pain relief and can help with muscular problems by loosening stiff muscles. It is a good idea to see a sports masseur if you have a muscle strain, especially in larger muscles such as the gluteals or hamstrings. Regular visits to a sports masseur, even before injury occurs, may help with flexibility and with recovery from training.

Podiatrist

Also known as chiropodists, podiatrists are thought of as foot specialists but will usually examine your gait from head to toe to determine the root of a running injury. They will usually watch you walk up and down or on a treadmill, and will perform a static examination to look for potential problems. They can refer you for X-rays and further tests. They also prescribe orthoses, special insoles to correct your gait, and can advise you on shoes. Again, it may be worth seeing a podiatrist before becoming injured to prevent problems before they occur.

Chiropractor

Sometimes known as 'back doctors', chiropractors focus on the back, particularly the spine, and will 'clunk' your back and neck back into the correct position. However, they also work on joints all over the body, so can treat a wide range of sports injuries, in particular lower back pain, ITB syndrome and hip problems.

Like physiotherapists, some chiropractors use ultrasound, and some use electromagnetic pulse therapy to encourage healing.

Below: Podiatrists will often perform static examinations of your feet to look for problems.

Osteopath

An osteopath may also 'clunk' your bones but the treatments they offer usually involve working on the muscles and tendons around your joints to balance your body. Osteopaths take a holistic approach to injury treatment, so they will examine you for weaknesses all over the body and may advise you on nutrition and cross-training. It may be useful to see an osteopath early in your running career, even if you are injury free, to determine any weak spots. Osteopaths may prescribe stretching

Below: Some runners swear by regular sports massage as an effective means of injury prevention.

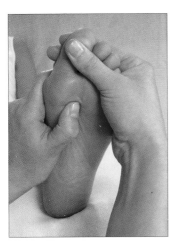

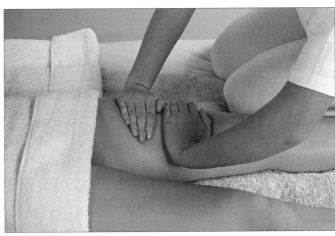

Alternative Injury Treatments

Sports injuries can often be very difficult to diagnose and even harder to treat, so it is no surprise that runners are often open-minded about the methods of treatment that they will try. Some may be sceptical, but the results speak for themselves.

Many of the methods of healing used on running injuries are on the fringes of conventional medicine, but for every one of these treatments there are thousands of runners willing to swear by its effectiveness.

Acupuncture

More and more health professionals are choosing to add acupuncture to their range of skills as it becomes more accepted in all areas of medicine. In traditional acupuncture, which comes from ancient Chinese medicine, very fine needles are inserted just beneath the skin at different points along meridian channels – the theory being that chi (energy) should run freely down the channels, and when they become blocked this is what causes physical problems.

Whether or not you believe in Chinese medicine, several studies have shown that acupuncture can help with pain relief, and with specific running injuries.

Below: A session of acupuncture could help to release muscle tightness, easing sports injuries.

In one piece of research, acupuncture was successfully used to treat plantar fasciitis, with needles placed along the arch of the foot and on different muscle trigger points on the calf. It is thought that acupuncture works on sports injuries both by reducing any tightness in the muscles and by prompting the brain to release painkilling chemicals.

Reiki

Another treatment based on an ancient Eastern philosophy, Reiki is a Japanese word meaning 'universal life energy'. Practitioners of Reiki are able to channel this life energy to promote both physical and mental wellbeing. In a Reiki session, they will place their hands on or over the problem area, with the idea being that by channelling the life energy they will help the body to heal itself. Reiki is used for a wide range of physical, mental and spiritual problems, and once you have been trained in Reiki, you can use it on yourself as well as on other people.

Right: The meridian channels used in acupuncture. Energy (chi) should be allowed to flow freely around the body.

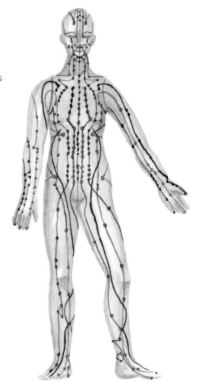

Electromagnetic pulsed field therapy (EMPT)

Like acupuncture, EMPT is employed by health professionals to treat sports injuries. As the name suggests, during treatment, electromagnetic pulses from a small machine are passed through the injured area (applied through a wrap around the affected limb). EMPT is said to work by realigning the ions in the cells of the damaged area; it also improves circulation and therefore oxygen delivery, helping speed the healing process. Regular users say it can reduce pain, swelling and muscle tightness to relieve injuries. Again, it is possible to use this treatment on yourself, as the machines are available either to buy or hire.

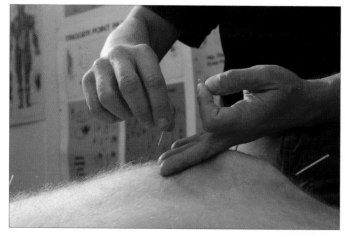

Simple self-help

Runners are used to being active and in control of their bodies, so injuries are always frustrating, especially when treatments involve so much trial and error. However, keeping a positive outlook can really help with your recovery, so keep these strategies in mind during any lay-off:

• Remember that the vast majority of runners recover fully from their injuries, and many are even better runners after the break

• Do something positive to help your recovery each day, whether it is a stretch, massage or icing your injury

• Do some activity every day: walking and swimming are usually safe for injured runners

• See your time off as a chance to meet up with non-running friends and have fun

• Set yourself goals in other areas of your life, so you don't feel bad about missing any running targets

Below: Staying positive by meeting up with friends helps you recover from injury faster.

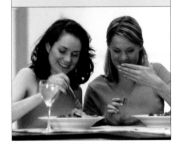

Hypnotherapy

For many people, the idea of being hypnotized still conjures up images of someone swinging a watch in front of your face. However modern hypnotherapy is more a method of programming your brain through visualizations and affirmations. This may help with sports performance but can also be useful for the treatment of injuries. Research has shown that athletes hold on to the memory of pain from an injury long after the physical

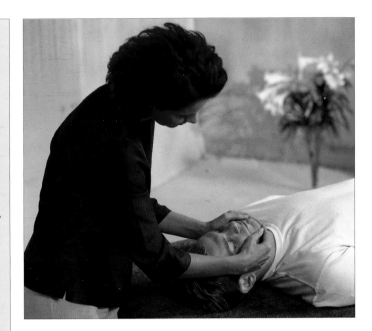

damage has disappeared. Hypnotherapy can use visualization of a positive outcome to overcome stress or anxiety about the injury, which may be at the root of residual pain.

SCENAR therapy

This treatment was originally developed in the former USSR to treat injury and illness on its space programme. Later it was used by the Soviet Olympic team, and is still used by many sports-people to treat injuries. SCENAR involves the stimulation of nerves using electrical currents via a small, handheld machine, operated by a health professional who will have trained specifically to use the equipment. The SCENAR (Self-Controlled Energo Neuro Adaptive Regulation) machine is used first to test nervous response and identify problem areas, and then to treat them. The theory behind it is that it 'reminds' the body of the original injury, stimulating the healing response – though the newer the injury, the quicker and more effective it is said

Right: You can use self-hypnosis and visualization to help your own recovery.

Above: Reiki practitioners are able to channel the body's life energy to help banish aches and pains.

to be. Where it is effective, just two or three treatments are enough to resolve the injury.

Reflexology

Though it is thought to have origins dating back thousands of years, reflexology as it is practised today was popularized in the early 20th century. The therapist applies pressure to different zones on the feet (and sometimes hands) which are said to correspond to other parts of the body. Its use for treating sports injuries is mainly for pain relief, and it should be used in conjunction with other forms of treatment.

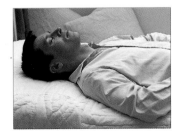

Running for Life

Running is a flexible sport. Not only can you adapt it to your changing circumstances, but it can help with challenging life stages. To make the most of what running can offer you at these times, be creative with the way you train.

It's easy to see why elite athletes run so well: all they have to do is train and recover, and they have teams of experts on hand to help with any changes that take place over time, such as having children, getting injured or just growing older. For the rest of us, exercise has to fit in around changing lifestyles, family and career. When your life alters the way you train, you may need to adjust your goals and expectations for running accordingly, but in return, running will help you cope with stressful changes, both physical and emotional.

When life becomes busy, running is often the first thing you drop. But staying physically fit helps you cope with pressure, changes and stress and running is known to benefit your mental wellbeing too. Make time for even a short run no matter what else is going on in your life,

Below: Having a baby does not have to mean the end of your running career – with the right kit you can run together.

and you'll feel stronger, calmer and better able to tackle some of these difficult periods.

Pregnancy
The days of doctors advising pregnant women to take things easy are long gone. Pregnancy is not the time to start running from scratch, but if you already run then you can carry on as long as your body will let you. Running can help alleviate many of the common, unpleasant symptoms of pregnancy, including mood swings, excessive weight gain and poor sleep. Staying fit through your pregnancy will also leave you stronger for labour when the time comes.

If you plan to run throughout pregnancy, you should tell your doctor or midwife from the outset – they will be able to advise you on how best to adapt your training. Drop intense training such as long runs and speedwork, and have a session with a personal trainer to adapt your strength and flexibility work. During the last half of

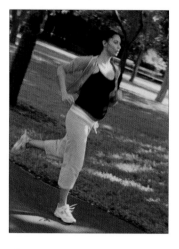

Above: It's safe to run at low intensity throughout your pregnancy.

pregnancy, your body produces a substance called relaxin, which makes your joints more flexible – this enables your pelvis to stretch during birth, but also leaves you susceptible to injury.

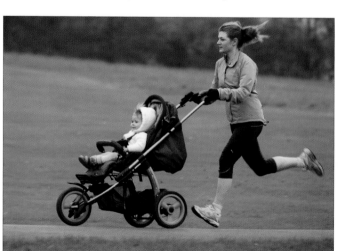

Pregnant runners' quick tips
- Try to keep your heart rate low (below 140 bpm) and your body temperature down
- Wear two sports bras for extra support and comfort
- Don't try to start or increase running during pregnancy
- After giving birth, don't try abdominal exercises until your rectus abdominis muscle has closed up again (it will separate down the middle of your stomach during pregnancy)
- Practise pelvic floor exercises regularly – stress incontinence is very common after giving birth and may be worsened by running

After giving birth, if there are no complications you can start low-intensity training within days if you feel comfortable. Wait until you can run pain free, and start at a low intensity. Don't try to jump back in to your pre-pregnancy training and don't try to lose weight too quickly – if you are breastfeeding, you will need the extra calories to produce milk. Once you begin training again you may be pleasantly surprised: pregnancy gives your cardiovascular system extra training, your pain threshold is higher and many women find they are more confident. As a result, you may find yourself a quicker runner.

Work stress

While runners who have successful work lives are often also very successful sportspeople, it is easy to underestimate the impact a busy career has on your ability to run well. Of course, lack of time is the main problem, but work stress also impacts on your general health through the release of hormones, lowering your immunity and making you feel too tired to run well.

Although running is an excellent way to cope with busy periods at work, you may need to revise the way you train. If you know you are facing a hectic few weeks, avoid

> **High flyers' quick tips**
> • Save time and stress by making your run part of your commute, taking you away from the hassles of road rage and public transport failures
> • Watch that your diet doesn't start to fall apart when you are working long hours. Take raw vegetables and fruit to snack on and make sure you don't miss meals
> • Think about changing your goals – for example, instead of going for a personal best at a marathon, aim to pace a first-timer
> • Make sure that you do not scrimp on your sleep, as it will impair your recovery from running as well as your ability to work efficiently

> **Veterans' quick tips**
> • Run on softer surfaces, which are easier on your joints
> • Stay motivated by switching distances, so that you are not chasing 20-year-old best times
> • If you take part in races, view your results in the context of your age category. Check your times against the World Association of Veteran Athletes (WAVA) age-grading tables
> • In training, focus more on flexibility as this will naturally decline, and will affect your speed
> • Allow yourself more time to recover from hard runs

setting ambitious running goals that will just put you under more pressure. Instead, dedicate short blocks of time (30–45 minutes) on set days of the week for running, leave your watch (and phone!) at home and just enjoy the break. Set these appointments in stone as you would an important work meeting; you may not feel you have the time to run, but remember that it will most likely lead to a more productive day, as well as an easier return to more structured training when your busy spell is over.

Ageing

Slowing down is of course an inevitable part of growing older and you will find that running becomes harder from your mid-30s onward. However, as long as you are prepared to change the way you train and race, you can still enjoy running and, if anything, the benefits can be even greater as you age.

Regular exercise will help you to fend off many age-related problems including high blood pressure, weight gain, loss of mobility and muscle tone, loss of bone density, and slowed metabolism. Runners also lose their VO2 max (the rate at which the body can use oxygen) around 50 per cent slower than non-runners – which means that you will stay fitter for longer.

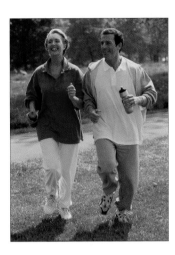

Above: Keep running as you grow older and you could avoid many age-related health problems.

However, no amount of training will enable you to completely out-run the ageing process. All of the processes listed above will still continue to take place, albeit at a much slower rate than if you were not running or doing any exercise at all. The consequence of ageing is that you will run slower for the same amount of effort, and accepting this fact is key to continuing to enjoy running. You may also find that you need more recovery time between hard runs, and that you are much more susceptible to injury. To avoid this, run less often and introduce some cross-training to reduce the impact on your body.

On the days that you do run, you will need to work hard to maintain your fitness, so aim for about three or four good quality sessions per week. Include at least one session of short, sharp speedwork to help maintain mobility in your joints, and be more diligent than ever about stretching out your muscles after you run. Weight training is also more important, as it helps to counteract loss of muscle mass and keeps your bones strong. Try to aim for about two sessions of weight training per week.

Children's Running

Almost as soon as a child can walk, he or she starts trying to run. With childhood obesity rates increasing, it is more important than ever to encourage children to engage in physical activity, and you may even find you have a champion in the making!

By the time they reach school age, many children have lost a lot of their initial energy, but if you show an interest in keeping your child active you can make the most of his natural urge to run around. That doesn't mean your child should be doing speed drills every morning, but by encouraging energetic play you can instill a lifelong love of exercise for the sake of it – and perhaps nurture a talent for formal athletics later in life. Here's how to involve your child in your sport from preschool to early adulthood. Remember, of course, that children have their own special needs, and that eventually they may not share your passion for running.

Preschool children

From when they learn to walk until the age of five, children should not do any structured running at all. They are still developing quickly, and have undeveloped vision, gait and co-ordination, so it is better to encourage active play rather than running. Luckily this comes naturally to most preschool children; all you need to do is provide a safe, ideally outdoor, environment for them to play in.

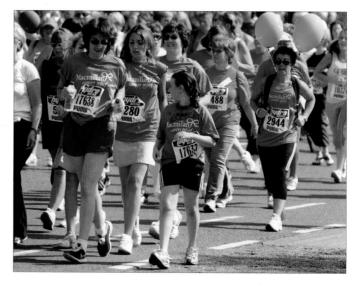

Above: As a child's age reaches double figures, she can train to run a mile at a time, but should not train too hard.

Age 6 to 11

Children should have developed a more controlled running motion by this age, but their natural tendency is still to run in short, fast bursts. They may have trouble running efficiently, as their limbs are out of proportion to their muscle mass. Incorporate running into physical games, and include ball skills to improve co-ordination. Think in terms of time spent on activity (aim for 20 to 30 minutes, three to five times per week) rather than distance covered.

As children near the end of middle school, their growth may begin to accelerate. This can lead to growing pains, and active children may suffer from a condition called Osgood-Schlatter syndrome. This causes sharp pain just underneath the kneecap, and is a result of strain being placed

Below: Preschool children should be encouraged to play actively rather than run seriously.

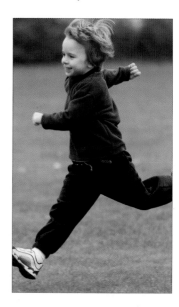

Keeping cool

Children are more prone to overheating (and to cooling too quickly) than adults. They are not as efficient at sweating, and have a greater skin surface to body weight ratio, which means they pick up and lose heat very quickly. Ensure they train in lots of thin layers that can be removed or put back on quickly, and don't allow children to train during the hottest part of the day. It is also important to ensure that they drink plenty of fluids, as many children will forget to do so themselves.

on the soft growth plate at the end of the leg bone just below the knee. The condition disappears once the child is fully grown but should not be ignored or run through. In fact, it is not advisable for children to try to run through any pain since they may be causing damage that may last into adulthood. Providing the child has no problems, they can start to run over longer distances (up to a mile) to learn endurance.

Age 12 to 16
As children grow into teenagers their training can become more focused. This is a good age to start competing over short distances (up to 5K), and is often when running talent becomes more obvious. Physically they may still have problems caused by their rapid development. Teenagers' limbs grow so quickly that they can seem clumsy, as the brain struggles to keep up, resulting in poor spatial awareness. It is a good idea to teach young runners good form at this age. Teenage girls need to become used to training through their menstrual cycle and with increased

Right: From age 12 upward, more structured training sessions can be introduced if the child wishes.

body fat, which will slow them down. At the same time it is important that they do not become concerned with keeping their body fat at a low level, as this will interrupt menstruation (as well as potentially leading to longer term body-image problems). For both sexes, bones are still developing and stress fractures are a risk; counter this by training on soft surfaces wherever possible.

In their mid to late teens, most children can cope with training sessions almost as intense as adults. However, it is still a good idea to maintain interest in other sports both to provide respite from the impact of running and to help the young athletes explore which activities they enjoy most.

Age 16 to 18
Most children are almost fully grown by this age and are able to cope with high mileage training. However, races should still be kept short and

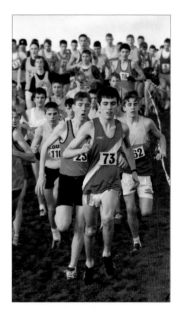

varied – up to 10K on cross-country courses, tracks and roads. As endurance does not develop until the mid to late 20s, it makes sense to concentrate on faster events at this stage.

Fussy eaters
Active children need to eat more than those who exercise less, but resist the temptation to calorie count for your child (they should definitely not become preoccupied with food). Instead try to pay attention to their appetite and energy levels, which should indicate whether they are eating enough. Don't allow your children to eat extra junk food to make up for training. Instead, ensure they have extra protein in their diet (research suggests 1.1 to 1.2g per kg body weight per day is the right amount for active children) for growth and repair, as well as extra calcium for growing bones and plenty of different vitamins to help them metabolize food.

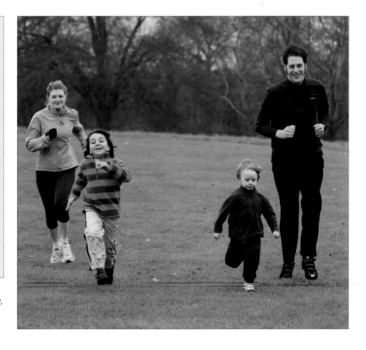

Right: Young children enjoy being active, so find open, safe environments for them to run around in.

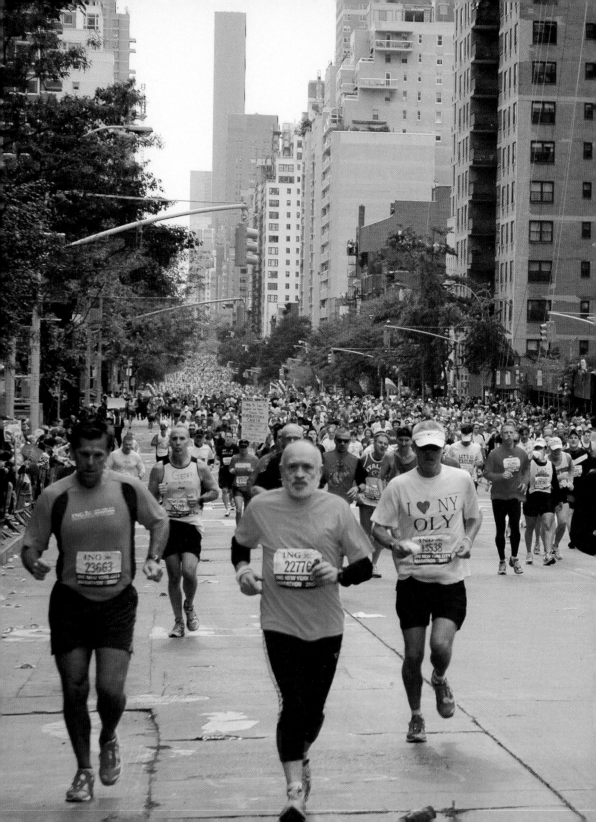

STARTING EVENTS

The word 'race' may bring you out in a cold sweat,
but competing adds a new level to your sport, no matter
where you finish. Your training will have a new focus,
and you will find motivation in trying to achieve more
from each run. The excitement, camaraderie and sense
of personal triumph of your first race will stay with you
forever. In this chapter you will find out how to race and
why you should do it, and there are examples of the
best beginner-friendly races running has to offer.

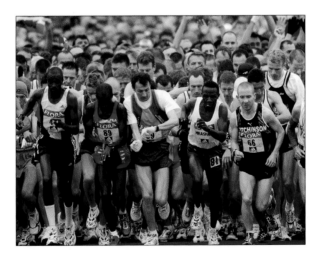

*Above: Once you start taking part in larger events you will soon see that running really
is for anyone and everyone.*
Left: The New York City Marathon, the original 'people's race', is a great event for first-timers.

Why Run an Event?

Although the idea of pinning on a race number and pitting yourself against others may seem daunting at first, once you have run in a race you will never look back. Taking part in organized events is a great way to make contact with the wider running community.

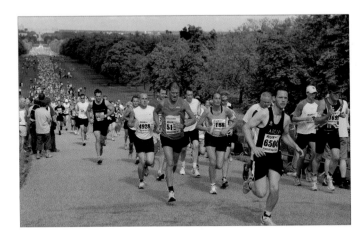

Left: Enter a race with a big field, and you'll see that running is a very inclusive sport.

performance. You will have achieved something millions of people never have the courage to experience.

Self-discovery

Every run tells you that you are a determined, disciplined person, but in a race you might shock yourself with your own strengths. Your ability to dig deep and push on, whether you are sprinting for the end of a 5K or pulling yourself through the 18th mile of a marathon, is something you will always be able to call on in difficult situations.

Community

Running can sometimes be a lonely sport. In fact many beginners choose to run alone, worrying that they will feel too embarrassed if they run with others or that they won't be

Below: Racing makes you push yourself to your limits and helps you learn about yourself.

If you are feeling nervous about filling in your first race entry, take a look at some of the great reasons to race:

More motivation

Running your first complete, non-stop mile gives you an incredible high. After a few months, however, covering the same route over and over again, that mile starts to feel like a chore. Entering a race gives you renewed focus and a reason to vary your training – in fact it might be when you start to think about training, rather than simply going for a quick jog.

Fitter and faster

Seeing the date of your race marked on the calendar will spur you on to think about running to a structured plan for the first time (you will find examples for the most popular distances in this chapter). This target alone is enough to transform your fitness, as the satisfaction of ticking off each session makes you push yourself harder and run faster than you thought possible. You will rediscover that 'first mile' feeling in no time.

Confidence

Many new runners don't even think of themselves as runners. They tell friends and family that they are just jogging or plodding around the block. As soon as you reach the start line of your first race, however, you will definitely know that you are a runner. If your training has gone to plan, you will exceed your own expectations as the atmosphere of the race and adrenaline rush boost your

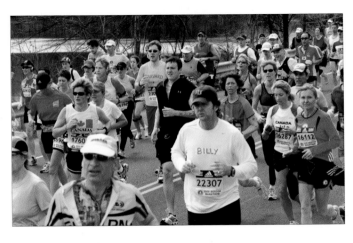

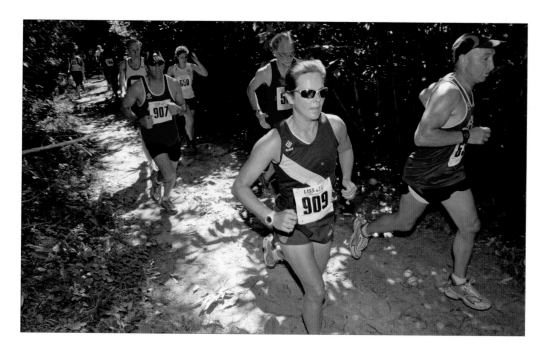

Above: Having a race to focus on helps you train harder and become fitter than ever.

able to keep up. Take a look around you at the start of any race – especially those with big fields – and you will see that the running community really does embrace people of all ages, shapes and sizes. Racing is a great way to meet other runners in your area, to chat about trainers, niggling aches and routes for the first time with people who understand, and

to experience the support and camaraderie of other runners. It is also a good opportunity to involve your friends and family in your new interest; bring them along to cheer you on and perhaps it may even inspire them to join you next time.

Rewards

Research has shown that people who compete for intrinsic rewards (for example, to build their confidence or achieve an ambition) do much better than those who compete for

extrinsic rewards (perhaps to please their friends). However, you can use these external rewards to help spur you on by ensuring they mean a lot to you. Use races as a way of seeing places you have always wanted to explore, or to raise money for a charity close to your heart; race for a medal to make up for missing out at school sports days.

Below: The more people there are taking place in a race, the less likely you are to finish in last place!

Beat the excuses

'I'm not competitive' Racing is not necessarily about competing against other runners, but about pushing yourself harder. Even the most mild-mannered jogger finds it hard to resist a sprint for the finish!

'Racing is too stressful' Take care of the logistics, and you can think of racing as just a chance to run in new surroundings with a few hundred like-minded companions. Relax!

'I can't afford to race' Big events run by professional organizers can be costly, but choose a smaller, local charity event and

you are sure to get value for money. Keep an eye on your local paper or library noticeboard for events.

'I'm scared I'll finish last' It is surprisingly difficult to finish in last place, especially in bigger races. Rest assured that even if you are last over the line, you will still have achieved more than most people just by completing a race – and there will still be plenty of cheering spectators waiting at the finish line to help you celebrate.

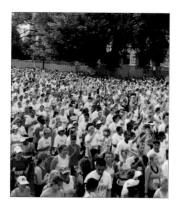

Choosing your Event

The image of thousands of people having a carnival in the London or New York City Marathon is enough to get thousands more people running. When considering your first race, a marathon may seem the obvious choice, but it is worth starting small and working your way up.

There are several factors to consider when choosing your first event. The big public events covered by the media have tens of thousands of finishers, and these are often good choices for first-time racers. Lots of runners (and media coverage) means there will be lots of supporters along the route, and the course is usually accessible to spectators so your friends and family can be there. As a participant you are far less likely to be left alone at any stage of the route as the field never truly spreads out. Facilities and organization are almost guaranteed to be

Below: If you want to use a race to raise money for charity, a well-known event might work best.

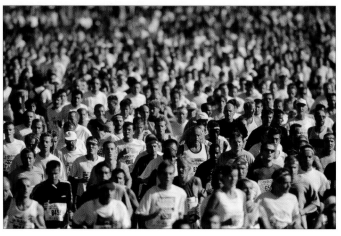

good in a big race, and the day feels more like an event than a race. This is not to say that smaller races should be avoided. Ask around local running clubs to find good, beginner-friendly races. If you are anxious about coming last, check last year's final finisher time and ask the organizer if there is a cut-off point. It is a good idea to find a race in a park or town centre where there are always crowds to cheer you on; rural races are beautiful but can be lonely.

Above: Big races are great if you want atmosphere, but are not so good for achieving fast times.

Finding inspiration
It is also important to consider your motives for running the race. You may have been inspired to race by the sight of club runners tearing through your local 10K, but if a fast time is not your goal then look around

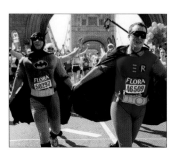

Most popular race distances					
Event	**Distance**	**Build-up**	**Minimum training (beginners)**	**Time to complete**	**Frequency and season**
5K	5km (3 miles)	6–12 weeks	3 walk/run sessions per week; one session at least 40 mins duration	25–40 mins	Traditionally a summer event; 5K weekly series run all year round
10K	10km (6.2 miles)	2–4 months	3 sessions per week; one session at least 1 hour long	40 mins to 1hr15	Take place most weeks of the year; more common in summer
Half-marathon	21km (13 miles)	4–6 months	3–4 sessions per week, running up to 90 mins at once	1hr35 to 3hrs	Often combined with big marathons; or one month before big marathons
Marathon	42km (26.2 miles)	1 year	3–5 sessions per week; long runs up to 3 hours plus one faster session	3hrs30 to 6+ hours	Take place all year round, but with spring and autumn peaks

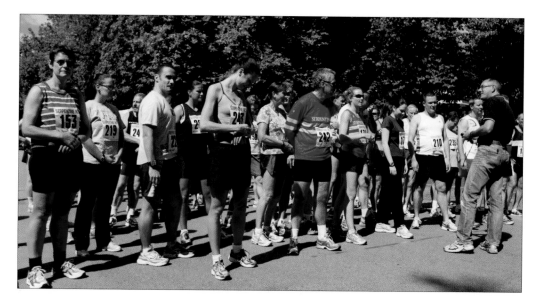

Above: Smaller races can be good build-up events for your main target race.

at other events. On the other hand, if you know you want to run fast, then a fun run with 2,000 joggers is not the best place to bag a personal best. If you would like to raise money for charity, find an event your friends and family will have heard of – they will be more inclined to support you. Think about what you would like to get from the day: do you want a medal for your efforts? Would you like to meet other runners over cake or a beer afterward? Do you want an event your whole family can take part in? Race organizers will be able to provide all the information about what is on offer.

Race distances

It is sensible for beginners to start their racing career with a short race, but many people do dive in with a half-marathon or even a marathon. The most popular race distances are listed in the table.

Below: Research your chosen race so you know what the terrain and crowd will be like.

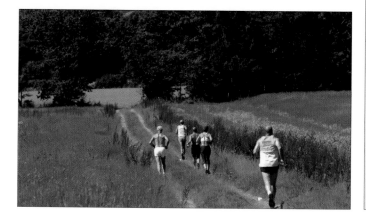

Know your field
Make sure you know what kind of event you are turning up to.

Road races: the most popular races are run on roads or tarmac, and these are usually the easiest races for beginners.

Track races: usually much faster than road races and may not always be open to the general public; it is important that you check before you go. Traditionally take place during the summer.

Cross-country races: avoiding footpaths, cross-country races traditionally take place during the winter months and are muddy, hilly and very tough. The start is often very fast, which can sometimes be intimidating for beginners.

Trail races: more laid-back than cross-country, these races are a great way to get back to nature and explore forests, nature reserves and parks on soft, forgiving ground. Not good for fast times.

Fell races: a specialist category for brave runners. Fell racers run up and down fells or mountains. The distance is often shorter than a road race but the terrain is far more difficult.

Great Beginnings

There are thousands of races on offer when you are ready for your first event. These are some of the biggest, brightest and friendliest, with great crowds, fun costumes and runners of all shapes and sizes taking part.

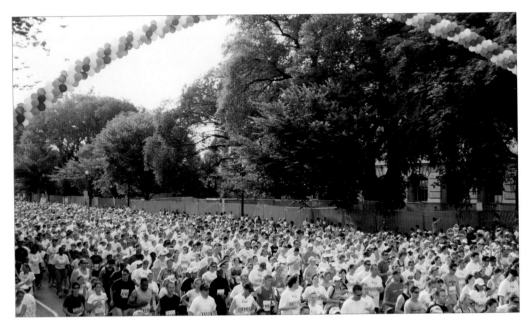

Race for the Cure, nationwide, USA; Race for Life, nationwide, UK
Distance: 5K
Date: May–July
Finish times: Not recorded; from 20 minutes to more than 1 hour

It is impossible to overstate the effect that these events have had on the whole running community, as well as in terms of charity fundraising. The charity Susan G. Komen for the Cure was set up in 1982 by Nancy G. Brinker, who promised her dying sister Susan Komen that she would fight to end breast cancer. The first Race for the Cure took place in Dallas, Texas, the following year, with just 800 runners. Now it is the biggest fundraising series in the world, with well over one million people running in the events every year. The charity's flagship event, the National Race for the Cure in Washington DC, is the world's biggest 5K run: more than 45,000 people took part in 2006, raising nearly $4 million in the process.

Although a much younger event, Cancer Research UK's Race for Life series has had as big an impact on women in the UK. Since the first event in 1994, more than two million women have taken part, with around 750,000 in 2007 alone taking part in nearly 300 events. In 2006, it set a new Guinness World Record for the biggest simultaneous stretch with 115,000 women performing identical stretches at 24 Race for Life events.

These events have inspired millions of women to take up running, in a welcoming, supportive environment. You can walk, race, or walk and run the 5K distance, and for most women involved, it is the first step toward a happy lifetime of running. If traditional 'serious' races intimidate you, try one of these.
www.komen.org; www.raceforlife.org

Above: The Race for the Cure series includes the world's biggest 5K, in Washington DC.

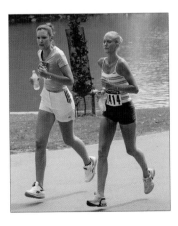

Above: The UK's Race for Life raises money for cancer research charities.

Great Santa Race, Las Vegas, USA; Santa Dash, Liverpool, UK

Distance: 5K
Date: December
Finish times: Not recorded; approx 18 minutes to 1 hour

The best way to ensure you don't take your first event too seriously is to dress up, but you are unlikely to stand out from the crowd at these 5K races. Competitors must wear the Santa suit provided, though you can customize it if you prefer. There are dozens of Santa runs around the world, but the Great Santa Race in Las Vegas and the Santa Dash in Liverpool are the biggest and enjoy a friendly rivalry, each aiming to set a record for the most Santas in one place. In 2007, Las Vegas retained the world record with over 7,000 Santas taking part, but competition is hotting up, with new races in Italy and Australia joining the race.

Both the Las Vegas and Liverpool events are great for first timers: the city-centre routes pass famous landmarks (admittedly very different), from the bright lights of Vegas to the historic waterfront and architecture of Liverpool. These events enjoy plenty of crowd support, and of course, the Christmas spirit imbues a party atmosphere. Both are run to benefit local charities.

Las Vegas: www.opportunityvillage.org
Liverpool: www.runliverpool.org.uk

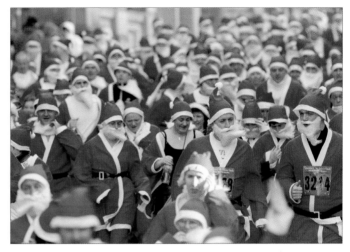

Above: The Liverpool Santa Dash runs through the city centre and past its famous waterfront.

Below: Friendly competition between Santa races keeps thousands of Santas returning to Las Vegas each year.

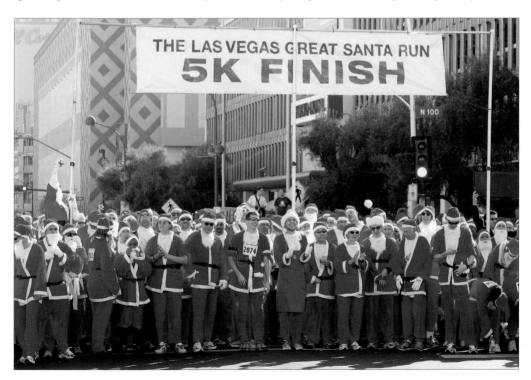

Men's Health Forum Scotland 10K, Glasgow, UK

Date: June

Finish times: 32 minutes to 2 hours

Despite the huge success of women-only races, it has been thought that men would not be attracted to single-sex events in the same way, but the fast-growing popularity of this 10K shows this might not be true. The event is part of a countrywide programme of jogging for health in Scotland which, so far, has been hugely successful. Scotland's men are among the least healthy in Europe but that is set to change. The first MHFS 10K in 2006 had 500 runners; that increased to 2,000 the next year and the organizers hope for 5,000 in future events. The race does as much to challenge stereotypes about Glasgow as it does for the image of Scottish men, running through beautiful (and undulating) Bellahouston and Pollock parks. It is run on Father's Day every year, so crowds of proud family and friends line the route.

www.mhfs.org.uk

Below: The MHFS 10K aims to replicate the success of women-only events in encouraging new runners.

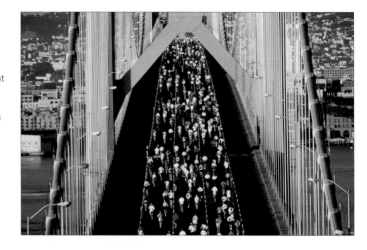

ING Bay to Breakers 12K, San Francisco, California, USA

Date: May

Finish times: 33 minutes 42 secs (record) to 4 hours

The world's biggest road race is also one of the oldest, having started in 1912 as the Cross City Race, a bid to raise morale in San Francisco following a devastating earthquake six years earlier. Today about 70,000 people take part every year, from international athletes to walkers, to costumed fun runners. There is even a separate 'centipedes' class:

Above: The Bay to Breakers race has some spectacular views, as well as some spectacular costumes.

groups of 13 runners who must have a set of feelers at the front and a stinger at the back. Runners also have to look out for the 'spawning salmon', who run from the finish to the start through the crowds. Bands line the route from the Embarcadero through Golden Gate Park to the ocean and although it is a hilly course, no one seems to mind.

www.ingbaytobreakers.com

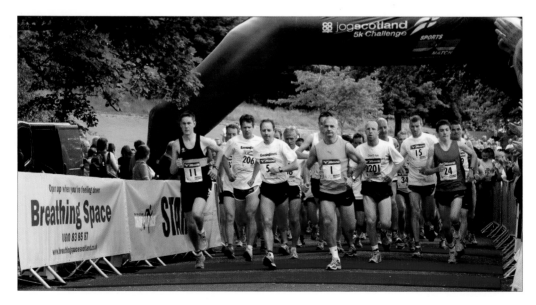

BUPA Great North Run, Newcastle, UK

Date: October

Finish times: 59 minutes 37 secs to 4+ hours

The Great North Run is a product of Britain's first running boom, and began in 1981. The race's founder, the Olympic 10,000m runner Brendan Foster, was inspired by running the Round the Bays race in New Zealand two years earlier. From 12,000 runners in that first event, it has become the biggest half-marathon in the world with more than 35,000 finishers each year. The fast course attracts top athletes and first-time runners alike, and now sells out many months in advance. The course begins just outside the city centre, with back runners taking 20 minutes just to reach the start line, before heading through cheering crowds in Newcastle itself. Running over the famous Tyne Bridge about a mile into the run is a great moment. The locals are rightly proud of this event and turn out in their thousands to support it, usually offering drinks and snacks to runners from their homes in the last few miles of the race. The last mile along the seafront is thronged with cheering spectators to spur you on to a strong finish. www.greatrun.org

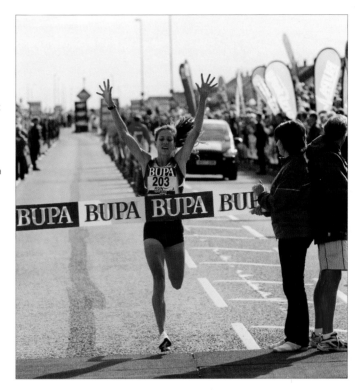

Above: Athlete Kara Goucher of the USA wins the Great North Run in Newcastle, England, 2007.

Below: The start of the 500 Festival Mini Marathon, which takes runners over the same course as the famous Indy 500.

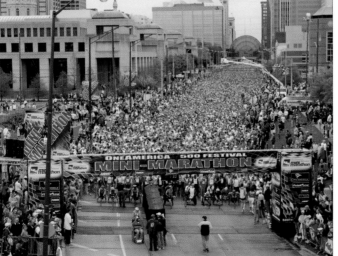
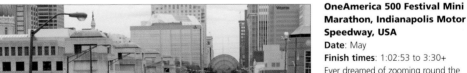

OneAmerica 500 Festival Mini Marathon, Indianapolis Motor Speedway, USA

Date: May

Finish times: 1:02:53 to 3:30+

Ever dreamed of zooming round the famous Indianapolis Motor Speedway, home to the Indy 500? This family-friendly event can make that dream come true. The half-marathon started in 1977 and two years later officially became part of the 500 Festival. It's now America's biggest half, with about 35,000 runners. In 2008, for the first time in the event's history, the finish was a dead heat, with Kenyan runners Lamech Mokono and Valentine Orare crossing the line neck-and-neck. Farther back in the field, the atmosphere is relaxed and support is great, with pre- and post-race parties including live music and food. www.500festival.com

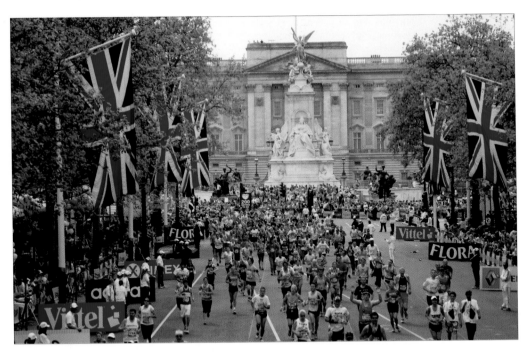

Flora London Marathon, London, UK

Date: April

Finish times: 2:07 to several days

Inspired by the New York City Marathon, the London Marathon first took place in March 1981 with 6,255 finishers. Now it is one of the biggest – and most oversubscribed – running events in the world, with 100,000 applicants competing for some 45,000 places, of which around 35,000 finish the race. The course has changed several times over the years, and now starts in Greenwich, south-east London, running through some of the capital's most deprived areas during the first half, where thousands of Londoners line the street to cheer runners on (many from pubs along the roadside). The second half of the race shows the other side of the city, crossing over Tower Bridge, heading

Above: The Mall outside Buckingham Palace provides an inspiring home straight for the London Marathon.

out to the skyscrapers of Docklands, then running back along the Embankment, past the Houses of Parliament to the finish on the Mall outside Buckingham Palace. Like most big city marathons, the front end of the race sees fierce athletic competition and world records set, but the race is most famous for the thousands of 'fun runners' competing against themselves, running in fancy dress, and raising millions of pounds for charity. In any case you are unlikely to be last, as one man has dedicated his marathon efforts to just that: Lloyd Scott has run the marathon in a suit of armour, and dressed as Indiana Jones pulling a 136kg 'boulder'. In one attempt, during which he wore an antique diving suit, Scott took more than eight days to complete the course.
www.london-marathon.co.uk

Left: Crossing Tower Bridge over the River Thames tells runners they are almost at the halfway point.

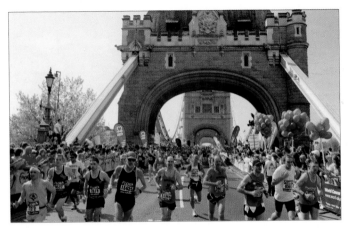

ING New York City Marathon, New York, USA

Date: November

Finish times: 2:09 to 10 hours

The original 'people's marathon' began in 1970 but really became a mass race four years later, when the course was redesigned to take in all five boroughs of New York City. Starting on Staten Island, runners cross the Verazzano Narrows Bridge and head on through Brooklyn and on to Manhattan, on a route that includes stunning views of the Empire State Building and the Chrysler Building. Throughout, the community spirit and support of all the diverse ethnic groups that make up the city's population show visitors what makes New York so special, and the finish in Central Park, with the cheers of thousands of spectators, stays with runners forever. In 2001, just weeks after the 9/11 terror attacks, the race was

Below: New York City Marathon runners enjoy crossing the famous Verazzano Narrows Bridge.

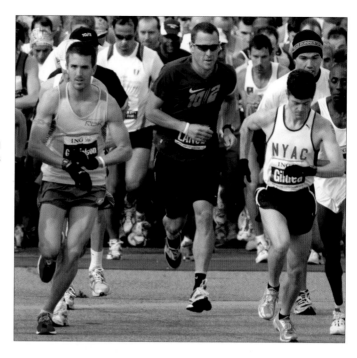

Above: American Tour de France legend Lance Armstrong (centre) joined the first-timers in 2006.

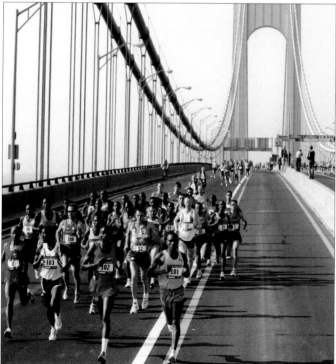

a poignant testament to the city's indomitable character. Like the Flora London Marathon, the race is hugely oversubscribed, and more than 700,000 people have completed the race over the years. The front of the race has seen some dramatic finishes, including a sprint between the Kenyan Susan Chepkemei and the women's world record holder Paula Radcliffe in 2004, which marked Radcliffe's triumphant return to form after dropping out of the Olympic marathon in Athens that year. Run this race and you will be in the company of celebrity runners too: in 2006, the legendary cyclist Lance Armstrong made his marathon debut here in a very respectable 2:59:36. It is a more challenging course than London, with the bridge crossings providing hills that can seem like mountains after miles of running, but being part of the event that introduced running to millions of people around the world makes the pain worthwhile.
www.newyorkcitymarathon.org

5K Event: Walk/Run Schedule

Five kilometres is an unimaginable distance for most of us when we first start running. But you will be amazed how easy it is to reach this milestone with a simple, structured training plan that will gently push your fitness to a new level.

Time target: 30 to 40 minutes
Starting point: Four 30-minute walk/run sessions per week for at least six weeks

You may feel intimidated before competing in your first 5K event, imagining hundreds of lithe, Lycra-clad runners tearing around the course at top speed. The reality is that 5K is the most beginner-friendly distance, and thousands of people choose to walk all the way round, especially in the larger events such as Race for the Cure and Race for Life. Even for more experienced runners, there are advantages to retaining walk breaks through your first race. It is a good way to break up the distance, to pace yourself, stretch out your body and give your legs a rest from the impact of running. Taking walk breaks doesn't necessarily mean a slow time, either – you can run as fast as you feel comfortable in the run sections, and you may find you finish quicker overall since you are less likely to tire.

Sessions

Walk/run pyramids. Speed sessions are not just for fast or non-stop runners. Picking up your pace during the run segments of your session helps to keep things interesting as well as improving your fitness. Try running a pyramid session: after a 2-minute warm-up, complete five sets of 4 minutes run, 2 minutes walk. Run the second run segment slightly faster than the first, and the third as fast as you can maintain for 4 minutes; the fourth slower again, and the fifth back at your easy pace. End with a 5-minute cool-down walk.

Event practice. As you approach your 5K, find out as much as you can about the practicalities: whether there will be water on the course, what time of day it starts, and the precise route of the run. Then try to have a dress rehearsal, going over the route at your planned pace, practising drinking every 15 minutes, and working out the best time to eat beforehand. This will help you to relax on the day of the event.

Long walks. Regular, long walking sessions are the best way to practise your strong walking technique for the event. We take walking for granted but it can be incredibly tiring, which leads to a drop in posture and pace. Use your once-a-week long walk sessions to think about walking briskly and with good form – it may help to set an alarm on your watch every

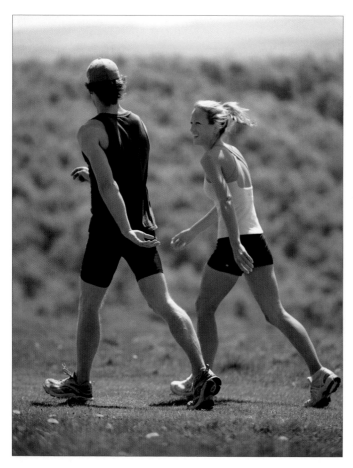

Left: Stay upright and strong during your weekly long walk sessions to make the most of them.

5K event: walk/run schedule

	Session one	Session two	Session three	Session four
Week one	Walk 10 mins; run 2 mins/walk 2 mins x 5; Walk 5 mins	Cross-train, 30 mins	As session one	Walk 30 mins at a brisk pace
Week two	Walk 10 mins; run 2 mins/walk 2 mins x 5; walk 5 mins	Cross-train, 30 mins	Walk 10 mins; run 3 mins/walk 1 min x 5; walk 5 mins	Walk 35 mins at a brisk pace
Week three	Walk 10 mins; run 3 mins/walk 1 min x 5; walk 5 mins	Cross-train, 30 mins	Pyramid session with run 3 mins/walk 1 min x 5	Walk 40 mins at a brisk pace
Week four	Walk 10 mins; run 4 mins/walk 1 min x 5	Cross-train, 30 mins	Pyramid session with run 4 mins/walk 2 mins x 5	Walk 45 mins at a brisk pace
Week five	Walk 10 mins; run 5 mins/walk 1 min x 4	Rest	Pyramid session with run 4 mins/walk 1 min x 5	Walk 40 mins at a brisk pace
Week six	Walk 5 mins; Run 5 mins/walk 1 min x 4	Cross-train, 30 mins	Pyramid session with run 5 mins/walk 1 min x 4	Event practice (dress rehearsal with drinks, on course if possible)
Week seven	Walk 1 min/run 5 mins x 6	Cross-train, 30 mins	Pyramid session with run 5 mins/walk 1 min x 5	Walk 40 mins at a brisk pace
Week eight	Walk 1 min/run 5 mins x 6	Rest	Walk 1 min/run 5 mins x 3	5K race

10 minutes as a reminder to check your posture. Don't think of it as a walk but as a fat-burning and all-over conditioning session.

Race day

If you are entering a 5K with a big field, you will need to think about the people around you as you change pace, especially if you are with a large group, as some races can be very crowded. At the start of the race, mention to those around you that you are planning to run for five minutes then walk for one, and if you are part of a group, call out, 'Walk!' or 'Run!' as you switch pace, to warn the crowds around you. Try to step smoothly from walk to run so that you don't cause any hold-ups.

Right: On the day of your first race, although it may be difficult, try to stay relaxed and stick to your walk/run plan.

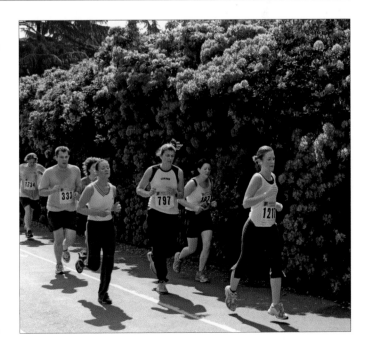

5K Event: Intermediate Schedule

Running or walk/running regularly should have given you confidence in your ability to build your own fitness. So why not put what you have learned to good use and test yourself with a more challenging intermediate routine.

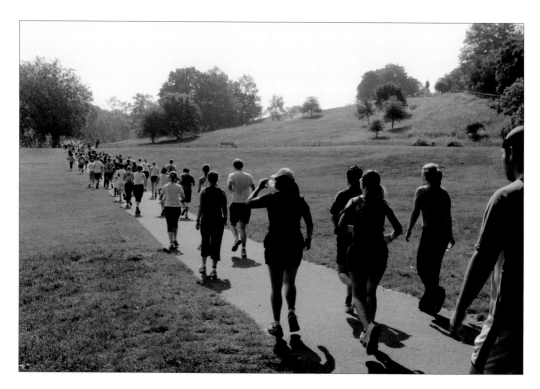

Time target: 25 to 35 minutes
Starting point: Four 20-minute runs a week for at least six weeks

If you are already able to run 5km comfortably without stopping, then entering a 5K event is likely to be more about testing yourself and meeting other runners than it is about completing the distance. There should be no room for complacency, however. Although relatively short, this is one of the most difficult race distances to get right, as it can be very tempting to sprint from the start, thinking you don't have far to run. This schedule should help you to get round the course comfortably and to the best of your abilities.

Sessions

Long intervals. To run a successful 5K, you need to learn to run fast for long periods of time. The best way to do this is to add threshold runs to your schedule, but you can start by simply running some long, fast intervals. The first interval of each set should feel fast but comfortable, so that by the last interval you are tired but still able to run at the same speed. It takes practice to get these intervals right, so don't be scared of them – you can always adjust your pace.

Long runs. When you are competing in a 5K event and aiming to run all the way round, the distance itself should not hold any fear for you. To make

Above: Practise for race day while you're training, running on the same route if possible.

sure you reach the start line feeling confident, once a week you should run 5km or farther in training, so that when the day of your event finally arrives, the distance will seem like nothing.

Race day practice. If you can, find the route of your chosen event and jog round it beforehand. Otherwise, practise running as precise a 5K as you can, dressed in your race-day kit and eating and drinking as you plan to do on the big day. Since you are not taking any walk breaks, it is especially important to work out when to eat,

5K event: intermediate schedule

	Session one	Session two	Session three	Session four
Week one	Run 20 mins	Run 25 mins	Run 20 mins	Run 30 mins
Week two	Run 20 mins	Warm-up 5 mins; 2 x 5 mins fast, 2 mins slow; cool-down 5 mins	Cross-train 30 mins	Run 30 mins
Week three	Run 25 mins	Warm-up 5 mins; 2 x 5 mins fast, 2 mins slow; cool-down 5 mins	Cross-train 30 mins	Run 35 mins
Week four	Run 25 mins	Warm-up 5 mins; 3 x 5 mins fast, 2 mins slow; cool-down 5 mins	Cross-train 30 mins with harder intervals	Run 40 mins
Week five	Run 25 mins	Warm-up 5 mins; 2 x 8 mins fast, 3 mins slow; cool-down 5 mins	Cross-train 30 mins with harder intervals	Run 45 mins/ Race day practice
Week six	Run 25 mins	Warm-up 5 mins; 2 x 8 mins fast, 3 mins slow; cool-down 5 mins	Cross-train 30 mins with harder intervals	Run 50 mins/ Race day practice
Week seven	Run 25 mins	Warm-up 5 mins; 3 x 6 mins fast, 2 mins slow; cool-down 5 mins	Cross-train 30 mins with harder intervals	Run 45 mins
Week eight	Run 25 mins	Warm-up 5 mins; 15 mins faster pace; cool-down 5 mins	Rest	5K event

as your risk of indigestion and cramp are higher the faster you go. Practise taking caffeine before you run, too – it could prove a big help.

Cross-training. When you start running, cross-training can help to build fitness, but as you move on you can use non-running sessions to help build your speed and stamina. Try making your cross-training sessions harder by increasing the resistance for 5 or 10 minutes. Alternatively, use the time to try yoga or Pilates classes, which will increase your flexibility and strength, helping you to stay injury free up to race day.

Warm-ups and cool-downs. If you have just moved up from walk/run training, the warm-up and cool-down parts of your hard sessions are really important as you won't have the walk sections to cushion your body. Get carried away

Right: Completing long runs in your training will make sure you're comfortable over the whole 5K distance when it comes to the event.

running fast from a standstill, and you could end up unable to complete your intervals or, worse still, injured. The cool-down is very important to loosen up your muscles and help you recover from the

hard work you've just done. Your warm-up and cool-down jogs should be very easy; you should almost feel that you're running too slowly, and you should be able to hold a conversation easily.

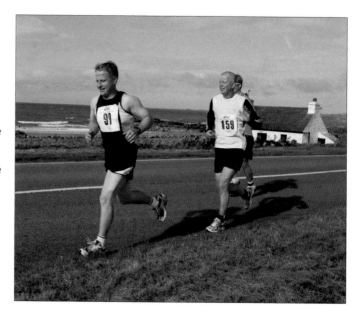

10K Event: Walk/Run Schedule

Conquering a 10K is something you can really be proud of. It takes real dedication to teach your body to keep going for an hour or more, but building up that strength will be worth it. It's a great base for tackling longer events and a popular distance in its own right.

Time target: 1 hour to 1:15
Starting point: Four 30-minute walk/run sessions a week for at least eight weeks

Whether you choose to take part in a 10K event as your first race or as a step up from the shorter 5K, the longer distance can feel extremely daunting, especially when you see the faster runners zipping around the course in 35 minutes or even less.

For a recreational walk/run participant, a 10K race is likely to take at least an hour, so it becomes more of an endurance than a speed event. The key factor in your training for this type of event is to concentrate on building up your overall strength and fitness so that you can finish

strongly and try to enjoy the race all the way round – soon those 10 kilometres (6 miles) won't seem like such a big deal after all.

Sessions
Hill walking. Just as hill running sessions are very beneficial for building up strength, walking up hills is also a good idea if you plan to spend a significant proportion of your 10K event walking. Hill walking will help to improve your overall strength, but its main purpose in your event preparation is to help you walk more powerfully, using your whole body, instead of slumping along between runs. As in hill running sessions, pump your arms to power up the hill. Try not to take long strides as they are less efficient and you

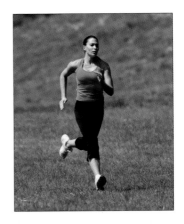

Above: Use your regular training sessions to find the walk/run ratio that will work best for you.

		10K event: walk/run schedule		
	Session one	**Session two**	**Session three**	**Session four**
Week one	4 mins run/ 2 mins walk x 5	4 mins run/2 mins walk x 2; 10 mins hill walking; 4 mins run/2 mins walk	4 mins run/2 mins walk x 4	Walk/run 35 mins
Week two	4 mins run/ 2 mins walk x 5	Walk/run fartlek, 20 mins	Cross-train, 30 mins	Walk/run 40 mins
Week three	5 mins run/ 1 min walk x 5	4 mins run/2 mins walk x 2; 10 mins hill walking; 4 mins run/2 mins walk	5 mins run/1 min walk x 5	Walk/run 45 mins
Week four	5 mins run/ 1 min walk x 6	Walk/run fartlek, 25 mins	Cross-train, 30 mins	Walk/run 50 mins
Week five	5 mins run/ 1 min walk x 6	5 mins run/1 min walk x 2; 15 mins hill walking; 5 mins run, 1 min walk	5 mins run/1 min walk x 5	Walk/run 1hr
Week six	5 mins run/ 1 min walk x 6	Walk/run fartlek 30 mins	Cross-train, 30 mins	Walk/run 1hr
Week seven	5 mins run/ 1 min walk x 7	5 mins run/1 min walk x 2; 20 mins hill walking; 5 mins run, 1 min walk	Cross-train, 35 mins	Walk/run 1hr15 mins
Week eight	5 mins run/ 1 min walk x 6	Walk/run fartlek, 30 mins	Cross-train, 30 mins	10K event

will tire easily. When you reach the top, jog down gently and walk back up again until you have completed the allotted time for your session.

Walk/run ratio. In this walk/run schedule, you will be working toward a walk/run split of 5 minutes running, 1 minute walking, but during your training try to experiment with different time splits to see which works best for you. If you are finding that you feel quite comfortable running continuously for more than 10 minutes at a time, it may be worth trying to run all the way round your event (in which case, you should follow the Intermediate Schedule for this distance).

Long walk/runs. Overcome your fear of the longer distance by trying to complete at least one longer walk/run each week – don't worry too much about the distance that you cover, but instead think about spending a long time on your feet. Use the time to practise your walk/run technique and to get into a good,

steady rhythm. One of the great advantages of a 10K event is that it is quite easy to pace because the distance is a nice, round number. So, if you can complete 1 kilometre with a 5-minute run/1-minute walk, you will finish the 10K race in an hour.

Walk/run fartlek. Your main aim in your first 10K event is to complete the distance, but some speedwork will still be very useful to you. Find a group of friends to train with, and take it in turns to call out, 'Run!' or 'Walk!' throughout your session. You can also vary the pace of your runs and insert short sprints between walk sections. These sessions will not only build your fitness, but will also help you cope during the race if you are unable to stick to your planned pace or walk/run splits because of the crowd.

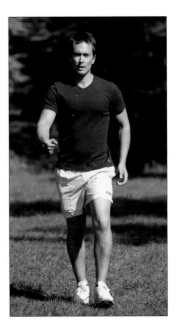

Below: Fartlek training with friends can help you cope with unexpected changes of pace on race day.

Above: You can use regular long walk/run sessions to practise pacing for your 10K race.

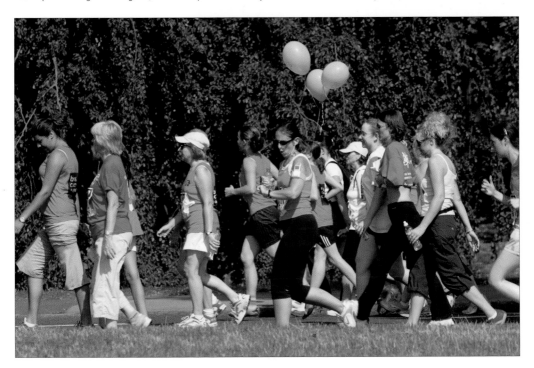

10K Event: Intermediate Schedule

It's easy to see why 10K races are so popular: the distance is long enough to be a challenge and short enough to run fast, once you're an experienced runner. The even kilometre splits also make it easy to pace – as long as you get your training right.

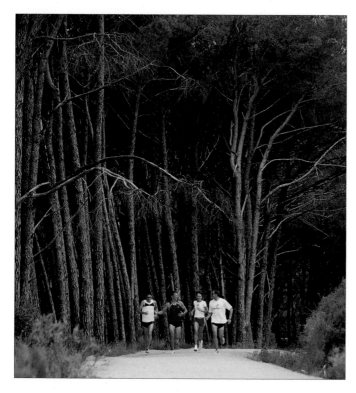

Left: Training for a fast 10K involves your first really long runs, so take friends along to make it easier.

Speed sessions. A 10K race is far from being a sprint but it is still very important that you have a good solid base of speedwork in your legs before you reach the actual event. This intermediate 10K schedule includes some longer fast intervals that are closer to the speed you will want to reach in your event, and some faster strides to work on your overall speed and running style.

If you haven't included any speedwork in your training before, you should pay close attention to how your body feels after these sessions, and cut back on your sessions if you feel any recurrent pain in the same place – speedwork is great for building fitness, but it can also lead to serious injuries if your body is not properly prepared.

Below: Use your long-run sessions to explore new areas while you build up your endurance.

Time target: 45 minutes to 1 hour
Starting point: Four 30-minute runs a week, including one longer run 45+ minutes, for at least six weeks

When you have been running regularly for a few months, there is every chance that you could complete a 10K event without too much extra training. To understand why this race distance is so popular, you need to try racing it instead of simply running it. Like the shorter 5K, it is a difficult distance to get right, as you need to run at a sustained, barely-comfortable pace. The beauty of 10K, however, is that you have much more room to pace. Provided

you don't set off too fast, you will be able to redeem your performance in the second half of the race.

Sessions
Long runs. You may think that it is unnecessary to run a distance farther than 10km in training for a 10K race, but doing so will in fact make you feel far more comfortable when you reach the start line. You want to finish the race feeling strong rather than exhausted and ready to collapse. Completing these longer training runs also builds your fitness base for after the race, so that you will be able to increase your race distance for future events.

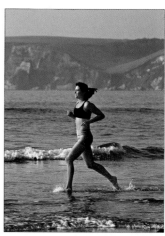

Right: Mentally divide your 10K into two halves and try to run the second half slightly quicker.

Out-and-back sessions. As well as being one the most basic (and the most fun) forms of speedwork, out-and-back sessions are perfect practice for a 10K event. You should think of the race in two halves: the first 5K is almost a warm-up, where you gradually come up to speed, while the second half is an all-out race. There should not be a huge difference in time between your first and second halves, a 51:49 split is usually recommended.

Racing the second half of the race faster is known as a 'negative split' and is a commonly used tactic by many runners. It may not be the best approach for everyone, but for beginners it is the easiest and safest option.

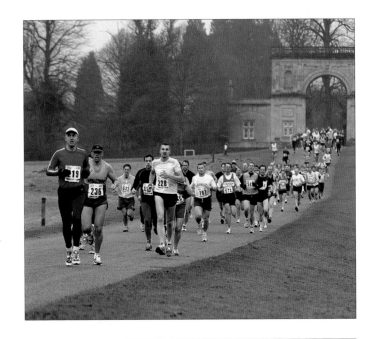

10K event: intermediate schedule

	Session one	Session two	Session three	Session four	Session five
Week one	Run 30 mins	Warm-up 10 mins; 4 x 800m/ 3 mins fast with 400m/90 secs recovery; cool-down 10 mins	Rest/cross-train 30 mins	Run 30 mins	Run 45 mins/ 6.5–9.5km (4–6 miles)
Week two	Run 30 mins	Warm-up 10 mins; three sets of 8 x 100m strides with 100m easy and 3 mins jog between sets	Rest/cross-train 30 mins	Run 30 mins	Run 55 mins/ 8–11km (5–7 miles)
Week three	Run 30 mins	As week one	Cross-train 30 mins	30 mins out-and-back run	Run 1 hour/ 9.5–13km (6–8 miles)
Week four	Run 30 mins	As week two	Cross-train 30 mins	40 mins out-and-back run	Run 1hr10/ 11–14.5km (7–9 miles)
Week five	Run 30 mins	Warm-up 10 mins; 6 x 800m/3 mins fast with 90 secs recovery; 10 mins cool-down	Cross-train 30 mins	30 mins out-and-back run	Run 1hr20/ 13–16km (8–10 miles)
Week six	Run 30 mins	Warm-up 10 mins; 15 mins fast with 8 x 100m strides at random; 10 mins cool-down	Cross-train 30 mins	40 mins out-and-back run	Run 1hr20/ 13–16km (8–10 miles)
Week seven	Run 30 mins	As week five	Cross-train 30 mins	50 mins out-and-back run	Run 1 hour/ 9.5–13km (6–8 miles)
Week eight	Run 30 mins	As week six	Cross-train 30 mins	30 mins out-and-back run	10K event

Half-marathon: Walk/Run Schedule

For obvious reasons, a half-marathon is often used as a warm-up for the full distance, but it's also a good goal to aim for in itself. You'll need commitment and patience, but having achieved it you can really call yourself a long-distance runner.

Time target: 2:15 to 2:45 hours
Starting point: Five 30-minute walk/run sessions per week; should be able to walk/run for 1 hour

Some runners might find the description of a race as a 'fun run' slightly offensive. Unfortunately 5K and 10K races, especially those with many thousands of participants, are often billed as fun runs. If you find that a little off-putting, then the half-marathon is a very good distance at which to start your racing life. Even the most flippant of spectators would have to concede that 21km (13 miles) of running and walking is about more than fun: it is about months of hard training and,

on the day of the event itself, a lot of willpower and determination. That's not to say you won't enjoy it, and as a walk/runner, you will have the advantage over your faster fellow runners, as the walk breaks provide a natural way of pacing for the longer distance. You will always have something left at the end of a half-marathon using this approach.

Sessions

Being a back marker. In a shorter 5K or 10K race, although walk/runners may feel like they are miles behind the winner, the truth is that you will finish within half an hour of them. As you hit longer race distances, however, the gap widens, so that

in a half-marathon you might finish an hour or more behind the leader. Be more careful about choosing your race, and make sure there are no stringent cut-off times. If you can, go for a half-marathon that is part of a full marathon event. These are often one lap of a two-lap course, so that you are guaranteed company all the way round. You will also have a really good opportunity to mix with the front runners and see some top-class running. Don't let the idea of being among the back markers discourage you in any way – runners of all speeds are generally very supportive of each other, and you should find an atmosphere of mutual respect at most races.

			Half-marathon: walk/run schedule		
	Session one	Session two	Session three	Session four	Session five
Week one	Walk/run 30 mins	Walk/run 30 mins	Cross-train 40 mins	Walk/run 30 mins	Walk/run 1hr
Week two	Walk/run 30 mins	Walk/run pyramid	Cross-train 40 mins	Walk/run 30 mins	Walk/run 1hr10
Week three	Walk/run 30 mins	2 x walk/run; hill walk 15 mins; 2 x walk/run	Cross-train 50 mins	Walk/run 30 mins	Walk/run 1hr10
Week four	Walk/run 30 mins	Walk/run pyramid	Cross-train 1hr	Walk/run 30 mins	Walk/run 1hr20
Week five	Walk/run 30 mins	2 x walk/run; hill walk 20 mins; 2 x walk/run	Cross-train 1hr20	Walk/run 30 mins	Walk/run 1hr30
Week six	Walk/run 30 mins	Walk/run pyramid	Cross-train 1hr40	Walk/run 30 mins	Walk/run 1hr45
Week seven	Walk/run 30 mins	Walk/run pyramid with 2 extra-fast runs in middle	Cross-train 2hrs	Walk/run 30 mins	Walk/run 1hr45
Week eight	Walk/run 30 mins	2 x walk/run; 20 mins hill walk; 2 x walk/run	Cross-train 2hrs20	Walk/run 30 mins	Walk/run 1hr30
Week nine	Walk/run 30 mins	Walk/run pyramid with 1 extra-fast run in middle	Cross-train 2hrs	Walk/run 30 mins	Walk/run 1hr45
Week ten	Walk/run 30 mins	Walk/run pyramid	Rest	Walk/run pyramid	Half-marathon

Time off. While you might be able to get away with struggling through a 10K event on very little training, the half-marathon is more than double that distance and most definitely requires some endurance practice. For a walk/runner, completing very long distances in training can take up huge chunks of time and can be very hard on your legs and feet, so use the longer cross-training sessions in your schedule to build up your endurance base while giving yourself a break from running and walking.

Cycling is the best alternative, as you will still be able to get out into the countryside, and you will be working your legs hard. However, any activity you feel comfortable doing for 90 minutes or more will help. Try hopping around all of the different types of equipment in your gym to keep your cross-training sessions interesting.

Speed and strength. Use the walk/run pyramid session from the 5K schedule, but take each pace down a notch – even your easiest run pace. Your slowest run should feel almost

Below: You may find it useful to do some training on your own in case you find yourself alone during the race.

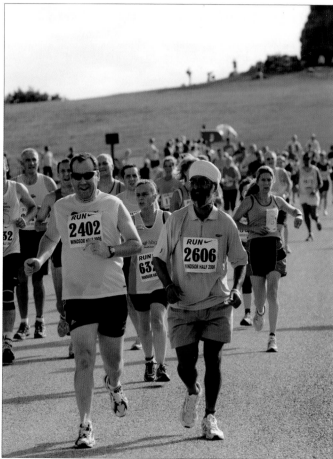

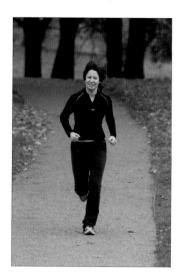

uncomfortably slow, and at your fastest you should still be able to talk in short sentences. In the later weeks of your training, repeat the middle, faster-run segments as directed in the plan, to challenge your fitness levels. Your schedule also includes hill-walking sessions to build up your strength in the lead-up to your race.

Your longest walk/run sessions. The half-marathon is a long distance that requires a much higher volume of training than you've been used to if you've only been running shorter events up to now. Your long walk/run session (session five on the table, opposite) will regularly take you over an hour of training in one go. The idea

Above: You may find yourself some way behind the leaders, but other runners are always supportive.

is to feel confident that you can complete 21km (13 miles) comfortably, so don't feel the need to push yourself too hard during these first long sessions. To begin with, plan routes that are made up of several short laps so that you can cut down if something goes wrong; ideally stay near your home at first so that you can pick up drinks or stop to use the toilet if you need to. As you become more confident with longer runs, you can go farther afield and use these training sessions to enjoy discovering new places and new scenery.

Half-marathon: Intermediate Schedule

Once you have gained some running experience and want to really push yourself, half-marathon training is a good place to start. This training plan is not too heavy-going and should get you ready to run a half-marathon time you can be proud of.

Time target: 1:45 to 2:15 hours
Starting point: Five runs a week including one speed session and one run of 1 hour

The biggest obstacle to running and enjoying a successful half-marathon is in its name. It is often regarded as a build-up race for the full marathon distance, and many people fail to train properly for 21km (13 miles) and are subsequently disappointed with their results. The race is placed awkwardly in a marathon training plan, and the runner is unable to think of the race as a whole. Make the race a goal in its own right, and you will find it a rewarding distance when you are ready to move up from 10K: it is long enough to really challenge you but short enough to run fairly fast without completely wearing yourself out.

Sessions
Pick and mix speed sessions. Running intervals of varying pace and length is a great way to build up to a half-marathon. Although your aim is to run at as even a pace as possible, you will need the strength to surge past others as gaps appear in the field and to put in a good sprint finish at the end. Longer speed sessions are good for developing your overall pace. If you have avoided training on a track until now, give it a try – you may find it helps you to focus on the session in hand, without having to keep looking at a watch or listening out for an alarm.

Long, long runs. As with shorter 10K events, it is not necessary to run farther than the race distance in training for a half-marathon, but doing so will definitely help you. Your long runs will quickly head past the 90-minute mark, but try not to view this as a chore. Set out early on a weekend morning, relax, take it slowly and enjoy the fitness you have built up. It is also a good idea to use these runs as race practice, so try to do at least one run at the exact time of day that your race will start, and practise eating and drinking before and during the run.

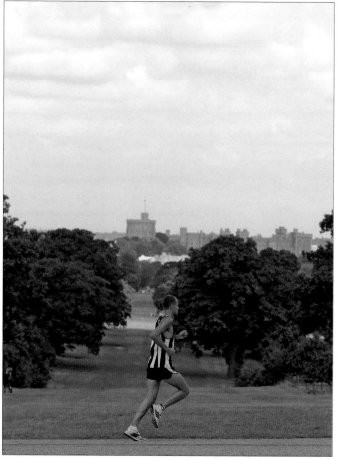

Left: It can be lonely, but a few early-morning long runs will really pay off.

Half-marathon: intermediate schedule

	Session one	Session two	Session three	Session four	Session five
Week one	Run 40 mins	Warm-up 10 mins; 4 x 800m fast, 400m slow; cool-down 10 mins	Cross-train 40 mins	Run 30 mins	Run 1hr/9.5–13km (6–8 miles)
Week two	Run 40 mins	Warm-up 10 mins; 1 x each 200m, 400m, 800m, 1,200m fast with 200m recoveries; cool-down 10 mins	Cross-train 40 mins	Run 30 mins	Run 1hr15/13–16km (8–10 miles)
Week three	Run 40 mins	Warm-up 10 mins; 20 mins faster with 5 x 200m sprints; cool-down 10 mins	Cross-train 40 mins	Run 30 mins	Run 1hr30/16–19km (10–12 miles)
Week four	Run 40 mins	Warm-up 10 mins; 6 x 800m fast with 400m recoveries; cool-down 10 mins	Cross-train 40 mins	Run 40 mins	Run 1hr30/16–19km (10–12) miles
Week five	Run 40 mins	Run 50 mins	Cross-train 50 mins	Run 40 mins	Run 2hrs/19–22.5km (12–14 miles)
Week six	Run 40 mins	Warm-up 10 mins; 1 x 200m, 400m, 800m, 1,200m, 600m, 300m; cool-down 10 mins	Cross-train 40 mins	Run 40 mins with 10 x 100m strides at random	Run 2hrs20/21–26km (13–16 miles)
Week seven	Run 30 mins	Warm-up 10 mins; 3 x 1,200m fast with 400m recoveries; cool-down 10 mins	Cross-train 40 mins	Run 40 mins	Run 2hrs30/ 19–22.5km (12–14 miles)
Week eight	Cross-train 30 mins	Warm-up 10 mins; 6 x 800m fast, 400m slow; cool-down 10 mins	Run 40 mins	Run 40 mins with 2 sets of 5 x 200m fast, 200m easy	Run 2hrs/ 19–22.5km (12–14 miles)
Week nine	Run 40 mins	50 mins fartlek	Run 40 mins	Cross-train 50 mins	Run 1hr30/16–19km (10–12 miles)
Week ten	Cross-train 30 mins	Run 30 mins with 5 x 100m strides at random	Run 30 mins	Rest	Half-marathon

Break it down. The half-marathon is an awkward distance and this often catches first-time competitors out. They will either approach it as a 10K and run far too fast early on, or worry about the long distance, run slowly and find that they could have run much faster.

The trick to pacing this event is to forget about running even splits. Rather than thinking of it as 21km (13 miles), break the distance down into two sections: a 16km (10-mile) easy run, with a 5km (3-mile) race at the end. When you are used to racing, or if you are very confident of your abilities, you can run fairly fast all the way through, but as a beginner it is much safer to run fairly comfortably for that first 16km (10 miles). Once you have reached that point, gradually increase your speed and feel yourself running smoothly and quickly toward the finish. As the distance is so much longer than 10K, some people find it easier to count down the miles than to count up.

Right: Even though race pace for a half-marathon is quite slow, fast speedwork will help you finish strongly.

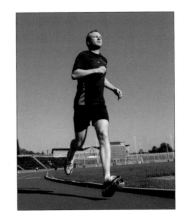

Facing the Marathon

The respect and trepidation with which athletes approach the marathon is not surprising. No matter where you fall in the race pack, the 42km (26.2-mile) distance of a marathon will test you to the limits of your endurance, both mental and physical.

The marathon requires not just months of dedicated training, but sound planning and deep thought before you even commit to that training. Asking yourself 'What's my motivation?' is as important for a potential marathon runner as it is for an actor. Willpower is the driving force behind the months of hard training you will need to put in as well as the gruelling event itself. Whether you are racing for a charity

Below: Many thousands of runners successfully complete marathons – and you could be one of them.

close to your heart, a landmark birthday coming up, or just a bet with a friend, the marathon must mean a great deal to you if you are to succeed.

At the same time it is important that you choose a race that you really want to do. Rather than picking a local event that is 12 to 16 weeks away (the minimum amount of time you will need to train), find an event that you can become passionate about: perhaps in a beautiful place that you have always wanted to visit, or a famous race that you have seen on television and would like to try.

Quick checks

Ask yourself these quick questions:
• Am I running pain-free all of the time?
• Can I give up my Saturday nights out for two or three months?
• Will my family be happy to cope without me some evenings?
• Is my diet balanced and healthy?
• Will I be free from major work projects for the next three months?
If the answer to all of these questions is 'yes', then you are ready to start marathon training.

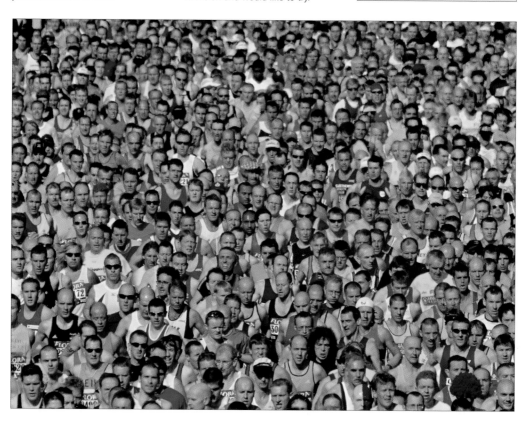

Right: If you are looking for that extra bit of motivation, choose an event in a place you have always wanted to visit.

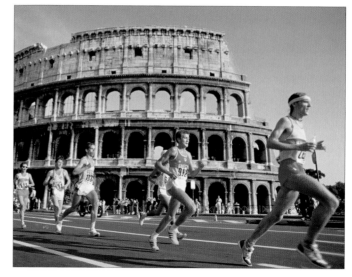

Build your base

Before you start any of the marathon schedules in this book you will need to have attained a good base of fitness. If you are a total beginner, a marathon is not an ideal first race as, ideally, you need a year to steadily build up your strength and fitness. Choose a goal race only when you feel really fit and strong. Similarly, if you become injured, don't use a marathon goal to force yourself to run again, but wait until you have fully recovered. Your body needs this build-up time to develop the systems that will support you through the race.

The rest of your lifestyle may need tweaking to support your training. If you have been running for months but still harbour bad habits, such as a poor diet, smoking or a stressed-out work life, you should concentrate on ironing out these issues before you think about increasing your exercise load. If you are prone to recurring injuries, look at why these happen – perhaps you have skimped on buying good shoes, or you need to have a gait analysis. Unlike shorter races, the marathon will find out

Below: Review your lifestyle and diet before you start training to iron out any potential problems.

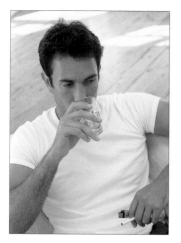

your weak spots, so limit them as much as possible. While you are thinking about your lifestyle, decide whether you really have enough time to train for a marathon. There is a big difference between squeezing in five 30-minute runs a week, and the 7 to 10 hours (maximum) training per week required for your marathon schedules.

Find your motivation

It may seem obvious, but a love of running is crucial. Setting yourself a marathon target to force yourself to run more, perhaps because you want to lose weight or test yourself, won't work if you find the act of running boring or repetitive, or if you would rather stay in bed on a Sunday than go for a long run. If the marathon is not for you, that's fine – plenty of people enjoy long running lives doing shorter events or not racing at all. At the same time, if you have become addicted to running, you need to be prepared to broaden your horizons. Cross-training, whether through stretching routines, weightlifting or just enjoying other sports to recover from hard running sessions, is an essential ingredient in marathon training.

Finally, training for a marathon requires strict honesty. You may be able to fool yourself about how many miles

you have run in training, but 29km (18 miles) into the event you will be faced with the stark truth. Stick to your schedule as much as you possibly can, and if circumstances mean you miss sessions, be honest and revise your targets. You also need to be honest with yourself about what you can achieve. By the end of your training, you may well find that you can go farther than you had ever dreamed.

Below: Nothing beats the pride and satisfaction you will feel on running your first marathon.

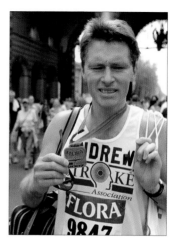

Marathon: Walk/Run Schedule

You may still feel like a beginner, and you may still prefer to take walk breaks while you train, but don't feel the marathon is beyond you. In fact, with the right training, you'll be in the perfect position to enjoy 'the big one'.

Time target: 4:30 to 6 hours
Starting point: Four sessions per week with one longer (1 hour) session, for at least six months

You may feel a little self-conscious about taking walk breaks during a race, but in a marathon you will find walk/runners often have the best experience. You can savour the atmosphere of the race, make new friends, and enjoy the sights and sounds on the course. However, the distance is a test no matter what your speed, so be aware that you may go through a rough patch toward the end of the race. Good, solid training can work wonders to reduce the

Below: As a walk/runner you'll have a better chance to soak up the atmosphere than the front runners.

impact of that low, and you can finish the race with a smile and a great sense of achievement.

The long walk/runs are the most important part of your schedule, as these sessions most closely resemble the marathon. You will never be out for longer than 3½ hours even though your race time might be 5 or 6 hours. This maximum is for practical reasons – it may be difficult to find time for a 5-hour session every weekend, and it will also avoid unnecessary damage to your body. Instead, intensive cross-training sessions will help supplement the long walk/runs.

You may feel pushed for time as your training increases, but don't neglect conditioning work. Your schedule includes hill-walking sessions but, if you can, fit in extra sessions of light strength work. It is a good idea

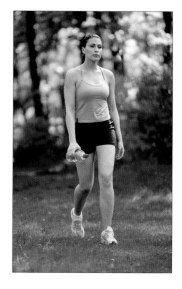

Above: You won't cover the full distance in training, but your long walk/runs are very important.

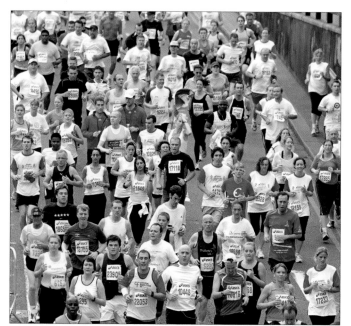

Walk/runners quick tips

• Practise carrying food and drink on your long walk/runs – find a small, comfortable day pack or waist pouch to carry food in

• Study the race route to find out where places like the toilets and water stations are beforehand

• Keep your feet comfortable with the right socks, shoe lacing and blister plasters in spots where you know your shoes rub

• Find out where the best spectator spots are, then ask your friends and family to come along and support you on race day

• If you are feeling strong during your last mile, you can skip the last walk break and sprint to the finish – it will feel fantastic!

Marathon: walk/run schedule

	Session one	Session two	Session three	Session four
Week one	Walk/run 30 mins	Walk/run 30 mins	Cross-train 30 mins	Walk/run 1hr
Week two	Walk/run 30 mins	Walk/run 30 mins with 10 mins hill walking	Cross-train 30 mins	Walk/run 1hr15
Week three	Walk/run 30 mins	Walk/run 30 mins with 10 mins hill walking	Cross-train 45 mins	Walk/run 1hr30
Week four	Walk/run 30 mins	Walk/run 35 mins with 15 mins hill walking	Cross-train 45 mins	Walk/run 1hr45
Week five	Walk/run 30 mins	Walk/run 35 mins with 15 mins hill walking	Cross-train 1hr	Walk/run 2hrs
Week six	Walk/run 30 mins	Walk/run 40 mins with 20 mins hill walking	Cross-train 1hr	Walk/run 2hrs15
Week seven	Walk/run 40 mins	Walk/run 40 mins with 20 mins hill walking	Cross-train 1hr	Walk/run 2hrs30
Week eight	Walk/run 40 mins	Walk/run 40 mins with 20 mins hill walking	Cross-train 1hr15	Walk/run 2hrs45
Week nine	Walk/run 40 mins	Walk/run 40 mins with 20 mins hill walking	Cross-train 1hr15	Walk/run 3hrs
Week ten	Walk/run 30 mins	Walk/run 30 mins	Cross-train 1hr	Walk/run 2hrs30
Week eleven	Walk/run 40 mins	Walk/run 40 mins with 20 mins hill walking	Cross-train 1hr15	Walk/run 3hrs
Week twelve	Walk/run 40 mins	Walk/run 45 mins with 25 mins hill walking	Cross-train 1hr15	Walk/run 3hrs30
Week thirteen	Walk/run 30 mins	Walk/run 30 mins with 10 mins hill walking	Cross-train 1hr	Walk/run 3hrs
Week fourteen	Walk/run 40 mins	Walk/run 40 mins with 20 mins hill walking	Cross-train 1hr	Walk/run 2hrs30
Week fifteen	Walk/run 40 mins	Walk/run 30 mins with 10 mins hill walking	Cross-train 45 mins	Walk/run 1hr30
Week sixteen	Walk/run 30 mins	Rest	Walk/run 30 mins	Marathon

to add some yoga or Pilates to improve your body awareness, so you naturally walk and run taller.

If you have been training by time rather than distance, find out how far you travel in each run and walk set using a running track. Find a run and walk pattern that fits evenly into a mile (approximately four laps of the track). This will help you pace yourself in the race, as well as to give you a finish-time estimate for the race.

After each intensive week, your training drops off slightly to allow your body time to recover and become stronger. At the end of the schedule you will notice that your training volume drops right off – this is known as tapering and enables your body to store much-needed energy for the main event.

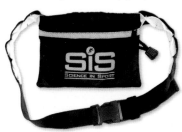

Left: Using a small waist pouch like this one makes it easier to carry fuel while you run.

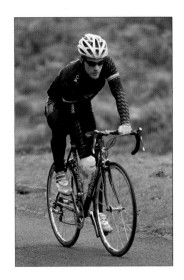

Right: Use intensive cross-training, such as cycling, to build up your fitness without impact.

Marathon: Intermediate Schedule

Running a marathon without walking is an ambition held by many beginners. If you can run for an hour at once then you're closer to achieving that dream than you might think. Your four-month training plan will build on that hour of endurance while increasing your speed.

Time target: 3:30 to 4:30 hours
Starting point: Five 30-minute runs per week including one speedwork; ability to run for 1 hour

Running a marathon in a time of less than 4:30 is not easy, but you will be in good company. In most marathons, the majority of runners finish between 3:30 and 4:30, so you will never be alone. This might feel like a disadvantage in the first half of the race, as the volume of runners holds you back, but in the tougher final stages the other people around you will keep you going. The marathon is all about the last 9.5–13km (6–8 miles) and avoiding the wall – the point 2 to 3 hours into the race

Below: In big-city events such as the Paris Marathon, you'll be in good company at 3:30–4:30 hours.

Quick tips
• As your training increases, place greater importance on sleep by adding 30 to 60 minutes per night
• If you become injured or over-tired, drop your speed sessions for a week. If you take time off, don't try to make up for it later
• On race day, if there are no official pacers, look for someone running a similar pace to you and use them as a marker to avoid starting too fast
• Split the race in two in your head; for the first 25.5km (16 miles), distract yourself with the views and fellow runners, then bring your mind back to the race and focus on finishing

Right: If possible, train with someone you can race with too – you can help to pace each other.

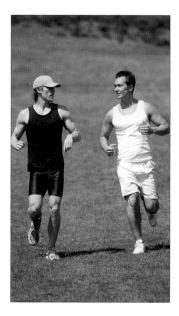

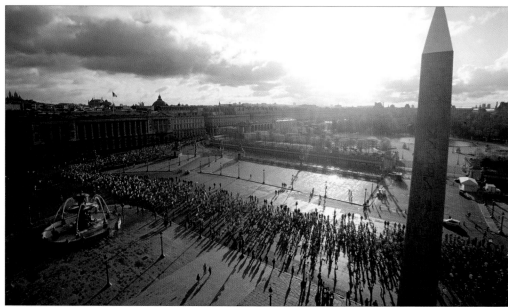

where your muscles run out of fast fuel. Nutrition, pacing, mental strength and honest training will see you through this tough time.

Over the following 16-week plan, you will run 29km (18 miles) or more five times. While these long sessions will seem daunting at first, they will fill you with confidence for your race. Don't be tempted to push yourself beyond a distance of 35km

(22 miles) in training – you will simply wear your body down before the race itself. As a beginner you should keep long runs at talking pace. At least once, you should use one of your long runs as a race practice: run in 4 or 5-mile loops and set up a water station at your home so that you can practise taking on sports drinks. This will boost your marathon performance, help you to avoid hitting

the wall, and protect your immune system from being dampened by the marathon. There are three different types of faster session in your schedule: threshold running, interval sessions to build your overall speed and increase fitness, and strides to help improve your form. Start these sessions with a 10-minute warm-up jog and then end with a 10-minute cool-down.

Marathon: intermediate schedule

	Session one	Session two	Session three	Session four	Session five
Week one	Run 30 mins	6 x 800m	Run 30 mins	Run 30 mins with 5 x 200m strides	9.5km (6 miles)
Week two	Run 30 mins	15 mins threshold	Run 30 mins	Run 40 mins	13km (8 miles)
Week three	Run 30 mins	8 x 800m	Run 30 mins	Run 30 mins with 5 x 200m strides	16km (10 miles)
Week four	Run 30 mins	15 mins threshold	Run 30 mins	Run 8 x 800m	19km (12 miles)
Week five	Run 40 mins	1 x 200m, 400m, 800m, 1,200m with 200m recoveries	Run 30 mins	Run 40 mins with two sets of 3 x 200m strides (200m in-between strides)	22.5km (14 miles)
Week six	Run 40 mins	20 mins threshold	Run 40 mins	Run 40 mins with two sets of 3 x 200m strides (200m recoveries)	25.5km (16 miles)
Week seven	Run 40 mins	8 x 800m	Run 40 mins	Run 40 mins with 8 x 200m strides	29km (18 miles)
Week eight	Run 40 mins	20 mins threshold	Run 40 mins	Run 8 x 800m	32km (20 miles)
Week nine	Run 40 mins	6 x 800m	Run 40 mins	Run 40 mins with 5 x 200m strides	25.5km (16 miles)
Week ten	Run 40 mins	10 x 800m	Run 40 mins	25 mins threshold	29km (18 miles)
Week eleven	Run 40 mins	2 x 200m, 400m, 800m, 1,200m with 200m recoveries	Run 30 mins	Run 40 mins with two sets of 5 x 200m strides (200m recoveries)	32km (20 miles)
Week twelve	Run 40 mins	8 x 800m	Run 30 mins	Run 40 mins with three sets of 5 x 200m strides (200m recoveries)	Half-marathon race/24km (15 miles)
Week thirteen	Run 30 mins	10 x 800m	Run 40 mins	Run 40 mins with two sets of 5 x 200m strides (200m recoveries)	35km (22 miles)
Week fourteen	Run 30 mins	6 x 800m	Run 40 mins	2 x 15 mins threshold with 10 mins recovery	26km (16 miles)
Week fifteen	Run 40 mins	8 x 800m	Run 40 mins	Run 40 mins with three sets of 5 x 200m strides (200m recoveries)	19km (12 miles)
Week sixteen	Run 30 mins	Rest	Run 30 mins	Rest	Marathon

The Perfect Race Week

Training for your first race is hard work. So hard that you might forget about the race itself until the week before, when it suddenly dawns on you that all your effort is about to be put to the test. A little organization will go a long way in keeping you calm on race day.

Some runners find themselves becoming consumed with nerves and thinking about the 101 things that could go wrong – but they won't. Thousands of people successfully cross the finish line of a race every week, and you will almost certainly be one of them, but what you do – and don't do – in the week before your race can make a difference to your race experience.

Hopefully you will have trained hard for 6 to 16 weeks, so don't work too much in the last week. The effects of your training on your muscles and cardiovascular system will already have taken hold, and little you do at this stage will make any difference. On the other hand, a last over-zealous speed session could give

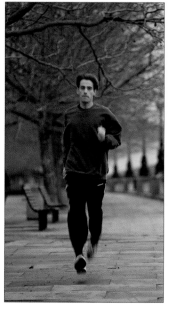

Below: Eating extra fruit and vegetables helps keep you healthy the week before your big race.

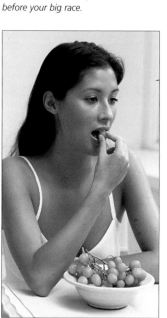

Above: Wind your training down to allow your body to recover in time for the big day.

you an injury, ruining your race chances. The longer your race, the more important it is to cut back (taper) your training this week.

Eat for success

Instead, pay a little extra attention to your diet and fluid intake during race week. This is not the time for a complete overhaul, so if you have made it through training on nothing but cake then so be it, but for most people it is a good idea to cut out junk food and make sure you have extra fruit and vegetables. If your race is longer than 10K, try carbohydrate loading: eat plenty of low-GI carbohydrates and increase your intake by 100 to 200kcal per

main meal. The idea behind this is that the extra carbohydrate will be stored in your muscles (as you will be training less hard than usual), ready for race day. Be careful to drink plenty of water, too, as hydration is cumulative: drinking gallons of water on the morning of your race will be of little use if you are dehydrated from the days before.

Be prepared

It may seem obvious, but ensure that the logistics of your race are sorted out, so you can relax. Double-check details such as directions to the start, what time you should arrive (usually at least an hour before the race start time) and whether you can park nearby. Make sure you have your

Below: Hydration is cumulative, so make sure that you drink more all week, not just on race day.

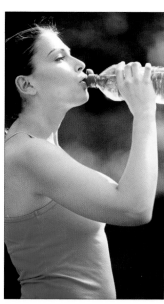

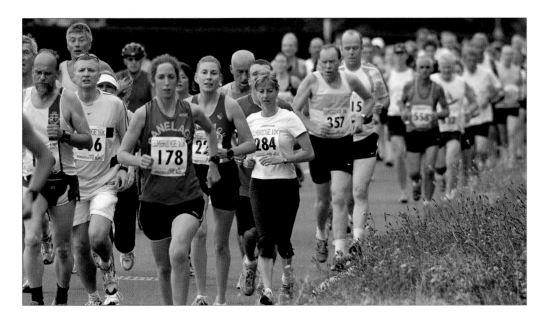

Above: Prepare yourself mentally for the race ahead, by trying to visualize a positive experience.

race number or know where to collect it from, and pack a bag for the race the night before. Try to persuade friends or family to come along with you, so they can help you remember everything and get there on time.

Once everything is in place, you will need to deal with your own final mental preparation – possibly the hardest element to get right at this stage. Allow yourself to think about the worst-case scenarios, but instead of dwelling on them, imagine how you might deal with them and bounce back. Spend 5 minutes every day visualizing yourself crossing the finish line strong, happy and in your target time, if you have one. If you have kept a training diary, look over it to remind yourself how well prepared you are. If you are still nervous on the morning of the race itself, simply think of it as a relaxed run with a few other people – and above all, try to enjoy yourself!

Below: Check that you have all your food, drink and equipment ready the night before your race.

Race week do's and don'ts

Do:
• Sleep well, especially during the two nights before the race
• Have a glass of wine every night if this is usual
• Relax and see friends to distract yourself from nerves
• Go for a few easy runs to keep your legs loose
• Have sex the night before the race if you want to – there is no evidence to suggest that it will affect your race performance on the day

Don't:
• Cram in last-minute miles or speed sessions, or try new sports
• Use the time off running to party every night
• Dwell on missed training sessions
• Buy new shoes for race day – stick with what you have trained in

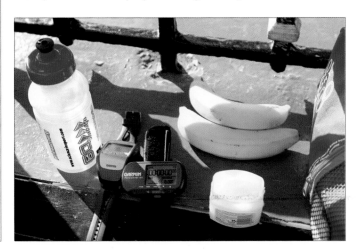

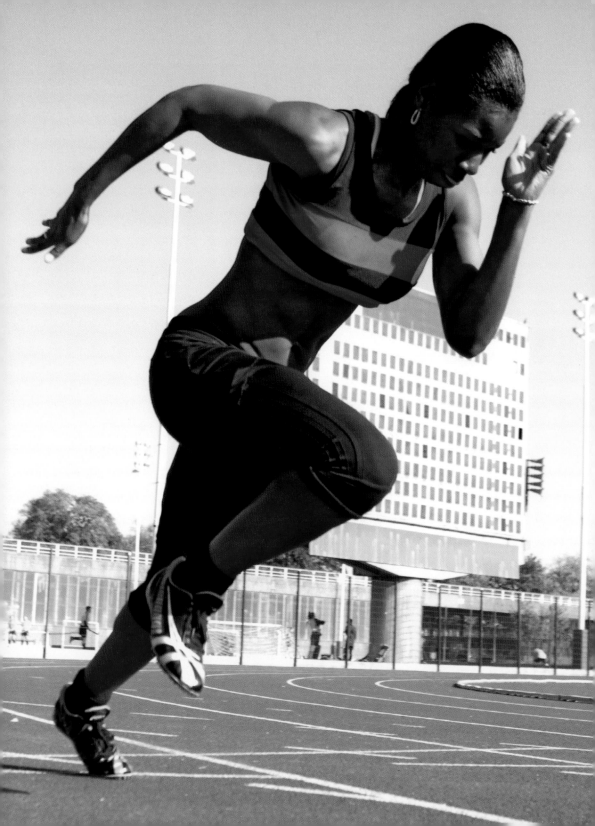

SPRINT AND MIDDLE-DISTANCE RACING

The advice given so far has largely centred on training for distance events of 5K and beyond, which is the most accessible type of running for most people. This chapter discusses some of the specialized training necessary to become a truly great sprinter and middle-distance runner, and the athletes that have inspired generations by pushing past accepted beliefs about how fast a human being can run.

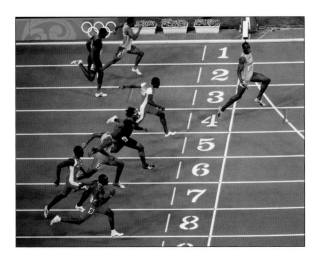

Above: Usain Bolt wins the men's 100m in the 2008 Olympic Games, earning the title 'world's fastest man'.
Left: More than any other form of running, sprinting requires sharp focus and concentration.

Sprint Form and Drills

Good form is very important for all runners, but especially so for sprinters. At speeds of up to 48kmh (30mph), where every hundredth of a second counts, every part of the body's movement must contribute toward moving forward.

A marathon runner might be forgiven for a tight shoulder or even a lopsided arm swing, but at the other end of the spectrum technique makes a much bigger difference. In sprinting there is no room for any wasteful side-to-side movements or energy spent tensing the neck, and biomechanical problems that seem minor in slow motion are exaggerated at speed. The key to great sprinting is relaxed speed.

The best sprinters make their motion look smooth and almost effortless, and the mistake many slower runners make is to 'try too hard' – running with

clenched fists, gritted teeth and hunched shoulders, which wastes energy and prevents a full range of motion. Watch a group of well-trained sprinters, and you will see that their style is often strikingly similar. This 'perfect' sprint form is developed over years of training using drills, visualization of correct technique and, crucially, the input of an experienced sprint coach.

Right: A sprinter in her starting blocks focuses on the track ahead of her, visualizing perfect form.

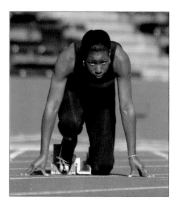

Sprint form

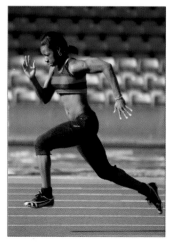

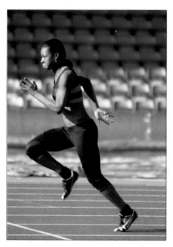

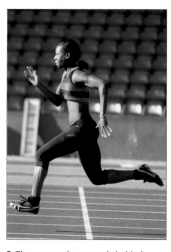

1 *The leading knee should drive high and forward, so the thigh ends up parallel with the ground. The toes of the lead foot should be pointed up, so that the foot is not allowed to 'drop' at any point during the cycle. Meanwhile, the back leg remains almost straight, not collapsing under the weight of the runner while on the ground, and extending right out behind the runner once off the ground.*

2 *The lead leg should land on the ball of the foot, in front of the runner but not so far forward as to produce an exaggerated stride, which leads to a braking effect. On striking the ground, the foot must pull the ground underneath the runner in a clawing action, without the heel dropping to the floor. As the other knee drives forward, the heel of that leg is brought up tucked under the runner before the lower leg is extended forward.*

3 *The support leg extends behind as before. Throughout the sprint, the torso should stay high and straight, the neck and face should be relaxed and the shoulders relaxed and down. The arms should both be bent at 90 degrees at the elbow, and should drive backward and forward, keeping in time with the runner's steps, helping to keep leg speed up.*

Starting from blocks

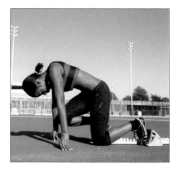

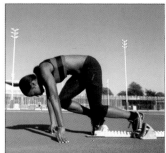

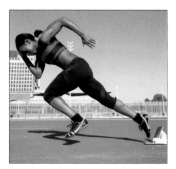

1 On your marks. *You need to experiment with the blocks to find the best position for you. Many sprinters find that a distance roughly equal to that from your ankle to your knee works well. You need to get the angle of the blocks right – the back block should be steeper. Start with your feet in the blocks, crouched, and your hands just touching the line, just wider than shoulder-width apart, with your thumb and fingers forming a bridge, and your arms straight but not locked.*

2 Set. *Keeping your hands where they are, with your thumb and fingers still in the bridge position, raise your hips up so that they are higher than your shoulders and you are leaning forward slightly – you should feel quite stable, but not exactly comfortable. Your front knee should be roughly at a right angle, while your back knee should make an angle of about 120 degrees. Push your feet hard into the blocks. Your face and neck should remain relaxed.*

3 Go! *Your reaction time here is crucial, but be very careful not to react before you hear the gun go off. Push hard out with your front leg, and drive the back leg forward at the same time, pushing up and forward, and leaning almost horizontally as you accelerate out of the blocks. Don't stride too far on your first step, or take steps that are too small; you need to move as quickly as you possibly can into your perfect sprint form.*

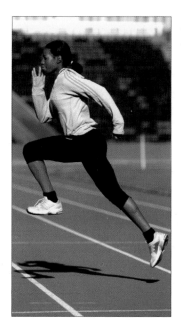

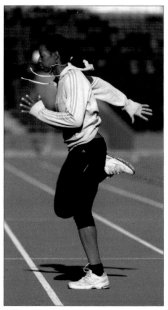

Above: Include sprint bounds in your training sessions and you will soon see an improvement in your form.

Above: Keep your back straight and head up to get the best results from exercises like heel flicks.

Sprint drills

Practice drills are as crucial for sprinters as they are for distance runners. Add these exercises to improve your sprint action.

Sprint bounds: over a distance of 50m (164ft), practise driving your lead knee forward and fully extending your back leg, using your arms to help the action as you would while running. Bound forward, slowly at first, speeding up as you perfect the technique. Over time, aim to cover the 50m (164ft) in fewer bounds.

Heel flicks: over a distance of 30–50m, (98–164ft) run forward on the balls of your feet, kicking your heel up to almost touch your bottom as quickly as possible. Ensure that your body stays upright and straight during the drill.

Harness runs: working in pairs, one runner holds the ends of a harness while the other walks forward in the harness until he feels resistance. Run forward against the harness, trying to keep as natural a gait as possible (instead of leaning right in to the harness).

Strength Training for Sprinters

You only have to look at a group of sprinters in the starting blocks to realize that strength training plays a huge part in their success. Compared with the lean, wiry build of a distance runner, sprinters look muscular and powerful.

While strength training plays an important role in all athletes' routines, for sprinters it is essential for developing the explosive power needed to drive them along at speeds of up to 10m (30ft) per second, and the control needed to ensure no energy is wasted along the way. Generally speaking, the shorter the specialist distance, the more strength is needed.

Top-level sprinters will push themselves through two or three weight-training sessions per week up to the competition phase of their year and, as with all training, they must be careful not to overload their muscles by strength training on the same days as their more intense running workouts. In race season, sessions are cut down and resistance is reduced.

There is some debate over how much emphasis should be placed on strength training. Some coaches feel that it plays too great a part in sprinters' training, to the detriment of out-and-out speed. Even at the elite level, sprinters should not spend more than an hour at a time on strength work, and should look on it as a complement to rather than replacement for specific running sessions. Too much strength work, particularly using weights, can increase bulk and body weight to a point where the athlete's power-to-weight ratio drops. Moreover, while resistance work increases the power of large muscle groups, research has shown that type IIb fast-twitch muscle fibres, which produce 'pure speed' (as opposed to type IIa which are not quite as fast), thrive when weight training is reduced. It is therefore important to include weight training and to reduce it just before the competitive season begins.

Press-ups

Works: chest, back, arms and core

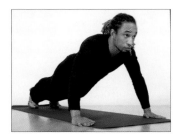

Press-ups may be performed quickly or slowly, but always take care to ensure good technique is held throughout, with the abdominals contracted, and a full range of movement down to elbows bent to right angles and up to fully extended arms. To increase intensity, perform press-ups with your feet up on a bench.

Squats

Works: This exercise trains the muscles used to drive the legs forward during a sprint, including the gluteals, hamstrings and calves

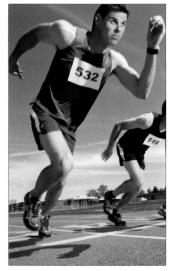

Above: Whole-body strength plays a huge part in a sprinter's explosive power on the track.

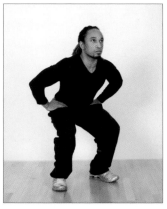

1 Increase the intensity by performing faster sets of half-squats (going down into a squat, but only coming halfway back up until the end of the set).

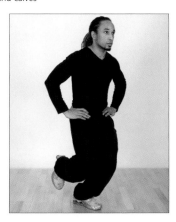

2 Single-leg squats work on core strength and balance. Keep your hands on your hips for balance, and lift one foot up off the ground before going into a squat.

Step-ups

Works: gluteals, hamstrings, calves, quads

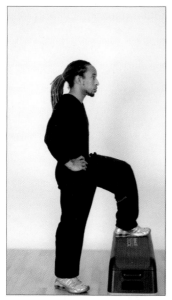 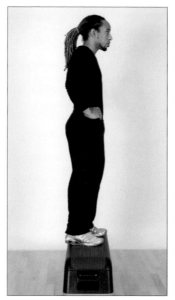 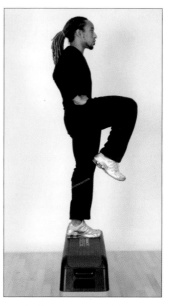

1 *Use a bench high enough that the lead thigh is parallel with the floor, with the knee bent at a right angle, just before stepping up. Put your hands on your hips or drive your arms up with your legs.*

2 *With your feet shoulder-width apart, step up with one leg and use that leg to push up on to the bench, bringing your other foot up next to the first, then step back down on the same leg.*

3 *Make the exercise more challenging and sprint-specific by driving the knee of the trailing leg high into the air before planting it on the bench. As you do so, rise on to the toes of your lead foot.*

Incline sit-up

Works: upper and lower abdominals, core and back

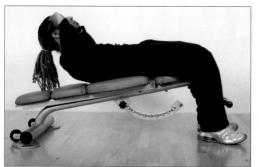

Using an abdominals board, perform sit-ups against gravity to increase their intensity, taking care not to pull your neck. Before you begin, ensure your spine is in a neutral position and engage your core muscles to avoid over-arching or flattening your back too much as you sit up. Try not to allow your feet to leave the floor or your quads to tense during the exercise.

Bridge

Works: gluteals, core

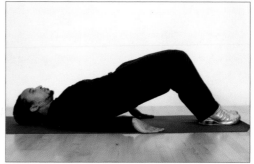

Lie on your back with your knees bent, feet flat on the floor. Push up through your heels, until your hips are in a diagonal line with your shoulders (which stay on the floor). Keep your abdominals tense, and hold the position for 10 seconds, then pulse up and down for 30 seconds, building up to 1 minute.

Weight Training for Sprinters

When training with weights, sprinters lift much heavier amounts than distance runners, but they should not attempt this kind of training without a general background in strength and conditioning.

Strength and fitness for sprinters might be achieved through special running workouts – for example, running on hills or sand; by using core strength exercises; or with regular bodyweight exercises. Plyometric sessions are also vital for sprinters. Strength training programmes need to be tailored to the individual sprinter, with particular attention to their specialist distance and training goals, but here are some of the basic exercises they might perform. It is important to have at least one spotter – a training partner to help you catch the weight if you become unsteady – during all weighted exercises. As you become stronger and the weights you use are heavier, this is especially important since there is a real risk of serious injury if you are unable to control the weight.

Weights and repetitions

It is important to have someone work out a weight-training programme for you: getting your weights wrong could lead to injury. The weights you lift and number of repetitions you perform will vary depending on where you are in your training year. Before you start it is useful to know your Repetition Maximum or 1RM: the heaviest weight you can lift once for a particular exercise. You need a spotter to help you work this out, an exercise professional who can make an estimate from your size and training history.

Once you know your 1RM, use it as a base measurement for deciding your workouts and for progressing to heavier weights.

Dumbbell arm swings

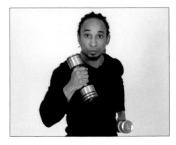

This will improve arm drive. With light dumbbells, watching your action in a mirror, stand up straight with your feet fixed and core engaged to hold your torso steady. Bend your elbows and pump your arms back and forth as quickly as possible, as if you were sprinting for 1 minute; rest 1 minute then repeat. Complete 4–6 sets.

Power clean

Watch points: Try to keep your abdominal muscles and back tight throughout this exercise to protect your back. Try not to push the weight out in front of you, instead jump it straight up.

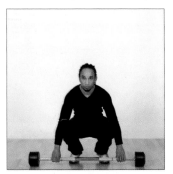

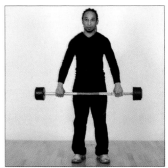

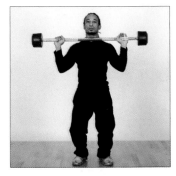

1 *Start the exercise with your feet hip-width apart and the barbell on the floor just in front of you. Slowly bend down to grip the barbell with both hands – you should have your hands over the bar (with your knuckles pointing down) and about shoulder-width apart.*

2 *Lift the weight at a controlled speed by straightening your knees and back, keeping the bar close to your legs. Once the barbell has passed your knees, accelerate your motion. As the bar reaches mid-thigh level, jump the weight up, taking care not to push it out in front of you, but straight up.*

3 *Flip your elbows forward so you have an under-bar grip, and bring your body under the weight, allowing it to rest on your shoulders at the top of the movement. Drop into a half-squat to take the force of the weight, before immediately straightening up. Lower the barbell back to the ground slowly.*

Snatch

Watch points: Make sure you are steady before beginning the lift. Make the final flip movement of the weight as quick and smooth as possible.

1 The start is very similar to the power clean: feet hip-width apart, bend down to grip the barbell with your hands just wider than shoulder-width. Lift the barbell in a smooth motion as before, keeping it very close to your legs.

2 When you are standing straight, continue to lift the weight, keeping the same grip and allowing your elbows to move out to the sides.

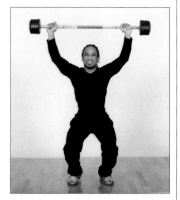

3 As the weight reaches shoulder level, quickly flip it and drop underneath the bar, extending your arms and dropping right under the weight into a squat.

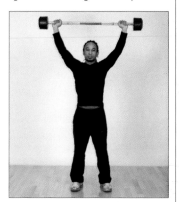

4 Slowly and steadily stand out of the squat to complete the lift.

Weighted step-up

Watch point: If the weight makes you lose control of the action, use a lighter one until you are able to step up straight.

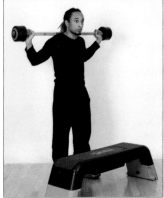

1 The step-up exercise described earlier in this section can also be performed using a barbell. Lift the weight on to the back of your shoulders, using a towel to protect your neck if necessary.

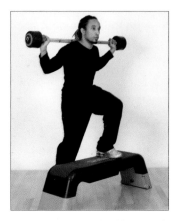

2 Ensure you are steady and in control of the weight, with your feet hip-width apart and core tense. Step up on to a strong bench, slowly bringing your lead leg up onto the bench.

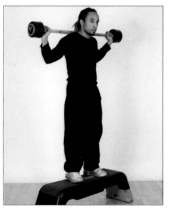

3 Slowly and steadily, bring your back leg up to stand square on the bench next to your lead leg.

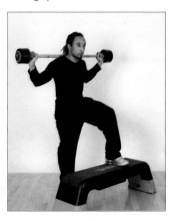

4 Finally, lower the same leg down followed by the lead leg, so that you are back in the starting position.

Other weighted exercises

Since general strength and good overall conditioning is very important to all sprinters, you will also find it useful to include some of the standard weighted exercises used by other types of runners in your regular training sessions.

Alternatively you may decide to use heavier weights and fewer reps. Try to include different general exercises like weighted squats, lunges, calf raises and bench presses in your regular training routine.

Sprinting: 100m and 200m

The 100m sprint is the classic athletic competition, while the more specialist 200m involves a level of technical skill that only the best sprinters can master. The best sprinters start training young but anyone can learn to enjoy running as fast as they can.

For events that are over in less than half a minute, the short sprints take years to perfect. Here are the basics of 100m and 200m training.

100m

Running the 100m is not simply a case of running as fast as you can. Good sprinters break the distance down into a series of phases. First comes the start and acceleration phase (which is sometimes called the 'drive' phase). Practising reacting to the starting gun is crucial. Coming out of the blocks, the sprinter should drive hard, looking down at the track. From 30m to 60m, they will come up slowly and smoothly into the full sprint stride, fixing their eyes on the lane ahead. This 'tunnel vision' is essential to remain relaxed and in control – you should not be thinking about the people behind you. At 60m, sprinters reach their top speed, and the aim now is to hold on

Below: The sheer determination shows on the face of Jamaican Shelly-Ann Fraser (centre) as she goes on to win the women's Olympic 100m final, 2008.

Great athletes: Carl Lewis (b. 1961, Alabama, USA)

From a young age, Carl Lewis (Frederick Carlton Lewis) was determined to be a great athlete, and by any measure he succeeded. In 1999 he was voted Sportsman of the Century by the IOC. Throughout the 1980s and early 90s, he dominated both sprint and long jump at international level. He won five Olympic gold medals for sprinting (100m, 200m and 4 x 100m relays), and was three times the world champion at 100m, the first time in 1983 and last time in 1991. Lewis openly stated his intention to match Jesse Owens' 1936 record of four gold medals at one Olympic Games, and in 1984 in Los Angeles, he succeeded, winning the 100m, 200m, long jump, and leading the 4 x 100m winning relay team. His career was not without controversy, and when he accused Canadian athlete Ben Johnson of using drugs following defeat at the 1987 World Championships, many people thought he was bitter. However, he was vindicated at the Seoul Olympics the next year, when Johnson, who had beaten Lewis to gold in the 100m, tested positive for steroids. Lewis was awarded gold. He retired in 1997.

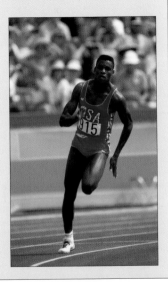

Right: In 1999, Carl Lewis was voted Sportsman of the Century by the IOC.

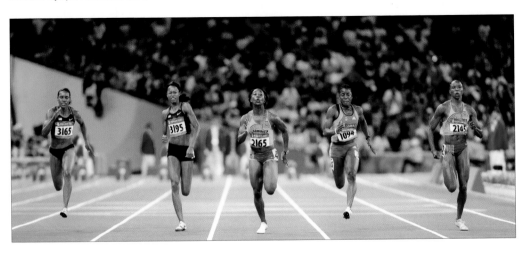

100m and 200m: training examples

Date	Training phase	Theme	Weekly sessions
Oct–Dec	Conditioning	Strength and base building; less speed. Outdoor and off-road sessions	Aerobic training e.g. 3–4 mile easy runs Hill sessions (inc. sand dunes) 3 weights sessions per week: bodyweight and max weight sessions Core and flexibility work 2–3 skills and drills/plyometrics sessions
Jan–Mar	Speed endurance/ indoor season (e.g. racing 60m)	Learning to deal with lactate build-up, working in speed	2–3 endurance sessions (100–200m runs e.g. 5 x 100m, 4 x 150m; Pyramids: 110m, 120m, 130m, 140m and back down with long recoveries) 3 weights sessions: slightly lower weights than in conditioning phase Hills (1 session) 2–3 skills and drills/plyometrics; greater emphasis on power moves
Apr–May	Pre-season/ speed phase	Sessions move on to track; event specific practice	2–3 weights sessions: lower weights 2–3 skills and drills/plyometrics 3–4 speed and start practice sessions e.g. reaction sessions (coach starts with no warning, run 10–15m from blocks only); curve start practice; accelerations sessions e.g. 3 x 30m, each faster than last; 2–3 sets of 2–3 x 30–60m (long recoveries) 1–2 speed endurance sessions as above
Late May–Sep	Competition phase	Much lighter training volume, with races every week	Max 2 weights sessions per week with light weights 1–2 skills and drills sessions 2–3 speed and start sessions as above, but longer recoveries (12–15 minutes) e.g. 50m, 150m, 50m, 150m x 3; ladders 50m, 60m, 80m, 100m, 120m

to that speed as long as possible – usually from 60m to around 85m. From 85m to 100m deceleration is inevitable but during this 'finish' phase, the runner should relax and try to hold form. The finish is measured by the torso crossing the line, so a good lean forward is essential, but time it right: leaning too early slows you down.

Sure starts

Getting sprint starts right can help you to win races. When you are in the 'set' position you will react to the first sound that you hear.

This, however, can sometimes be a problem, as competition rules state that any reaction time faster than 0.10 seconds is a false start (because scientific research has shown that this is the fastest any human can truly react). In a race, one false start puts all the athletes on a 'yellow card', and the next athlete to commit a false start is disqualified, even if the first false start was not theirs.

200m

Most good 100m sprinters can also run a decent 200m, and vice versa, but the 200m is more technical. The first complication, which both 200m and 400m runners must deal with, is the curve start. It will take practice to find the right positions for your blocks (make sure no part of the blocks is in any other lane than your own). On the curve you cannot start at full speed, but you must learn to take it as fast as possible. Stay as far toward the inside of your lane as possible, bearing in mind that your speed will push you to the outside. As you come out of the bend, turn your right shoulder slightly to face the direction you want to run in (toward the finish), using the 'swing' effect of the curve to move up to full speed. Energy conservation is also crucial, as you have farther to run and need to limit your deceleration from 150m. Unlike in the 100m, a very small amount of lactic acid will build up, which is perhaps why 400m runners can excel at this distance.

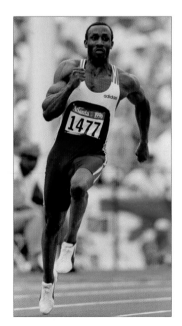

Above: British 200m runner Linford Christie uses the curve in the track to accelerate up to full speed.

Sprinting: 400m

Running one lap of a track may not look difficult, but the longest of the sprint distances is uniquely tough. Pacing must be finely tuned as lactic acid builds up from 300m onward, resulting in heavy legs and inevitable slowing.

The special challenge of the 400m – not quite short enough to be a true sprint, not long enough to be a middle-distance run – is such that great 400m runners can come from a short sprint background (such as Michael Johnson – see box) or from a background of good 800m running.

At the elite level, the 400m is over in less than 50 seconds (less than 45 for male athletes), and there are a number of technical details to get right over that short space of time. Like 200m runners, athletes running the 400m need to practise curve starts, but they also have to

negotiate a second bend at full speed (accelerating again at 200m), staying upright and not compromising form.

Endurance is another important aspect of good 400m running, and something that doesn't really come into the shorter sprints. Physical speed endurance is clearly crucial, and 400m runners need a strong aerobic base as well as plenty of lactate-threshold-level training to learn to deal with the discomfort of running with lactate build-up. Mental endurance is just as important, since athletes will have to 'dig in' over the last 100m to win the race; they need to be able to shut off from the other lanes and run their own race.

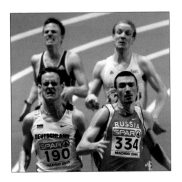

Above: Toward the end of the 400m, athletes need to stay strong and mentally focused on their own race.

			400m: training examples
Date	**Training phase**	**Theme**	**Weekly sessions**
Oct–Dec	Conditioning	Building aerobic base and strength	20–45-minute off-road runs 2–3 sessions weights (moderate, not as heavy as for 100m/200m training) 1–2 sessions skills and drills/plyometrics Hill and stair running session Long, slow intervals e.g. 4 x 600m, short recoveries (2–3 minutes)
Jan–Mar	Speed endurance	Learning to cope with race pace over long periods	Hill/stair running session 2 weights sessions 2–3 plyometrics/skills and drills sessions Speed sessions of 5–10 reps of 100–600m e.g. 8 x 150m, 2 x 600m; 4 x 450m close to race pace; negative split runs 200m, rest 200m x 3–4 (total distance should be not be more than 3–4 times race distance)
Apr–May	Speed/pre-season	Moving almost all training on to track	2 weights sessions, reduced intensity 2 skills and drills/plyometrics (shorter sessions) Curve-start practice sessions Pure speed sessions as for 100m/200m e.g. 50m fast, 50m relaxed fast x 6 with long recoveries Event sessions: completed at race pace, but with race distance broken down e.g. 2 sets of 3 x 350m with 50m fast, 150m relaxed, 150 as fast as possible
Jun–Sep	Competition	Regular racing, reduced training volume	1–2 weights sessions, light weights 1–2 skills and drills sessions Event sessions e.g. 200m, rest, 200m at race pace 320m as race practice; add 10–12 seconds for predicted time (used by Clyde Hart, Michael Johnson's coach)

Great athletes: Michael Johnson (b. 1967, Texas, USA)

From 1991, when he won his first World Championship title over 200m, until his last international competition at the Sydney Olympics in 2000, where he won gold at 400m and as part of the 4 x 400m relay team, Michael Johnson won a total of five Olympic golds and nine World Championship golds. His 200m world record of 19.32 seconds, set at the Atlanta Olympic Games in 1996 was the biggest improvement ever over the previous record, which he had also set earlier that year. His record was only broken in 2008 by Jamaican Usain Bolt. Johnson achieved what many thought was impossible, winning gold at the 200m and 400m in the same Olympics. His 400m world record, still standing in 2008, was set in more remarkable circumstances. Coming into the 1999 World Championships in Seville, Johnson had suffered injury problems, which meant he had barely raced that season, and only qualified by virtue of being the defending champion. He won in 43.18 seconds, and went on to lead home the American 4 x 400m team to gold. Throughout his career, Johnson's strange running style puzzled onlookers: his stiff, straight back and short strides going against ideal sprint form, but with seven of the ten fastest-ever 400m times to his name, few would argue that it worked against him.

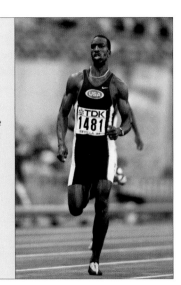

Right: Michael Johnson was extremely talented, winning gold in 200m and 400m at the same Olympic Games.

Pace the race

Different athletes develop different strategies for pacing the 400m. As with longer races (right up to the marathon) they are faced with a choice between running out fast and 'holding on' – which is always a risky plan – or starting the race relatively slowly and gradually speeding up. When considering the second approach, it is worth bearing in mind that it will be impossible to run a negative split (the second 200m faster) in a good field, and it can be mentally very demoralizing to watch the field run away from you at the start. Ideally, athletes should train to run with as even a pace as possible. This is incredibly difficult and requires acute awareness of your own limits and your pace. The last 100m of the race is inevitably always the slowest, as your body simply cannot cope with the level of oxygen debt, but great 400m runners will learn how to minimize this slowing down – a perfect example being Michael Johnson's world-record run in 1999: he ran the first 200m in 21.22 seconds, and the second in just 21.96 seconds.

Below: Jeremy Wariner (centre) of the USA, on his way to winning the men's 400m at the IAAF World Championships in Athletics, 2007.

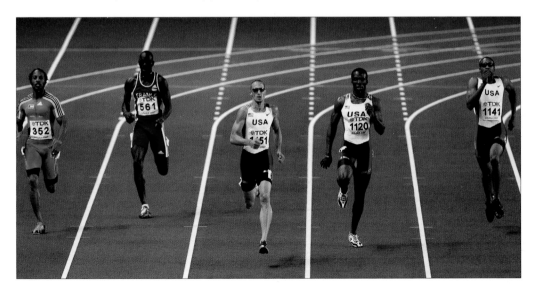

Hurdles

For schoolchildren trying clear them for the first time, hurdles is probably the most fearsome athletic event. Even in later life we use hurdles as a metaphor for barriers and difficulties in our lives. A good hurdler will almost literally take the hurdle in his stride.

Hurdle races should be seen as sprints with added low obstacles rather than a series of 'jumps'. In fact, much of the power, speed and strength required of a hurdler crosses over with straight sprinting, and many athletes will be proficient at both (hurdlers often start out as promising sprinters). The main differences are that a hurdler needs excellent rhythm, and advanced flexibility. Losing your rhythm in a hurdling race can cost valuable hundredths of a second. As well as building basic speed and power (using similar training to sprinters), hurdlers must learn to fix their stride rate: over 110m (or 100m for women), they'll take 8 strides from the start to the first hurdle, then 3 strides between hurdles; over 400m, 20 strides should reach the first hurdle and they'll aim for 13–14 strides between barriers. Throughout the race, the aim is to keep as close to sprint form as possible so that the forward action remains fast and smooth.

Right: The short distances between the hurdles mean that getting into a good rhythm is essential for athletes.

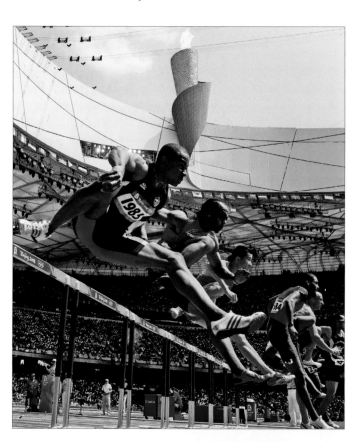

Great athletes: Ed Moses (b. 1955, Ohio, USA)

The career of American 400m hurdler Ed Moses started abruptly, but his incredible run of good form lasted for almost ten years. Having trained as a straight sprinter, Moses had only raced the 400m hurdles once up until March 1976, but using fewer strides between hurdles than his rivals (12–13), he was able to take his personal best over the 400m event from 50.1 seconds at the start of 1976, to 48.30 going into the Montreal Olympics that summer. He went on to win the gold medal at the Games, at the same time setting a new world record of 47.64 seconds. The following year Moses began an incredible winning streak that lasted up until 1987, winning 122 races consecutively including another Olympic gold and two World Championships titles. Moses ended his career with an Olympic bronze medal in Seoul in 1988.

Right: American hurdler Ed Moses won 122 consecutive races in just under 10 years.

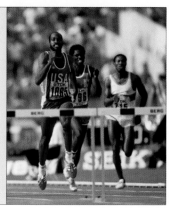

Hurdle sequence

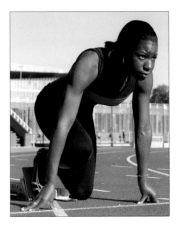

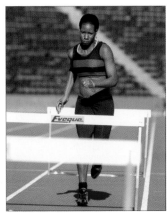

1 *At the start, the lead leg should be in the back block. The start is identical to a sprint start, driving hard out of the blocks with the body almost horizontal. However, hurdlers must come up into full sprint stance (running upright and 'tall') sooner, within four or five strides, in order to take the first hurdle well.*

2 *On take-off, the athlete drives the lead leg up and forward knee-first (as in sprinting and hurdle drills), extending but not fully straightening it. The knee should not lock, as this makes it difficult to land smoothly and keep running. At the same time she drives her opposite arm forward for balance.*

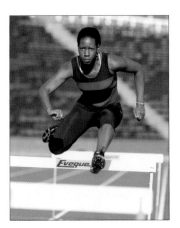

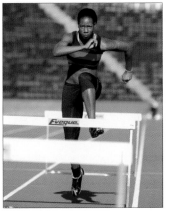

3 *Coming over the hurdle, the hurdler leans her torso forward at the hips, keeping her centre of gravity as low as possible. Remember the aim is to clear the hurdle efficiently rather than 'jump' over it. The trail leg should be tucked up and pulled through as tightly as possible, ready to drive forward for the next step after landing.*

4 *There is no pause on landing, as the lead foot touches down and 'claws' the ground (as in sprinting). The hurdler pulls upright again as she lands, to continue sprinting. As in straightforward sprinting, twisting and side-to-side movements are wasteful and disrupt running rhythm, so the aim is to keep the hips and shoulders square on to the hurdles throughout.*

Relays

The sprint relays offer more than an extra chance for a podium finish. Sprinters' success usually depends on their ability to block out other athletes, so the relays are a completely different kind of running, based on team training and team success. Athletes who can perform smooth, fast handovers can sometimes beat those whose actual sprint speed is faster.

The 4 x 100m relay is perhaps the trickiest as the baton changes must take place without looking (turning back to look at the team-mate before you leads to too much slowing). It is crucial that athletes get to know each other's speed and style. The handover takes place inside a 20m box, and the runners are allowed to begin running up to 10m before that box (in the 4 x 400m, they cannot start outside the 20m change zone). In training, they will work out where they need to start from and where their team-mate will hand over. To avoid running too far with the arm out waiting for the baton, the preceding athlete should call out when they're ready to hand over. At handover, the baton should be held at the very end so there is plenty for the next runner to take hold of. Handing the baton down into the upturned palm of the next runner allows for the fastest change, but is not as secure as handing 'up' in to a down-turned hand. In the 4 x 400m, the receiving athlete turns to look at their preceding team-mate to receive the baton, but has a harder task judging when to start running, and accelerating away from their inevitably slowing predecessor.

Below: The baton handover is slower in the 400m relay.

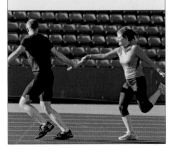

Speed Endurance for Middle-distance Running

In races up to 400m, the athlete's focus must always be on speed and on 'true' speed endurance. Middle-distance track races may look pedestrian in comparison, but running a sub-2-minute 800m or a sub-4:30 mile are as much about the 'endurance' as the speed.

The first time a runner races as fast as he can around two or four laps of a track, and experiences the shattering fatigue of the last few hundred metres, it becomes clear just how important tough training is to run these distances well.

To understand this unique challenge, it is important to be aware of the different energy systems that give runners the power to propel themselves forward at different speeds. Broadly speaking there are two energy pathways: the aerobic system, which uses oxygen to produce energy from the fuel in your muscles, and the anaerobic system, which does not use oxygen. (The anaerobic system can be broken down further into the alactic or immediate anaerobic system – which

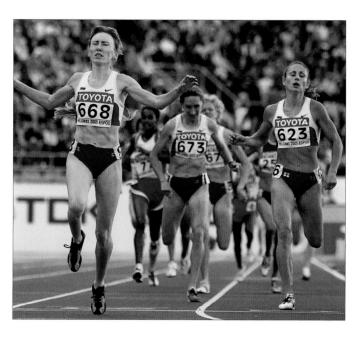

Right: Tatyana Tomashova of Russia wins the women's 1,500m race at the World Athletics Championships, 2005.

Great athletes: Maria Mutola (b. 1972, Maputo, Mozambique)

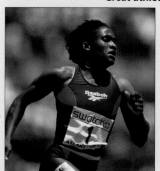

Above: Maria Mutola was a reluctant runner at first, but went on to win nine world titles at 800m.

A somewhat reluctant athlete at first, Maria de Lurdes Mutola has become one of the most successful female 800m runners ever, with 11 world titles to her name (including 7 indoors) and 2 Commonwealth golds. Mutola had been a keen footballer at school and, even when persuaded to try track running, initially found the training too intense. However, her talent for middle-distance events quickly became obvious and, at just 15 years old, she competed in her first Olympic Games (in 1988) – though she was knocked out in the first heat of the women's 800m. Mutola gained funding from the IOC and moved to the USA to train, and it was after this that she began her domination of the event. She finished fourth

at the World Championships in 1991, and went on to win five Championships medals from 1993 to 2003 (including three golds). She won Olympic gold at the Sydney Games in 2000, but was beaten to the title in 2004 by her training partner Kelly Holmes. Over the next two years, Mutola suffered injury problems, but in 2006 she again won gold at the World Indoor Championships, and she competed at the World Championships in Osaka in 2007, finishing third in her semi-final. Mutola's only world-record performance was over 1,000m in 1995, but while she may not be the fastest 800m runner ever, her consistency and longevity as an athlete are matched by few.

provides intense bursts of energy for up to 4 to 6 seconds – and the lactic or short-term anaerobic system, providing energy for up to about 90 seconds of intense exercise.) While sprinting predominantly uses the anaerobic pathway, middle-distance runners make much greater use of the aerobic systems so need more aerobic training. The real difficulty, though, is getting the balance right – more than for any other running events, speed and endurance are of equal importance.

Building a base of aerobic training is essential for 800m and 1,500m runners, and during the winter months their training may not be dramatically

Below: Rashid Ramzi, 800m winner at the 10th IAAF World Championships in Athletics, knows that this race is as much about endurance as it is about speed.

Use of energy systems over different distances

Race distance	Aerobic	Anaerobic
100m	8%	92%
200m	14%	86%
400m	30%	70%
800m	57%	43%
1,500m	76%	24%
Marathon	99%	1%

different to that of long-distance runners. Long, slow runs and relatively slow intervals with short recoveries help to condition the body ready for the serious speedwork that takes place in the lead-up to competition.

Anaerobic training could take up two or three sessions per week, though the total distance covered at this level would not amount to many miles (doing too much anaerobic training

leads to fatigue and an increased risk of illness and injury). Middle-distance runners race at or close to their maximum heart rate, and well beyond the lactate threshold, so they must train their body to adapt to these stresses. Use a mixture of very fast, fairly short reps – 200m to 400m – with long recoveries, and longer intervals at race pace or slightly slower, with shorter recoveries. The British athlete Sebastian Coe and his coach and father Peter believed that not quite allowing the heart rate to recover between intervals, so allowing lactic acid build-up, was a good way to help the body adapt. Speed endurance sessions from both sprint programmes (400m) and from 5K programmes are useful, as the middle-distance runner needs the pure power of the sprinter combined with the endurance and lactate tolerance of the longer-distance athlete.

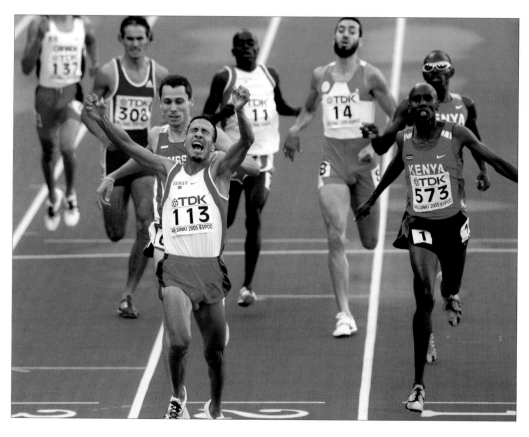

Middle-distance Racing: 800m and 1,500m/Mile

The mile was long regarded as the 'classic' distance in athletics, a baseline measure of an athlete's speed and skill. These days, thanks to the metric system, it is rarely raced – certainly at international level – and the 1,500m has taken its place.

Sitting in between the 'metric mile' and the sprint events are the tough two laps of the 800m. Athletes who are able to compete well in one middle-distance are usually able to compete well in both distances, though they may choose to specialize in one or the other.

Both the 800m and the 1,500m require impeccable pace judgement, so participating athletes must know precisely how fast they can run each lap – the aim being to run as evenly as possible, with a 'kick'

over the last lap. However, in a race situation, of course, you may not always be able to run the race exactly as you would choose to do. Runners with a stronger endurance base might choose to push the pace early on, while those with a sprint finish might prefer to head straight to the front of the pack and try to keep the pace down.

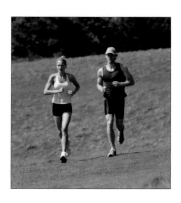

Right: Some long-distance, easy running to develop aerobic fitness is vital for middle-distance running.

Middle-distance racing: 800m & 1,500m schedule			
	Session one	**Session two**	**Session three**	**Session four**
Week one	4 x 400m Race Pace (RP); 6–8 mins rest; repeat	8 x 200m faster than race pace, with 200m easy between; then 2 x 600m RP with 2 mins recovery	5K/3-mile time trial or race	60 mins easy
Week two	6 x 300m just faster than RP, 3 mins recoveries	150m, 200m, 250m, 300m, faster each time, then back down, with 200m recoveries	5K time trial	60–80 mins easy
Week three	5 x 400m RP with 2 mins recoveries; 6–8 mins rest; repeat	2 x 1,000m just slower than RP, with 3–4 mins recovery	1,500m/1-mile time trial	60 mins easy
Week four	5 x 400m RP with 1 min recoveries; 6–8 mins rest; repeat	800m, 1,000m, 800m at mile pace with 2–3 mins recoveries	15–20 mins at lactate threshold pace	60–80 mins easy
Week five	4 x 400m at RP, 50 sec recoveries; 5 mins rest; repeat	150m fast, 50m easy x 6; then 2 x 800m at RP with 2 mins recovery	1,500m or 800m time trial	60 mins easy
Week six	8 x 300m at RP with 1:30–2 mins recoveries	2 x 1,000m at mile pace with 3–4 mins recovery	5K time trial	60 mins easy
Week seven	4 x 400m at RP with 1 min recoveries; 6-8 mins rest; repeat	200m fast, 200m easy x 6; then 2 x 800m at mile pace with 400m recovery	1,500m/1 mile time trial	60 mins easy
Week eight	As week 7	2 x 1,200m at mile pace, 5–6 mins recovery	15 mins lactate threshold, then 4 x 200m RP with 400m recoveries	1,500m or 800m race

Great athletes: Sebastian Coe (b. 1956, London, UK)

For British athletics fans, Sebastian Coe is an icon of a golden era of running, along with his 'rivals', Steve Ovett and Steve Cram. Though an 800m specialist, Coe's two Olympic gold medals were at 1,500m and he remains the only man to successfully defend this title at consecutive Games.

Coe won his first major competition at the 1977 European Indoor Championships, taking gold in the 800m. His first (much-hyped) race against Ovett, the European Championships 800m in 1978, was an anti-climax. Ovett won silver, Coe bronze. The next year, Coe set world records at 800m, 1,500m and the mile. In total he set 11 world records during his career.

The Moscow Olympics in 1980 saw Coe and Ovett winning each other's events – Ovett won the 800m, leaving Coe with silver; then Coe won the 1,500m, with Ovett in third place. In 1984, despite having been ill most of the previous season, Coe defended his 1,500m title, beating Steve Cram. Cram, four years his junior, eclipsed Coe the following year, beating his mile world record. In 1986 Coe was ranked number one in the 800m for the fourth time but he was not picked for the 1988 British Olympic team.

On leaving athletics, Coe went into politics but nevertheless remained heavily involved in sports. Most recently he led London's successful bid to host the 2012 Olympic Games.

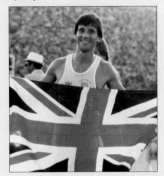

Above: Sebastian Coe holds up the Union Jack after winning the Olympic men's 1,500m final, 1984.

The best way to prepare for this is to include regular time trials or low-key races in your training. Training in a group can, of course, help you to work on your speed and tactics, but only running against a group of real competitors can teach you how to run your own race.

Below: The 1,500m can be a very tactical race as competitors must decide where to position themselves in the pack.

And don't just race the distance you've chosen to specialize in: 800m runners should try the odd 400m sprint and 1,500m or even 3,000m race, while 1,500m runners should have good 800m speed and endurance up to 5,000m.

Middle-distance race schedule

Runners should have a solid base of aerobic training, hill running, weight training, plyometrics and

perhaps also some cross-country racing, built up over the winter months. Note that only the four key sessions are given in the schedule, on the other days athletes should use easy aerobic running, plus some weights or plyometrics sessions if desired.

Below: Wilfred Bungei (centre-right) of Kenya wins in the men's 800m final at the 2008 Beijing Olympics.

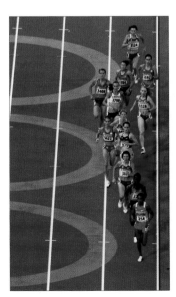

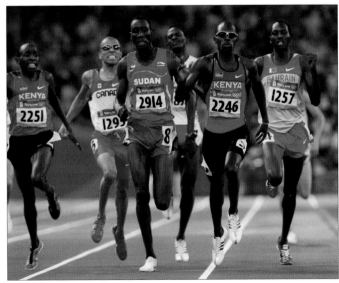

Middle-distance Racing: 3,000m and 5,000m

The 5,000m and the less common 3,000m are a natural step up from the classic middle-distance races. For young athletes, learning real endurance on the track in these races provides a solid background for moving on to the 10,000m and on to long-distance events.

The training for 3,000m and 5,000m track races is very similar to training for a 5K race on the road (the obvious difference being that almost all sessions take place on a track). However, the difference between a 5,000m and a 5K race is marked and each setting requires a completely separate mental approach. In a road-based 5K, the front runners might not see anyone else after the first few kilometres, but on the track the athletes are never far away from each other, and this makes the whole race much more intense. Moreover, unlike a

Right: In a 5,000m event, concentration and planning are important to ensure that you don't get boxed in by other athletes.

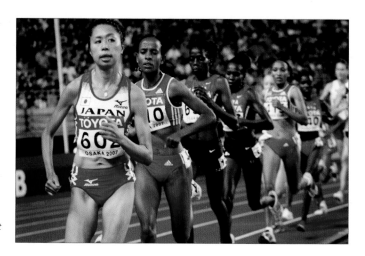

	Monday	Tuesday	Wednesday	Thursday	Friday	Saturday	Sunday
				5K: advanced schedule			
Week one	3 easy	2 x 1,000m with 3 mins recoveries	5 easy with 4 x 100m strides at end	4 x 800m with 2 mins recoveries; 8 x 200m with 200m recoveries	Rest	6km (4 miles) inc. hills	10–13 km (6–8 miles)
Week two	4 easy	3 x 1,000m with 3 mins recoveries	5 easy with 150m hard, 50m easy x 4 at end	6 x 400m with 90 secs recoveries; 1,200m x 1	Rest	8km (5 miles) inc. hills	13–15km (8–9 miles)
Week three	4 easy	1,000m; 1,600m; 1,000m with 3 mins recoveries	4 easy with 6 x 100m strides throughout	6 x 800m with 90 secs–2 mins recoveries	Rest	6km (4 miles) inc. hills	13–16km (8–10 miles)
Week four	4 easy/ cross-train	1,200m, 1,600m, 800m with 3 mins recoveries	5 easy with 150m hard, 50m easy x 6	200m, 400m, 800m x 2 with same distance recovery	Rest	6 km (4 miles) inc. 10–15 minutes easy fartlek	13–15km (8–9 miles)
Week five	4 easy/ cross-train	1,200m x 3 with 2 mins recoveries	5 easy with 4 x 100m strides at end	6 x 400m with 90 secs recovery; 4 x 200m with same recovery	Rest	8km (5 miles) with 6 x 100m strides at end	10–13km (6–8 miles)
Week six	3 easy	3 x 1,000m with 2 mins recoveries	Rest/cross-train	6km (4 miles) with 150m hard/50m easy x 4 at end	Rest	3 easy/rests	5K race

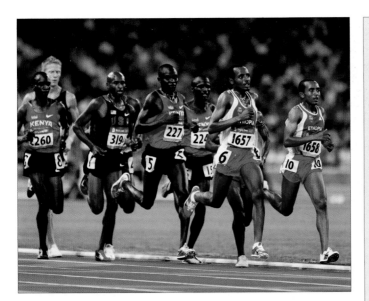

Above: Tariku Bekele and Abreham Cherkos of Ethiopia lead the field at this stage in the 5,000m 2008 Olympic final.

road race, there are no distractions on the track: with lap after lap of running, athletes are forced to concentrate on the task in hand. A 5,000m or 3,000m runner needs to think about where he sits in the pack for most of the race; run to the front too soon, and you risk 'blowing up' in the last few laps, but stay too far back and you risk being boxed in by other athletes, unable to break away from the pack.

Track races can become quite aggressive, and runners can expect to be elbowed, tripped over and spiked as the

competition heats up. The pace is usually faster than on the road, because of the flat, smooth surface of the track, the close proximity of the other competitors, and the relatively sheltered environment. Because of this, even for the longer track distances, runners should work on leg speed, training at mile or 800m pace two or three times per week.

5,000m and 3,000m: advanced schedule

To train for these distances, follow the Advanced 5K Schedule, but do all of your speedwork on the track and aim to race once or twice a week. Even low-key races with relatively small fields will give you the competition practice you need to become accomplished at the distances.

Include some of the following sessions to build leg speed and confidence on the track:
- 6–8 x 400m at mile speed with 90-second recoveries
- 6–8 x 300m at 800m speed with 2-minute recoveries, reducing recovery if these become too easy
Longer speed ladders at 3K pace:
- 1,000m; 1,200m; 1,400m; 1,600m and down again with 2-minute recoveries
- 150m hard, 50m easy, to exhaustion.

Great athletes: Wang Junxia (b. 1973, Jiaohe, China)

Wang Junxia's brief career as an international runner came to an end at the age of just 23, but some of her best performances on the track remain unbeaten. Having won the 10,000m at the world junior championships in 1992, her best year was 1993, when she became the world champion at 10,000m in Stuttgart. She went on to break the world record at the distance by 42 seconds, running 29:31.78. A month later, she set a world record at 3,000m (8:06.11).

However, Wang's career was not without controversy: her then-coach, Ma Junren, was criticized for his harsh treatment of his athletes, which included forcing them to run a marathon a day at altitude; he was later (in 2000) expelled from the Chinese Olympic team after six of his athletes tested positive for illegal substances. Some have claimed that Wang's world records, in particular her 10,000m time, could not have been possible without drugs, though Wang maintains this is not the case.

In 1994, she left Ma behind, and at the 1996 Olympics she won gold in the 5,000m in 14:59.88 and silver in the 10,000m in 31:02.58. However, years of intense training had taken their toll, and Wang retired the following year on a doctor's advice.

Below: Wang Junxia's track career was brief but brilliant, with a 10,000m record of 29:31.78.

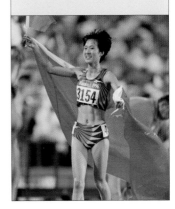

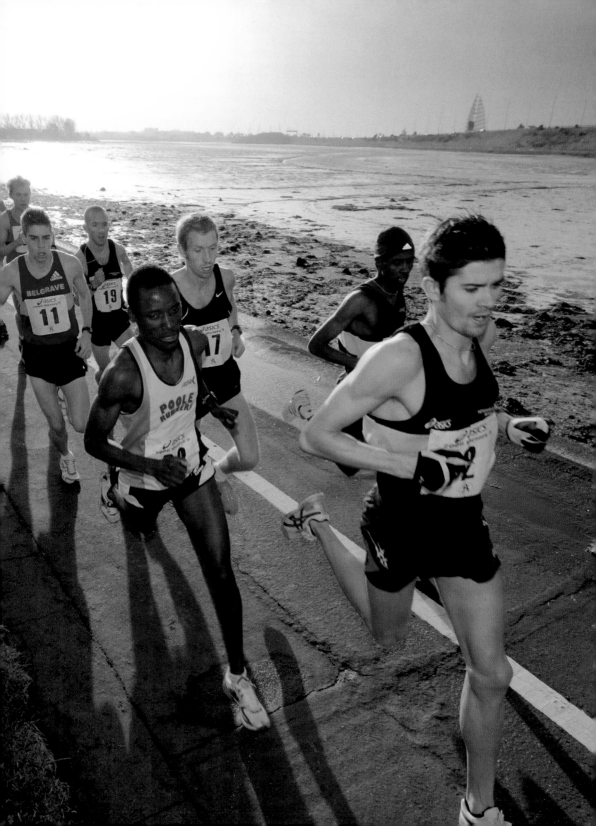

ADVANCED LONG-DISTANCE RUNNING

When you have been running for several years, the idea of covering 5K or even 32km (20 miles) in one go does not seem daunting. However, there is a huge difference between completing long distances comfortably, and actually racing them. This chapter looks at how to race long distances successfully, covering everything from perfecting your pre-training nutrition, to training your mind to deal with the loneliness that comes with long-distance running.

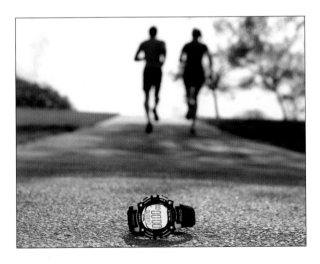

Above: Once you know you can conquer a distance comfortably, you'll be racing against the clock.
Left: At the front of the pack, long-distance races are fast and tactical.

Perfect Nutrition Planning

The diets of elite athletes are almost as legendary as their 240km (150-mile) training weeks. As an amateur you don't need to start eating egg-white omelettes for breakfast, but if you want to maximize your potential, then nutrition planning is as important as the training itself.

If you decide to completely devote yourself to your sport, then unfortunately you will need to accept a few difficult facts. Heavy training sessions mean that you will burn more calories than the average person, but this does not mean that you can eat whatever you want. In fact, it is more important than ever to cut out unhealthy junk food and ensure that every mouthful you eat has some nutritional benefit for your body. It is also worth noting that the best athletes are slightly underweight – research has suggested that sprinters and hurdlers are 5 to 6 per cent lighter than the average 'ideal' weight, while long distance runners should be about 15 per cent lighter. However, runners need to balance the need to stay lean with a tendency to become obsessive (which can lead to eating disorders) and the need to eat enough to fuel their training.

Below are some guidelines for planning what you eat. If you are committed to taking a detailed approach to your diet, you will need to keep a precise food diary and plan what you are going to eat each day (research has shown that people who keep long-term food diaries are more

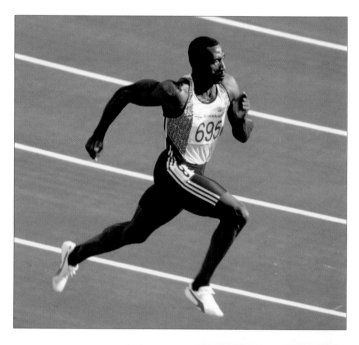

Above: Even though sprinters like Linford Christie look bulky, they are 5 to 6 per cent lighter than the average ideal weight.

Right: Marathon runner Paula Radcliffe has a very low BMI of 18, thanks to careful nutritional planning.

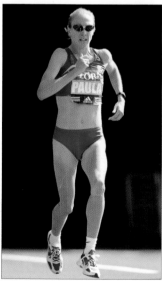

Featherweight champions

There do seem to be different ideal body types for different kinds of sport, and for different forms of running – on the whole, the longer the distance, the smaller and lighter the athlete should be, but what is really important is the athlete's power-to-weight ratio. It is no good being extremely light if this means that you have no muscle. The great athletes listed below would all be considered light by average standards.

Athlete	Distance	Height	Weight	BMI
Herb Elliott	Mid distance	1.79m/5'10.5"	66.6kg	20.8
Seb Coe	Mid distance	1.78m/5'10"	54.4kg	17.2
Linford Christie	Sprint	1.89m/6'2.5"	77kg	21.6
Paula Radcliffe	Long distance	1.73m/5'8"	54kg	18.0

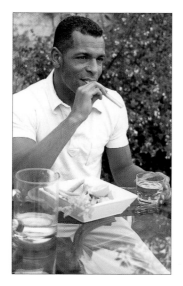

Above: You can work out how many calories you need to maintain or lose weight easily.

successful at losing weight and maintaining their ideal weight). Weigh and measure your portions, and check the packaging of any pre-packed foods to note what they contain. When working out how much to eat, remember to account for all the exercise you do or don't do – you may need to alter your intake if you become injured and miss sessions.

How much should you eat?
Whether you want to maintain your current weight or lose weight, you need to know approximately how many calories you burn every day. First, work out your resting metabolic rate (RMR).
For men aged 18 to 30:
(weight in kg x 15.3) + 679
For men aged 31 to 60:
(weight in kg x 11.6) + 879
For women aged 18 to 30:
(weight in kg x 14.7) + 496
For women aged 31 to 60:
(weight in kg x 8.7) + 829

Right: The men's finalists in the 2008 Olympic marathon knew the value of strict dietary planning.

Remember, your RMR is the lowest number of calories your body needs simply to function. Any activity you do during the day must also be accounted for, so if you have a sedentary job (for example you work at a desk or behind a store counter), multiply your RMR by 1.4; if you do some activity, such as walking around, multiply it by 1.7; or if you are very active (outside of your sports training), multiply it by 2. Then, add to this figure the approximate number of calories you burn during your training. You can measure this using a heart-rate monitor (you will need to input details such as your weight, age and maximum heart rate); if you work out in the gym, you can use the read-outs on the machines' consoles as a rough guide.

If you want to lose weight, reduce the number of calories you consume by 10 to 20 per cent, aiming to lose around 0.5kg (just over a pound) each week. Lose weight any faster and you risk slowing down your metabolism and losing muscle mass. You should aim to cut calories from fat – one gram of fat contains nine calories, so it is energy-dense food. Restrict your carbohydrate intake to

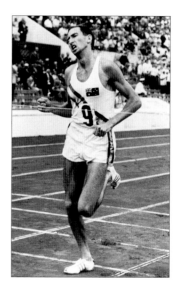

Above: Middle-distance runner Herb Elliott weighed just 66.6kg at the peak of his athletics career.

about 60 per cent of your calories, reduce your fat intake to around 20 per cent of your daily calories, and at the same time aim to slightly increase your protein intake to 1.6g per kg of body weight.

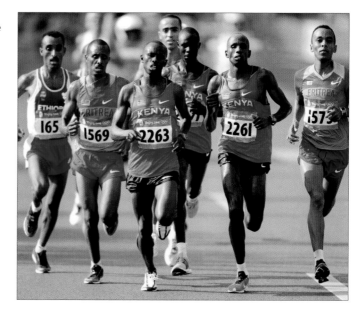

High Protein Diets

Running and controlling your body weight go hand in hand – running is a great way to lose weight, and losing weight is a good way to improve your running. It is no surprise that many runners will diet at some point, and high protein diets are an obvious choice.

Athletes know that they need more protein than the average person to build muscle; they may also have heard that high-protein diets are a fast and effective way to lose unwanted fat. However, to avoid having a detrimental effect on your running, you must be careful about what kind of high-protein diet you follow.

High protein vs low carbohydrate

The recent popularity of high-protein, low-carbohydrate diets such as the Atkins model stems from the idea that dieters can eat as much as they want (in terms of calories) and still lose weight fast. The theory behind these diets is that cutting down carbohydrates reduces insulin resistance, which in turn stops the body from storing energy as fat. High-protein, low-carbohydrate diets force the body into a state of ketosis, in which fat is broken down and

Below: American sprinter Carl Lewis followed a vegan diet, showing you don't need meat for protein.

chemicals called ketones are released into the bloodstream. In the initial stages of the diet, carbohydrate intake drops to around 20g (¾oz) of carbohydrate a day (remember that athletes usually get 60 per cent of their calories from carbohydrates – at least 250g/9oz a day). After the first two weeks, small amounts of carbohydrates are gradually reintroduced.

These diets are highly controversial. Some scientists say they work only by creating a calorie deficiency, largely because the choice of foods is so restricted. Others go as far as to say they are dangerous, leading to kidney and heart problems. What is certain is that these diets are not suitable for athletes. Studies have shown that people on low-carbohydrate diets have far lower endurance levels than those on diets with a high or standard level of carbohydrate. Dehydration is also a risk on low-carbohydrate diets, a clear disadvantage for runners. So, runners wishing to lose weight and gain muscle should think in terms of high protein rather than low carbohydrates.

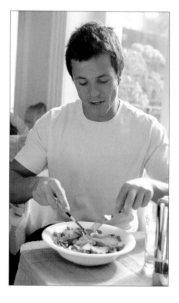

Above: As a serious runner, you should view food as fuel, and consider the nutritional benefit of every meal.

The benefits of protein

It has been suggested that a sports person requires more protein than the average person regardless of their weight goals. An averagely active person needs around 0.8g protein per kg of body weight, but that rises to 1.2 to 1.4g/kg for middle- and long-distance runners. If you are trying to lose fat, that figure rises again to around 1.6g/kg. It is useful for several reasons. For long-distance runners, protein can be a useful extra fuel when your carbohydrate stores (as glycogen) run down. It helps build muscle, making you a more powerful, stronger athlete, and to repair damaged muscle, not only when you are injured but after any tough or long run. Protein is useful for athletes trying to lose weight, as foods that are high in protein are more difficult to digest, thus

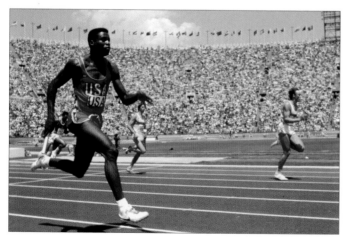

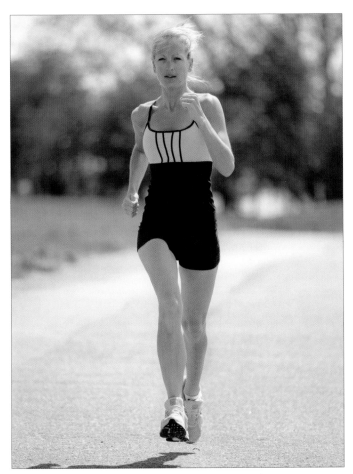

Left: Be careful not to cut down on your carbohydrate intake, since it gives you energy for fast running.

raising your metabolism slightly. It also makes you feel full for longer: some scientists believe this is due to a hormone, PYY (peptide YY), being released into the blood by cells lining the gut when you eat protein, which tells your brain you are full. Protein also helps prevent you from losing muscle when dieting (a common side effect).

Eating enough protein

Keep a detailed food diary for a week, and work out how much protein you currently eat. The chances are you will be far short of your required amount as an athlete. It can be difficult to work out how much protein you are eating at every meal, so if you don't have time to plan every gram, try adding protein: sprinkle nuts and seeds on your breakfast cereal, or have a low-fat yogurt with your usual snack of fruit. If you need to cut calories from elsewhere, try to cut down on fatty foods rather than protein or carbohydrates.

Contrary to popular belief, vegetarians do not suffer from lack of protein or poor quality protein (the great sprinter Carl Lewis was a vegan), but you may need to plan your meals more carefully. In fact, whether you are vegetarian or not, you should aim to get your protein from a range of sources. Different foods contain different types of protein, so a combination is best.

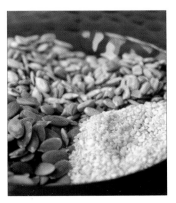

Below: Sprinkle sunflower, pumpkin or sesame seeds on to cereals or salads to instantly increase your protein intake.

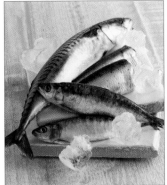

Below: A 100g (3¾oz) serving of oily fish provides one-quarter to one-third of your daily protein requirement.

Protein-rich food:	
Food	**g protein/100g**
Lightly roasted turkey meat	33.6
Lean grilled (broiled) beef	29.5
Grilled (broiled) mackerel	29.5
Sunflower seeds	18.8
Walnuts	14
Quorn	12
Kidney beans	8.3
Tofu	8
Medium egg (per egg)	8
Low-fat yogurt	5.5
Baked beans	5

Perfect Light Meals

Most professional sportspeople have nutritionists to carefully plan their diets, from breakfast first thing in the morning through to the smallest snacks during the day. The rest of us have limited expertise to draw on, but these simple meals should help keep you on top form.

In an ideal world you would spend hours every day training, and the hours in between planning the rest of your life around your training, including a meticulous diet. The reality for most amateur athletes is that life – and work – gets in the way, and food is often the first aspect of our lifestyles to suffer. Your light meals are often more rushed than your main meal of the day, so it's easy to grab a pre-packed salad or bagel without checking what's in it. Unfortunately these convenient meals aren't designed with runners in mind, so you'll often find them full of hidden fats and refined carbohydrates, and lacking in the essential nutrients you need to run well and stay healthy.

But it doesn't take much time or effort to make your own healthy light meals; soups can be prepared in large batches and frozen in portions so you won't need to spend time on them on busy working days. These recipes are all low in fat but high in protein and slow-release energy; serve them with wholegrain bread for the extra carbohydrates and calories you'll need for training. Each of the following recipes makes four modest portions (for which the values are given) or three more generous servings.

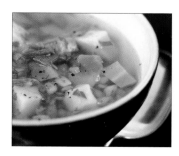

Lean Scotch broth

200g/7oz pearl barley
1 onion
2 carrots
1 small swede (rutabaga), peeled and chopped
1 leek, washed and chopped
115g/4oz/1 cup cabbage, shredded
75g/3oz/½ cup boiled lean gammon (smoked or cured ham), cubed
salt and pepper

Put the pearl barley in a pan with 1.5 litres/2½ pints/6¼ cups of water. Bring to the boil, cover and simmer for 45 minutes. Add all the remaining ingredients and simmer for 30 minutes.

Nutritional information per portion: Energy 280kcal/1176kJ; Protein 11.3g; Carbohydrate 50.4g; Fat 5.3g.

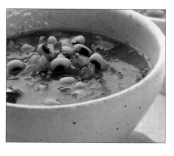

Hearty bean soup

15ml/1 tbsp olive oil
1 onion, finally chopped
1 clove garlic, peeled and crushed
2 large carrots, peeled and chopped
2 x 400g/14oz cans mixed beans, drained and rinsed
400g/14oz can chopped tomatoes
15ml/1 tbsp tomato purée (paste)
5ml/1 tsp dried oregano
5ml/1 tsp dried basil
1 bay leaf
150ml/¼ pint/⅔ cup red wine

Heat the olive oil in a large pan, and then fry the chopped onion and garlic together in the oil until soft. Add the chopped carrots and continue to cook gently for 4 or 5 minutes, until the carrots start to soften. Next, pour in the mixed beans and the chopped tomatoes, stirring, then add the tomato purée, dried oregano, dried basil, bay leaf and red wine, and stir well.

Gently simmer the soup for 10 to 15 minutes, then remove the bay leaf. At this stage, you can either transfer the soup to a food processor and process until smooth, or if you prefer a chunky texture, serve as it is.

Nutritional information per portion Energy 238kcal/1000kJ; Protein 17g; Carbohydrate 52g; Fat 4.1g.

Eating on the run

In an ideal world, everyone would eat a homemade lunch every day, but life gets in the way, often forcing us to grab a pre-packed lunch. If you have to do this, make sensible choices:

• Good sandwich fillings are lean proteins such as chicken or fish, or eggs or falafel for vegetarians. These will keep you full and help to keep your muscles healthy.

• Try to avoid buying over-complicated sandwiches or those which contain an obvious dressing – this will probably contain mayonnaise and will increase the fat content

• Go for wholemeal (whole-wheat) or seeded bread rather than white for slow-release energy

• If you choose a soup or pasta dishes with sauce, go for tomato-based or cream-free varieties.

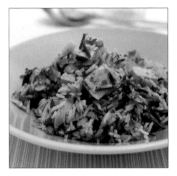

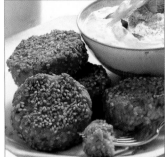

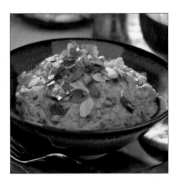

Tofu and wild rice salad

175g/6oz/1 cup basmati rice
50g/2oz/generous ¼ cup wild rice
250g/9oz firm tofu, drained and cubed
25g/1oz preserved lemon, finely chopped
30ml/2 tbsp fresh parsley, chopped

For the dressing:
1 garlic clove, crushed
10ml/2 tsp clear honey
10ml/2 tsp of the preserved lemon juice
15ml/1 tbsp cider vinegar
15ml/1 tbsp olive oil
1 small fresh red chilli, finely chopped
ground black pepper

Cook the basmati rice and wild rice in
two separate pans. Whisk together
the dressing ingredients in a bowl.
Add the tofu, stir to coat and marinate
for 20 minutes. Fold the tofu, marinade,
preserved lemon and parsley into the rice,
check the seasoning and serve.

Nutritional information per portion:
Energy 284Kcal/1185kJ; Protein 9.6g;
Carbohydrate 47.6g; Fat 5.8g.

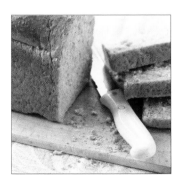

Homemade falafel

2 x 400g/14oz cans chickpeas in water,
* drained and rinsed*
1 small onion, chopped
2 garlic cloves, peeled and crushed
30ml/2 tbsp fresh coriander (cilantro),
* finely chopped*
30ml/2 tbsp flat leaf parsley, finely
* chopped*
5ml/1 tsp ground cumin
5ml/1 tsp garam masala
salt and pepper
10ml/2 tsp vegetable oil
sesame seeds, for sprinkling

Place all the ingredients except for the
salt and pepper and vegetable oil in
a blender and blend to a dough-like
consistency (you may need to add a dash
of oil to help the mixture stick together).
Season, making sure that you mix the
seasoning in well. Take the falafel 'dough'
out and roll it into golf-ball sized rounds,
then pat down so they are flat. Sprinkle
with sesame seeds.
  Heat the oil in a pan over a medium
heat and fry for 2 minutes on each side,
until they are crispy. Serve with a leafy
salad, tomato salsa and low-fat plain
yogurt as a dip. You can keep the falafel
for up to two days in the refrigerator
before the frying stage, fry them as
required and use them in sandwiches.

Nutritional information per portion:
Energy 183kcal/768kJ; Protein 9.7g;
Carbohydrate 22.9g; Fat 6.5g.

Left: Wholegrain bread is a great source
of the extra carbohydrates your body
will need while in training.

Tomato and lentil dhal

30ml/2 tbsp vegetable oil
1 large onion, finely chopped
3 garlic cloves, chopped
1 carrot, diced
10ml/2 tsp cumin seeds
10ml/2 tsp mustard seeds
2.5cm/1in fresh root ginger, grated
10ml/2 tsp ground turmeric
5ml/1 tsp mild chilli powder
5ml/1 tsp garam masala
225g/8oz/1 cup split red lentils
800ml/1½ pints/3¼ cups vegetable stock
5 tomatoes, peeled, seeded and chopped
juice of 2 limes
60ml/4 tbsp chopped fresh coriander
* (cilantro)*
ground black pepper
25g/1oz/¼ cup flaked (sliced) almonds,
* toasted, to serve*

Heat the oil and cook the onion for
5 minutes. Add the garlic, carrot, cumin
and mustard seeds, and ginger. Cook for
5 minutes. Stir in the ground turmeric,
chilli powder and garam masala, and cook
on a low heat for one minute, stirring.
Add the lentils, stock and chopped
tomatoes, and season with ground black
pepper. Bring to the boil, then reduce the
heat and simmer, covered, for 45 minutes,
stirring occasionally.
  Stir in the lime juice and 45ml/3 tbsp
of the coriander. Cook for a further
15 minutes until the lentils are tender.
Sprinkle with the remaining coriander
and the flaked almonds.

Nutritional information per portion:
Energy 326Kcal/1372kJ; Protein 16.9g;
Carbohydrate 43.8g; Fat 10.5g.

Perfect Main Meals

Complicated cooking is probably the last thing you feel like doing after a hard day at work or looking after your family, but let low energy stop you from eating well and you'll get caught in a vicious circle. You need to eat well to refuel no matter how long your day has been.

There is no need to spend hours and hours slaving away in the kitchen to cook the perfect main meal that will help you recover from both your chores and your training. And you certainly don't need to cook separate meals for yourself and your family; in fact children are likely to benefit from a well-balanced runner's diet, although of course you will need to make smaller portions of food for younger children.

These healthy versions of classic family main meals are low in fat, but high in protein and slow-release energy to help you recover from a hard day's work and training.

The portions in these recipes are all quite modest, but if you have worked out your nutritional requirements you can adjust the recipes to provide you with more energy if necessary.

Below: When you are training hard it is important to find the time to sit down and eat a healthy, balanced meal.

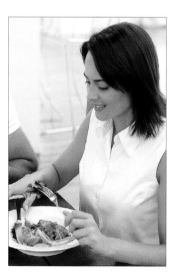

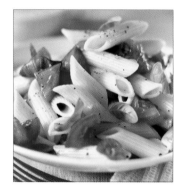

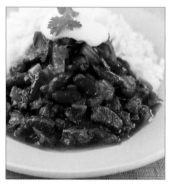

Pasta with fresh tomatoes and basil

500g/1¼lb dried penne
5 very ripe plum tomatoes
1 small bunch fresh basil
60ml/4 tbsp extra virgin olive oil
salt and ground black pepper

Cook the dried pasta in a large pan of lightly salted boiling water for 12–14 minutes, or according to packet instructions, until tender.

Meanwhile, roughly chop the tomatoes and tear up the basil leaves. When it is cooked, drain the pasta thoroughly and return it to the clean pan. Add the tomatoes, basil and olive oil, and toss to mix together thoroughly. Season with salt and freshly ground black pepper and serve immediately.

COOK'S TIP

If you cannot find ripe tomatoes, roast those you have to bring out their flavour. Put the tomatoes in a roasting pan, drizzle with oil and roast at 190°C/375°F/Gas 5 for 20 minutes, then mash roughly.

Nutritional information per portion:
Energy 552kcal/2336kJ; Protein 16.3g; Carbohydrate 96.9g; Fat 13.8g.

Low-fat chilli con carne

15ml/1 tbsp vegetable oil
1 onion, finely chopped
1 garlic clove, peeled and crushed
300g/11oz lean beef steak, cubed
100g/3¾oz/scant 2 cups mushrooms
1 red (bell) pepper, chopped
400g/14oz can tomatoes
400g/14oz can red kidney beans
15ml/1 tbsp tomato purée (paste)
5ml/1 tsp paprika
5ml/1 tsp ground cumin
5ml/1 tsp chilli powder
500g/1¼lb sweet potatoes
200g/7oz/scant 1 cup low-fat natural
  (plain) yogurt

Heat the oil in a large pan. Fry the onion and garlic in the oil until soft. Add the beef, mushrooms and pepper and continue to cook until the meat is browned. Add the canned tomatoes, kidney beans, tomato puree and spices. Simmer for 20 minutes. Meanwhile, cut the sweet potatoes into wedges and bake in the oven at 200°C/400°F/Gas 6 for 20 minutes. Serve the chilli with the wedges, topped with the yogurt.

Nutritional information per portion:
Energy 380kcal/1596kJ; Protein 31.1g; Carbohydrate 45.6g; Fat 9.4g.

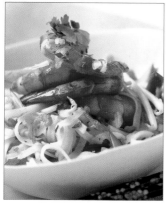
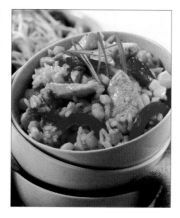
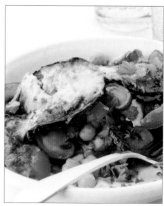

Stir-fried prawns with noodles

130g/4½oz rice noodles
30ml/2 tbsp groundnut (peanut) oil
1 large garlic clove, crushed
150g/5oz large prawns (shrimp), peeled
15g/½oz dried shrimp
15ml/1 tbsp Thai fish sauce
30ml/2 tbsp soy sauce
30ml/2 tbsp palm sugar (jaggery) or
    light muscovado (brown) sugar
30ml/2 tbsp fresh lime juice
90g/3½oz/½ cup beansprouts
40g/1½oz/⅓ cup peanuts, chopped
15ml/1 tbsp sesame oil
chopped coriander (cilantro), 5ml/1 tsp
    dried chilli flakes and 2 shallots,
    finely chopped, to garnish

Soak the noodles in a bowl of boiling
water for 5 minutes, or according to
the packet instructions. Heat the
groundnut oil in a wok. Add the garlic,
and stir-fry over a medium heat for
2 minutes, until golden brown.

Add the prawns and dried shrimp
to the pan and stir-fry for a further
2 minutes. Stir in the fish sauce, soy
sauce, sugar and lime juice. Drain
the noodles, then add to the wok
with the beansprouts, peanuts and
sesame oil. Toss to mix, then stir-fry
for 2 minutes. Serve immediately,
garnished with the coriander, chilli
flakes and shallots.

Nutritional information per portion:
Energy 312Kcal/1299kJ; Protein 11.8g;
Carbohydrate 35.8g; Fat 13.3g.

Chicken fried rice

30ml/2 tbsp groundnut (peanut) oil
1 small onion, finely chopped
2 garlic cloves, chopped
2.5cm/1in piece fresh root ginger,
    peeled and grated
225g/8oz skinless chicken breast fillets,
    cut into 1cm/½in dice
450g/1lb/4 cups cold cooked white long
    grain rice
1 red (bell) pepper, seeded and sliced
115g/4oz/1 cup drained canned corn
5ml/1 tsp chilli oil
5ml/1 tsp hot curry powder
2 eggs, beaten
spring onion (scallion) slices,
    to garnish

Heat the oil in a wok, and stir-fry
the onion for 1 minute, then add the
garlic and ginger and cook for
2 minutes more. Push the onion
mixture to the sides, add the chicken
to the centre of the wok and stir-fry
for 2 minutes more.

Add the rice and stir-fry for
about 3 minutes, until the chicken is
cooked through. Stir in the red pepper,
corn, chilli oil and curry powder.
Toss over the heat for 1 minute.
Stir in the beaten eggs and cook
for about 1 minute more. Serve in
bowls and garnish with the spring
onion slices.

Nutritional Information per portion:
Energy 356kcal/1500kJ; Protein 21g;
Carbohydrate 46.4g; Fat 10.9g.

Low-fat meat-free moussaka

15ml/1 tbsp olive oil
1 garlic clove, peeled and crushed
1 onion, finely chopped
1 red (bell) pepper, chopped
250g/9oz/generous 1 cup red lentils
100ml/3½fl oz/scant ½ cup red wine
400g/14oz can tomatoes
10ml/2 tsp dried oregano
2 large aubergines (eggplants)
40g/1½oz unsalted (sweet) butter
600ml/1 pint/2½ cups skimmed milk
150g/5oz/1¼ cups plain (all-purpose) flour
200g/7oz half-fat Cheddar cheese, grated

Fry the onion and garlic in half the oil
until soft. Add the pepper and cook for
1 minute. Add the lentils, red wine
tomatoes, and oregano and bring to the
boil, then reduce the heat and simmer for
20 minutes. Slice the aubergines and
brush with the remaining oil, then grill
(broil) for a few minutes until soft.

Melt the butter, then add the flour and
fry for a few minutes over a low heat.
Gradually add the milk, stirring. Slowly
bring to the boil to thicken the sauce,
then add most of the cheese, keeping a
handful back. Layer the lentil mix and the
aubergine in a baking dish, ending with
an aubergine layer. Pour the cheese sauce
over the top and sprinkle with the
remaining cheese. Bake for 30 minutes at
220°C/425°F/ Gas 7 until brown on top.

Nutritional information per portion:
Energy 527kcal/2213kJ; Protein 31.1g;
Carbohydrate 57g; Fat 18.9g.

Sports-specific Fuel

Ideally, the fuel needed to run well and recover quickly would come from natural sources. However, consuming enough energy and nutrients from normal food is not practical, particularly for longer races: special energy drinks, bars and gels are designed for this.

To overcome the problems of eating on the run, manufacturers have come up with a huge range of drinks, energy gels and bars to help athletes take on food and fluids as easily as possible. Many runners struggle with these products at first, as they often taste sweet and artificial, which can be difficult to tolerate when two hours of running has left you feeling nauseous. However, it is well worth practising taking on energy foods as you run, because they will help you perform better and protect you from illness and injury afterward.

Your muscles' preferred choice of fuel is glycogen, a quickly-accessible form of carbohydrate. However, you can only store enough glycogen for between two and two and a half hours of running. For an amateur marathon runner that will only take them 29–32km (18–20 miles). At this point, as the body switches to fat for fuel, many runners

Below: Take advantage of drink stations along the race route to ensure that you don't become dehydrated.

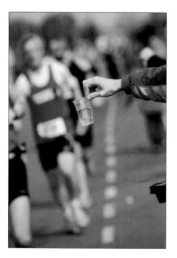

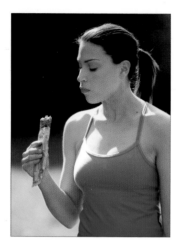

Above: Energy bars will provide plenty of calories but are best eaten before a race rather than during.

'hit the wall' – they temporarily run out of energy as the body works to convert fat into usable energy. The aim of sports fuels is to feed your body carbohydrate so that it doesn't need to switch to fat burning (you can also help yourself by training your body to use fat as fuel – for example using long, slow runs – so that your glycogen stores are preserved for longer).

When running a long-distance race, you should aim to consume about 40 to 60g of carbohydrate per hour. It can be difficult to stomach carbohydrates on the run, so you should never try eating them for the first time during a race. Practise taking on carbohydrates in training, using whatever brand you plan to use during the race. Sports products fall into three categories:

Energy bars
These are the most energy-dense form of sports foods, but as such they are more difficult to digest. They

are best used before a race, or during long, slow races, such as ultramarathons or stage races. (However, studies have shown that eating an energy bar and taking on water with it is as effective in delivering energy as sports drinks or gels.) Typically they provide carbohydrates from rice, oats and maltodextrin. Beware of bars with high levels of glucose, which can cause a spike in your blood sugar, and fructose, which can have a laxative effect. Many bars also contain some protein (for recovery, and slow-release energy), and may also include nuts, chocolate or toffee to make them taste better. From a functional point of view, the simpler the better – more than 5g of fat, 5g of fibre and 10g of protein will make the bar difficult to digest. They usually provide 30 to 60g of carbohydrates per bar, which is enough for an hour of exercise.

Below: You can buy powdered sports drinks and add water – some races will allow you to leave these at water stations.

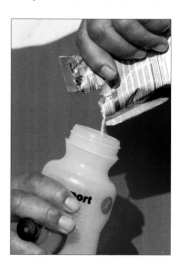

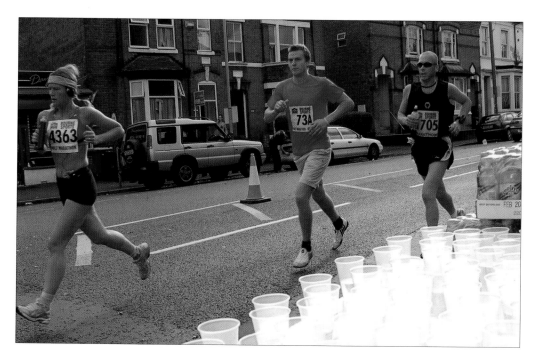

Above: All races must provide water, and many bigger events will also have sports drinks on offer.

Energy gels

A good compromise, energy gels are a more compact way of carrying your fuel and are easier to digest than bars. The downside is that they can be messy

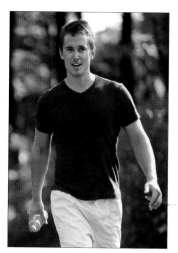

Left: Practise using your chosen food and drink during training to make sure you react well to it.

to take, and you usually need to drink some water with them (to make the mixture isotonic and easily absorbed). However, they only provide around 15 to 30g of carbohydrates per portion, so you will need at least two for each hour of exercise. On a marathon that could add up to six to ten gels, which is a lot to carry and a lot to stomach. Gels usually contain fast-release carbohydrates from sugars, so it is important to take them at regular intervals (every 20 to 30 minutes) to keep your blood sugar levels steady.

Sports drinks

Faster athletes usually choose drinks over gels and bars because they are much easier to take on at high speeds. At many big races, sports drinks are available around the course so you don't have to carry anything – check which brand will be used and practise drinking it in training. Otherwise, see if you can make up your own drinks and

have them placed at water stations around the course. Most sports drinks, mixed up correctly, provide an ideal 6 to 8g of carbohydrate per 100ml – you will need to drink between 750ml and 1 litre per hour.

Preventing illness

Many athletes complain that they are more likely to catch colds and bugs in the days just after a big race. This is because the harder you train and race, the more your immune system is suppressed. Part of the reason for this is that the stress hormones which are released when your body switches to fat burning for energy block the action of some types of white blood cells, which form part of your body's defences against illness. By keeping your body's carbohydrate levels topped up, you will reduce the need for fat to be used as fuel, and also help prevent stress hormones from being released, so fuelling your run will not only help you run well on the day, but will aid your recovery afterward.

DIY Training Fuel

Runners tend to have a better awareness of what they put into their bodies than other people, so it is strange that many of them come to rely on manufactured training fuels, which can be full of highly refined sugars, especially when these recipes are so easy.

Even energy bars and drinks that contain only natural ingredients – and there are plenty of examples of these on the market – can taste artificial. For this reason many athletes prefer not to use them at all, sticking to water. In doing so they are missing out on the hugely important benefits of staying well-fuelled during tough training sessions and long races. However, if you are prepared to invest a little time, you can easily make your own energy snacks and drinks at home.

All of these recipes deliver more than 30g of carbohydrates, roughly the same as a store-bought energy gel, but because of their slightly higher fat content (in most cases), they will take a little longer for your body to digest. As such they are better for eating before you begin a training session rather than while you are out running, with the exception of the natural isotonic drink, which will provide you with an almost instant energy hit.

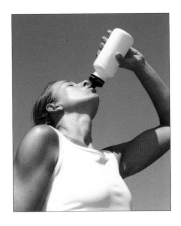

Above: Mixing your own natural energy drink from fruit juice and water at home is cheap and easy.

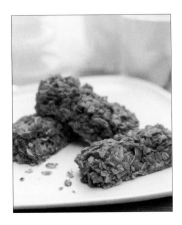

Fruit flapjacks
The oats in this bar should help to calm pre-race nerves; the sultanas and honey give a moderate-GI energy release, while the ground ginger (which is optional) should help to stave off nervous nausea.

200g/7oz/scant 1 cup butter or margarine
225g/8oz soft light brown sugar
30ml/2 tbsp clear honey
300g/11oz/2½ cups jumbo oats
150g/5oz/1 cup sultanas (golden raisins)
2.5ml/½ tsp ground ginger

Melt the butter, sugar and honey together in a large pan over a low heat, stirring constantly, until the sugar and honey have dissolved. Mix in all the other ingredients. Press the mixture into a lightly greased baking tray and bake at 190°C/375°F/Gas 5 for 15 to 20 minutes, until golden brown. While it is still hot, cut into 16 portions, but leave to cool in the tin, as the flapjack remains soft until it has cooled slightly.

Nutritional information per portion:
Energy 250kcal/1050kJ; Protein 2.5g;
Carbohydrate 34.1g; Fat 11.6g.

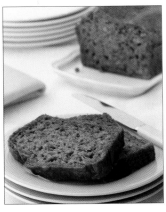

Banana bread
Bananas are the classic runner's fuel and this soft loaf should be easy to eat before a run. Adding cinnamon may help control your blood sugar levels, avoiding a crash after the initial burst of energy.

100g/3¼oz/scant 1 cup butter
200g/7oz/1 cup caster (superfine) sugar
2 eggs, beaten
225g/8oz/2 cups wholemeal
  (whole-wheat) flour
2.5ml/½ tsp baking powder
5ml/1 tsp cinnamon
200g/7oz ripe bananas, mashed

Cream the butter and sugar together. Beat in the eggs, then fold in the flour, baking powder and cinnamon. Add the bananas and mix thoroughly. Pour the mixture into a greased loaf tin (pan) and bake at 180°C/350°F/Gas 4 for 50 minutes, until risen and golden brown on top (note the consistency of the loaf may remain soft because of the bananas; you can firm it up by refrigerating it later). Slice into ten pieces.

Nutritional information per portion:
Energy 265kcal/1113kJ; Protein 5g;
Carbohydrate 39g; Fat 10.3g.

Natural isotonic drink

This natural isotonic drink delivers the same amount of carbohydrates as a store-bought energy drink – around 6g per 100ml, so it can be absorbed easily on the run. It is very easy to make and cost effective too, as store-bought energy drinks can be expensive. To save time on early-morning runs, make up a bottle the night before and keep chilled in the refrigerator overnight.

Makes 1 litre/1¾ pints/4 cups

500ml/17fl oz/generous 2 cups
* unsweetened apple juice*
500ml/17fl oz/generous 2 cups water
pinch salt

Pour the apple juice and the water into a 1-litre (1¾-pint) sports bottle, then add the pinch of salt. Shake the bottle thoroughly to mix.

Nutritional information per portion
Energy 190kcal798kJ; Protein 0.5g;
Carbohydrate 55g; Fat 0.5g.

Low-fat fruit loaf

Lack of fat in this loaf makes it easier to digest on the run. It provides enough energy for about an hour of exercise, but be careful of the high fibre content, which could unsettle your stomach.

115g/4oz/1 cup raisins
115g/4oz/1 cup sultanas (golden raisins)
115g/4oz/1 cup currants
25g/1oz/2 tbsp soft dark brown sugar
150ml/¼ pint/⅔ cup hot black tea
10ml/2 tbsp thick-cut marmalade
2 eggs, beaten
175g/6oz/1½ cups wholemeal
* (whole-wheat) flour*
5ml/1 tsp mixed spice (apple pie spice)
30ml/2 tbsp skimmed milk

Soak the fruit and sugar in the tea overnight. Stir in the other ingredients and mix. Pour into a greased and lined loaf tin (pan) and bake at 180°C/350°F/ Gas 4 for 1½ hours until firm.

Nutritional information per portion
Energy 249kcal/1045kJ; Protein 6.3g;
Carbohydrate 50.9g; Fat 2.7g

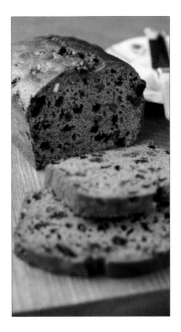

Above: This fruit loaf has a very low fat content and so is easy for your stomach to digest as you run.

Instant energy

If you don't have the time to spare to make your own training snacks, just grab some natural quick-release energy in the form of:

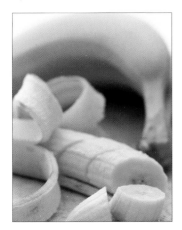

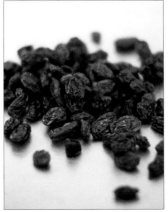

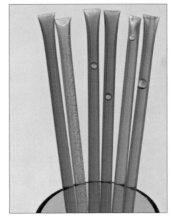

A medium banana: *this will give you enough energy for around 30 minutes of running, as well as potassium to keep your muscles from cramping. Choose very ripe bananas, which are easier to digest.*

Raisins: *this high-energy dried fruit packs a powerful 135kcal/567kJ and 35g of carbohydrates for every 50g (handful). It also contains high levels of antioxidants, which help combat some of the damage done by intense exercise.*

Honey: *clear honey in a squeezy pack (sometimes called a honey stick) makes the perfect natural energy gel. Research suggests it is just as effective as store-bought energy gels for fuelling exercise.*

5K Event: Advanced Schedule

It is a tough distance to get right, but learning how to run 5K to the best of your ability will stand you in good stead for longer distances. It's a great test of speed, stamina and strength of character and is short enough to be raced once a month.

In some ways a 5K road race is more daunting for an experienced runner than for a complete beginner. In training, there are three main areas to work on.

Style
You will need to develop a faster stride for the 5K, especially if you have become used to running farther and slower. Working on your form will help your legs to move quickly and will keep you from wasting energy during the race. Most people find that their style naturally improves when they run a bit faster, but you can work on it. Including regular skills and drills sessions to work on your flexibility, reactions and style will help, as will performing fast strides at the end of some runs.

Below: Working on your running form is important for 5K racing. Include some hill walks and runs in your sessions.

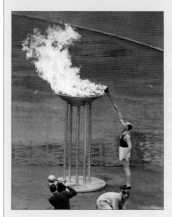

Great athletes: Paavo Nurmi (b. 1897, Turku, Finland, d. 1973)
One of the earliest examples of a strong tradition of Finnish distance runners, Paavo Nurmi won nine Olympic gold medals and three silvers and set countless world records across a huge spectrum of distances, making him a national hero in his home country. At his first Olympic Games in Antwerp, 1920, he won gold in the 10,000m, two cross-country events, and silver in the 5,000m. He was a determined athlete and his tough training is legendary. He went on to compete at two more Olympics, but in 1932 was not allowed to take part as officials ruled he had accepted too much money for expenses, breaking the strict rules on amateurism. He won his last major race in 1933. In 1952, when the Olympics came to Helsinki, Nurmi carried the torch at the opening ceremony, and there is a statue of him outside the Olympic stadium there.

Left: The Finnish great, Paavo Nurmi, lights the Olympic flame at the 1952 Games in Helsinki.

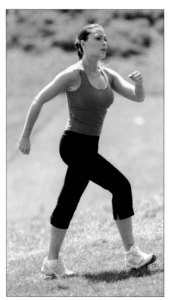

Pacing
There are two approaches to pacing a 5K. The traditional approach is the negative split – the safer option – where the first half is run slightly slower. However, recent research suggests that the best approach is actually to head out fast and try to hang on. Whichever tactic you choose, you need to develop an instinctive feel for your goal 5K pace, and longer intervals (over 1,000m) can help with this.

Coping with pain
It sounds dramatic, but if you don't feel strong discomfort for at least the last 2km of your 5K race, you are probably not working as hard as you can. Unfortunately it takes practice to learn to deal with this, which is where your mile pace and longer

Right: Running fast intervals of 1,000m and longer is a good way for you to learn pace judgement.

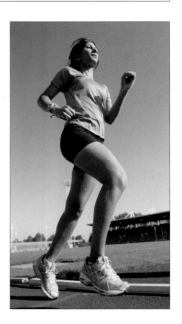

intervals come into play. As you get more experienced you can cut down recovery times between repetitions, which brings you closer to the race experience. For these sessions it is especially useful to train with faster athletes; if you train alone it will be very difficult to force yourself to run this fast for any length of time.

Example six-week schedule

Before starting this schedule, you should be running at least five times a week. Your long run should be at least an hour, and you should be doing one or two speedwork sessions. For longer intervals here (1,000m and beyond) you should aim to run at 3 to 5 seconds faster than a 5K pace; for shorter repetitions aim to run at your mile pace. Speed sessions should include a 10-minute warm-up jog and 10-minute cool-down. Your race goal is faster than 24:30 (8-minute miling); if you are aiming to run sub-20 minutes, reduce the recovery periods between long intervals.

Right: Train with someone slightly faster than you to make sure you push yourself hard enough.

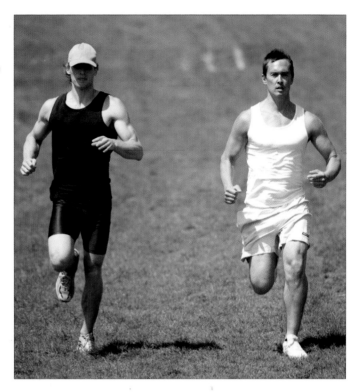

5K event: advanced schedule

	Mon	Tue	Wed	Thur	Fri	Sat	Sun
Week one	3 easy	2 x 1,000m with 3 min recoveries	5 easy with 4 x 100m strides at end	4 x 800m with 2 min recoveries; 8 x 200m with 200m recoveries	Rest	6km (4 miles) inc. hills	10–13km (6–8 miles)
Week two	4 easy	3 x 1,000m with 3 min recoveries	5 easy with 150m hard, 50m easy x 4 at end	6 x 400m with 90 sec recoveries; 1,200m x 1	Rest	8km (5 miles) inc. hills	13–15km (8–9 miles)
Week three	4 easy	1,000m; 1,600m; 1,000m with 3 min recoveries	4 easy with 6 x 100m strides throughout	6 x 800m with 90 secs–2 mins recoveries	Rest	6km (4 miles) inc. hills	13–16km (8–10 miles)
Week four	4 easy/ cross-train	1,200m, 1,600m, 800m with 3 min recoveries	5 easy with 150m hard, 50m easy x 6	200m, 400m, 800m x 2 with same distance recovery	Rest	6km (4 miles) inc. 10–15 minutes easy fartlek	13–15km (8–9 miles)
Week five	4 easy/ cross-train	1,200m x 3 with 2 min recoveries	5 easy with 4 x 100m strides at end	6 x 400m with 90 secs recoveries; 4 x 200m with same distance recovery	Rest	8km (5 miles) with 6 x 100m strides at end	10–13km (6–8 miles)
Week six	3 easy	3 x 1,000m with 2 min recoveries	Rest/cross-train	6km (4 miles) with 150m hard/50m easy x 4 at end	Rest	3 easy/rests	5K race

10K Event: Advanced Schedule

For the experienced runner, the 10K has a particular draw. It is a fairly short race, so you can recover quickly from it and have several attempts at a personal best over a season, and the nice round 10 kilometres makes it perfect for pace practice.

It is a distance that eludes some of the best professional athletes, but the 10K is worth revisiting several times a year; in the winter as a means of keeping your speed up, and in the summer to ensure you can still cover a decent distance. If you're training for a 5K or for a longer event, then you should be able to run a good 10K time, but if you are training

specifically for this distance you'll need to fine-tune your sessions. The key sessions involved in running a 10K are:

Race pace
Some coaches believe that 10K race pace is the most efficient speed for most athletes. However, that is true only if you can get it right. You will use long stretches of 10K pace in your speed

sessions to get used to the pace. If you are training for a longer event, the 10K pace will stand you in good stead, as it forms the basis for faster sessions for a half-marathon and longer. If instead you are aiming to knock a huge chunk off your personal best, try these sessions at your current best pace and if they feel easy, step up to your 'dream' pace to see how you cope.

	Mon	Tue	Wed	Thur	Fri	Sat	Sun
			10K event: advanced schedule				
Week one	Rest	6 x 800m with 400m recoveries	8km (5 miles) with 5 x 100m strides at end	3 x 1.5km (1 mile) at race pace with 4 min recoveries	Rest/ cross-train	8km (5 miles) easy	13–16km (8–10 miles)
Week two	Rest	4 x 200m hard/200 easy; 10 mins easy; 4 x 800m with 400m recoveries	8km (5 miles) easy	1,000m; 1,200m; 1,600m; back down at race pace with 2 min recoveries	Rest/ cross-train	8km (5 miles) easy with 5 x 100m strides	13–16km (8–10 miles)
Week three	Rest	As week 1	6.5km (4 miles) neg split run	4 x 1.5km (1 mile) at race pace with 4 min recoveries	Rest	6.5km (4 miles) easy	16–19km (10–12 miles)
Week four	Rest	As week 2	4km (2.5 miles) neg split run	2 x 1,600m race pace, 4 min recs; then 6 x 200m hard/200m easy	Rest	8km (5 miles) easy	16km (10 miles)
Week five	Rest	6 x 800m (just faster than race pace) with 400m recoveries	8km (5 miles) easy	10K neg split run (on race course if poss.)	Rest/ cross-train	8km (5 miles) easy	13km (8 miles) with 3 x 10 mins 10K pace plus 5 x 100m strides
Week six	Rest	2 x (200m, 400m, 800m, back down); with 200m recoveries	6.5km (4 miles) neg split	5 x 1.5km (1 mile) at race pace with 2 min recoveries	Rest/ cross-train	10km (6 miles) easy	13km (8 miles) with 2 x 10 mins at race pace
Week seven	Rest	As week 5	8km (5 miles) neg split	4 x 1.5km (1 mile) at race pace with 90 sec recoveries	Rest/ cross-train	8km (5 miles) easy	16km (10 miles) easy
Week eight	Rest	6 x 800m, with 400m recoveries	8km (5 miles) neg split	8km (5 miles) easy	Rest	5km (3 miles) easy with 4 x 100m strides	10K race

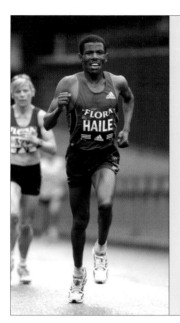

Great athletes: Haile Gebrselassie (b. 1973, Arsi Province, Ethiopia)

In an international career that began in the early 1990s, Haile Gebrselassie has earned a deserved reputation as one of the greatest distance runners ever. He has set 26 world records, won two Olympic gold medals and four 10,000m golds in four consecutive World Championships.

His first real international breakthrough came at the World Junior Championships in 1992, where he won the 5,000m and 10,000m. He was not without close rivals, mainly fellow African runners, and at the 2000 Olympics in Sydney he beat the Kenyan runner Paul Tergat in the closest 10,000m in Olympic history: the margin was just 0.09 seconds. His next Olympics in Athens was a disappointment; he had hoped to retain his 10,000m title but lost to countryman Kenenisa Bekele. Since that Games,

Left: Haile Gebrselassie running the London Marathon. He set a new world record at the distance in 2008.

Gebrselassie has focused on road races, with impressive wins over 10K, and world records at 10 miles and half-marathon. In 2005, he won all his road races. The one record that seemed to evade him was the marathon. Despite wins at Amsterdam and Berlin, his performances at the Flora London Marathon in 2006 and 2007 ended badly – he pulled out at 18 miles in the latter race. However, later that year, Gebrselassie was vindicated with a new marathon world record, 2:04:26. The following year proved disappointing: having decided not to race the marathon at the Beijing Olympics – he feared the city's pollution would aggravate his asthma – Gebrselassie could only reach sixth place in the 10,000m. He has now turned his attention back to road racing, and broke his own record in 2008, running 2:03:59 in Berlin. He maintains that he will run a marathon in less than 2:03 before the end of his career.

Negative splits

A 10K event is the perfect distance to use the negative split. Practise this in slightly shorter training sessions so that you are able to get used to the feeling of running relaxed then speeding up. Gradually you will build up to a 10K 'time trial', so find a route that is as close as possible to 10K (you can use a track or a treadmill to measure the distance accurately if necessary).

Example eight-week schedule

Before beginning this eight-week schedule you should be running at least five times per week, covering a minimum of 48km (30 miles). You should be able to run for 1 hr 30 mins comfortably, and ideally you will be doing one or two speed sessions per week. All speed sessions should have a 10-minute warm-up jog and 10-minute cool down. Your target race time is 35 to 45 minutes.

Long runs

It may seem strange to run almost to half-marathon distance during a 10K schedule, but without this comfortable

Right: Some coaches believe that 10K pace is the most efficient speed.

level of endurance you won't be able to sustain a fast pace. It's also worth bearing in mind that the 10K can be the stepping stone to great

marathons – as it has been for many an elite athlete, such as the great Gebrselassie – so you won't regret maintaining your long-run base.

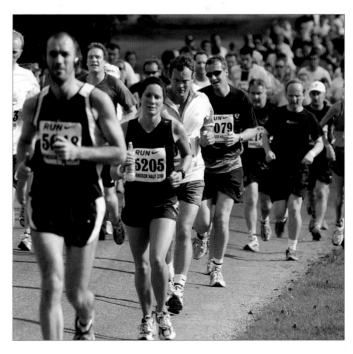

Half-marathon: Advanced Schedule

Half-marathon training is not dissimilar to training for the full distance, and most runners train for both concurrently. The noticeable difference is in the pace, which, if you are racing well, should be considerably less relaxed than at marathon level.

Half-marathons tend to be run just below lactate threshold pace, so you need to practise this more often in training. You can only estimate your exact lactate threshold without being tested, but for most people it is around 80 to 85 per cent of their maximum heart rate. Some of your sessions will be longer runs with periods of threshold and race pace running built in.

The mileage needed for a half-marathon almost matches that of a marathon schedule. You can run a half-marathon with fewer really long runs, but to be able to push the pace you will need to be comfortable over much longer distances. In fact, if you have

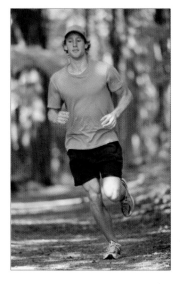

Below: Over 24,000 participants competed in the 28th Berlin half-marathon in April 2008.

time to build up to running twice a day, then you should add an extra 30 to 40 minute easy run to every day (separate from the sessions listed on the plan).

Example 12-week plan

To follow this plan you must have been running five or six times a week for several months, with one long run of 1hr 30 mins and two speed sessions per week. For intervals over a mile (5 to 8 minutes) in length, run at threshold or race pace; for one-mile repetitions use 10K pace; for 400 to 800m use 5K pace. Each speedwork and threshold session should begin with a 10-minute warm-up.

Left: To run a fast half-marathon, your mileage will need to almost equal full marathon training.

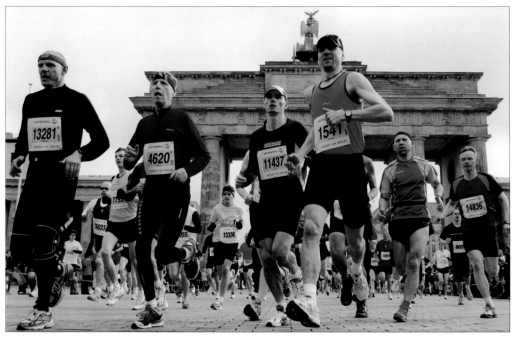

Half-marathon: advanced schedule

	Mon	Tue	Wed	Thur	Fri	Sat	Sun
Week one	5km (3 miles) easy/cross-train	6 x 800m with 400m recoveries	8km (5 miles) easy with 5 x 100m strides throughout	2 x 10 mins threshold, 5 mins recovery	8km (5 miles) easy	Rest/cross-train	16–19km (10–12 miles)
Week two	5km (3 miles) easy/cross-train	400m, 800m, 1,200m, 1,600m then back with 400m recoveries	8km (5 miles) easy with 5 x 100m strides throughout	15 mins threshold; 10 mins recovery then 5 x 200m fast but relaxed	8km (5 miles) easy	Rest/cross-train	19–22km (12–14 miles)
Week three	5km (3 miles) easy/cross-train	8 x 800m with 400m recoveries	10km (6 miles) easy with 5 x 100m strides throughout	15 mins threshold; 10 mins recovery then 5 x 200m fast but relaxed	8km (5 miles) easy	Rest/cross-train	22–25km (14–16 miles) with 2 x 10 mins at race pace
Week four	8km (5 miles) easy/cross-train	4 x 1 mile with 2–3 min recoveries	10km (6 miles) easy with 8 x 100m strides throughout	3 x 10 mins threshold; 5 min recoveries	10km (6 miles) easy	Rest/cross-train	26–29km (16–18 miles) with 3 x 10 mins at race pace
Week five	8km (5 miles) easy/cross-train	8 x 800m with 400m recoveries	10km (6 miles) easy with 8 x 100m strides throughout	2 x 15 mins threshold with 5 mins recovery	10km (6 miles) easy	Rest/cross-train	32km (20 miles) with 2 x 20 mins at race pace
Week six	Cross-train/rest	2 x 800m, 1,600m, 2,000m with 3 min recoveries	10km (6 miles) easy with 5 x 200m fast but relaxed	2 x 15 mins threshold with 5 mins recovery	10km (6 miles) easy	Rest/cross-train	22–25km (14–16 miles) with 3 x 15 mins at race pace; or race 10K
Week seven	8km (5 miles) easy/cross-train	2 x 800m, 1,600m, 2,000m with 3 min recoveries	10km (6 miles) easy with 5 x 200m fast but relaxed	30 mins threshold	10km (6 miles) easy	Rest/cross-train	32km (20 miles) with 40 mins at race pace
Week eight	5km (3 miles) easy/cross-train	5 x 1 mile with 2–3 min recoveries then 5 x 150m fast/50m easy	6.5km (4 miles) easy	30 mins threshold	10km (6 miles) easy	Rest/cross-train	29km (18 miles) with 3 x 15 mins at race pace
Week nine	8km (5 miles) easy/cross-train	10 x 800m with 400m recoveries	10km (6 miles) easy with 8 x 100m strides	2 x 20 mins threshold with 5 mins recovery	10km (6 miles) easy	Rest/cross-train	22–25km (14–16 miles) with 2 x 20 mins at race pace; or race 10K
Week ten	8km (5 miles) easy/cross-train	5 x 1 mile with 2–3 min recoveries then 5 x 150m fast/50m easy	10km (6 miles) easy; gradually accelerate over last 2 miles	30 mins threshold	10km (6 miles) easy	Rest/cross-train	22–25km (14–16 miles) with 2 x 20 mins at race pace
Week eleven	8km (5 miles) easy/cross-train	6 x 800m with 400m recoveries	8km (5 miles) easy with 8 x 100m strides	2 x 15 mins threshold with 5 min recovery; 5 x 200m fast but relaxed	10km (6 miles) easy	Rest/cross-train	16km (10 miles) easy
Week twelve	5km (3 miles) easy/cross-train	Rest	Rest/cross-train	5 miles easy	Rest	5km (3 miles) easy with 5 x 100m strides	Half-marathon

Marathon: Elite Schedule

The traditional and most widely accepted method of marathon training is to run a high mileage, six or seven days a week, reaching more than 160 kilometres or 100 miles per week in training. This training is not just the preserve of top marathon runners.

Running an elite schedule is hard on your body and should not be attempted unless you have gradually built up a base fitness for this distance. However, if you can handle it, you will be using a similar schedule to the world's best marathon runners.

The key sessions for this schedule are similar to other approaches, but it requires running twice a day from Monday to Friday, with a second semi-long run halfway through the week. Your long runs are also slightly longer, reaching 37–38km (23–24 miles) at their peak.

The 12-week schedule

The easy runs are not listed in the table as they remain constant throughout: run 6–10km (4–6 miles) each morning from Monday to Friday. Remember to

Right: Following a high-mileage schedule is tough but is the surest way to reach the front of the pack.

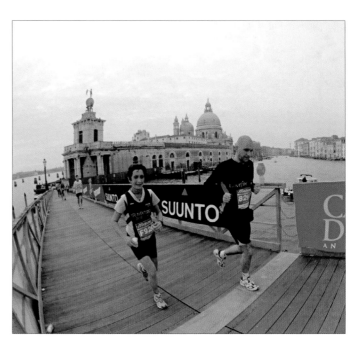

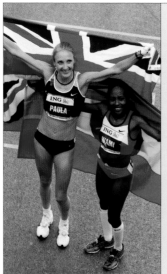

Great athletes: Paula Radcliffe (b. 1973, Davenham, Cheshire, UK)

In the early stages of Paula Radcliffe's career, it seemed that she would be another young athlete full of never-realized potential. She broke into elite running in 1992 with a convincing win in the junior race at the World Cross-country Championships. However, a series of injuries, illnesses and – many thought – a weak sprint finish left her out of the medals in track races at major competitions. Radcliffe finally found her distance in 2002 when she ran the fastest ever debut marathon, winning the London race in 2:18:56, a women-only record. She went on to break the women's world record in Chicago later that year, then took her time down again to 2:15:25 at the 2003 Flora London Marathon.

Left: Paula Radcliffe after winning the New York City Marathon in 2007, pictured with second-placed Gete Wami.

The following year saw the lowest point of her career to date, when exhaustion and injury caused her to pull out of the Olympic marathon in Athens, where she was favourite to win. There was some consolation that autumn when she won the New York City Marathon in a sprint finish against Susan Chepkemei, and then in 2005 when she won gold in the marathon at the World Championships in Helsinki. Radcliffe took time off in 2006 and most of 2007, when she had her first child. Following victory in the New York City Marathon in November 2007, more disappointment followed when her training for the Beijing Olympics was ruined by a stress fracture; determined to finish the marathon, she struggled home in 23rd place. However, she is still aiming for an Olympic gold medal before she retires.

Marathon: elite schedule

	Mon	Tue	Wed	Thur	Fri	Sat	Sun
Week one	10km (6 miles)	8 x 800m with 400m recoveries	10–13km (6–8 miles)	2 x 10 min threshold, 5 mins recovery	10km (6 miles) with 6 x 3 mins hill reps	6km (4 miles)/ rest	19–22km (12–14 miles)
Week two	10km (6 miles)	800m, 1,200m, 1,600m then back with 400m recoveries	13–16km (8–10 miles)	2 x 10 min threshold, 5 mins recovery	10km (6 miles) with 6 x 3 mins hill reps	6km (4 miles)/ rest	19–22km (12–14 miles)
Week three	10km (6 miles)	8 x 800m with 400m recoveries	13–16km (8–10 miles)	2 x 15 min threshold, 5 mins recovery	10km (6 miles) with 6 x 3 mins hill reps	6km (4miles)/ rest	22–26km (14–16 miles)
Week four	10km (6 miles)	5 x 1 mile with 2–3 min recoveries	10–13km (6–8 miles)	1 x 15 mins threshold	10km (6 miles) with 5 x 100m strides	6km (4 miles)/ rest	26–29km (16–18 miles)
Week five	10km (6 miles)	10 x 800m with 400m recoveries	16–19km (10–12 miles)	2 x 15 min threshold, 5 mins recovery	10km (6 miles) with 8 x 3 mins hill reps	10km (6 miles)/ rest	32km (20 miles)
Week six	10km (6 miles)	2 x 800m, 1,600m, 2,000m with 3 min recoveries	16–19km (10–12 miles)	25 mins threshold	10km (6 miles) negative split run	10km (6 miles)/ rest	35km (22 miles)
Week seven	10km (6 miles)	2 x 400m, 800m, 1,200m with 3 min recoveries	19–22km (12–14 miles)	30 mins threshold	10km (6 miles) fartlek session	10km (6 miles)/ rest	29km (18 miles)
Week eight	10km (6 miles)	5 x 1 mile with 2–3 min recoveries then 5 x 150m fast/50m easy	19–22km (12–14 miles)	30 mins threshold	10km (6 miles) with 4 x 5 mins hill reps	10km (6 miles)/ rest	35–38km (22–24 miles)
Week nine	10km (6 miles)	8 x 800m with 400m recoveries	19–22km (12–14 miles)	35 mins threshold	10km (6 miles) with 6 x 3 mins hill reps	10km (6 miles)/rest	29km (18 miles)
Week ten	10km (6 miles)	3 x 1 mile with 2–3 min recoveries then 5 x 150m fast/50m easy	16–19km (10–12 miles)	20 mins threshold	6km (4 miles) negative split run	10km (6 miles)/ rest	26km (16 miles)
Week eleven	10km (6 miles)	6 x 800m with 400m recoveries	10–13km (6–8 miles)	20 mins threshold	6km (4 miles) fartlek session	10km (6 miles)/ rest	19km (12 miles)
Week twelve	5km (3 miles)	Rest/cross-train	5km (3 miles)	Rest/cross-train	Rest	5km (3 miles) easy/rest	Marathon

run two miles as a warm-up and cool-down for all speed and threshold sessions. You'll notice that there is the option to run every single day with this plan, but you should only run the Saturday session if you feel really strong and full of energy. Many elite runners will train every day but it takes years of conditioning to cope with this, so if you want to play it safe, stick with six days' training per week.

Try to run some of your longer efforts at race pace – perhaps just 40 to 50 minutes in the middle – to get used to how it feels. Also, if you have time, add two weight training sessions per week (on easy run days), and two Pilates sessions to maintain core strength – the higher your mileage, the more important this is to help you avoid injury.

Marathon Training the Easy Way

Logging hundreds of miles might be the best way to train for a front-of-race marathon performance, but it doesn't suit everyone. The good news is that for the average runner, great results are possible from running just three times a week, if you make the sessions count.

If you find that your training is always interrupted by impact-related injuries, or family and work commitments mean you simply don't have time to run 160km (100 miles) per week, then you can still run a good marathon with just three running sessions per week. In fact, for a marathon runner with a few years' experience, this type of training plan can bring the kind of results that win smaller races.

Sometimes high-mileage training programmes are criticized for containing too many junk miles – easy, aimless running which, some would argue, simply put you at higher risk of overtraining or picking up an injury. The key with lower-mileage training is to make sure that every run you do really counts. Your three runs per

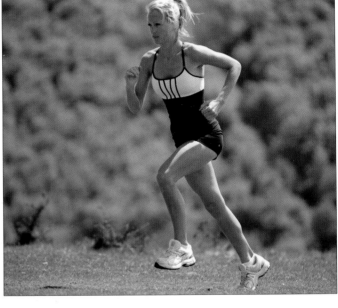

Above: In this type of schedule, your long runs should be quite fast – at target marathon pace.

Below: Hill training and other quality training sessions build your strength and speed without injury risk.

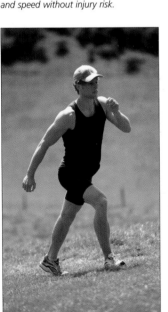

Low-mileage training tested

It takes a leap of faith for any marathon runner to cut down to three runs a week, but science is on your side. In 2003, a group of scientists and runners at Furman University, South Carolina, USA, formed the Furman Institute of Running and Science Training (FIRST). They trained a group of 25 volunteers using a rigid three-runs-per-week schedule. Of the 21 runners who finished the target marathon, 15 ran personal bests. Laboratory tests showed that their oxygen uptake had gone up by 4.2 per cent, their lactate threshold speed had increased by 2.3 per cent, and their body fat had gone down by an average of 8.7 per cent. For further details of their programme visit their website at www.furman.edu/FIRST.

week are a speed run, a tempo or hill run, and a long run. In addition to the three runs per week, you should aim to cross-train for two sessions a week to keep your fitness levels high and weight down. Some runners even find that they gain fitness using this method; you can train harder on your cross-training days than you would running, as the change of activity uses different muscles and usually has no impact, so your running muscles get the rest they need. Your overall fitness should improve, your body fat should reduce (making you a more efficient runner), and your risk of injury should be lower, putting you in great shape to tackle the marathon.

Marathon: easy schedule

	Day one	Day two	Day three	Day four	Day five
Week one	6 x 800m with 400m recoveries	Cross-train 30 mins	2 x 20 mins tempo with 5 mins recovery	Cross-train 30 mins	16–19km (10–12 miles)
Week two	3 x 1,600m with 3–4 min recoveries	Cross-train 30 mins	5 miles with 6 x 2 mins uphill effort	Cross-train 30 mins	19–22km (12–14 miles)
Week three	3 x (400m, 800m) with 400m recoveries	Cross-train 40 mins	40 mins tempo run	Cross-train 40 mins	22–26km (14–16 miles)
Week four	6 x 800m with 400m recoveries	Cross-train 30 mins	40 mins tempo run	Cross-train 30 mins	16–19km (10–12 miles)
Week five	4 x 1,200m with 600m recoveries, then 4 x 400m with 200m recoveries	Cross-train 40 mins	5 miles with total 10–15 mins uphill effort	Cross-train 40 mins	26–29km (16–18 miles)
Week six	8 x 800m	Cross-train 40 mins	50 mins tempo run	Cross-train 40 mins	29–32km (18–20 miles)
Week seven	4 x 1,600m with 3 min recoveries	Cross-train 45 mins	1hr tempo run	Cross-train 45 mins	32km (20 miles)
Week eight	4 x 1,200m with 600m recoveries	Cross-train 45 mins	5 miles with 4 x 2 mins uphill effort	Cross-train 45 mins	19km (12 miles)
Week nine	10 x 800m	Cross-train 45 mins	1hr 10 mins tempo run	Cross-train 45 mins	29km (18 miles)
Week ten	4 x 1,400m with 600m recoveries, then 4 x 400m with 200m recoveries	Cross-train 40 mins	1hr 10 mins tempo run	Cross-train 40 mins	26km (16 miles)
Week eleven	6 x 800m	Cross-train 40 mins	50 mins tempo run	Cross-train 40 mins	16–19km (10–12 miles)
Week twelve	Rest	Cross-train 30 mins	5km (3 miles) easy/ easy cross-train	Cross-train 30 mins/rest	Marathon

The 12-week schedule

There are only three runs a week in this schedule, but you must complete them all (if you like you can add a fourth easy run) and you must put effort in. On your long runs, stay close to your target marathon pace, even adding bursts of half-marathon pace running. Do your tempo runs at 10K pace (just faster than threshold pace), long intervals (1,000 to 1,600m) at 5K pace and 800m or less at mile pace. Choose an activity you enjoy for your cross-training and treat your cross-training sessions as high-quality workouts, adding faster intervals and higher resistance for extra fitness gains. Scientists (see box opposite) have found that runners can see much greater improvements in marathon times when they take the cross-training sessions as seriously as they would a speed workout or long run, so decide before each session what kind of training you will do and make the sessions progressively harder as the weeks go by.

Right: You can cross-train hard once or twice a week, building fitness and reducing body fat.

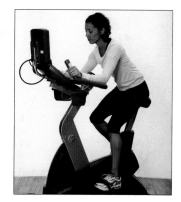

Marathon: Heart-rate Training

It can be difficult to tell how hard you are training, as your mood, the weather and even illness all have an effect on your perception of effort. What's more, until you are experienced at racing over a range of distances, it can also be hard to judge your pace.

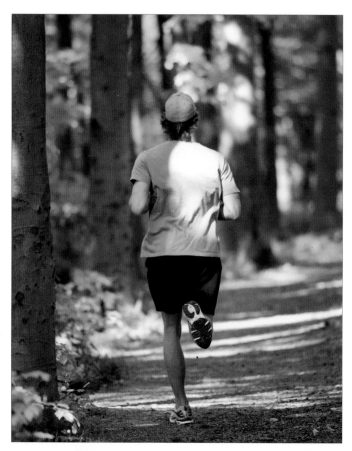

Above: When you first begin heart-rate training, you may find it frustrating running slower than usual.

be able to stay below your lactate threshold, which in turn means you are less likely to hit the wall.

Finding your target zones

You can choose to have laboratory tests to find your different heart-rate training zones, but if you don't have the time or money for that, use these simple sums.

First of all, you need to find out your maximum heart rate (MHR). You can do this using the formula 214 – (0.8 x age) for men, or 209 – (0.9 x age) for women. For a more accurate figure, however, use this test (which you should not attempt if you are very unfit or new to exercise): warm up, then run for 4 minutes as fast as you can on a treadmill; take a 2-minute recovery jog, then repeat the hard run. You should hit your MHR toward the end of your second fast interval.

Below: A basic heart-rate monitor is enough to tell you when you're in the right training zone.

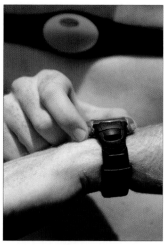

This is where introducing objective science, in the form of heart-rate training, can be useful. Switching to heart-rate training can be frustrating for runners used to pushing themselves as hard as they can. Running at your target heart rate feels incredibly slow at first. Your body – and your willpower – allow you to train much harder than is beneficial, often leading to overtraining or injury. To begin heart-rate training from scratch, you will need to spend a period building a base, training at less than 60 per cent of your working heart rate (WHR, see below) and excluding speedwork. You will gradually be able to run faster at the same heart rate, and after this you can add speedwork and tempo runs. The advantage of training this way is that your heart rate should be lower in marathons, so you should

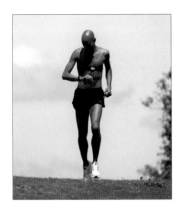

Find your resting heart rate (RHR) by wearing the heart-rate monitor to bed. In the morning it will tell you the minimum heart rate achieved during sleep.

Work out your WHR like this:
1 MHR − RHR = x
(for example 205 − 44 = 161)
2 Take the effort level you need to achieve, say 60 per cent, and multiply this by your WHR
(for example 161 x 0.6 = 97)

Left: Once you've found your working heart rate, use it to plan sessions.

3 Add this figure to your RHR to find your target heart rate
(for example 97 + 44 = 141 bpm).

Applying zones to training: 12-week schedule
Follow this schedule after building up your base using a heart-rate monitor. You can use the alarm on your monitor to tell you when you have hit your target rate. Figures are percentage WHR. Before and after each speed session (Days Two and Four) do 10 minutes at 60 per cent WHR.

Marathon: heart-rate training

	Day one	Day two	Day three	Day four	Day five
Week one	40 mins at 60%	5 mins at 70%; 4 mins at 85%; 3 mins at 85–90%; then run all-out for 1 min; then back down	40 mins fartlek at 70%	2 x 10 mins at 80% with 3 mins recovery	1:30 at 60–70%
Week two	40 mins at 60%	2 x 10 mins at 85–90%, recovering to 55% in between	40 mins fartlek at 70–85%	15 mins at 80%	1:45 at 60–70%
Week three	40 mins at 60%	As week 1	40 mins fartlek at 70–85%	3 x 8 mins at 80% with 3 mins recovery	2:00 at 60–70%
Week four	40 mins at 60%	3 x 5 mins at 85–90%, recovering to 55% in between	50 mins fartlek at 70–85%	20 mins at 80%	2:15 at 60–70%
Week five	40 mins at 60%	As week 1, but repeat sequence	50 mins fartlek at 70–85%	25 mins at 80%	2:30 at 60–70%
Week six	40 mins at 60%	8 x run up to 90%, recover to 55%	1 hour fartlek at 70–85%	30 mins at 80%	3:00 at 60–70%
Week seven	40 mins at 60%	4 x 4 mins at 85–90%, recovering to 55% in between	40 mins fartlek at 70–85%	20 mins at 80%	2:30 at 60–70%
Week eight	40 mins at 60%	As week 5	1 hour fartlek at 70–85%	35 mins at 80%	3:00 at 60–70%
Week nine	40 mins at 60%	10 x run up to 90%, recovering to 55%	1 hour fartlek at 70–85%	40 mins at 80%	2:45 at 60–70%
Week ten	40 mins at 60%	6 x 4 mins at 85–90%, recovering to 55%	50 mins fartlek at 70–85%	40 mins at 80%	2:30 at 60–70%
Week eleven	40 mins at 60%	As week 1	40 mins fartlek at 70–85%	20 mins at 80%	1:45 at 60–70%
Week twelve	40 mins at 60%	Rest	30 mins fartlek at 70–85%	Rest	Marathon

Key Race-training Sessions

Every workout you do helps you to reach the start line of your race in peak condition.
But just as specific running training is the only way to become a better runner, putting
in a few race-specific sessions is the best way to be competitive on the big day.

Race training sessions are not the
same as speedwork; though many are
fast, the point of these workouts is
always to replicate race-day conditions
in some way. The following workouts
will help you feel confident and
ready to race.

Race-day warm-up
You'll need a thorough warm-up
before your race, and you should
practise this before some of your
training sessions. Run gently for
5 minutes. Then, find some flat,
even, soft ground and do 20–30m
(65–98ft) of high knees (skipping

*Below: Group fartlek sessions, where
you take it in turns to dictate pace,
are great race practice.*

forward, on the balls of your feet,
kicking your knees high in front);
cover the same distance with some
heel kicks ('running' forward kicking
your heels right back to your bottom).
Use your arms throughout, pumping
them back and forward. Finish the
warm-up with a few more minutes'
light running.

Race pace practice
Even if you've chosen to do most of
your long runs at a slow pace, you
should add a couple of race-pace
sections during the hardest point of your
training (usually 6–8 weeks before the
race). Work out your mile pace based
on your target race time, but be flexible
– if you can't talk after 30–40 minutes at
this pace in training, or if your heart rate

is consistently above 85 per cent MHR,
it's too fast (if you're aiming for a
marathon or half, your race pace should
feel very comfortable over a short
distance). You can find your ideal
training pace, and work out a predicted
race pace, using the tables at the end of
the book.

At the sharp end of a race, there
are likely to be several surges in pace
as different people try to establish a
lead. Sometimes people may even
deliberately slow the pace, which can
be off-putting (and is meant to be!).
Learn to cope with this using group
fartlek sessions. Gather a group of
friends of different paces and abilities,
and draw numbers out of a hat.
Don't tell anyone else which number
you have. After 10 minutes of easy

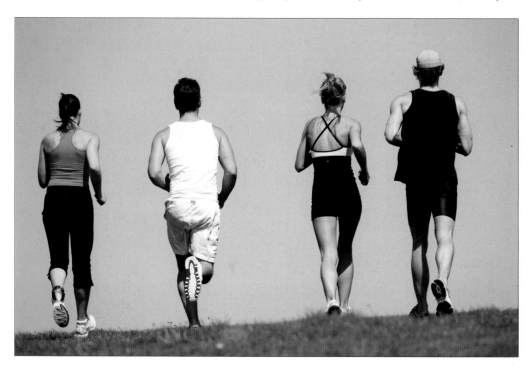

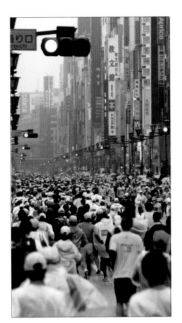

Above: It's impossible to know how you'll feel on race day but visualizing the event will help.

jogging, the person with number one goes to the lead, running as fast as they like for any length of time from 1 to 5 minutes, then shouts "End!" The group jogs to recover and regroup for 2 or 3 minutes, then the next person takes the lead without warning; and so on until everyone in the group has led an interval.

Negative split
This is by far the safest approach to pacing long events (10K or more), so it makes sense to practise it in training (it features strongly in our 10K Schedules). The simplest way to do this is to find a short, fairly straight out-and-back route and run the return leg faster, but remember you're aiming for a very close split, so don't crawl the first half and sprint the second. Go for a time that is just a minute or two faster over the second leg.

Right: Try running hard at the end of sessions, when you're already tired, to toughen yourself up.

Fast finish
Even if you're not a naturally fast finisher, you can train to develop a good final kick, which will often put you at an advantage, especially in races of 10K or less. Short, sharp speed sessions will develop the basic leg speed you need for this, but you should also try sprinting when you're already tired. At the end of a threshold or race-pace section, without a recovery break, accelerate smoothly into a 200m sprint. Recover for 30 seconds, then repeat. Build up to three or four sprints over a few weeks.

Dress rehearsal
Try to visit your race course before race day. If you can, have a run out over the course the week before, practising your pace and fuelling strategy (but relaxing toward the end of the route). If you can't get to your course, then choose a route with similar characteristics (e.g. gradient and surface), and run it at the same time of day as your race will be.

Races are perhaps the best kind of specific race training you can do. Up to 16km (10 miles), you can even race the same distance in your build-up, but treat it as a practice run so you don't wear yourself out. For the marathon or half, shorter races are a good progress check and help you to cope with race-day nerves, practise your warm-up and nutrition strategies, and even find out which kit you're most comfortable in.

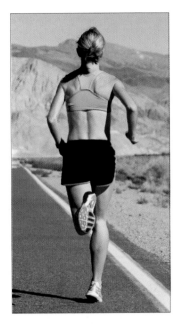

Above: When you're running well, hold on to the feeling for race day.

Try to set aside some time in the few weeks before your race to think through your race day and visualize everything going according to plan, right up to crossing the line in your target time. You can also use training sessions: when you feel you're running smoothly and strongly, tell yourself 'I will run this well on race day.'

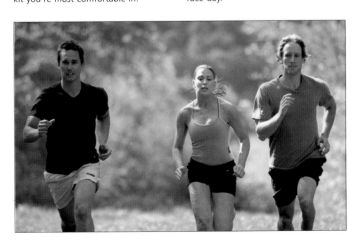

Race Tactics

You might think race tactics are only for athletes at the very front of a race, but a little planning is useful for anyone hoping to perform well. Well-rehearsed tactics can shave seconds off your time or just boost your confidence with a higher placing.

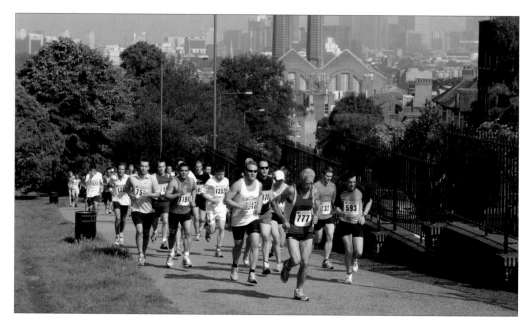

The most important decision you will have to make is how to pace your race. Confident and well-trained runners run as evenly as they can. However this is a difficult approach to take, as other runners will try to influence your pace. Runners who have a strong sprint finish will try to hold the pace slow to keep something for the end of the race, while those who don't have this strength may force the pace early on to create a gap between themselves and the rest of the field. Paula Radcliffe uses this tactic to good effect in most of her marathons. Forcing surges in pace also exhausts sprint finishers, so they are unable to use their end kick.

Assessing the competition

Your choice of pacing strategy may depend on who else is running. If you are at the sharp end of a race and know some of the other fast athletes, try to

discover who are the main threats beforehand, working out what kind of runners they are, what times they have run recently, and how they are likely to respond to your tactics.

You can use other runners to help you through your race, particularly in longer road events. Psychologically it is difficult to run alone for long periods of time: you will become too focused on your own discomfort and may lose perspective and find it difficult to judge your pace. Staying with a group of runners means you can use them as pacers, and you can use them either to distract yourself (perhaps by chatting as you run if they are willing and able to talk), or to help focus you on the race pace. You can also draft behind groups of runners, effectively using them as a windblock to minimize resistance to your own forward motion. For this to work, you need to stay close behind the other runners.

Above: You can use the other runners taking part to help you stick to your pace in crowded events.

Using earphones

Earphones have become an increasingly common feature at long-distance road events, and it is true that music can be useful to help keep you on pace as you run. However, the running community is divided over whether they should be allowed at large events, some feeling that it is rude and anti-social to wear them, others arguing that it is simply a safety issue. If you choose to run wearing your earphones, don't put them on until you have started so that you don't miss any announcements. Keep the volume low enough so that you can hear someone if they are trying to get your attention.

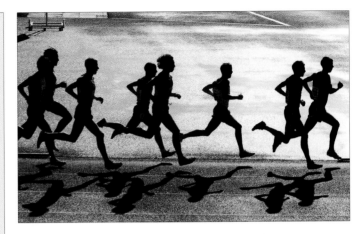

Race etiquette

Emotions can run high on race day, so try not to tread on anyone's toes – literally or figuratively – by following these six simple guidelines on race day etiquette:

1 Start in the right area for your predicted finish time, not in front of faster runners. If there are no start pens, ask a few runners what time they are aiming for to help you gauge where to stand.

2 During the race, don't side-step, stop suddenly or start walking unexpectedly. Call out to those behind you first so they don't trip over you.

3 Don't over-draft. Staying behind someone all the way then dashing out to beat them at the finish is very bad form. If you're running at the same pace as someone else, take it in turns to lead so you can both conserve energy, up to an agreed point. Then race them!

4 Help people who are in distress. If another runner has collapsed, don't assume that someone else will find them soon.

5 Make sure that you thank volunteers around the route.

6 Try to stay for the medal presentations and to cheer on the slower runners, finishing after you, even if you have had a bad race yourself and just feel like going home.

Above: Take it in turns to lead a pack of runners, as it's harder to run at the front all the way.

Crowd control

Ensure the crowd doesn't work against you. Don't waste energy weaving in and out of others to move forward – run to the outside and sprint around the group. Water stations are prime spots for losing places, so be prepared. If possible, have your friends and family hand out drinks to you slightly apart from the official water station, so you

don't end up in a scrummage, and have your water in bottles rather than cups. Also, don't be pushed into running on the outside of a group, as courses are measured along the shortest route possible (in big races this is sometimes marked by a line painted on the road).

Whatever your race plan, it will be effective only if you stick to it. Don't allow yourself to be distracted by others' tactics – after all, this may be precisely what they are relying on to gain an advantage.

Below: Be courteous to runners around you and if you need to change pace, warn them by calling out.

Below: Over longer distances your race tactics may not come into play until the final few miles.

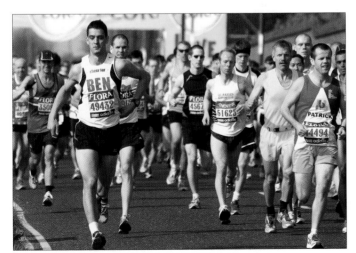

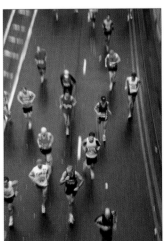

Mental Training: Long-distance Strategies

Any sports event requires as much mental strength as physical fitness, but the mind plays a far greater role for long-distance runners. In a marathon, whether a first-timer or about to set a world record, your body will be aching and your instincts telling you to stop.

The last few miles in any long-distance event are extremely gruelling. At this point, the only thing that will keep you going is a strong mind.

Disassociation vs focusing

There are two main approaches to getting through long-distance events. The first, disassociation, is where the athlete tries to distract himself from the discomfort, fatigue and sometimes boredom of the race. For recreational runners, listening to music while racing is a good example of this (some experts also believe that music can help you run

Below: Focusing on the positive, perhaps by remembering good training sessions, helps to keep you strong.

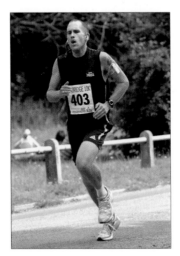

faster). Other techniques might be playing mental games – trying to remember a list of past winners of the race, or something completely unrelated such as your top ten favourite films.

Focusing is the opposite approach, and is tough to do in a marathon – it takes practice. With this approach, you concentrate intently on the task in hand. Be careful not to focus on the negative (aches and pains, loss of confidence) and instead focus on your breathing, your style, and the feel of the pace. Think about all the training you have put in and the goal you have for the race.

Left: Some scientists believe that listening to music while you run can actually make you faster.

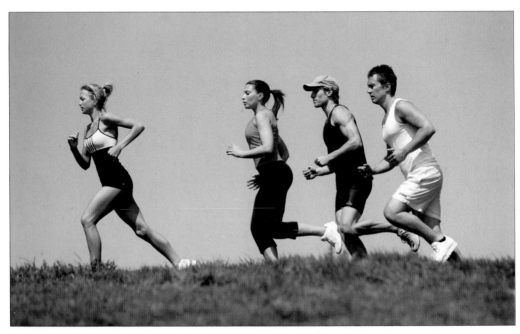

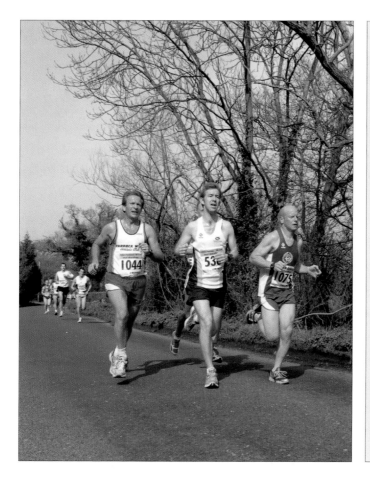

Above: When you are competing in a race, learn to focus on your tactics and competitors to stay on target.

If you are at the competitive end of the race, think about your tactics and the opponents around you. Research has shown that the focusing approach is more successful, so it is worth practising, however unpleasant – try it in shorter races first.

Motivation

To train for a long race, you will have had strong motivation. Keep that in mind as you race. Remind yourself what you want to get from it, whether it is a specific time, to beat a particular opponent, or to win. Studies have shown that people who race for intrinsic rewards (to feel good about themselves, to achieve a new personal best) are more successful than those who compete for extrinsic rewards (their coach's approval, prize money). Whatever your goal was, it should be strong enough to push you to the finish when the going gets tough.

Visualization

This technique is widely used by elite athletes and can be applied to your life in general. The idea is to visualize running a successful race over and over again and in as much detail as possible. Think about your smooth, strong running style, hitting each mile bang on target pace, and finishing strongly and in your desired time. Just thinking about these actions produces the same effect on your brain as if you had actually done them, and so creates a pattern of success. Practise visualization two or three times a day, in a quiet, calm space, and run through your success just before your race and when you hit bad patches.

Enjoyment

Toward the end of your race, it is easy to feel tired and grumpy, particularly if you have missed a mile time by 30 seconds and start to believe you are failing. Try to focus on your enjoyment of the sport: appreciate the strengths of your body and the success you have had in training. Try not to count down the miles; if it helps, slip into your race pace, trust yourself to stay on target by intuition, and promise yourself not to look at your watch for three or four miles.

Central Governor Theory

For years it has been generally accepted that long-distance athletes become fatigued because their body runs out of fuel or is not strong enough. However, the Central Governor Theory, supported by the respected sports scientist and runner Professor Tim Noakes, opens the possibility that this fatigue is all in the mind. The theory goes that our ancient ancestors had to keep back some of their energy for emergency situations, and our bodies still hold on to this legacy, so that when fuel stores are running low, a central governing mechanism in the brain tells the muscles to slow down to conserve energy. If you can show your brain that you are not going to die from excessive effort, the theory goes, you can keep running.

Supporters argue that this theory is proven by the fact that so often runners feel they have nothing left to give, only to put in a final spurt when they know they are about to stop. You can retrain your brain with race-specific, stressing sessions, such as very long runs for marathons, or 5 x 1,000m at 5K pace for a 5K event. In theory, surviving the stress should show your brain that it is feasible to go the distance.

Mental Training: Winning Strategies

In any race, at any distance, it could be argued that essentially, winning comes down to mental toughness. Two competing athletes who have exactly the same ability and training must use all their mental powers to gain victory.

The elite athlete is often portrayed as an aggressive opponent, 'destroying' other competitors, but there is far more to winning than fighting talk, and whether you are aiming to win or just to perform to your very best, these strategies can help you.

Toughness

Mental toughness is an important quality for endurance runners in particular, but there is a great deal of debate over whether runners are born with it or learn it. The truth is probably somewhere in between. You can help yourself to become mentally strong by using 'character building' workouts: run at race pace in training, pit yourself against faster athletes, train in difficult

Below: Try to think like a winner, no matter what your speed, to help you to achieve your goals.

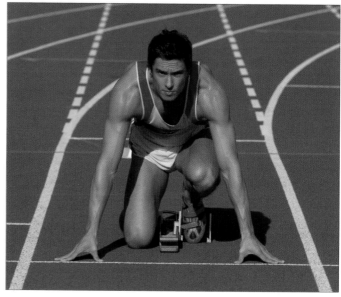

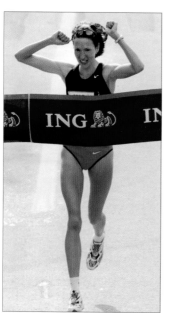

conditions. Coaches will sometimes teach their athletes to cope with stress by arranging for interruptions to training, or changing plans at the last minute. This helps runners deal with unexpected problems and stay focused on their race.

Self-confidence

There is a fine line between self-confidence and unfounded arrogance, but it is an important distinction: the latter will lead to complacency, disappointment and ultimately loss of confidence. Self-confidence is crucial, however, as positive 'self-talk' is a valuable tool in helping you to maintain your pace through rough patches in a race. Use affirmations in training that you can call on again on race day – say out loud, 'I am strong', 'I can achieve my target', or train yourself out of weaknesses (for example 'I will run smoothly' if you know you have a problem with erratic style).

Above: Sprinters are known for their focus, but relaxation techniques will help runners over any distance.

You can also build up your confidence by thinking about past successes, by going through your training diary to reassure yourself that you have done all you can, and by asking other people (such as your coach or training partners) what they feel are your strengths.

Focus

Watch top-class sprinters before a 100m race, and you will see them go through their own rituals to help them focus on the task ahead. Focus and 'getting in the zone' is also crucial for longer-distance runners. You need to calm any pre-race nerves without becoming so calm that you breeze through the race without putting full effort into it. Relaxation techniques such as deep breathing, or energizing techniques such

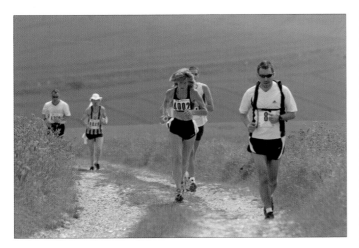

Left: If a race is going to be physically tough, you will also need to be mentally tough and should train for this.

can do to prevent it from happening again, and move on. Otherwise the memory of your disappointing race will spoil future performances.

Analyse your performances
If you have a coach, he will be able to give you feedback, but it is also useful to become more self-aware so that you're constantly assessing your own strengths and weaknesses. Sports psychologists sometimes teach athletes to use a technique known as performance profiling. The runner draws up of a list of traits they think are important in their sport (for example relaxation, focus, enjoyment); rates the relative importance of each trait for a 'perfect' athlete; and then rates their own performance for each of the attributes. This is a good way of objectifying yourself to determine which areas you need to work on.

Below: Your training partner can build your confidence by reminding you of your strengths.

as thinking intently about your target or an opponent, can be useful in achieving the right balance.

Think like a winner
You may have heard gold medallists saying that if they didn't think they would win, they wouldn't race. You may not

Below: Events with different elements, such as triathlon or adventure racing, require renewed focus for each stage.

expect to come first, but you can adopt this approach. Instead of heading to a race and thinking 'I'll see what happens' or 'I'll do my best', be determined to achieve your target time or the position you want. Do not allow doubt to take over your mind at any time. However, if your race does not go to plan, don't waste time punishing yourself. The best athletes make mistakes sometimes, and sometimes conditions are against them. Work out what went wrong, what you

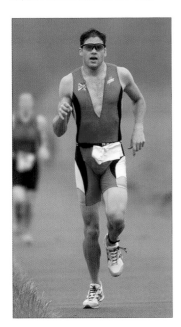

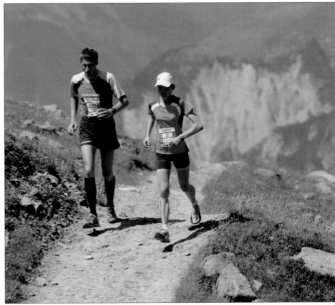

Advanced Racing Kit

At the start of any running race, it is clear which people are going to be the front runners. The difference can be seen not just in their lean, muscular physiques, but also in the pared-down clothing they wear.

Choosing special kit for a race may not take much off your finish time, but it could give you an extra edge. Light, comfortable kit should be barely noticeable, enabling you to fully focus on the clock and your opponents as you run. Wearing the right kit is about more than the science of running faster, however: racing kit should make you feel confident, strong and psyched up, and this psychological benefit will be more noticeable to you than any reduction in weight or drag.

If you buy special kit for a race, make sure that you have worn it beforehand (especially your shoes); this is not the time to test new styles, as something as seemingly innocuous as a badly placed seam could chafe and ruin a good run. At the opposite end of the spectrum, if you have been wearing the same

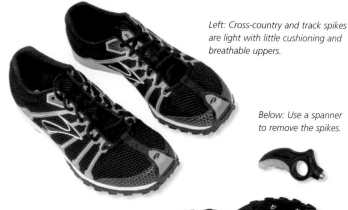

Left: Cross-country and track spikes are light with little cushioning and breathable uppers.

Below: Use a spanner to remove the spikes.

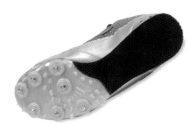

Right: As the name suggests, the shoes have removable spikes that add traction.

'lucky' T-shirt for five years, perhaps it is time to treat yourself to something better suited.

Performance shoes

Most shoe manufacturers now make a range of shoes especially designed for fast training and racing. These typically weigh less than 300g (for a men's UK size 8/US size 9), and have been stripped of most of the technical features found in standard training shoes. They have less cushioning, fit more snugly, and may have a more curved shape for faster running.

Heavy runners or those with serious gait problems should avoid these shoes. For track and cross-country races, you can wear 'spikes' or 'racing flats', which look like old-fashioned running slippers. As the name suggests, some have spikes that screw into the outer sole for better traction on the ground.

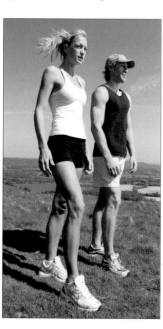

Left: Good technical kit can give you a powerful psychological edge when it comes to your race day.

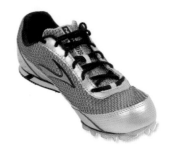

Above: These track shoes have shorter spikes and are made for middle-distance running.

Shorts and tights

In a race situation, you want to carry as little weight and bulk as possible, so many people go for traditional, very short, vented shorts, which allow your legs a fuller range of movement (although they are not for the self-conscious!). Tight shorts are another good option as they minimize the risk of chafing on the insides of your legs. In winter, it is worth wearing full-length tights to keep your muscles warm and to avoid cramp. Whichever you choose, unless you are on a very long race, keep pockets to a minimum – you need only a small internal key pocket.

Tops

Fast runners tend to opt for sleeveless tops, but be careful that the armholes don't chafe. Sleeveless tops not only reduce the weight of your outfit but keep you cool, which is essential at the front-end of a race. Loose-weave tops are a good choice as you will need to use safety pins to attach your race number.

It is not really worth wearing a jacket to a race, even on a cold day. It is very difficult to pin your number to it, it becomes too hot after a few minutes' running, and the extra bulk can slow you down. If the weather is poor, stay inside as long as possible before the start or wear a bin-liner (trash bag), which you can throw away once you get going Make sure you have some warm clothes to put on straight after the race.

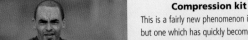

Compression kit

This is a fairly new phenomenon in sportswear, but one which has quickly become popular. Compression kit is always very tight, and some types have plastic webbing to support muscles. Originating in team sports and power sports (such as sprinting), the idea behind this kit (worn as a base layer) is that it increases bloodflow and therefore oxygen delivery to your working muscles. As such, it is also said to help with recovery. The best compression kit has graded pressure to help keep blood circulating. Research suggests that good compression kit is genuinely effective at improving endurance and aiding recovery, but it is more likely to give an edge to a good athlete than to transform an average runner. In fact, one of its biggest selling points is that it gives you a psychological boost by making you more aware of your muscles.

Left: Compression kit is very tight to support the muscles.

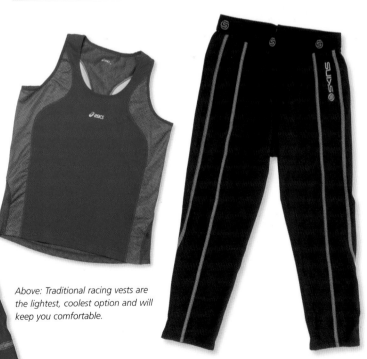

Above: Traditional racing vests are the lightest, coolest option and will keep you comfortable.

Left: Tight shorts minimize chafing – these trail shorts also have handy loops to hold energy gels.

Above: Compression kit boosts bloodflow to your muscles and makes you aware of your body.

Advanced Equipment

While top-end apparel and shoes are essential for fast racing, investing in some essential equipment will give your training an edge – and having splashed out a week's wages to buy a new watch, you will certainly feel motivated to use it.

Once you've started measuring your training it's easy to find plenty of gadgets to help you out, from simple stopwatches to the most advanced GPS speed and distance monitors.

Watches

Time is very much of the essence for runners. The more you run, the more detail you will want to know – which is why that old plastic watch you have had since you were 12 will no longer be good enough. Sports watches can have a bewildering array of functions, but the ones you need to look out for are:

Chronograph. The chronograph or stopwatch mode is the most basic requirement for a sports watch. Most will be capable of recording far longer times than you will ever be running in one go, but make sure the display is detailed enough: if you enjoy doing fast sprints on the track, you will want to know your time down to hundredths of a second.

Lap timer. Recording your lap times or mile splits is a useful way of tracking your progress and training yourself to pace runs evenly. Some watches store up to 300 split times, which sounds excessive – but if you want to review a few weeks' training, it is surprisingly easy to use up the watch's lap memory.

Interval and countdown timers. If you can, buy a watch with two interval timers – this is especially useful for speedwork if you don't have access to a track. You can set one timer to countdown 3 minutes for a hard 800m, then the other for 90 seconds' recovery time. An alarm will sound every time you need to change pace, and you can usually record splits and total time as well.

Pacing alarm. Some top-end watches have an alarm that beeps to keep you on pace, which is especially useful if you are trying to work on your cadence.

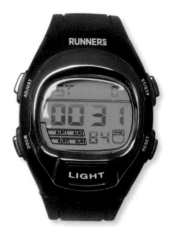

Above: Few advanced runners train without a basic chronograph (or stopwatch) to time themselves.

Basics. Make sure your watch has a big, clear display – some are angled to make them easier to read when you are running; a durable strap; scratch-proof glass; a backlight for running in the dark; and is a good fit on your wrist (women may need to look for a female-specific watch, as men's watches may slip).

Heart-rate monitors

Once a tool for obsessives only, heart-rate monitors are now a fairly standard piece of kit for runners. Monitors range from a basic model that shows your heart rate and has a stopwatch, to top-end versions with 'virtual coaching'. Heart-rate monitors consist of a chest strap with electrodes (you need to wet these for the monitor to work well) and a transmitter, and a wrist unit, which picks up the signal and tells you your heart rate. Functions might include:

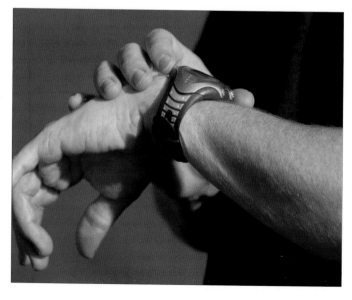

Left: The bigger and clearer your watch display, the more useful you will find it.

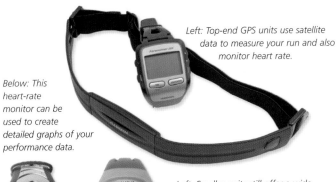

Left: Top-end GPS units use satellite data to measure your run and also monitor heart rate.

Below: This heart-rate monitor can be used to create detailed graphs of your performance data.

Left: Smaller units still offer a wide range of functions, the most basic being current heart rate.

with heart-rate data to give an estimate of how many calories you have burned during a session.

Heart-rate zones. You will be asked to set up heart-rate zones for different levels of activity (for example lower than 60 per cent of your maximum heart rate; 61 to 75 per cent; 76 to 90 per cent). The monitor then sounds an alarm to let you know how hard you are working, and you can use this to plan your interval training.

Calories burned. You can usually input personal details such as your weight and gender, and the monitor will combine this

Memory. Some monitors can store information about several workouts at once, including total time, splits, time in each pre-set heart-rate zone, average, minimum and maximum heart rate.

Software. Top-end models come with software for your home computer, which enables you to download and analyse information from your monitor, creating graphs and charts of your heart-rate data. This can be useful for evaluating and planning your training.

Above: Non-GPS speed and distance monitors use footpods like this one to give accurate measurements.

Speed and distance monitors
Often combined with a heart-rate monitor, speed and distance monitors (SDMs) fall into two categories. The less expensive models work with a footpod that attaches to your shoes, which sends information to the watch unit – you need to calibrate these models to get a more accurate reading, and they can lose accuracy on hills or uneven ground when your stride changes. The second type uses global positioning system (GPS) technology to give an accurate pinpoint of where you are and how fast and far you are running. The disadvantage with GPS-based monitors is that, in urban areas especially, you can lose contact with the satellite and be unable to take any measurements. SDMs usually come with the same features as a heart-rate monitor, but can combine this with data on your average speed, maximum and minimum speed, distance travelled, and sometimes cadence (on footpod models).

Left: They may be cumbersome, but GPS monitors are the easiest way for you to gauge your pace.

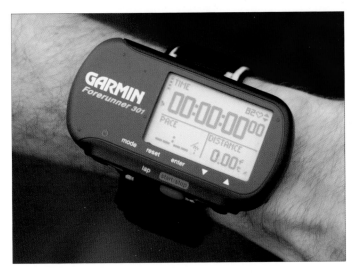

Periodization and Self-coaching

Great running performances always involve a little bit of luck. Weather conditions, catching a bug or tripping over could all spoil what would have been a perfect race. What really matters is the condition of the athlete on the day of the race.

The goal of runners at any level or distance is to be in their absolute peak condition – highly trained, but not overtrained – and that is the result of careful long-term planning or 'periodization'.

Track athletes almost always use periodization, as sprinting and middle-distance running have distinct seasons, but it is also a useful concept for long-distance runners, and one widely used by those at the top of the sport. The idea is to divide your training into different periods. First, the whole training year (sometimes called a macrocycle) is divided into broad phases lasting from a few weeks to a few months. Within this big picture are mesocycles of three to

Below: Dividing your training sessions into cycles ensures that you reach a peak when it comes time to race.

four weeks and microcycles of one or two weeks. Specific sessions don't need to be planned a year in advance, but the general theme is decided and, as you approach a particular period, specific days can be allocated to work on different areas of your training. The idea behind this planning is to allow your body to adapt to hard training, to bring yourself to a peak of fitness and speed in time for a particular race goal, and to recover and progress your training. Learning how to plan your own training year is essential if you are coaching yourself (as many recreational athletes do).

Successful self-coaching
A coach is a valuable asset for any runner (see box), but sometimes time and money mean we have to plan our own training. In this case,

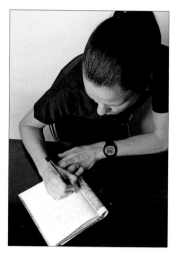

Above: A training diary enables you to plan ahead and is a very valuable self-coaching tool.

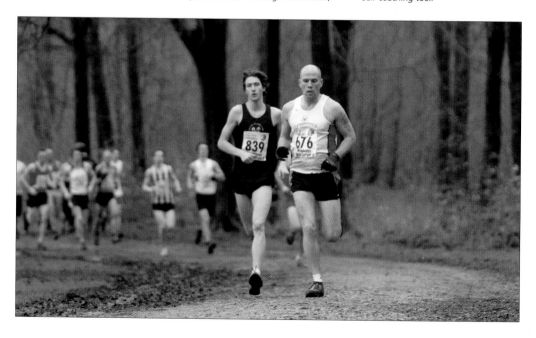

you must learn to be as objective as possible about your running. A good coach will not simply hand you a training schedule. He will look at your lifestyle, how factors such as your career, family life or even your personality will affect the kind of training that is realistic for you. He will be able to listen to your problems and worries and adapt your training as necessary. If you are coaching yourself, you need to be aware of this and have the confidence to go with your instinct – for example if you have been feeling tired for weeks on end, recognize the need for a recovery week.

Planning, patience and progression

The secret to successful self coaching is the 'three Ps': planning, patience and progression. If you don't plan your training, you will become aimless and either do too much, too soon, or you will have the opposite problem and find that you never run any faster, which

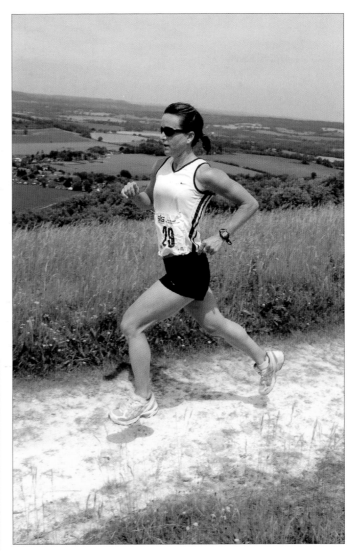

Finding a coach

There is no doubt that any athlete will run better with than without a coach. The question is which coach, because working with someone who does not understand your needs is more likely to have a negative effect on your training.

A good coach should have an understanding of elite training – he may have been an international athlete himself – but should also be confident and happy coaching people at all levels and appreciating their individual limitations. When choosing a coach, remember that each one will have his own individual approach: some coaches favour lots of long, slow running; some believe in training with very high mileage; while others put an emphasis on cross-training. Make sure that you are happy with your coach's approach before you start training together. If you are looking for a coach for the first time, a good place to start is your local running club, or the athletics governing body in your area.

---

saps your motivation. Lack of patience is the quickest route to injury and frustration. Any lack of progression in your training means you are unlikely to achieve your long-term goals.

If you are coaching yourself and are serious about improving your running, your training diary takes on a new level of importance, too. Instead of simply writing down your achievements at the end of each day, work out your training periods: when planning the year, write themes across the top of each week in

Above: It's vital to plan progressive training so that you continue to see improvements in your running.

pencil. Then map out your three to four-week cycles (for example, weeks one and two might be moderate, week three hard, week four easy) and your short-term goals. Plan your specific sessions a week or two in advance, so that you can be flexible and adapt your training if something isn't working (or working better than you expected!).

Planning your Training Year

Planning your training a long time in advance should, in theory, make your training easier and more successful. With a clear plan to follow you will be less tempted to throw yourself into last-minute training for a race or, on the other hand, to avoid stepping up your training.

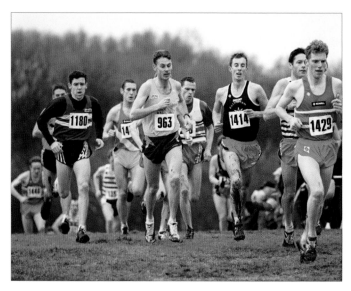

The basic concept of periodization is built around the idea of training for a particular event, so before you plan your year, you will need to decide on your primary goal.

Setting a goal

For many distance runners the goal will be a marathon, which you can only race well once or twice a year;

Above: You can run short 'practice' races in your sharpening phase to fine-tune race speed.

if your goal is a shorter distance you may be able to race it several times over, but should aim to peak at a particular race. In order for periodized training to work well, you should choose a goal more than six months away so that you have time to build the foundation of your fitness (see below). Once you have chosen your goal race, you can work your planning backward from that date. You should also think about setting mini-goals – these might be shorter races (for example a half-marathon four to six weeks before a full marathon), or simply realistic time and distance targets for training.

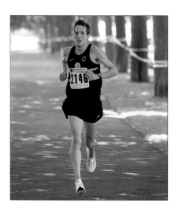

Left: Before planning your training periods, you need to prioritize races for the coming year ahead.

Single and double periodization

If you have been running for several years, your body will have adapted to exercise and will not need such a long base phase. Some runners choose to have a double peak in their training year. This is normal for track and field runners, who want to peak for the indoor season in winter then the main season in summer; long-distance track runners might also aim to peak for the winter cross-country season. For road runners, especially those whose main event is the marathon, there are usually two peaks, in spring (March–April) and autumn (September–October). The training year might look like this:

January	Strength
February	Speed end/speed
March	Speed
April	Peak 1
May	Recovery
June	Base/strength
July	Speed endurance (inc. short races)
August	Speed
September	Speed
October	Peak 2
November	Recovery
December	Base

Training phases

Typical training phases over a year might be:

Base or foundation phase. There is no intense running during this phase. You are simply building up the number of miles you do slowly. The aim of this phase is to allow your body to make the physiological changes it needs to support the demands of more intense training: your muscles and tendons become stronger and your body becomes more efficient at transporting oxygen. The length of time spent in this phase is probably the most variable: a beginner or someone returning from injury could spend up to six months base building, while someone with many years of healthy running behind them could spend six to eight weeks in this phase.

Strength and conditioning phase. This is an important stage to go through to avoid injury and build the power of your muscles ready for faster running. You will maintain moderate mileage built up during your base phase, but start to add hill training, weight training and training on soft ground. Your stronger muscles will propel you forward faster, stabilize your joints and help alleviate fatigue in the late stages of a long race. You might spend one or two months in this phase.

Speed endurance phase. This phase can be incorporated into your strength phase, and experienced runners do some sort of speed endurance work all

Below: Running on soft ground during your strength and conditioning phase helps stabilize your joints.

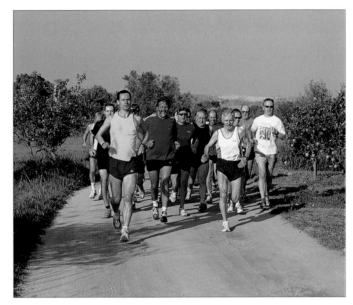

year round. It is worth spending some time working on this area; think of it as a mini base-building phase for your shorter, quicker speedwork. During this period you will introduce threshold runs and long intervals once or twice a week, and you should spend anything from four to six weeks in this phase.

Speed or sharpening phase. This is when you bring all your preparations together, adding the leg speed that will make you a faster racer. You will add two or three faster speed sessions – ideally on a track – and reduce the amount of strength work you do, while maintaining a high mileage. During this phase you might also run some short races as a guide to your progress. This is the phase covered by most training schedules – the 8 to 16 weeks of true race preparation, and your goal race comes at the end of this period.

Recovery phase. Too often overlooked by runners, who may feel guilty about skipping training, this phase is crucial to racing well in your next training year. After your race, you might take a few days off running altogether, then ease back in with short, easy runs and cross-training.

Above: In the base or foundation phase, you'll work on building volume without intensity.

Below: Your fastest speed sessions, on a track, will take place just before you complete your goal race.

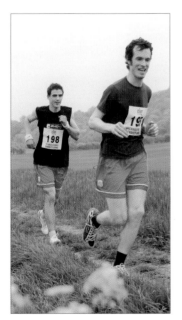

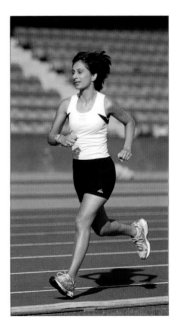

Race Recovery

We have all heard stories about how hard elite runners train, but perhaps the most common mistake made by recreational athletes is thinking this means training as hard as you possibly can, as often as you can. Sometimes, not running is just as important.

Top athletes work just as hard at not running when necessary as they do at putting in 240km (150-mile) weeks. Missing out on essential recovery time will, at best, leave you exhausted and unable to run as fast as you would like; and at worst, ill or seriously injured. Taking easy weeks or weeks off should be part of your training on a cyclical basis (periodization), and it makes sense to put your longest recovery period after your hardest race of the year. There is a great deal of debate about the best way to recover from a race, but no doubt at all that it is necessary. Ideally, race recovery begins before you even reach the start line.

Before your race
The work you put in before a race, especially when that race is a marathon, is crucial to recovering well. If you have planned your training carefully and have had a long build-up with no interruptions from injury, then your muscles will be much better

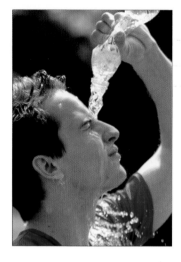

Above: If weather conditions are tough on race day, you'll need to take longer to recover.

Below: In the weeks immediately before a race it's important to cut down on your training.

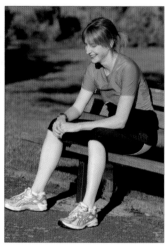

Above: When your training session hasn't gone to plan, sitting down and reconsidering your race goals will help.

prepared to cope with the demands of the race. Damage will be limited and recovery much quicker. It follows that if your training has not gone according to plan, you should revise your race goals to avoid placing undue stress on your body. Failure to do so leads to a downward spiral: your training goes badly, so the race goes badly, you skip recovery to get back into training and race better next time; then you become injured again and your next race is even worse. Treat your race as a high-quality training run, take some time out afterward and start from the beginning again.

The training you don't do is also very important. Before taking part in any race it is important to have a period of 'tapering', where you cut down your training to around 30 to 40 per cent of your highest workload for between one and three weeks

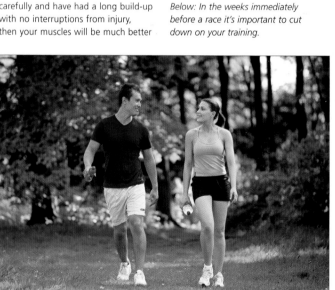

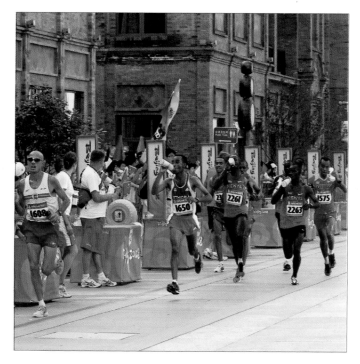

Left: Research has shown that the right nutrition and hydration before and during your race improves recovery time.

stress hormones that lower your immunity, and potentially causing damage to your undertrained muscles.

Nutrition is also essential to keep you well after the race. Countless studies have shown that marathon runners in particular report far higher than average rates of illness (usually colds) than the rest of the population (even athletes who have trained but do not complete a race). There are no definite explanations for this, but some studies have shown a link between carbohydrate consumption during the race (from sports drinks) and risk of illness afterward. One theory is that when your body switches to using fat for fuel, the stress hormone cortisol is released during the process; this blocks the actions of some immune responses. If you can keep your glycogen stores topped up throughout by drinking about one litre per hour of sports drink, then your body will not need to use as much fat for fuel, so less cortisol is released.

Below: Fit in extra time for rest and relaxation before you race, to reduce the impact of stress hormones.

before you race. The longer your goal distance, the more important the taper, so the week before a marathon you barely need to train at all. This taper period ensures your muscles have time to repair any minor damage from your intense training, and they can store enough fuel for your run. Some runners don't believe in tapering, but research has shown that runs of more than 16km (10 miles) two weeks or less before a marathon are detrimental.

Eating, drinking and sleeping well will also help your body meet its race demands. The female marathon world-record holder, Paula Radcliffe, eats around 3,000kcal (12,600kJ) per day and sleeps for 12 hours. You may not have time for 12 hours of sleep, but the principles that work for her will also work for you.

During the race

Try not to get carried away when you race. If you have put in the training, you should have an idea of the fastest pace you can realistically

aim for; stick to that. Running beyond your limits will ultimately lead to a poor race performance, which could take months to recover from psychologically. It also puts you at greater risk of injury and illness, raising your heart rate too high, releasing

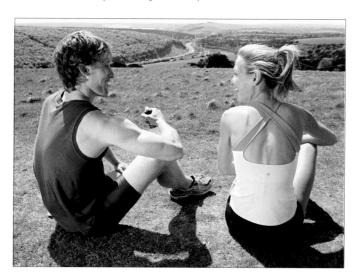

After your Race

You may just feel like collapsing on the ground as soon as you finish a race, but try hard to resist the temptation. What you do in the first few minutes and hours afterward can have a real impact on your recovery.

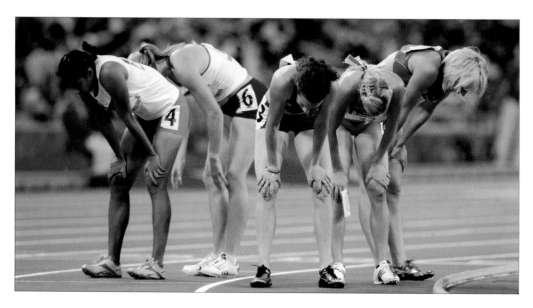

When your race is finally over, however tempting it might be, don't stop moving. Walk around for at least 10 minutes immediately after finishing your race, staying tall and stretching out your arms and legs as you walk. This will help to keep your circulation up, starting the process of removing waste products that have built up (such as lactic acid). It is also a good way of gently stretching out your muscles – static stretching after a long, fast race is a bad idea, as your muscles will be riddled with tiny tears that could be worsened by intense stretching.

While you're walking around, start the process of refuelling your body with a light snack. It is not uncommon to feel nauseous after a race, but try to force some carbohydrates and protein down now and you will reap the benefits later. The ideal ratio for recovery is to eat 4g of carbohydrates for every 1g of protein, and recent

Above: Fight the urge to collapse after a race; have a gentle walk and try to refuel as quickly as possible.

research suggests that the protein will be used by the body more effectively if it is eaten immediately rather than a few hours later. The good news is that when your appetite returns later in the day, you can keep eating – you will have burned around 2,500kcal and used up 30 to 70g of protein during a marathon so you need to replenish those stores.

Reducing inflammation in your legs early on could also help with your recovery. You can take anti-inflammatory drugs to help with any aches and pains you have. Another (much-debated) treatment is ice baths, an idea popular with elite athletes. The obvious benefit is cooling and numbing your sore legs, and some say that the icing boosts circulation, again helping to remove

Mental recovery

Many athletes have a sense of anticlimax after taking part in a big race, and taking time off running can make matters worse. Try to use the time off positively – remind yourself that you worked hard for your race and deserve some time to yourself. You can use the time to refresh your training; review your training diary and analyse your performance in the race. Look at areas of your training that you think could be improved – perhaps if you had done more strength training, for example, you could have stayed more upright at the end of the race.

When you are training again, use the recovery period as a chance to try new activities or start work on an area of weakness, such as core strength. This will keep you feeling positive and give you a strong basis for your next training period.

waste products from the body. A massage might seem like a tempting prospect after 26.2 hard miles, but save it for a few days later – your legs will be too sore to be handled, and you risk causing further damage to your muscles.

Returning to running

Different athletes have very different approaches to returning to training after a race. Some jump straight back into speedwork, while others wait for weeks before pulling their trainers (sneakers) on again. The best path is somewhere between these extremes.

You might start to get itchy feet a few days after your race (especially if the result was good), but refrain from any running for a week after your race. At this stage there is no such thing as 'active rest' (cross-training to give your body a break); your muscles need to rest and refuel. After that, you can start to reintroduce gentle running and cross-training.

Below: Your body will cool down quickly after a race, so make sure that you wrap up warm.

Post-race problem-solving

Here are some of the most common post-race problems, and possible solutions

Problem	Before race	During race	After race
Muscle tears and sprains	Train well, taper well; work on strength and flexibility	Keep to your steady, pre-planned pace	Do not stretch; ice; rest
Colds	Taper	Take on 60–70g carbs per hour	Rest, sleep well, avoid sources of infection
Feeling down	Set realistic race goal, plan activities for the weeks after	Stick to your race plan and trust in it	Be proactive: analyse your race, then plan ahead
Poor, slow running	Taper	Keep to your planned pace; take on carbs	Eat carbs and protein; take a full weeks rest; sleep well

Treat the three or four weeks after your race as a reverse of your taper, starting at 30 to 40 per cent of your highest workload, and building

Below: Some runners have a sense of anticlimax after their goal events, but planning ahead helps with this.

back up slowly to what you would consider a full but light week of training. Avoid racing again until you are completely recovered – a good rule of thumb is to take a day off racing for every mile raced (so that is around a month off for a marathon).

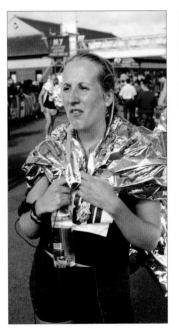

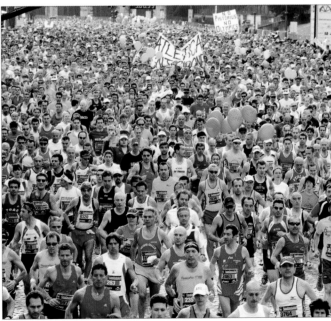

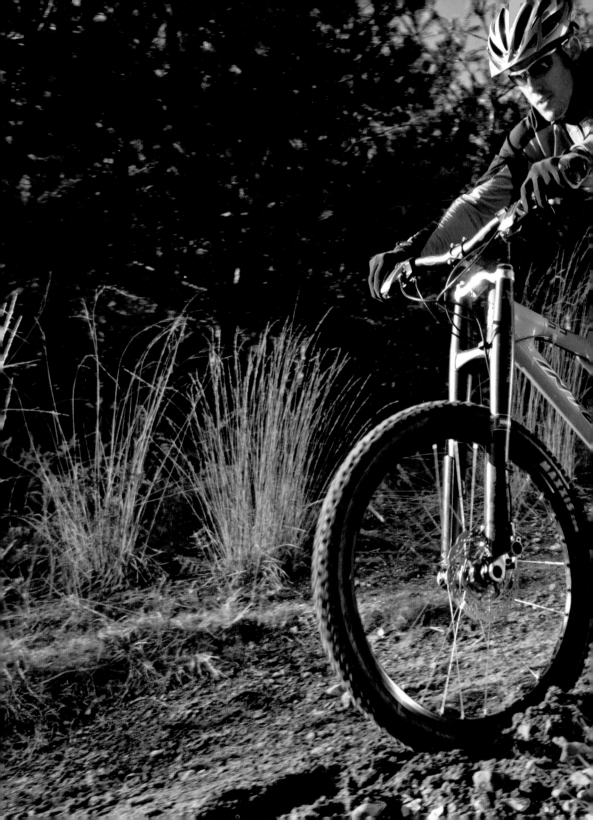

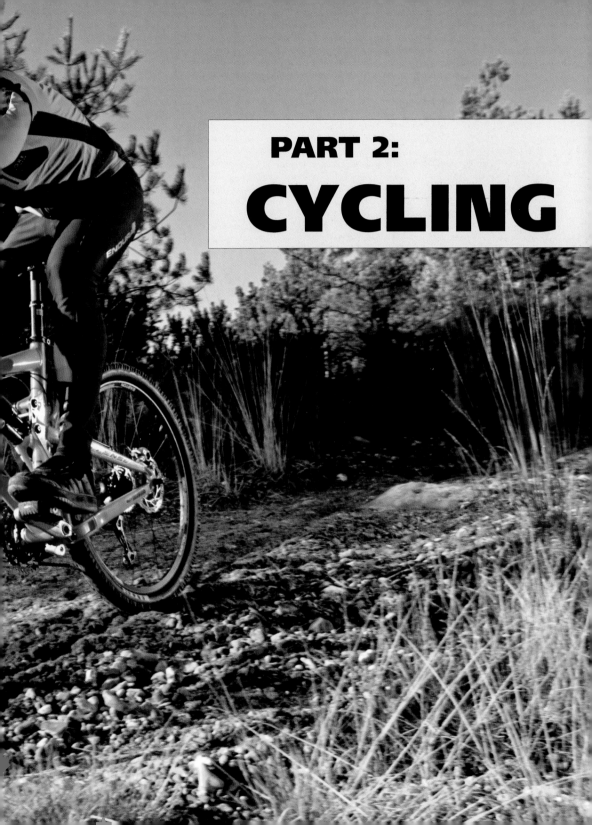

PART 2:

CYCLING

Introduction to Cycling

The bicycle symbolizes freedom, mobility, independence and self-sufficiency. It is far more than a mode of transport – it is a recreation, a means to lifelong health and fitness, and the most environmentally friendly and efficient way of getting from A to B.

The beauty of cycling is that you can participate at any level, be it for practical reasons such as commuting, to compete seriously, or simply just for fun. For many people, the bicycle is the first step to independence and exploration. On foot, children can explore to the end of the road or perhaps a little way beyond, but on a bike, their freedom grows exponentially. Millions, perhaps billions, of children around the world have grown up with their bike as their companion. Many leave the bike behind when they enter adulthood, but increasingly we are seeing bicycles with fresh eyes, and more and more people are starting to ride again.

Cities around the world are following the lead of European capitals such as Amsterdam, incorporating bike lanes into their transport policy. There is no cheaper, cleaner, greener method of getting around town. Bikes are also fast. In competition with a car in a gridlocked city, the bike wins every time.

With the invention of the BMX and its popularization in the 1980s, and the explosion of interest in mountain biking in the 1990s, cycling has been one of the fastest-growing leisure activities in the Western world. Cycling has also become one of the most effective methods of keeping fit. If you cycle, you are exercising, and by doing it you will become fitter, healthier and happier. Just taking a 30-minute bike ride every one or two days will have a marked effect on the fitness of a sedentary individual.

Many leisure cyclists find that these increased fitness levels inspire them to take it more seriously, finding events to provide a challenge and sense of achievement. From local children organizing BMX races, through 'weekend warriors' who are competing locally, to the winner of the Tour de France, the sport of cycling is attracting a broad audience.

When you start to ride your bike, you have deliberately chosen a fitter and healthier lifestyle. You have chosen to be practical and self-sufficient. What's more, you have chosen to have fun.

Right: However, and wherever, you choose to cycle, it is the ideal activity to combine fun, fitness and adventure, and a great way to spend time outdoors.

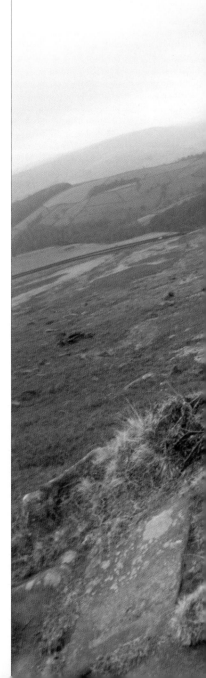

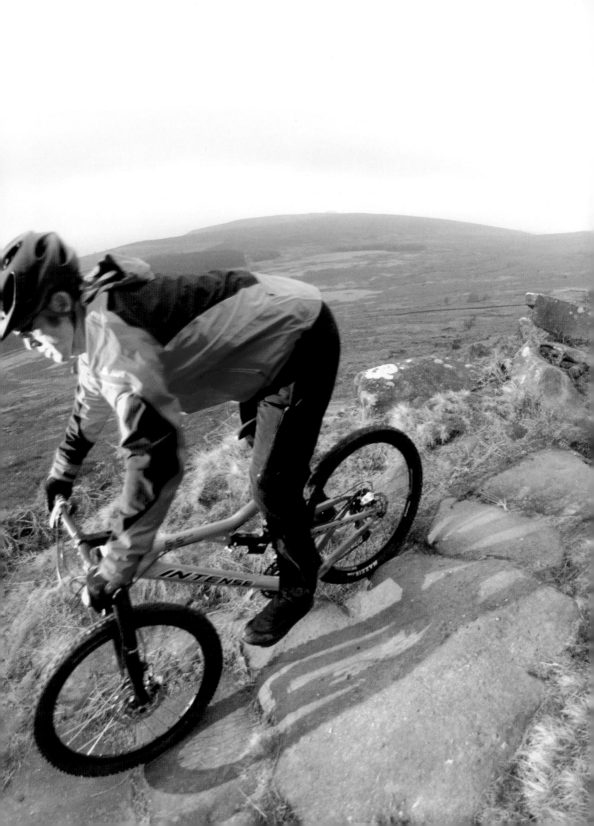

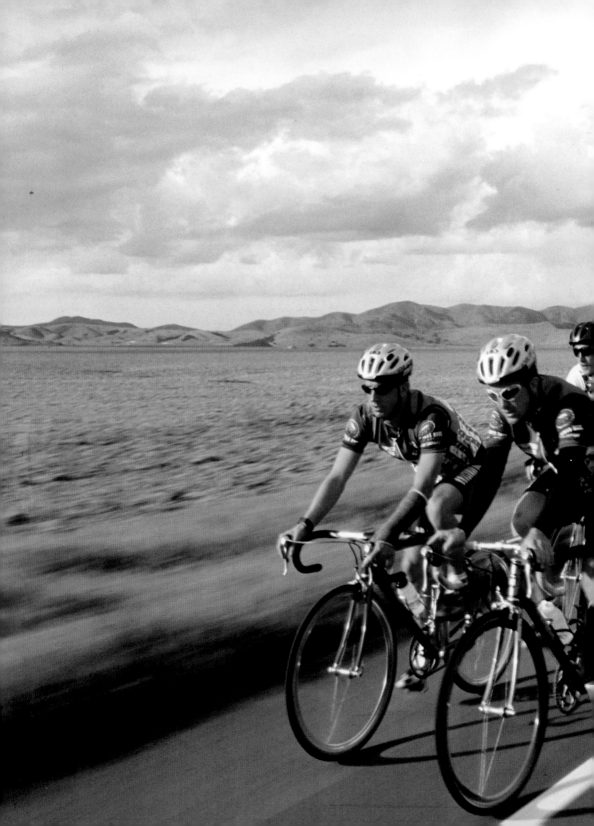

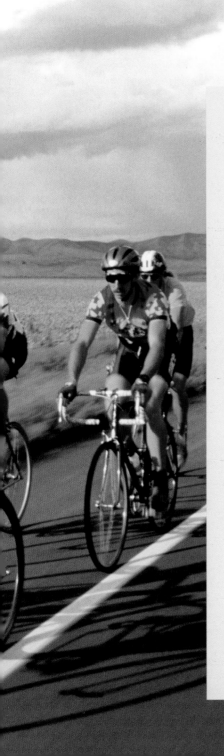

RIDING FOR PLEASURE

There are two things you need to start cycling: a bicycle, and a lot of enthusiasm. Then you are ready to take advantage of all the opportunities cycling can offer. Getting started, you may just want to ride around town, but you will need to consider which bike to buy, what to wear and how to ride in an urban environment. Or you may want to strike out farther afield, and embark on a cycling tour. Good planning and preparation are essential to ensure that cycling is a positive experience for you.

Left: A sociable group of cyclists take to the road.

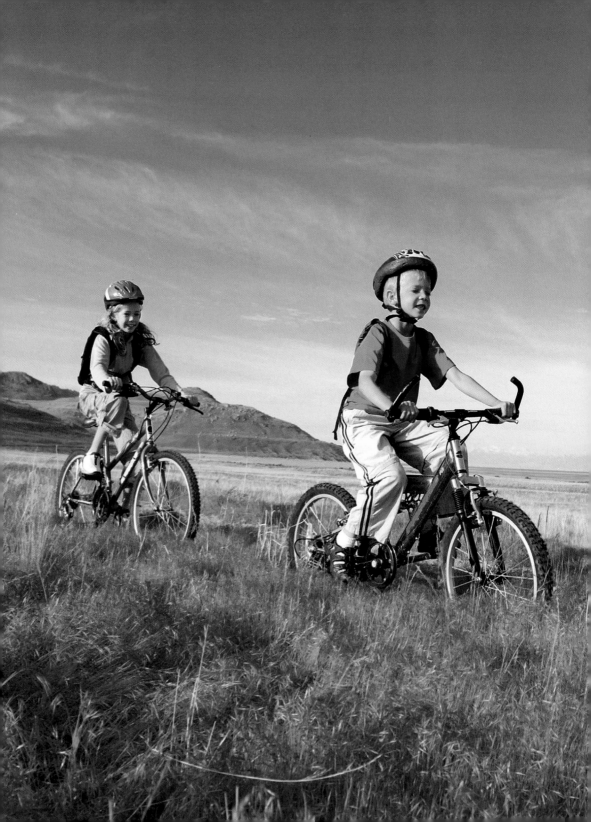

LEISURE RIDING

You don't have to start cycling with the aim of participating in the Tour de France. For most people, the simple practicalities of getting around town, commuting, or embarking on a short off-road leisure ride with family and friends are all that interests them. Even when cycling aims are this simple, just working on a few key skills and boosting confidence will enable you to get the most out of your cycling experience. Improving fitness will also make cycling easier and more effective.

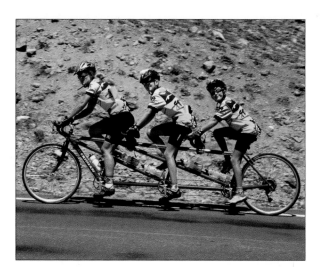

Above: A family ride a three-seater bike through a national park in Oregon.
Left: Children ride through a field in the country.

The Hybrid Cycle

A compromise between the speed of a racing bike, and the comfort of a mountain bike, the hybrid bike is the perfect bike for the leisure cyclist who wants to get around town, but maybe strike out farther for rides in the countryside or on bike paths.

Hybrid bikes resemble mountain bikes. While mountain bikes are built to withstand punishing rides off-road, hybrids don't need to be so resilient. They have narrower wheels, and usually come with slick tyres, which offer less rolling resistance on the road. This makes them faster. Flat handlebars and an upright position mean that riding is both safe and comfortable. Some even have suspension, which makes them still more comfortable to ride.

Most hybrid bikes are also set up so that panniers can be attached to carry luggage, making them the perfect all-round bike for short and middle distance leisure riding.

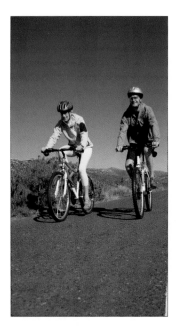

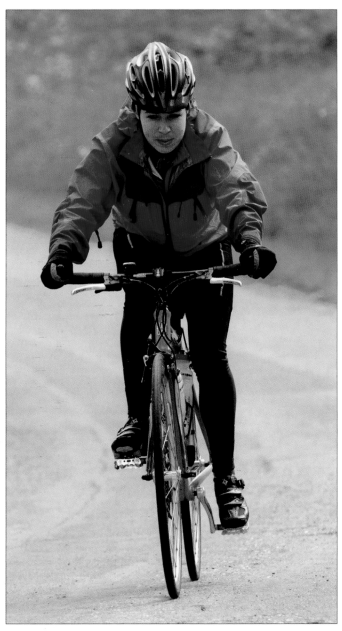

Above: Hybrids are equally practical for off- and on-road cycling, and are built for comfort and speed.
Right: Hybrid bikes suit cyclists at all levels of achievement.

Anatomy of a hybrid bike

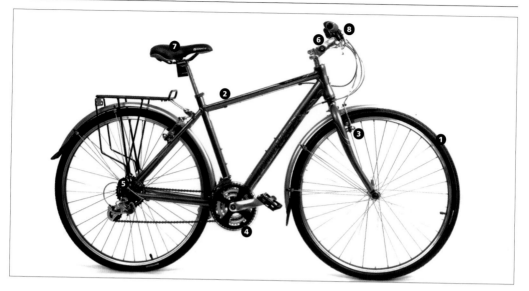

❶ Wheels: size 700x28c, which is the same as a racing bike, slightly larger than the 26in wheel standard on mountain bikes. Slick tyres for urban riding.

❷ Frame: Lighter and faster on the road than a heavy-duty mountain bike frame. Geometry is tailored for an upright position.

❸ Brakes: Calliper brakes.

❹ Chainrings: Either two or three, depending on the model. Three chainrings offer a larger range of gears, useful in hilly areas.

❺ Sprockets: There are usually eight or nine gears.

❻ Gear changers: These are mounted on the handlebars for ease of changing. Many gear changers are attached to the brake levers for good accessibility.

❼ Saddle: The saddle on a hybrid bike is wide and padded for extra comfort for the rider.

❽ Handlebars: Flat handlebars give the rider comfortable steering and an upright position.

Folding Bike

One of the most practical ways of getting around in big cities is using the folding bike.

For most city-dwellers, lack of storage space is a problem. Buses and trains often refuse to carry bikes, or restrict them to off-peak times. Once you have reached your destination, parking may be a problem.

These problems are solved by a folding bike, which are easy to carry on public transport, and can be stowed under a desk. However, they are not designed for long distance or fast cycling and they lose in comfort and speed over long distances.

Right: The Brompton has 40cm (16in) wheels, and collapses to a neat portable package.

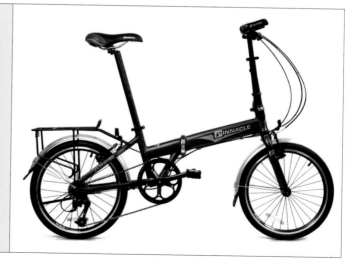

Clothing for Leisure Cycling

For very short distances, in temperate weather, it is possible to cycle in any clothes, but if you choose practical, comfortable gear, suited to the prevailing environment, your cycling experience will be a more positive and comfortable one.

The farther you cycle, and the more extreme the weather conditions, the more you have to think about what to wear. Suitable clothes and shoes will help you enjoy your cycling, no matter what the weather conditions.

Summer wear

Staying cool is the most important consideration when cycling in hot weather. For the leisure cyclist, overheating will spoil what would otherwise be a pleasant ride. For the office-bound commuter, there is nothing worse than arriving at work covered in sweat with the prospect of sitting at a desk wearing formal work clothes.

Modern, breathable fabrics ensure that cycling clothes are light and comfortable, and importantly, wick the perspiration away from your skin. On a hot day, it is a good idea to wear a pair of Lycra cycling shorts, a lightweight undershirt and a cycling top.

A good quality pair of cycling shorts is one of the first things you should consider buying when taking up cycling. Cycling shorts have a padded, seamless insert, which makes a huge difference in comfort levels. Normal trousers are impractical for cycling – the seam will be very uncomfortable after only a few minutes' riding, and the weight of the fabric is also a problem. In the past, inserts were made of chamois leather and needed regular treatment from creams to prevent them hardening. However, modern cycling shorts come with synthetic antibacterial inserts that require no special care.

It is also possible to buy shorts or long trousers, which are not skin-tight but still have a chamois insert.

Undershirts, or base layers, are recommended to keep the sweat away from your skin. On hot days, when you are sweating, a long downhill freewheel or a breeze can cause you to catch a

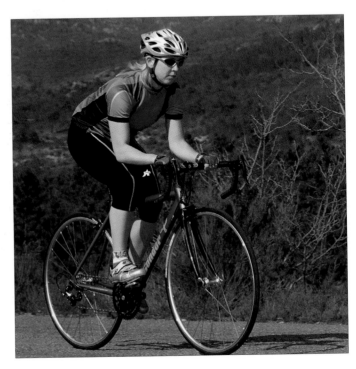

chill. Over the base layer, you can wear a cycling jersey. These are also lightweight and help to keep the sweat away from your body. They also have pockets sewn into the lower back, which are ideal for carrying small objects such as keys and money.

Protect yourself

Wearing two tops while cycling will help to protect you in the event of a crash. The two shirts will slide against each other, protecting your skin to a certain extent from abrasions.

It is also a very good idea to wear cycling mitts, which have padding on the palm of the hand and cut-off fingers to prevent you from overheating. Mitts absorb sweat and so ensure that you can keep a good grip on the

Above: When cycling in summer, it is important to wear comfortable lightweight, breathable clothes.

handlebars. In the event of a crash, they will also protect your hands from painful injuries.

In more humid areas it is necessary to invest in a good raincoat. You can get special raincoats designed for cycling, which are waterproof, extremely light, and are extra-long in the back to protect your lower back from the rain when you are in a cycling position.

During spring and autumn, when the weather can be unpredictable, it might be worth considering a gilet, which is a sleeveless top, over your cycling top. This will help keep you warm in the cooler evenings.

Winter wear

The real test of your commitment to cycling comes in the winter months, when cold and wet weather can try the resolve of even professional cyclists. However, with the right mental attitude and a sensible choice of clothing, you can be as comfortable in the cold and wet as you are on a warm summer's day.

On your legs, you need to wear thermal leggings, available from bike shops. These often have bibs attached, which stretch over the shoulders to add an extra layer of insulation to your upper body without restricting your movement. These are ideal to wear in cold weather.

As in summer, a base layer is essential. Even in cold weather, your body can heat up while cycling, so it is even more important to wick the sweat away from your body. In extremely cold weather, a thermal base layer will help you keep warm. Over your base layer, a windproof long-sleeved jersey will protect you from the cold but still allow ventilation to prevent overheating. In freezing temperatures, a base layer and windproof jersey should keep you warm enough once you have started moving.

If you suffer particularly from the cold, or if the temperature has dropped below freezing, there are several ways of

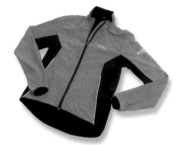

Above: A thermal jacket is necessary for cycling during the winter.

adding lightweight layers for further insulation. Cycling shops sell detachable arm warmers made of Lycra, which can be rolled up or down according to what is comfortable. They are extremely compact, and when you are not wearing them they can be stowed in the back pocket of your cycling jersey.

In cold weather it is also essential to cover your head – many thermal cycling hats and headbands are designed to be worn under a helmet without compromising safety and comfort. The feet and hands need to be protected, too. Buy a pair of waterproof, thermal overshoes and thermal gloves, and you are ready to go.

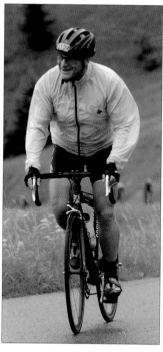

Above: A warm and waterproof lightweight jacket over a base layer and long-sleeved jersey is essential when conditions turn very cold or wet.

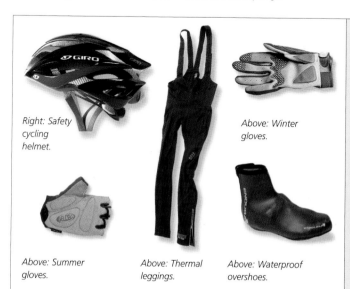

Right: Safety cycling helmet.

Above: Summer gloves.

Above: Thermal leggings.

Above: Winter gloves.

Above: Waterproof overshoes.

Cycling gear

In general, the better the shoes are for cycling, the worse they are for walking. The most efficient cycling shoes have stiff soles, with shoeplates screwed in for the pedal attachments. They make you cycle faster, but once you are off the bike, at best they make you walk like a penguin.

It is inconvenient to have to carry two pairs of shoes, one for walking, one for cycling, so a solution for the leisure cyclist and commuter is to buy cycling shoes that can also be used for walking, for example, Shimano's SPD (Shimano's Pedalling Dynamics) system. These still have plates to clip to pedals, but they are flush with the sole, which is also more flexible.

Safety is paramount, especially in the city. Wear a well-fitted helmet and high-visibility gear at all times, as well as a mask if you are concerned about pollution.

General Riding Skills

It is impossible to 'unlearn' riding a bike, and just about every adult in the Western world has a head start in cycling through learning to ride when they were a child. To regain confidence, practise on a quiet traffic-free road.

Most adults who want to take up cycling again, or even those who have kept riding throughout their lives, can benefit from refreshing their skill set. The more relaxed and assured you are about your cycling and your ability to deal with challenges and obstacles, the more enjoyable your cycling will be.

The most important thing when cycling is to feel comfortable, at ease and relaxed on your bike. Nervousness makes your body tense and affects the handling of your bike, especially the steering. On a busy road, this can prove to be very dangerous.

If you have not ridden a bike for a few years, it is a good idea to find a quiet road or a car park to rediscover the feeling of balance and flow that comes from confident bike handling. You don't have to spend weeks doing this – just ensure that you can manage the basic skills of starting, riding in a straight line, riding around a corner, and stopping. The rustiness will not take long to disappear, but it is better for this to happen away from busy roads.

Moving on

Once you are confident that you are used to riding your bike again, there are still some aspects of your cycling you should take care to work on.

Cornering should be smooth, consistent and safe. Depending on whether there is traffic around, and how tight the corner is, there are several different ways of getting around a corner efficiently.

For a shallow bend, it should be possible to just keep the line you have been following already.

For a sharper corner, take a wider approach to maintain as much speed as it is safe to have. If there are cars following behind, do not swing out into their path, but if you are certain that the road is clear, you can approach the

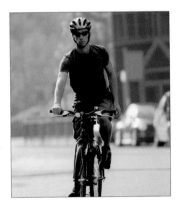

centre of the lane before turning as you reach the corner. What you are aiming for is to be more efficient and to go around the bend losing as little speed as possible, while remaining upright and safe.

Practising skills

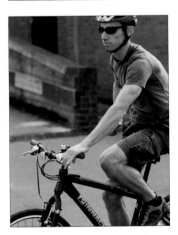

Riding one-handed: Find a quiet bit of road or a car park and practise riding one-handed, using both left and right hands. For the ambitious, it doesn't hurt to learn to ride no-handed, but don't practise this in traffic.

Left: Practise riding one-handed to improve your balance on a bike.

Two other factors need to be taken into consideration when cornering – the weather, and the road surface. In dry conditions on a smooth road, it is natural to lean with the bike as you go round a corner, though when you do this you should keep your head level. But in wet conditions, especially if there are drain covers in the road, or on loose surfaces such as gravel, leaning the bike too far will result in the wheels sliding out from under you. There is no need to slow right down unless the corner is very sharp, but to compensate for the lack of grip, try leaning your body while keeping the bike as upright as possible. This will ensure your safety, while maintaining speed around the corner.

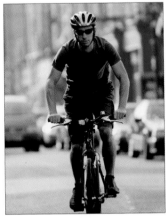

Looking ahead: *Once you are confident of your riding skills, get out on the road and cycle. Practise predicting what is going to happen consciously, before trying to make it a subconscious part of every ride you do.*

Drills to improve your skills

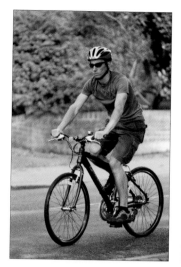

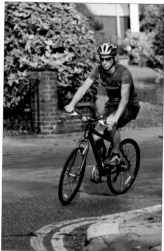

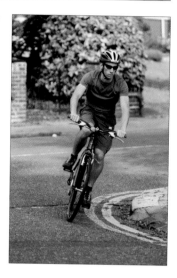

Cornering 1: *Find some quiet roads, and practise riding a loop. Plan your route through the corners and learn what your safe speed is. Push your limits, but be careful and sensible.*

Cornering 2: *Find a downhill section of road with good visibility and corners going left and right. Ride down a few times, learning to look ahead and plan your route through the corners.*

Cornering 3: *Once you have ridden around the route, try getting around the corner in a smooth and consistent way. Try not to lose speed but stay upright, relaxed and safe.*

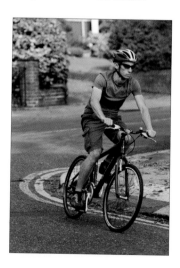

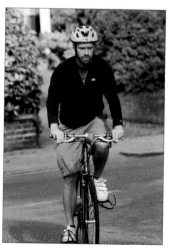

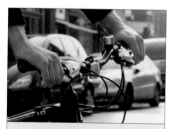

Go with the flow

Once you are cornering confidently and riding at an efficient speed, you are more in control of your bike. And the good news is that the more time you spend cycling, the more natural these processes will become.

Once you have got used to the way your bike handles, and the way you react to it, you will notice that you will stop thinking of yourself and the bike as separate entities, but don't relax too much – you still need to be ready to react to surprises.

Above: The more cycling you do, the more you will be focused.

Cornering 4: *Once you have got around the corner, maintain your speed and cycle confidently on. Always be aware of other road users such as cars and buses or heavier vehicles and be prepared to take avoiding action.*

Braking: *Find a quiet downhill bit of road. Ride at various speeds and work on getting your stopping distance down to a safe minimum. Start with the back brake to check speed and maintain control, then the front brake to stop.*

Braking, Gearing and Riding Safely

Once you have spent some time cycling on the roads, you will become aware that the average bike ride throws up hazards, obstacles and challenges when you least expect it. Learning to anticipate these things is key to becoming a more proficient rider.

Awareness is seeing what is going to happen on the road ahead a few seconds before it actually does. By watching the behaviour of others, you can learn to predict even the seemingly unpredictable. If a car is about to turn across you, it is safer to slow down. Pedestrians may wander into the road, assuming that if they cannot hear a car, there is nothing coming. Cars can pull out directly into your path. If you anticipate, you can avoid problems. Always be aware of what is going on around you.

Braking

Reacting to an obstacle can involve one of two things – evasive action, or braking. If you have the time and space to swerve around a pothole, pedestrian or other obstacle you can maintain your speed without wasting energy.

More often, you need to check your speed or even stop suddenly, and there is a technique to this. Slamming on both brakes can cause a rear-wheel skid, or worse, a front-wheel lock, which is as potentially painful as it is embarrassing. The aim is to be in control of the bike at every moment, and controlled and assertive braking is part of this.

The correct technique for braking is to rely more on the rear brake at high speed, and then the front brake as you decelerate. As weight is transferred forward during braking, there is a

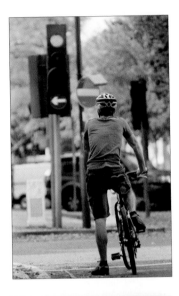

Right: When waiting at a stop light, keep one foot on the pedal, ready to accelerate away.
Below: Build the confidence to ride safely in traffic – anticipate what is ahead, be aware of what is behind.

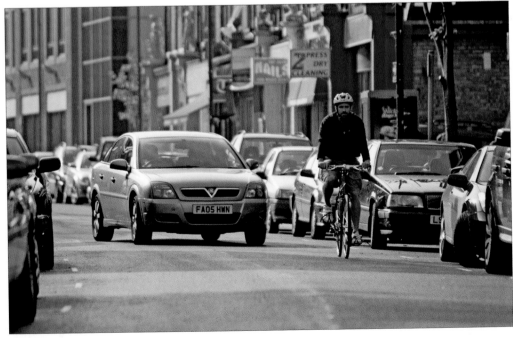

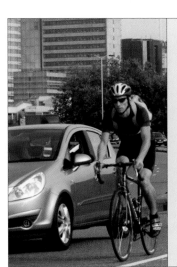

Left: Cars should give cyclists plenty of room. When one comes past, stay focused and relaxed.

tendency for the back wheel to skid, so try and push your own weight backward on the bike to compensate for this. It is a lot to think about for something that has to happen in a split second, but practise it until it is second nature. In most cases, the anticipation you have been developing will enable you to see hazards unfolding well in advance, and you will be able to slow down while remaining in control.

Sometimes you have to perform an emergency stop. Try never to panic and just grab at the brake levers, but stay

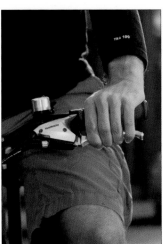

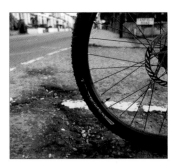

Above: Potholes can be a danger for cyclists. If possible, look ahead and avoid them, but don't swerve into the road.
Left: When braking, maintain a firm grip on the handlebars and squeeze the brake gently to control speed.

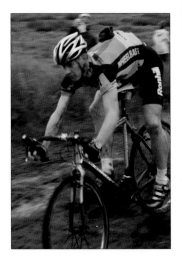

relaxed and calm and be confident that a well-maintained set of brakes and the correct techniques will enable you to stay safe.

Using gears efficiently

Cycling effectively is not about getting from A to B as fast as you possibly can. If you start a ride sprinting, you won't last long. The important thing is to ride

Left: Cyclo-cross riders keep their weight far back when braking, so that they can maintain control and traction.

at an efficient speed. Choose a gear that you can comfortably turn at 60–80 revolutions per minute, just over one per second, or whatever feels comfortable. Racing cyclists prefer a faster rhythm, but for leisure riding and commuting the main aim is economy of movement.

If you are going up an unexpected steep hill, you need to get the timing right. Lighten pressure on the pedals so you can shift down a few gears. Change up if you are going downhill. On varied terrain; uphills and downhills, the aim is to keep the same cadence.

Urban Cycling

The bicycle is the perfect mode of transport in an urban environment. A bike can squeeze through a gap when the road is blocked with traffic. There are health and fitness benefits too, and cycling is a great stress reliever.

Cars get stuck in traffic jams, and once they arrive at their destination, there is scarce space for parking. Buses and trains and even underground systems are better, but you are forced to go where they go. You also have to pay for the privilege.

If the closest train station is a 10-minute walk away from your destination, you often have no option but to walk. Cabs? More flexible, but the costs quickly mount up.

Cycling offers the best of all worlds – it's free, once you have bought a bike. It's fast. You can go exactly where you want to. And it is environmentally friendly.

More and more big cities around the world are starting to realize that congestion is a major problem, both economically and practically. It is also suspected that there are major health risks involved in having to breathe the emissions from cars stuck head-to-tail on the city's streets. So, following the lead of cities like Amsterdam in Holland, bike lanes are being laid and provision for bikes is being included in many metropolitan transport plans.

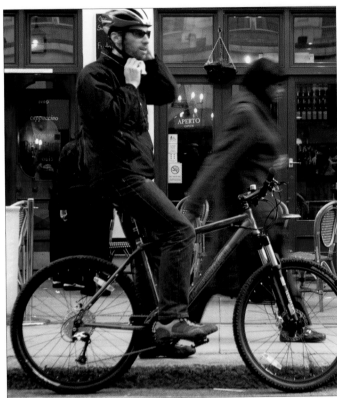

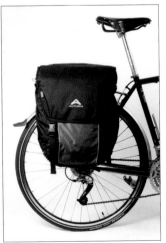

Getting around

So why not go by bike? For city dwellers, most journeys are made within a small radius, well within cycling distance. If you calculated the typical journeys you make in the course of a week, along with the mode of transport you use, you might realize that many hours spent on buses or trains could be spent cycling instead. You'll save money as well as getting fitter. It's not just going to and from work that might be

Left: Panniers fit on a bike and let commuters and urban cyclists carry their gear without a destabilizing backpack.

Above: Finding a parking space for a car if you want to go for a coffee is difficult in most cities, but cycling can take you right to the door of the café.

better by bike. Weekend day trips to a museum or exhibition could be even more fun by riding there and back. If you are a member of a sports, music or social club of any description, the act of cycling could become part of the routine of your hobby.

For a night out on the town, though, the bike is not the best mode of transport unless you stick to non-alcoholic drinks.

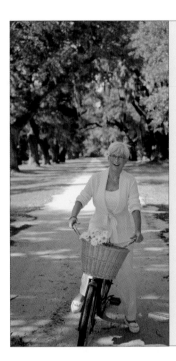

Shopping by bike

While it is easy to imagine travelling more within cities by bike, the idea of shopping by bike still puts some people off. Getting to the shop on a bike is straightforward, especially when it is not too far away. But getting back laden down with food or fragile goods can be difficult, or even dangerous, if you're not properly equipped.

The main problem is how to transport heavy shopping on your bike without affecting your ability to ride safely. With small loads it is possible to ride with a comfortable backpack. Backpacks are not ideal for cycling – they over-insulate your back and make you sweat uncomfortably. They also affect the handling and balance of your bike. If they are not fitted correctly, it's possible for them to slide off to one side and unbalance you. If you are riding with a backpack, make sure it is secure.

Left: Cyclists can conveniently carry light shopping in a basket fixed to the handlebars of the bike.

With most hybrid and leisure bikes, there are attachments on the frame for panniers, and for heavier loads, these are ideal. A pair of bags on a rear pannier should be able to accommodate a substantial amount of shopping. You can also attach an ordinary bag to the top of the rack with bungees, but check it is secure. The weight does affect the handling of your bike, but it is easy to get used to, and once you adjust to the extra weight, it won't slow you down too much.

Once you have got used to this, it is by far the easiest way to go shopping. Your bike is taking the load for you – even when you drive to the shops, you have to carry your shopping to the car, and then again at the other end. For very large loads, it is worth considering a detachable trailer. These hook on to the back of your bike, and can be pulled along. If you are cycling to keep fit, the extra work involved in pulling a laden trailer will have a substantial effect on your fitness levels.

When you start to cycle more, the planning of journeys becomes a major part of the exercise. Plot an interesting route down roads that avoid the main traffic arteries of the city, and you will discover new areas, streets and buildings. Exploration doesn't have to take place in the wilderness to be fun.

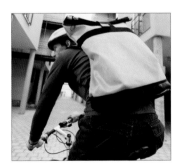

Above: Bikes are the ideal form of urban transport – cities are too congested for most people to consider driving.
Right: A young child can be transported by bike, strapped in a seat on the back. You may not want to risk cycling in heavy traffic, though.

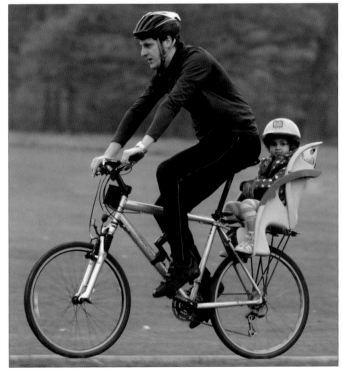

Commuting by Bike

If you live close to your office, there are many reasons to choose cycling as your method of transport. Door to door, cycling to work can save you time and you also do not have the expense of a bus or train ticket.

Cycling 16km (10 miles) a day will have a massive effect on your fitness level if you have been leading a sedentary lifestyle. If you cycle five times a week, there is no need to take out an expensive gym membership, which will save you time and money. Add this to the saving on travel tickets, or petrol and parking, and you will have substantially more money in your pocket. You will arrive at work fresh and invigorated from the exercise and the fresh air, even when it is raining. This will have a positive effect on your performance at work.

There is evidence suggesting that cyclists are less affected by pollution from car emissions than the drivers of the cars themselves. Cyclists' heads are above the level where the air is most polluted, while car ventilation systems take in all that polluted air and feed it straight into the vehicle. Of course, vehicle emissions are still a problem for cyclists, and you can buy lightweight face-masks that cover the mouth and nose and filter out pollutants and dust.

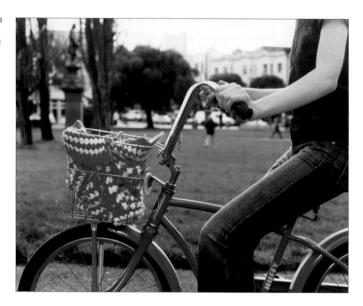

Above: Cycling to work keeps you fit, is faster than driving and allows you to enjoy the fresh air.

If you live up to 16km (10 miles) away from your office, commuting by bike is worth trying – your journey time might increase to somewhere between half an hour and an hour, but this is still less time than many people spend on public transport.

If you are starting from scratch, it is advisable not to try cycling to and from work five times a week. Suddenly going from no exercise to 160km (100 miles) in five days is a big jump. It is a good idea to plan a system whereby you ride to work one day, then get the train home. The next day you take the train in, and cycle home. You can build up from there.

If you live farther than 16km (10 miles) away, commuting by bike is still a viable option. Build up to the greater distance

Left: By riding to work you can save money on transport and gym membership – you'll get all the exercise you need.

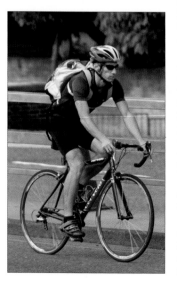

slowly, and take days off if you are tired. You could consider splitting your journey by cycling part of the way and using public transport for the other part.

Arriving at the workplace
Once you have taken the decision to start commuting by bike, it helps if your office or workplace has a shower so you can wash and change before work. Many employers provide showers these days, which is the first concern of many would-be bicycle commuters. If yours has not, start to press for one to be installed. The practical benefits for the cyclist will far outweigh the initial investment in time and money. Second, you will need somewhere secure and preferably dry to store your bike during the day. Some workplaces have bike-locking facilities. If yours does not, ask

for some to be installed. If you have a folding bike, however, you can fold it quickly and store it neatly out of the way under your desk.

Lock it up

Finally, invest in a heavy-duty bike lock. The thicker and stronger your lock is, the harder it is for thieves to cut through it. Cable locks, or simple chains, will deter some attempts at theft, but a rigid D-lock is more secure. These items are bulky, but bike security is essential. Leave a lock at work if you don't want to carry it back and forth every day. For peace of mind, some cyclists even use two locks.

Make sure you lock your bike to something secure – a set of railings or a purpose-built bike stand. Some bike stands have brackets screwed to the wall – beware of thieves unscrewing the brackets and taking away your bike, heavy-duty locks and all.

All change

Now that all the facilities are in place for you to cycle to work, the key thing is to be organized. Given that arriving at work in sweaty cycling gear and then doing a day's work is probably unviable

Below: Parking problems will become a nuisance of the past when you commute by bike. Just lock up your bike at a dedicated cycle rack and go.

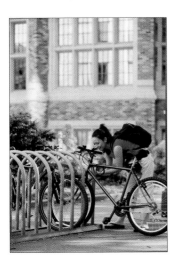

in most offices, you'll have to make sure that you have clothes to change into. Some bike commuters carry enough clothes for a week in on a Monday morning, then take it all home again on Friday. Others prefer to take fresh clothes in every day.

If you take fresh clothes in to work every day, experiment with the best way of folding your shirts to keep them pressed and the rest of your clothes crease-free. Carefully fold ties, or pay the consequences.

The less you have to carry, the easier your cycle ride will be. Pack a spare set of clothes, perhaps a laptop computer and diary. A good idea is to pack all your clothes and other items in plastic bags within your panniers or backpack to keep them dry in wet conditions.

On your bike

Now you are ready to go. In time perhaps you can start experimenting with different routes – a short deviation might add a mile or so to your journey, but may lead you to discovering new areas and finding a more scenic route. How many people who take the train get that opportunity?

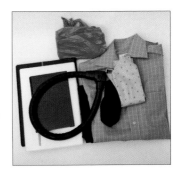

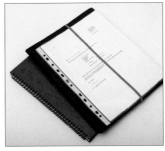

Above: What to pack when commuting to work by bike: clothes, your laptop, bike lock, and plastic bags (top) and work papers and notebook (above).

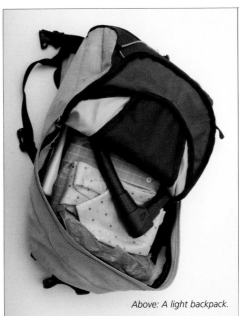

Above: A light backpack.

Checklist
What to wear
Cycling shoes
Cycling shorts
Base layer
Cycling jersey
Helmet
Mitts
What to pack
Laptop
Diary
Papers
Underwear
Trousers/skirt and shirt
Tie
Secure bike lock
Plastic bags
What to keep at work
Shoes
Towel
Toiletries
Spare cycling kit in case
of rain during ride

Mountain Biking: Getting Started

At some point, the ambitious leisure cyclist will want to broaden his or her horizons and take on the challenge of going for an off-road ride. Mountain biking is fun and user-friendly: you can ride the bike on and off the road.

Mountain biking off-road confers two immediate benefits. First, there is no traffic, save other cyclists, walkers and horse riders, and in general these three groups of people have learned to coexist harmoniously. (When riding on the trails, ride with tolerance and consideration, and everybody else should do the same.)

Second, in the unfortunate event of a crash, there is a higher likelihood of having a soft landing.

Unless you are riding on steep terrain, the same rules apply to off-road riding as to riding on the road. The specific skills of trail riding will be explored later in the book, but the main skill set is the same as for road riding, with the loose surface of most off-road paths taken into account.

Mountain biking in the countryside is one of the greatest pleasures of cycling, and it is a genuine social activity. If you are a recent convert to leisure cycling or commuting, mountain biking is a great way to get even more out of your bike.

Getting started is as easy as it is for road cycling. You need a bike and a healthy dose of enthusiasm. You can even use the same clothes and equipment, although you will need some proper mountain-biking shoes, which are good for walking, but that also clip in to your pedals.

The rough and the smooth

The biggest difference between road cycling and off-road cycling is obviously the surface on which you ride. Gravel and potholes aside, roads are uniform as well as predictable, while country paths are precisely the opposite. On a single ride, the surface can be soft mud, hard earth, gravel, rocks, grass or any combination of these surfaces. Learning to cope with the change in the surface, and the way it affects the handling of the bike, is important if you want to improve.

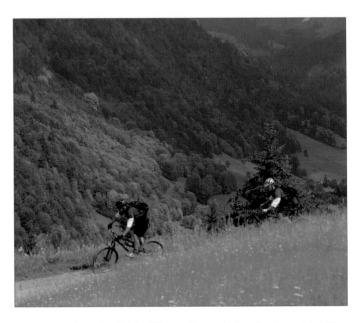

On most surfaces, the thick knobbly tyres on mountain bikes are capable of offering more grip than slick road tyres. On gravel, rocks or soft wet surfaces, however, cornering can still be hazardous. Approach bends with caution, and treat them as you would on a road bike, maintaining as much speed as possible, while staying within the bounds of safety.

Because of the bumpy surface on most off-road bike rides, mountain biking is more tiring. It is important to save energy by relaxing as much as possible, holding the handlebars in a firm but relaxed grip, and allowing the arms to be used as shock absorbers. If your bike has suspension forks, or is a full-suspension model, your ride will also be far more comfortable.

Braking also has to be treated with more caution, because of the tendency of wheels to lock up on loose surfaces. The front brake is the more powerful,

Above: The benefits of mountain biking are clear: it's just you, your bike and a spectacular landscape.

but use the back brake to control your speed, and the front brake to slow down more quickly.

Lastly, gearing is an important consideration. Because the hills tend to be steeper and more unpredictable, you can easily grind to a halt if you don't change down soon enough. If you see a hill coming, try to assess the steepness, and as you hit the bottom, change into a gear you know you will be able reach the top in. It's much better to err on the side of caution – if you stall, it is hard to get going again.

Above all, the best way of improving your cycling technique and to enjoy off-road riding more is to practise regularly and get used to the way your bike reacts on the different terrain.

Drills to improve your skills

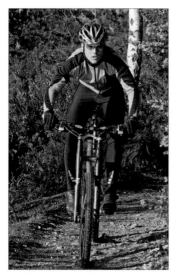

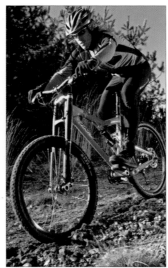

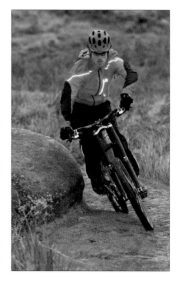

Braking 1: *Find a slightly downhill section with a loose surface. Build up a little speed, then bring yourself to a fast but controlled stop using both brakes.*

Braking 2: *On a steeper downhill path, repeat. Push your weight back, start to slow down with the back brake then the front brake once deceleration is controlled.*

Reactions: *Riding on a downhill path with a loose surface and corners, keep the same speed and avoid rocks. Be sensitive to the way the bike reacts.*

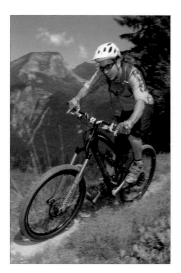

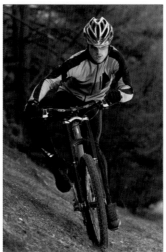

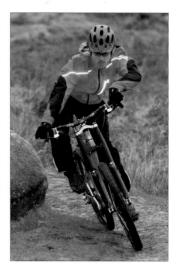

Gearing: *Find a section of path that goes up and down hills in quick succession. Change gear for the uphill section as you reach the bottom, and continue with no loss of momentum.*

Balance 1: *Ride along a camber, that is, across the slope of a hill, holding out your 'uphill' leg for balance if necessary. Prevent your bike from slipping downhill as you ride along the camber.*

Balance 2: *Ride on a very loose or unpredictable surface, making quite exaggerated turns on corners to test your reactions and balance. Try this on a flat surface first.*

Cycling for the Family

Riding a bike needn't be a solitary activity – it is one of the cheapest and most sociable ways of enjoying an outing for families and friends. In fact, if children get involved in cycling it will help them to learn a new skill and enjoy a healthy lifestyle.

Children enjoy cycling, both when they are very young and can ride as a passenger on their parents' bikes, and later, when they learn to ride themselves. The speed, freedom and fun of cycling gives children all the stimuli they need to develop, and it encourages them to explore other places.

All it takes is the attachment of a child seat, and you and your family are ready to ride. Once your children are riding their own bikes, the family ride takes on a new dimension – they can learn about independence, within the boundaries of spending time with the family.

Right: Cycling is a fun way for a child to learn independence.
Below: Going out on a ride is a cheap and enjoyable activity for a family.

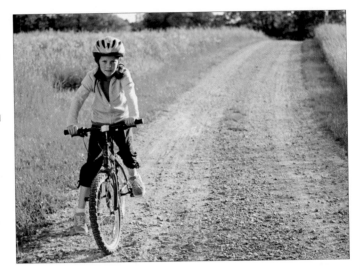

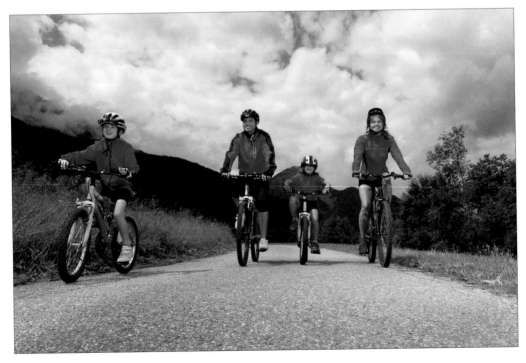

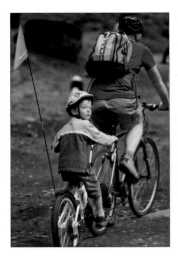

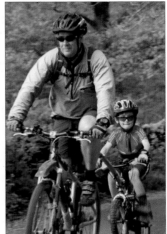

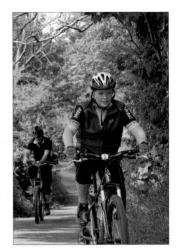

Above: A flag warns that there is a child on the back of an adult's bike.

Above: A child can gain confidence by riding a bike attached to a parent's bike.

Above: Cycling is a healthy activity that families can do together.

Starting young

If you have young children who are not old enough to ride bikes, there are several ways of including them in your cycling activities. One way is to attach a child seat to your bike. Most of these fit above the back wheel, but models exist in which the chair attaches to the top tube and the child sits between your arms. Both are safe, but handling and steering are affected by the weight above the back wheel with a rear-mounted seat. The main consideration, however, is safety. First, children should always be fitted with helmets and must wear them when they are cycling.

Rear-mounted seats should have safety guards to prevent the child's feet from touching the back wheel. Another way is to get a trailer with child seats. These are designed for one or two children, and can take a great deal more weight than a bike-mounted seat. If you use one of these, visibility to other road users is very important. Attach high-visibility strips and lights to the rear, and a flag to draw attention to the presence of a trailer.

Always check the manufacturer's guidelines for the minimum age for children to be carried in their products.

For older children, who are already competent at cycling and aware of the dangers on the road, you can buy a half-wheeler, which adds an extra wheel, seat and frame to the back of your bike. Your child can even help with the pedalling!

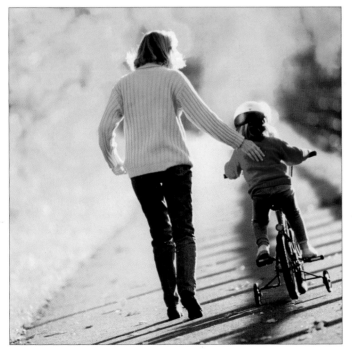

Left: Stabilizers attached to a child's bike will help him or her to achieve good balance before attempting to ride a two-wheeler bike.

Cycling for Kids

To children, the urge to explore, test their boundaries and broaden their horizons is as natural as wanting to eat or sleep. A bike is an ideal way of allowing them to do this. And once cycling is mastered, there is a satisfying sense of achievement.

It is important to give children their independence, but at the same time teach them that safety is paramount. Children should be encouraged to get around by bike, but responsible parents should explain which roads are safe to cycle on and which are too dangerous. They should be taught not to expect danger, but to be able to deal with it on

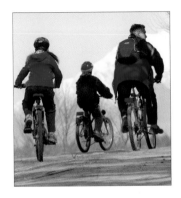

Above: Taking children on bike rides will keep them healthy and eager to explore their surroundings and the wider world.

the rare occasions it does come. The two most dangerous hazards are other road users, and children themselves. Children should be taught to be aware of approaching traffic and to avoid busy roads. Most car drivers will adjust their driving to take into account a child or indeed any person on a bike. But for the small minority who behave unpredictably, children need to be able to anticipate danger before it happens.

Once all the safety issues have been explained to children, most of the danger comes from their desire to find their limits. In doing so, they may pass their limits and crash, or fall off. In most cases, a few painful cuts and grazes are the consequences, as well as a more definite knowledge of their skill level.

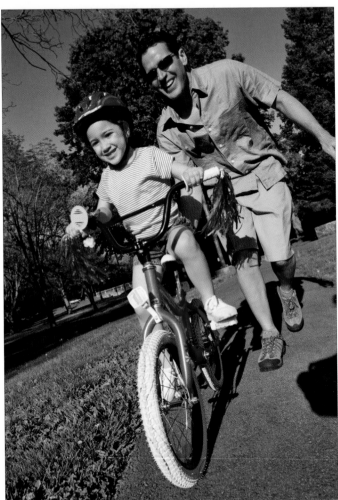

For family rides together, it is best to avoid busy roads. Keep to quiet roads with good visibility, or take the children off-road and ride on designated bike paths.

For children below the age of 13 or 14, be particularly careful about planning a ride, and make sure the

Above: Get involved in teaching your child to ride a bike. Giving a helping hand can help instil confidence.

distance is manageable. A few miles at a time is enough. Plan plenty of rest stops with healthy snacks, and don't forget to take food and water.

Learning to ride

There are two ways of learning to ride a bike. The first is by experience. The second is by analysing the techniques and attempting to explain them verbally. Experience wins every time. Take your child, along with his or her new bike, to a park, preferably with grass to ride on. Explain how the brakes work, and warn them not to turn the handlebars too sharply. You can then sit back and watch as they experiment with how to keep

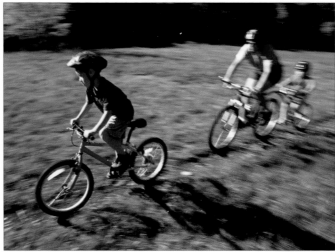

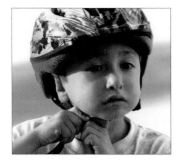

Above: Encourage your child to wear a helmet to protect his or her head.
Below: Once your children are proficient at cycling, take them on longer, more adventurous rides.

the bike upright. Only help if they ask for it, and be willing to hold them upright as they start, but otherwise, cycling is a skill best learned by trial and error. It will take a few goes, sometimes a few days, but eventually they will get the hang of it. Once they have mastered wobbling along in a reasonably straight line and can work the brakes well enough to stop, you can encourage

Above: Take children on rides away from roads to build their confidence and develop their skill at cycling.

them to work on more advanced techniques – turning left, turning right, speeding up and slowing down. Before long they will be fully fledged bike riders, and there will be no holding them back.

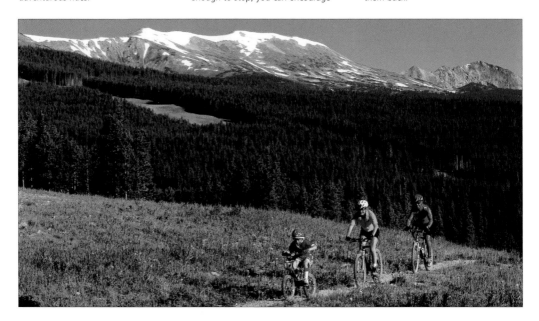

BMX for Kids

BMXs are ideal for children. They are designed for getting around without looking in the slightest bit sensible, for riding fast and for having fun on. They are perfect for riding on specially designed BMX dirt tracks, which will improve the child's bike handling ability.

Several Tour de France riders, including some of the best sprinters in the world, grew up riding BMX bikes.

BMXs are also great for stunts and tricks, either in BMX parks, which are similar to skateboarding parks, or on the street. Doing stunts is fun and safe, within certain boundaries, for kids. It is also great for learning co-ordination and balance, and building strength.

BMX tracks

It will take a while for your children to develop the appropriate skills. Encourage them to ride the BMX as much as possible without trying stunts. Once they are used to the way it handles, you can take them to a BMX track to start developing the skills to ride around it fast and safely.

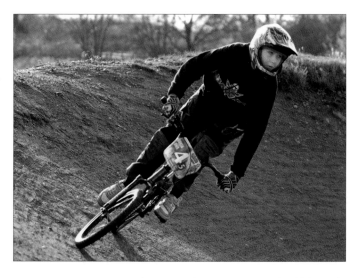

Above: You can maintain a high speed riding around berms on the race track.

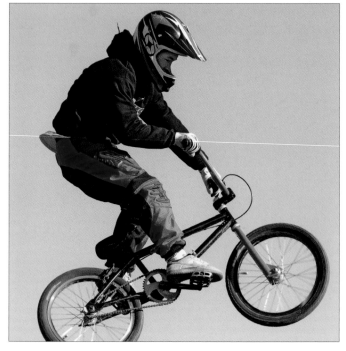

BMX tracks have a dirt surface and consist of a series of jumps, bumps, sloping corners or 'berms' and straights.

Good technique and balance are needed. When riding fast, the steepness of the jumps causes the bike to become airborne. Keep the BMX straight on the approach, stay straight on the jump, and land straight. Landing at an angle will cause the bike to veer and it may crash. Bumps should be ridden over, with the legs and arms bending to absorb the shock. The BMX should stay on the ground or it will lose speed.

Riders should aim for the centre of the berm for maximum speed. It's sometimes possible to pedal all the way through, but you may need to keep the outside foot at the bottom of the pedal stroke, or even to put the lower foot down, for balance.

Left: BMXs are good for developing agility, strength and balance.

Jumps and tricks

The easiest trick to perform on a BMX is a bunny-hop. These can be practised at low speed.

Stop pedalling, in a position where both your feet are at the same height, and 'crouch' over your BMX. The momentum for the bunny-hop comes from the action of the arms pulling up. Pull the arms up first, so that the front wheel comes off the ground, then pull the heels back and up (without coming off the pedals), and the back wheel will also come up. With practice, it is possible to co-ordinate these two movements so you can make them almost simultaneous.

Pulling wheelies is also fairly straightforward. As with learning to ride in the first place, trial and error is the best way to work out and maintain the correct balance.

Sitting down, pull up on the handlebars while pushing down on one pedal (this is called a power stroke). On an adult bike, the gears are generally too high to generate enough momentum, but BMX bikes have low enough gears to allow you to carry out the manoeuvre.

Extend the arms, and pull the handlebars up towards the chest. If you go too far, you can fall backwards. If you don't go far enough, the front wheel will come back down.

Bunny-hop

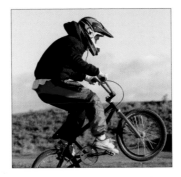

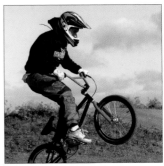

1 *To bunny-hop the bike, pull the arms up so that the front wheel comes up off the ground.*

2 *Pull the heels back and up. Pedal, and be prepared to jump the back wheel up.*

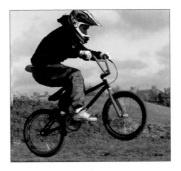

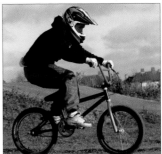

3 *Pull heels back and down to attempt to bring the back wheel into the air.*

4 *Land back on the ground with the handlebars straight.*

Wheelies

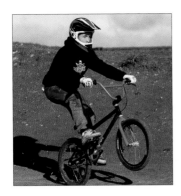

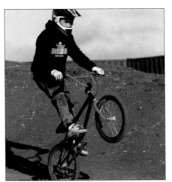

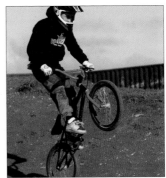

1 *To pull a wheelie, pull up on the handlebars and push down on one pedal.*

2 *Next, pull up the handlebars in the direction of the chest.*

3 *Keep pedalling while the bike is balanced on the back wheel.*

Improving Your Health by Cycling

Riding a bike is a healthy activity. Regular exercise in the form of cycling will make you fitter and stronger, help you reduce your fat levels and look in better shape, boost your energy and generally improve your mood.

Most everyday cycling is an aerobic activity, when muscles generate energy for movement using oxygen. Sprinting or riding up hills is anaerobic exercise, when the muscles burn energy supplies without using oxygen, because not enough is available. Aerobic activity is sustainable for long periods; anaerobic exercise is only possible for short bursts.

Unless you are training to race your bike, it is best not to get too hung up on whether you are exercising aerobically or anaerobically. Just getting out and riding will be enough to boost your fitness levels far above those of the average member of the population. You may want to push yourself sometimes, but be careful not to overreach yourself.

Effects of cycling

Cycling mainly works the legs, but the arms, back and core muscles also get a significant workout during a ride. More importantly, the cardiovascular system works hard and becomes more efficient. After just a few weeks of regular cycling, you will be less out of breath when you climb stairs, and able to sustain longer periods of activity.

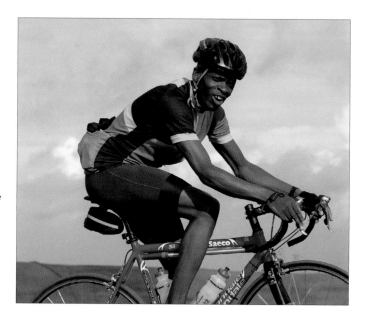

Depending on how hard you go, an hour-long bike ride can burn between 300 and 800 calories. If you ride at a moderate intensity, your body will gradually burn its fat stores. If you are

Top: Regular training and riding has a beneficial effect on health and fitness.

overweight, you will lose weight cycling, but the most important thing is not necessarily to lose weight, but to reduce fat to a healthy level. Cycling burns fat, but also builds muscle, so your lean body mass may increase after a few months' cycling. This is perfectly healthy.

Incorporating the bicycle into an organized exercise routine is easy. You may wish to ride 8km (5 miles) to and from work every day, which takes no organization. Or you can set aside two evenings a week and go for an hour-long ride, plus an extra ride at the weekend. The only limiting factor is your schedule, so work with it, not against it.

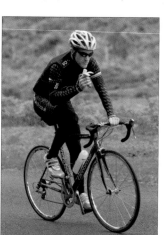
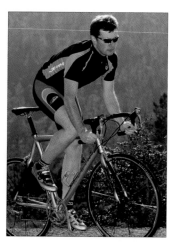

Far left: Bananas are easily eaten while cycling and are a good energy source.
Left: The faster and harder you ride, the fitter you will become.

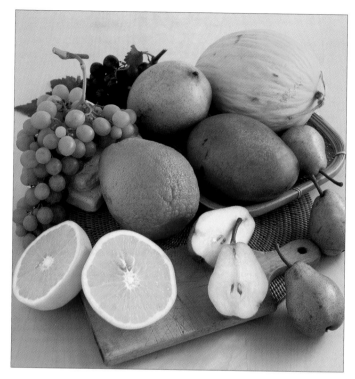

Above: Eat a variety of fresh fruit regularly as part of a healthy diet.

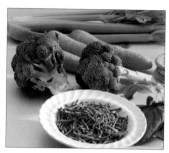

Above: Use plenty of fresh vegetables and grains to make your meals varied, interesting and tasty.

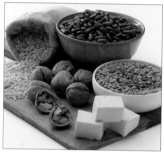

Above: Nuts, pulses and cereals will provide you with energy to keep cycling.

Cycling is great exercise, but it will have a far more positive effect on your body and health if you eat and drink properly as well. A balanced diet, with natural foods and sensible levels of hydration, will fuel your body much more effectively than TV dinners and junk food. By putting better fuel into your body you will have enough energy to continue cycling and also reap the health benefits.

If you are commuting to work, or planning on a leisure ride, it's essential to have a healthy breakfast, with cereal and fresh fruit.

If you can find a cheap source of fresh fruit, it can become extremely economical to make your own juice or smoothies. Bananas are perfect fuel for cycling. Dried fruit is good, too.

While you are cycling, it is important to eat extra food on rides longer than about an hour, to prevent an energy crash. Bananas, sandwiches, dried fruit, and cereal bars are practical. If you want to stop for a cake, go ahead – you've earned the privilege.

Eat well

After a long bike ride, replenish your body's energy supplies, or the tiredness will discourage you from going out again. There are more tasty and healthy combinations of lean meat, poultry and fish, eggs and cheese, or nuts and pulses, along with carbohydrates in the form of rice, bread or pasta, and steamed or raw vegetables than there are days in a month. Go for variety, fresh ingredients, seasonal produce and home-made sauces and dressings.

Finally, hydration is important for your general health. Cycling can dehydrate you quite badly on a hot day, so drink plenty of water. There is no correct amount of water to drink in a day – it varies enormously depending on the temperature and how much you exercise – but in hot weather, when you

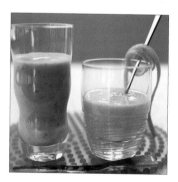

Above: Make your own juices and smoothies from fresh fruits.

have been out for an hour-long ride, you may need at least 2 litres (3.5 pints) of water. If you are not urinating often, you are dehydrated, but there's no need to consume huge volumes of water in a day if you're not thirsty.

Getting fit

As we have discovered, cycling has beneficial effects on your fitness levels. Regular cycling makes you fit and healthy, and for many, this is enough. But why stop there? If you design a long-term training plan and work on improving steadily in the long term, your fitness will continue to improve, with all the benefits that involves. It is a good idea to build a strong foundation of fitness, then progress further by adding time on the bike, or going a little harder.

The main principle involved in gaining fitness is overload. By stressing your body's muscles the cells within the muscles break down on a microscopic level, which explains the tiredness and stiffness you feel after exercise. However, your body will rebuild those cells stronger than they were before. You will become fitter.

In turn, as time progresses and you continue to ride, you will be capable of going just a little bit harder or faster than you could before. The muscle cells will break down again, and be rebuilt stronger than before.

The fitter you get, the closer to your capacity you will get, and the rate of improvement may slow. If you are just starting out in cycling you will be amazed at how fast your body adapts to the workload you are placing on it.

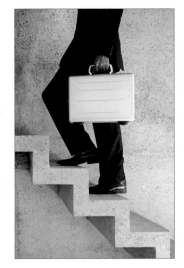

Above: Use the stairs at work whenever you possibly can, to give yourself a free daily workout.

It is easy to get carried away with an exercise regime when you first start out. The training plan below will suit anyone taking up cycling for the first time, but for unfit or overweight individuals, it is best to consult a doctor before taking up physical exercise. If the most you can handle is half the time on the schedule below, then that is the correct level for you to start at.

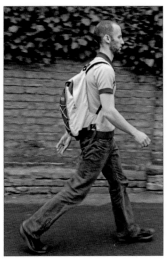

Above: Instead of taking public transport, briskly walk – this will burn calories and raise energy levels.

In only two months it is possible to make big changes in the level of your fitness, but at this stage the most important impact on your life will be to create the long-term habit of regular cycling. If you look on a training plan as a closed period of time that is only done once, you run the risk that when it is over you will sit back, relax and let your hard work go to waste.

Stick to the programme

Follow the training plan. Swap days around if urgent appointments get in the way of the schedule. Be flexible, and keep a record of each successful ride to spur you on. After one month, assess your progression, move on to month two, and then plan month three. This way, you will have the motivation of knowing that you are fitter than you were when you started, and you have a long-term plan beyond the initial two-month period. The most important thing is to establish cycling as a regular part of your life. The fitness benefits will come hand-in-hand with that.

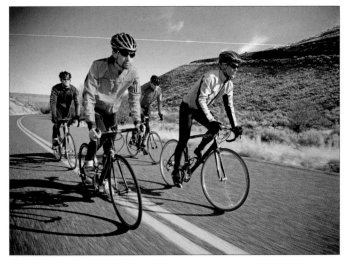

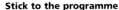

Left: By gradually making your training harder, your body will adapt to become fitter, stronger and more flexible.

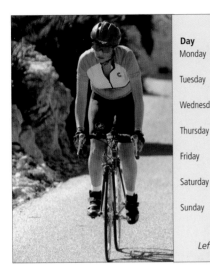

Day	Weeks one to four	Weeks five to eight
	Basic two-month training plan	
Monday	Rest day but if you wish do some gentle walking	Rest day with some gentle stretches or walking
Tuesday	Ride for about 30 minutes, slow and steady	Ride for about 1 hour at a moderate pace
Wednesday	Rest day, take it easy but if you wish do some gentle stretches	Rest day but do some gentle walking
Thursday	Ride for about 45 minutes, slow and steady	Ride for 1 hour at a moderate pace; go harder up the hills
Friday	Rest day with some gentle stretches and walking	Rest day but do some gentle stretches or walking
Saturday	Ride for about 1 hour, slow and steady	Ride for 1½ hours, slow and steady
Sunday	Ride for up to 1 hour, slow and steady (optional)	Ride for 1 hour, slow and steady (optional)

Left: Make cycling part of a healthy life by riding three or four times a week.

Lifestyle choices

In our basic two-month training system, there are three or four rides a week. Just this much exercise will help you reduce fat in your body to a healthy level. The maximum amount of time you will be on your bike in a week is only 3¼ hours at the start, which still leaves more than 164 hours over the rest of the week to sleep, eat, live and work!

There are some very easy changes you can make to your daily routine to make the most of your improved fitness levels and ensure that your healthy lifestyle doesn't stop when you get off the bike.

Stretch regularly to help to loosen muscles and improve flexibility.

Walk a little faster Pick up the pace a little, so you are conscious of your body working harder.

Take the stairs Cycling builds strength in the legs – make the most of it by taking the stairs whenever possible. Yes, even if you work on the 10th floor! Walk down, too, adding to your daily exercise.

Don't use motorized transport Popping to the supermarket for some shopping? Go by bike. Attach a basket or panniers to your bike to carry the shopping.

Right: Training regularly will reduce your vulnerability to injury.

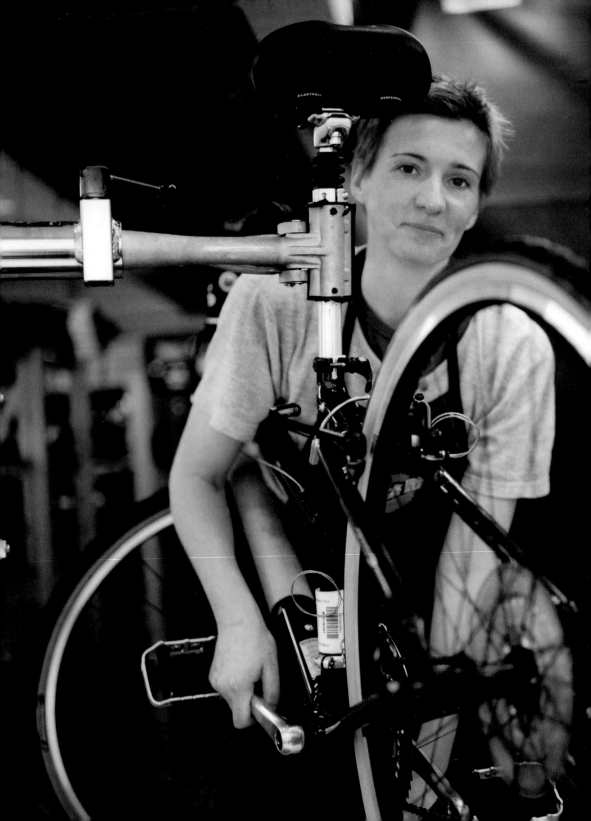

BIKE TECHNOLOGY

Maintaining a well-running bike is part of the enjoyment of cycling. It is easy to forget to look after your bike – they are so well-designed and engineered that it is possible to run them for long periods without maintenance or even cleaning. However, failing to look after your machine could lead to breakages, inefficient running and possibly even crashes. If you do a few small jobs regularly – some every time you ride, some on a weekly basis, and some once a month – your bike will continue to run as well as it did when it was new.

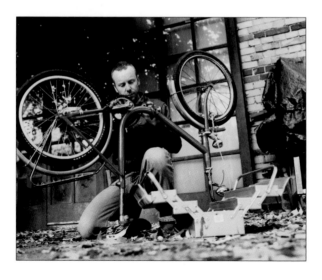

Above: Set aside an area in which to work on cleaning and repairs.
Left: To ensure its smooth running, learn how to maintain your bike.

Frames and Forks

The frame and forks are the heart of your bike. The material they are made out of, the angles of their design and the quality of the joins have more of an effect on the way your bike rides than any other component.

Bicycle frames need to be light and strong. The lighter the frame, the easier it is to ride up hills. The stronger the frame, the more reliable it will be. Both these factors depend on the material used and the thickness of the tubes. There is a third attribute, which affects how efficiently power is transferred from your legs into forward motion: stiffness. A stiff frame will respond better to accelerating forces, because less power is lost in the tubes flexing, but it can sometimes mean an uncomfortable ride over long distances – there is no shock absorbency, and the rider feels every bump and rut.

The geometry of the frame also affects the way the bike handles. The relaxed geometry of a touring frame makes for a comfortable ride, but acceleration is more sluggish. A steep-angled racing frame is much faster and more responsive, but over long distances is not as comfortable.

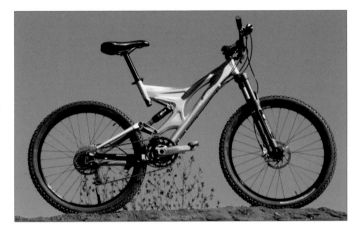

Above: Modern bike frames are available in all shapes and sizes. This one is a lightweight mountain bike with full suspension for shock absorbency.

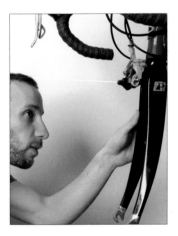

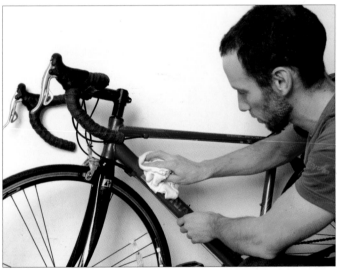

Above right: Wipe your frame clean every few days to prevent dirt building up.
Above left: It's important to inspect your frame and forks regularly to check for damage and denting.

Frame care		
Task	**Frequency**	**Time taken**
Wipe frame clean	Every 3 days	2 minutes
Check frame and fork for damage	After a crash	3–5 minutes

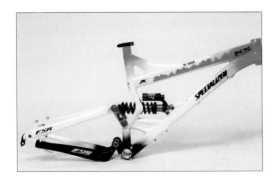

Above: A full-suspension mountain bike frame.

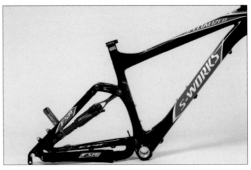

Above: A mountain bike frame with the suspension at the rear.

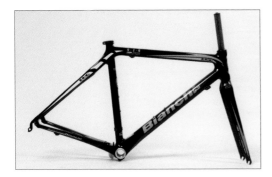

Above: A carbon fibre racing frame, which is stiffer than frames made from other materials.

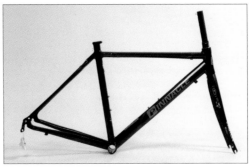

Above: A steel racing frame, which is more comfortable than carbon fibre.

Looking after the frame and fork

Unlike many parts of your bicycle, which can be stripped down into their constituent elements, the frame and the fork require very little in the way of maintenance. It is impossible to take the frame apart and put it back together again.

It is important to keep your frame clean because dirt and grit can quickly build up where the tubes join, and this can lead to scratches on the paintwork. After every ride in the wet, or every few days if the weather is dry, wipe your frame and forks with a damp cloth. This takes about two minutes and is well worth the time.

Another important task is to inspect your frame and fork regularly, especially if you have had a crash. Small dents and misalignments can eventually result in structural failure.

Materials

Frame materials have come a long way since the 1980s. Steel was the most popular and the best material for bike frames for most of the 20th century. Then, in the 1980s and 1990s, bike manufacturers started using carbon fibre, aluminium, titanium and even magnesium to make frames.

Steel is strong and easy to work with. Frames made of steel are very durable – if you avoid damaging them in crashes, they can last for a lifetime.

Aluminium is a more popular choice for racing bikes and serious tourers – it flexes less than steel, weighs far less and is cheap and easy to work with but it is not as durable. Aluminium frames seem to have a 'sell-by' date after which they wear faster than steel frames.

Carbon fibre is a popular material for high-end racing frames. It is as strong as steel and aluminium, and weighs even less than aluminium. Carbon fibre is moulded into shape, so that unusual frame designs such as monocoque time-trialling bikes can be made.

Titanium is strong and light, but is expensive and therefore a less common material for bike frames.

Suspension

For mountain bikes, it is not just the materials used for the frame and fork that have changed over the years. The development of suspension has radically altered the design of mountain bike frames and the way they handle. A suspension frame will be significantly more comfortable to ride on bumpy surfaces, but the suspension absorbs energy from the rider, resulting in a slower ride. There is also a payoff in having to maintain extra moving parts.

Wheels

Your bike is not going to get very far without these vital pieces of equipment. As with frames, the lighter and stronger the wheels are on your bike, the faster you will go. A little bit of maintenance of the wheels will give you a smoother ride.

Most wheels are designed along an arrangement of spokes radiating outward from the hub to the rim. The spokes are kept in tension, which makes the structure extraordinarily strong for its weight. Some specialized bikes for time trialling use solid carbon fibre bodies for superior aerodynamics, but the basic design of bike wheels has remained remarkably constant.

The two attributes of wheels that will affect the speed of your cycling the most are aerodynamics and weight. Even on a thin racing wheel there is a significant slowing effect from the spokes passing through the air. Manufacturers try to get around this by making the rims deeper.

Bike wheels are not particularly heavy compared with other parts of your bike, but the rotational movement increases their 'weight' through a phenomenon called gyroscopic inertia, whereby the momentum of the wheel resists changes to its orientation. In short, the less material there is in the wheel, the less energy it takes to brake and accelerate.

Racing-bike wheels are narrow and light, often containing 32, 28 or even 24

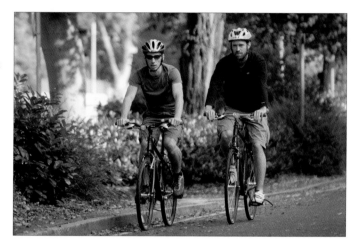

spokes – weight saved by cutting the number of spokes is significant, but the compromise is in the strength of the unit. Touring bikes, which carry much heavier loads, have 36- or 40-spoke wheels. Mountain bike wheels have a slightly smaller diameter, and they range between 28 and 36 spokes.

Spokes can be arranged in different patterns, which maintain lateral stiffness.

Above: Hybrid bikes need stronger wheels – they have an increased number of spokes, which add strength.

Looking after your wheels
Wheels are your bike's point of contact with the road and they consequently take a great deal of abuse, especially from rough road surfaces. Potholes, ruts and bumps in the road can put your

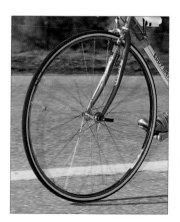

Above: Narrow-section racing wheel.

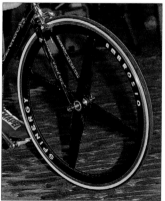

Above: Carbon fibre racing wheel.

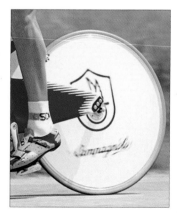

Above: Solid wheel for time trialling.

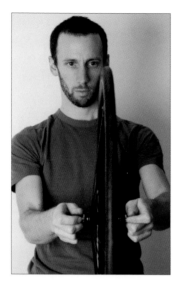

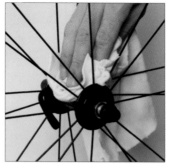

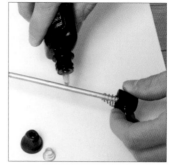

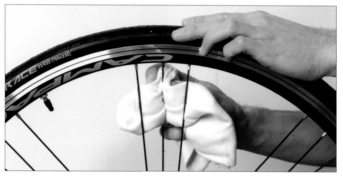

Above: Check your wheels for alignment by spinning them and watching the rim – if it moves, you may need to straighten your wheels.
Top middle: Prevent dirt building up on the hubs by wiping them every few days.
Top right: Apply grease to the axles on a regular basis.
Right: Wipe spokes down regularly.

wheels out of alignment, which affects your speed and leads to uneven braking. Learning to make wheels straight again is one of the great arts of bike maintenance. It involves mounting the

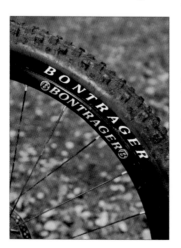

Wheel maintenance		
Task	**Frequency**	**Time taken**
Clean rims, hubs and spokes	Once a week	5 minutes
Check alignment	Once a week	30 seconds
Take axles out to clean and lubricate	Once a month	3 minutes
True your wheels (if you know how)	When misaligned	30 minutes+

wheel on a jig and tightening or loosening the spokes with a spoke key – called 'trueing' the wheel. When all of the spokes are at the correct tension, the wheel will be true, or straight, again.

Tyres
The fatter your tyres, the more comfortable the ride. The thicker your tyres, the less likely you are to suffer from punctures. But these benefits come at the cost of speed.

When choosing tyres for your bike, you must decide which kind of tyres best suit your needs. A racing bike needs slick, narrow tyres, although

Left: Thick tyres with a deep tread are used on mountain bikes.

punctures are more frequent. A touring bike needs slick tyres too, but wider, to fit wheels designed to take heavier weights. Mountain bikes need knobbly, thick tyres. These are good for puncture resistance, but much slower on a smooth surface.

Tyres are designated by size. Racing and touring tyres come in sizes between 700 x 20C and 700 x 28C (where 700 is the diameter of the tyre in millimetres and the second figure the width of the tyre in millimetres). But mountain bike wheels are generally 26in in diameter. Tyres are designated 26 x 1.5 (26in diameter x 1.5in wide) and upwards.

Always make sure you are buying the right size of tyre for your wheels, and choosing the right tyre for your needs.

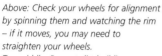

Drivetrain and Gears

The first bicycles had a single gear – good for riding on the flat but hard going up hills. Gears can make all the difference to whether your bike ride is easy or difficult. Understanding your gearing system will help you improve your cycling efficiency.

Racing bikes from the early 20th century managed to add a gear by putting one sprocket on either side of their back wheel – one for uphill sections, the other for flat roads. To change gear, the riders would dismount, unbolt their back wheels and turn them around.

Then Tullio Campagnolo, an Italian racing cyclist, came up with the idea of the derailleur gear, where the chain runs through a movable device and can change on to different sprockets while the bike is in motion. This is the gearing system used on most leisure bikes today.

The early derailleur gearing system had two or three sprockets on the back wheel. As technology evolved, it became possible to have two, then three chainwheels at the front, and in the case of modern bikes, 10 sprockets at the back, giving 30 possible gear ratios.

Gear ratios are what make it possible for you to ride your bike efficiently.

In a big gear, one revolution of the pedals causes more revolutions of the wheel, but it is correspondingly harder to push the pedals around. Smaller gears make it easier to ride up hills.

The more teeth on the chainwheel (at the front), and the smaller the sprocket (at the back), the bigger the

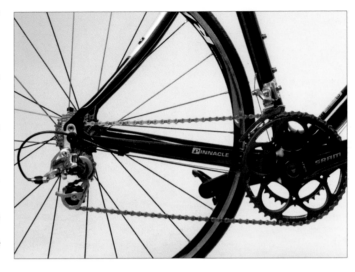

gear. On a typical racing bike, the front chainwheels have 42 and 52 teeth, although depending on the terrain, many riders change these for slightly smaller or larger numbers of teeth. At the back, sprockets range from 11 teeth (a high gear used only on steep downhills and in sprints) to 23 or 25 teeth, enough to get up long, steep hills. When selecting a gear, keep the chain as

Above: The drivetrain consists of chainrings, which are attached to the pedals and cranks at the front, and a range of sprockets at the back.

straight as possible. Riding in the big chainwheel, which is on the right-hand side, with the largest sprocket, which is on the left-hand side, puts the chain at an angle, which will quickly wear out both chain and cogs. On a 30-gear bike, there is enough crossover between gear ratios that you can change to the middle chainwheel and a smaller sprocket to find a similar gear.

Try to avoid overgearing – professional racing cyclists can cruise along in a 52-tooth chainwheel and 14-tooth sprocket, but trying to push big gears puts a strain on the knees. Aim instead to spin the pedals faster.

Looking after your drivetrain

The chain, chainwheels, sprockets and front and back gear changers are the parts of your bike that are most prone to dirt accumulation.

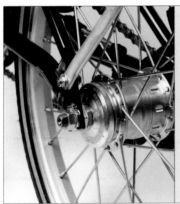

Hub gears

Shopping and town bikes sometimes come with three- or five-speed hub gears, where the changing mechanism lies in a sealed unit within the back hub. These do not offer as many different gear ratios as racing or leisure bikes and they are not as power efficient. If you are too busy to maintain your bike regularly, and only want your bike for riding around town, it is worth considering buying a bike with hub gears.

Left: Hub gears require just a squirt of lubricant every few weeks.

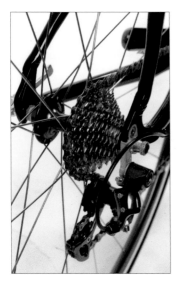

Above: The rear mech shifts the chain from side to side along the sprockets on the back wheel.

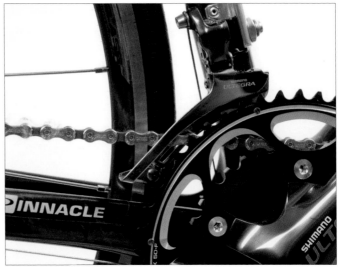

Above: The front gear mechanism shifts the chain from one chainring to another.

Keeping a smooth-running and clean drivetrain is crucial for the efficient performance of your bike. If you do not clean your gearing system, dirt and grit sticks to the lubricant and forms a thick, sticky black coating that wears down moving parts, makes changing gear inefficient and generally gets everywhere. Once this has built up, it takes a lot of time and effort to clean it off. It is far better to spend 15 minutes once or twice a week to clean and lubricate your gears than to leave it for a month, then have to spend an hour up to your elbows in dirty grease while

risking damage to your drivetrain. To clean the chain, you can use a chain-breaking tool to take it off the bike. An easier way is to attach a chain-cleaning bath to the bike. These are made of plastic and contain brushes and a reservoir of cleaner. Bike shops sell degreasers and solvents that will loosen the dirt on your chain.

To clean sprockets and chainwheels remove them from the bike and scrub out the dirt with a hard brush and cleaner. When cleaning sprockets that are still on the back wheel, be careful not to let grease drip on to the rims. You can buy a brush called a cassette scraper to clean between the sprockets. Finally, the derailleurs also need careful cleaning and attention. You can

generally wipe a front derailleur clean, but most dirt build-up occurs in the rear derailleur. Remove it from the bike and clean all the moving parts, paying special attention to the jockey wheels.

Once everything is clean, use a light lubricant. Too much lubricant will result in more dirt build-up.

Cleaning little and often, with a major stripping-down every month or two, will keep your bike in perfect, efficient working order.

Below: Modern racing bikes have their gear changers built into the brake levers.

Drivetrain care		
Task	**Frequency**	**Time taken**
Clean chain using a chain bath	Once a week (more in wet conditions or winter)	5 minutes
Clean sprockets	Once a week	15 minutes
Clean rear derailleur	Once a week	15 minutes
Clean front derailleur	Once a week	5 minutes
Take entire drivetrain apart for deep cleaning and lubricating	Once a month	30 minutes
Clean hub gear	Once a month	10 seconds

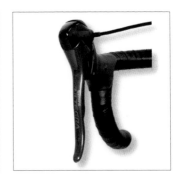

Brakes

A well-maintained set of brakes is one of the most important components of your bike. While an inefficient drivetrain or slightly untrue wheel will affect your speed and make cycling hard work, a badly worn set of brakes is potentially a killer.

Until the advent of mountain bikes, most bikes came with simple calliper brakes. By pulling a cable attached to the brakes, the brake blocks came into contact with the rim of the wheel, and the friction slowed the bike down. With narrow rims and lightweight wheels, not much surface area is needed on the brake blocks, meaning stopping performance with calliper brakes is generally very good.

Calliper brakes come in a variety of designs. Dual-pivot brakes are common on racing bikes and leisure bikes, and consist of two arms, one of which pivots around a point above the wheel, while the other pivots at the side. The arms grip the rim. They are light and useful for around-town use and longer rides, but should not be used on mountain bikes, where greater stopping power is needed, and the thick tyres get in the way.

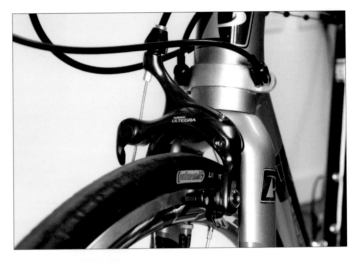

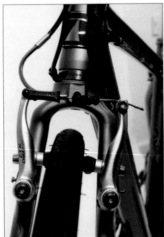

Above: Racing bikes are fitted with dual-pivot calliper brakes, which are lightweight and provide good stopping power.

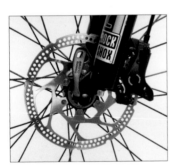

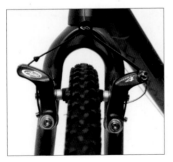

Above: Cantilever brakes are a good option for mountain bikes if disc brakes are not practical.
Above left: Modern mountain bikes are fitted with disc brakes, which provide good stopping power in poor conditions.
Left: V-brakes are fitted to hybrid bikes, and mountain bikes for urban use.

Cantilever brakes have each arm attached to a pivot point on the forks or seat stays. These have greater clearance than side-pull brakes, so they can be used on mountain bikes for riding around town, or light-duty off-roading. These brakes have generally been replaced for urban use by V-brakes, which have the cable housing on one arm, and the cable wire on the other. The longer arms of cantilever brakes provide more stopping power than V-brakes: they are also easier to maintain.

For serious mountain biking, especially on steep hills, traditional cable brakes are not strong enough to control speed effectively. Mountain bikes have heavier, wider wheels, and disc brakes, similar to those used in motorbikes and cars, can be used for greater stopping power. Disc brakes are heavier than traditional calliper brakes, but they work far better, and are easy to look after.

Brake maintenance

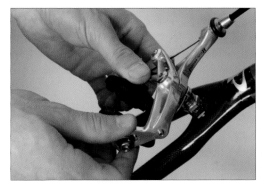

Alignment: *Check brakes for alignment regularly.*

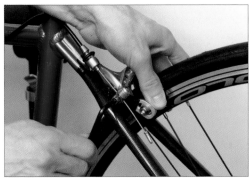

Cables: *Maintain stopping power by keeping cables tight.*

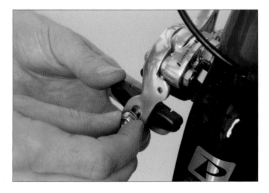

Blocks: *Replace worn brake blocks.*

Clean: *Keep your brakes clean and oil-free by wiping often.*

There is a metal disc attached to the hub, and brake pads squeeze the disc to slow the bike down. The benefit of disc brakes is that they work as well in wet as in dry conditions. Disc brakes are used for touring, when heavier loads make stopping difficult.

Brakes wear out fast, especially calliper brakes in poor conditions, and it is important to keep an eye on the rate of wear of the rubber brake blocks. When you notice blocks getting worn, replace them – unscrew the old ones from the brake arms and put the new ones on. Never replace just one brake block, and be careful to align it with the rim, so that the whole surface of the block is in contact with the rim when the brake lever is pulled. Brake levers are low maintenance, and do not need

to be stripped and cleaned often. You should also check your cables. Brake cables stretch, with a marked effect on performance. When you notice braking is less efficient than before, loosen the cable where it passes through the brake arms, then pull it through so it is tight again. The brake arms are exposed to all the dirt and grit that flies up off the

wheel, so keep them clean. Don't clean your disc brakes too often, as tiny bits of brake pad embedded in the disc surface improve performance, but it is important to keep the disc and callipers aligned – just loosen the callipers, line them up, and tighten again. Do not allow oil to get on to the surface of disc brakes – this will affect their performance.

Brake care		
Task	**Frequency**	**Time taken**
Check brake blocks	Once a week	30 seconds
Replace brake blocks	When they are worn	5 minutes
Tighten brake cables on calliper brakes	Once a week	5 minutes
Clean calliper brake arms	Once a week	1 minute
Check alignment of disc brakes	After every ride	30 seconds
Realign disc brakes	When they are out of true	5 minutes

Bike Maintenance

You have a choice when it comes to looking after your bike. You can invest small, convenient amounts of time on a regular basis, or you can pay for inaction with large amounts of time every few months, by which time your bike is dirty, worn and inefficient.

Although you do not need to clean your bike after every ride, it will save you trouble in the long term if you clean it after riding off-road, in muddy conditions or in rain. If you leave mud or grit on your bike, the parts are liable to rust or wear more quickly. In the winter, salt from roads can affect the smooth working of the bike and lead to rust.

Keeping your bike clean
The tools you will need are a bucket of warm water with detergent, a cloth and a brush. As a general rule, try to clean your bike once a week, and less in the summer months. To hold the bike firmly, attach it to a stand. Using a brush or a cloth, wash the frame, forks, wheels, including the spokes, hub and rims, the cranks, seatpin, handlebars and stem (where they are not covered by handlebar tape), brake levers, brakes and cable housings. Rinse the parts with clean water then polish with a clean dry cloth.

Replacing handlebar tape
If your handlebar tape becomes very worn and dirty from use, or if you scuff it in a crash, it is time to replace it. This is a fairly easy task, requiring only some sharp scissors or a knife and a roll of new handlebar tape.

Take the bar end plugs off; you may need to use a screwdriver or other tool to loosen them. Fold the edges of your brake lever hoods forward so they are out of the way and expose the old bar tape. Unwrap the old bar tape, cutting off pieces here and there and discarding them. Remove any leftover glue.

Replacement bar tape usually comes with two short lengths of tape – these are for covering the brake lever clamps. Stick these two lengths on first. Then start winding tape from the bottom of the handlebars, making sure that there is enough tape at the start to tuck into the handlebar ends.

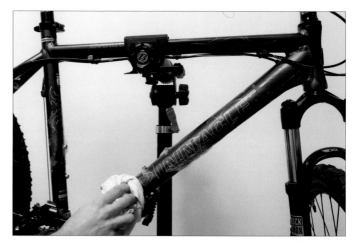

Above: Use a soft, clean cloth and detergent to wipe your frame, paying particular attention to corners where dirt can accumulate.

Keep winding round, overlapping up to half the width of the tape each time round. Pull on the tape as you are wrapping, to maintain the tension and avoid slackness, which will quickly come unstuck as you are riding.

When you get to the brake levers, work around them, making sure not to leave any part of the bars uncovered, then continue to wrap the tape around and around all the way to the tops of the handlebars.

Cut off any excess tape, and use black electrical tape to secure the end of the tape at the centre of your handlebars and tuck the other ends into the hollow end of the handlebars. Replace the bar end plugs, ensuring that the end of tape is tucked inside, and you are ready to go.

It's important to make sure the bar end plugs are firmly pushed in. Riding without these can be dangerous if you crash, and hit the bars with your leg.

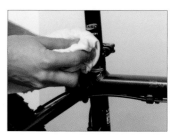

Above: Brush off any grit or mud before rubbing the frame with a damp cloth, then polishing with a clean cloth.

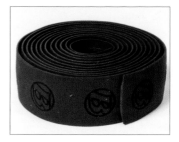

Above: When the handlebar tape becomes worn and uncomfortable to hold, it can be easily replaced.

Replacing a tyre and tube

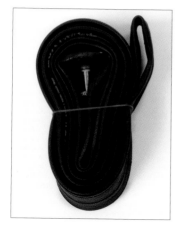

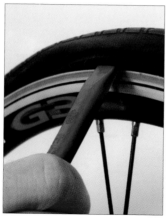

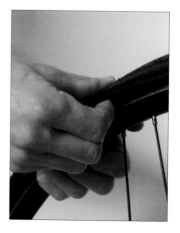

Tube: *Keep spare inner tubes in case you have a puncture that you cannot repair.*

1 *To remove tyre, insert a tyre lever. Keep it wedged there and insert the next. Then, lever along the rim to get the rest out.*

2 *Once you have got one side of the tyre away from the rim, use your fingers to remove it completely.*

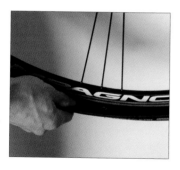

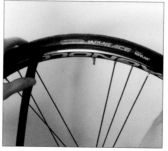

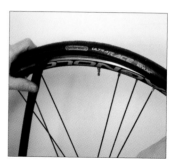

3 *Put one side of the new tyre inside the rim, then be ready to insert inner tube.*

4 *Put the valve through the hole in the rim, put the inner tube inside the tyre.*

5 *Continue working the inner tube inside the tyre, around the wheel.*

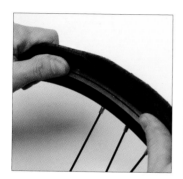

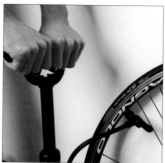

Basic maintenance equipment
Surgical latex gloves
Full set of Allen keys
Pliers and adjustable spanner (wrench)
Tyre levers
Track pump (upright with pressure gauge)
Screwdrivers and chain breaker
Degreaser
Chain lubricant
Freewheel remover with chain whip
Spanners (wrenches)
Bike stand
Cable cutter
Repair kit

6 *Press the other side of the tyre inside rim. Take care not to puncture the tube.*

7 *When the tube is inside the tyre and the tyre is inside the rim, pump it up.*

Preventing Problems

Bike maintenance can be broken down into a few basic tasks, which, if done on a regular basis, will keep your bike running smoothly. Rather than waiting for problems to develop, it is a good idea to pre-empt these by regular, careful maintenance.

Sticking to a few golden rules will help you to keep your bike in good order. Just by getting into the habit of regularly cleaning your bike, you will familiarize yourself with all its parts and will be alert for anything that is out of order.

Drivetrain maintenance

The drivetrain (chainwheels, chain and sprockets) is the part of your bike that is most vulnerable to dirt build-up and damage. Over time, dirt from the road or bike path will stick to the chain lubricant to form a thick black coating. If this is not cleaned off, the moving parts can be damaged by the grit being ground in. Every week, if you ride your bike regularly, it's a good idea to use a chain bath to clean the chain. This is an

Disassembly, cleaning and maintenance

1 Break the chain using a chain breaker. These push a rivet through so that the links can be pulled apart (never push a rivet all the way through, as you will not be able to get it back in). Some chains, called powerlink chains, have a single link that can be unhooked manually.
2 Take the back wheel off. Using a chain whip and freewheel remover, take the sprockets off the back wheel.
3 Undo your chainrings with Allen keys.
4 Scrub all sprockets, chain rings and chain using a degreaser. If very dirty, leave them to sit in a tub of degreaser.
5 Loosen cables and remove front and rear mechanism. Scrub with detergent. Use

degreaser for a large build-up of dirt.
6 Replace cables if they are stretched by running them through from the handlebars down to the mechs.
7 Reattach front and rear mech. Pull cables through so they are taut. Tighten.
8 Put freewheel back on wheel. Replace wheel. Run chain through front and rear mechs, and reattach chain using chain tool.
9 Use a rag to apply a light but even layer of lubricant to the chain.
10 Double-check that indexing of gears is accurate (such that a single gear change moves the chain one sprocket). Adjust using the barrel adjuster on the rear mechanism.

Cleaning bike parts

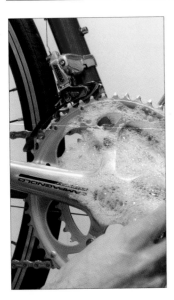

Chainwheel: *Use warm water with detergent to clean your chainwheels regularly and prevent dirt building up.*

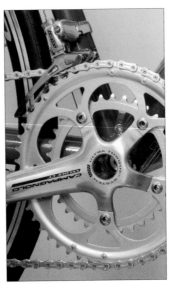

Chainset: *Examine the alignment of your chainset regularly to ensure that the chainwheel has not been damaged.*

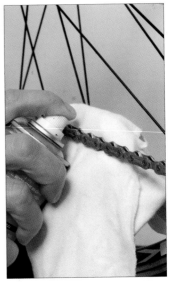

Lubricate: *Clean your chain regularly by spraying it with a chain cleaner and lubricant, then wiping with a cloth.*

Maintaining your bike

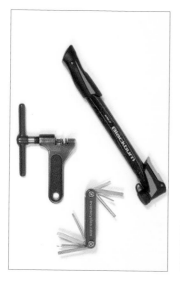

Toolkit: *Always carry a toolkit that contains basic equipment.*

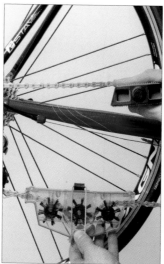

Chain cleaner: *Run your chain through a special bath, filled with cleaner.*

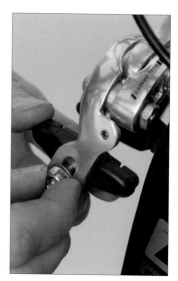

Brake blocks: *Replace brake blocks when worn, as they can be hazardous.*

attachment which fits around the chain, and contains brushes and a bath which can be filled with degreaser or cleaner. Simply run the chain through a few times, and the dirt will be scrubbed off.

You should also pay attention to the chainwheels, by scrubbing with detergent and water, and also the sprockets, by removing the rear wheel and scrubbing with degreaser or detergent. Then use a rag to apply a small but consistent layer of lubricant to the chain.

Golden rules

If you keep your bike clean, and lubricate the moving parts on a regular basis, it will work more efficiently, and last much longer without breaking down. This will save you money in the long term, and also ensure that your bike remains safe to ride. Worn brakes are hazardous. Always replace worn parts before they become dangerous. A poorly maintained chain can snap, with dangerous repercussions. A well-maintained bike is a safe bike.

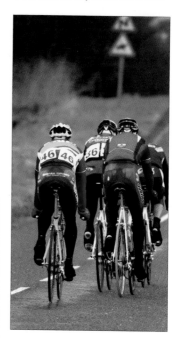

Above: In wet and muddy conditions, your bike builds up a lot of dirt and grease that can damage small parts.

Adjust your brakes

1 When brake blocks are worn, remove them and put new ones in, checking they are aligned with the rim.
2 If cables are stretched, replace them. Pull the cable through to the brake arms.
3 Tighten the cable. Check that the brake arms are centred. Adjust using the adjustment screw on the calliper.
4 Check that brakes are tight. If not, hold the brake blocks almost to the wheel rim, pull the cable through and tighten the bolt holding the cable.

Clean your drivetrain

1 Attach a chain bath containing degreaser to your bike, and run the chain through until the dirt has come off.
2 Remove the back wheel from your bike. Using a brush and degreaser, scrub the freewheel clean of dirt.
3 Scrub the chainwheels with detergent and water for light dirt. Use degreaser if necessary.
4 Put the back wheel in, and use a rag to apply a small but consistent layer of lubricant to the chain.

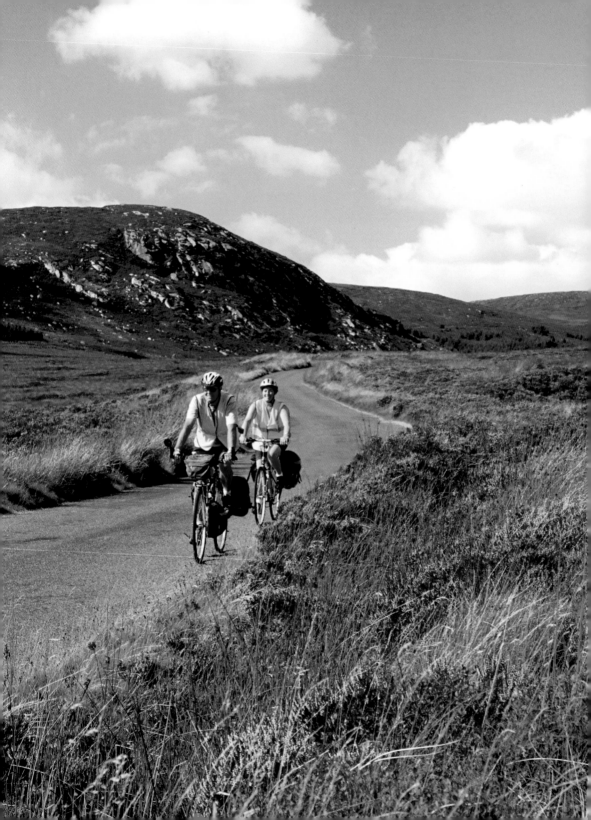

TOURING

Touring on a bike is a rewarding cycling experience.
Whether it is a day-trip, a weekend away, a week-long
tour in a foreign country or a full-scale off-road
expedition, bicycle touring is the ultimate in self-
sufficient, independent and environmentally friendly
tourism. Planning a trip is part of the fun, and designing
an interesting route can add to the enjoyment. Keeping
your baggage light is also an important part of touring.
And for those with a spirit of adventure, there is the
challenge and fun of camping with the bike.

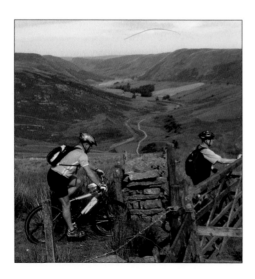

Above: Travelling light is essential when touring for long distances.
Left: Touring is one of the best ways to explore the countryside.

The Touring Bike

It is technically possible to go cycle touring on any bike. The fact that you own a mountain bike or hybrid bike should not prevent you from planning short-distance tours. However, it will be better to invest in a fully equipped touring bike.

For touring, especially long distances, buying a specialized bike is a great idea. Touring bikes are light but strong: self-sufficiency is the basis of cycle touring, and the bike must be durable enough to carry a heavy load for long periods of time.

The classic touring bike resembles a racing bike, but with several subtle differences that make it ideal for the purpose. The frame has more relaxed geometry than a racing bike, which makes it more comfortable over long distances. This sacrifices a bit of speed, but bike tours are not races. The wheels are strong, with heavy-duty tyres to prevent punctures. The fewer punctures you have on a long tour, the more you can enjoy the experience of the trip.

There are fittings for panniers over the rear wheel, and often over the front wheel as well. For a long tour, it's sometimes necessary to carry a lot of equipment, and if the load is spread evenly, it is easier to carry. Many cycle tourists attach bags to the handlebars, for maps, money and anything you need easy access to, with a basic toolkit in a bag under the saddle. Mudguards are essential – they add very little to the

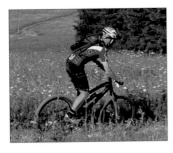

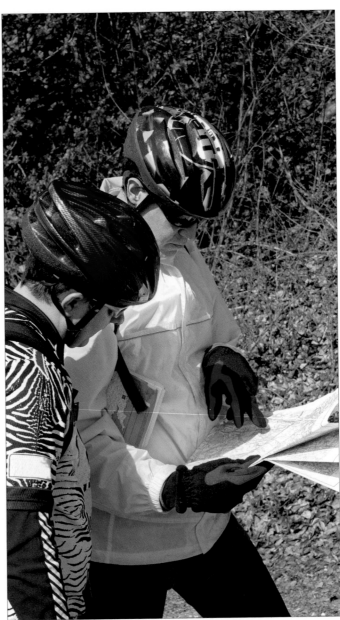

Above: A mountain bike is also suitable for a touring trip.
Right: Planning your route and following it is one of the enjoyable challenges of cycle touring.

weight of the bike, but keep you and your clothes drier in the case of rain (and your spare clothes will be limited).

When buying a touring bike, take time to think about which model will be best. If the longest tour you are going to do is a weekend of 50km (30 mile) rides, a hybrid bike with pannier fittings will be adequate, and good for riding around town as well.

If you are planning full-scale expeditions, covering up to 160km (100 miles) a day for a week or two, it is important to invest in a resilient, reliable and comfortable bike.

Make sure you give the bike a good test ride before you buy it, to see whether the saddle is right for you.

If your tours will include off-road riding, choose a hybrid or mountain bike, adapted and equipped so you can carry your luggage.

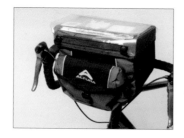

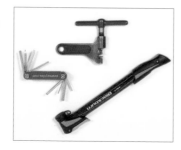

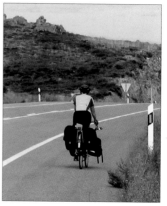

Above: Panniers fitted over the rear wheel can store your equipment on tour.
Top left: It's practical to keep money and maps in a handlebar bag.
Left: Allen keys, chain breaker and pump.

Anatomy of a touring bike

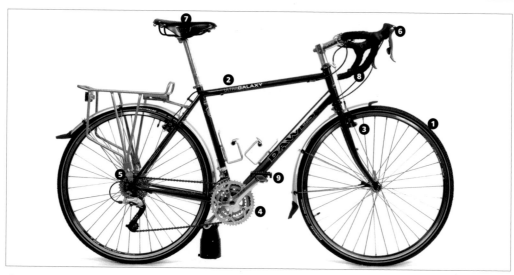

1 Wheels: Strong and durable, with 36 spokes to help take the weight of luggage and rider. The tyres are thick, with a good tread that will help to prevent punctures.

2 Frame: Comfortable, light and strong with relaxed geometry for riding long distances. The frame has attachments for rear panniers, pump and water bottles.

3 Brakes: Cantilever brakes for general touring. Some models have disc brakes, although maintenance is difficult with these.

4 Chainrings: A triple chainset offers low and high gears. With a heavier load, lower gears are needed to climb hills.

5 Sprockets: Nine gears at the back for all gradients.

6 Gear changers: These are attached to the brake levers to allow for good accessibility.

7 Saddle: Wide and padded for comfort during long rides.

8 Handlebars: Drop handlebars give a wide variety of hand positions, for comfort.

9 Pedals: Clipless pedals for combined walking/cycling shoes.

Touring Equipment 1

Develop the art of travelling light when touring on a bike. If you limit yourself to the bare essentials, you can go anywhere. Stick to a few guidelines and eliminate all the heavy unnecessary gear that will just weigh you down.

The number one rule in bike touring equipment is to take as little as you possibly can. That's not to say that you can leave the sleeping bag or map book at home, but superfluous equipment and items in your panniers have to be hauled everywhere – if you don't need to use something, leave it at home.

Pack a tool kit

For every trip, whether it's a day-long ride or an expedition, a toolkit is essential. You will need spare inner tubes and a patching kit in case of punctures. Allen keys for loosening and tightening bolts on the bike are useful.

A chain breaker is also necessary – breakages are rare, especially if you maintain your chain properly, but when it happens the only way to repair the chain is with a chain breaker. Perhaps more importantly, you will also need it every time you have to remove a wheel. Optional extras include a spare spoke, spoke key, screwdriver, spare cables and brake pads. It would be possible to carry a great deal more, but the compromise

Right: Always take a map on tours to keep track of where you are.
Below: If you're well equipped, you can relax and enjoy your tour.

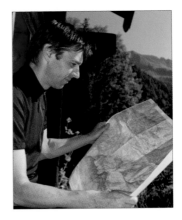

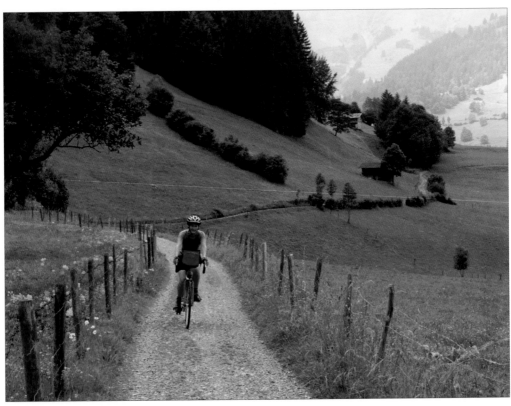

between travelling light and covering all possible eventualities has to be made. As a self-sufficient cyclist, you are responsible for deciding how to manage the risks of mechanical failure. But never go anywhere without a chain breaker.

Cycling clothing

Sensible clothing will make touring easier. Ordinary cycling clothing is perfect – it is light, warm, and keeps the sweat away from your skin. Shoes should be combined walking and cycling shoes, with a cleat to clip into the pedals. You will need clean clothing every day for cycling, and clothes to wear in the evening when it is cooler and you are not cycling. The longer you spend away, the more you have to consider how to ensure clean clothes every day. Hardened cycle tourists work along the principle that two sets of clothing will suffice – one to wear, one to wash. This keeps weight down, but it is worth considering a small number of spare garments in case washing facilities are impossible to find.

If you are washing your cycling kit on the go, remember to bring detergent. Clean kit is essential on a long tour, because riding in dirty shorts increases the chances of a nasty and probably painful infection. Some cycle tourists wash their clothes, then they attach them securely to the outside of

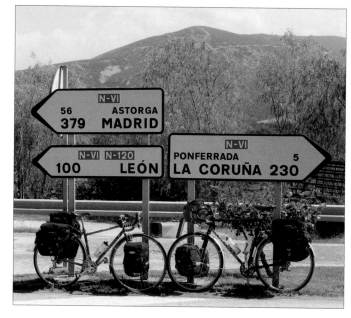

Above: Bike touring is one of the best ways to see and understand other countries and cultures.

their panniers, so they don't flap into the wheel. The motion of the bike wheeling smoothly along through moving air, combined with the heat of the sun, dries and freshens their clothes in no time.

Books and other essentials

Purists would say no to carrying books – after all, they're not essential. But a little extra weight for the sake of sanity and something to do in the evening is a payoff that most people would find reasonable.

You will also need a few essential items. Buy a detailed map of the area you are visiting before you leave home. In order to save weight, rather than taking an entire map book, you can detach the pages you need and only carry them. It's also a good idea to put map pages in waterproof sleeves, to prevent damage in wet conditions. Take a wallet with credit cards, identification and spare cash. Lastly, pack a mobile phone in case of emergencies. If you are staying in hotels or hostels, that is all you will need. If you are camping, you will also need to make space in your panniers for a tent, roll mat, sleeping bag, camping stove, plate, cup and cutlery. Suddenly the third set of clothing looks like a less practical idea.

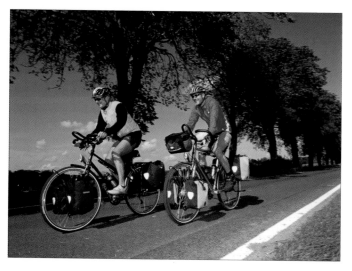

Left: Touring bikes are heavily loaded with conventional panniers at the back, as well as having capacity for extra baggage over the front wheels.

Touring Equipment 2

Modern cycling and camping gear means that you can go on a full-scale expedition without hauling several kilograms of extra weight up every hill. Over the course of an 800km (500 mile) tour, this makes a huge difference.

If you are going away for fewer than five days or if you are staying at hotels or hostels there is no need to attach front and back panniers to your touring bike. Back panniers and a handlebar bag have enough space for all the equipment you might need for a few days' cycling. If you cannot fit it all in, unpack and try again!

Panniers and tents

Front panniers become useful when you are carrying camping equipment. The main challenge is to balance all your kit equally on both sides of the bike. If your bags are heavier on one side, it will affect the handling of your bike.

A lightweight one-person tent generally weighs about the same as a sleeping bag, so a good idea is to put these on opposite sides at the back. Then cooking equipment can be split,

Below: A winding road in the Rocky Mountains, through beautiful scenery, is ideal for cycle touring.

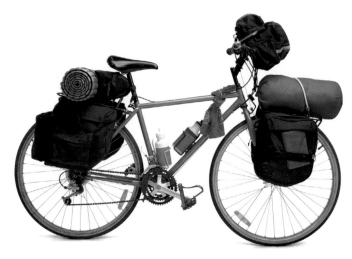

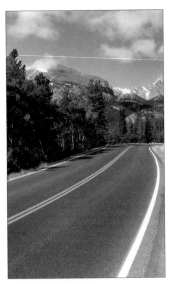

with spare clothes going in the front panniers. Roll mats are bulky but don't weigh much – they can stay on the outside, in a waterproof bag in case of wet weather. Sometimes tents are heavier than any other piece of equipment, but it should be possible to carry tent poles on one side, and the body of the tent on the other, then various items can balance.

Try to keep heavier items at the back, while light but bulky things are fine in front. Too much weight at the front will make steering more difficult.

Things become more efficient if you are camping with a group of people. Communal equipment like tents and cooking utensils can be shared out between everybody, with individually owned items such as sleeping bags and clothes in one's own panniers.

What if it rains?

Bad weather is the last thing the cycle tourist wants to experience but it is always a possibility. Soaking wet kit will cast a real dampener on a holiday, especially if you are camping and have

Above: A fully loaded bike with a handlebar bag, panniers, tent, sleeping bag and water bottles.

no means of drying it out. Unless the weather forecast is for an immovable ridge of high pressure over the area you are camping in and bright sunshine

Below: On a cycling tour, a global positioning system (GPS) will locate your position accurately. It is ideal if you are travelling long distances.

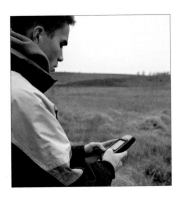

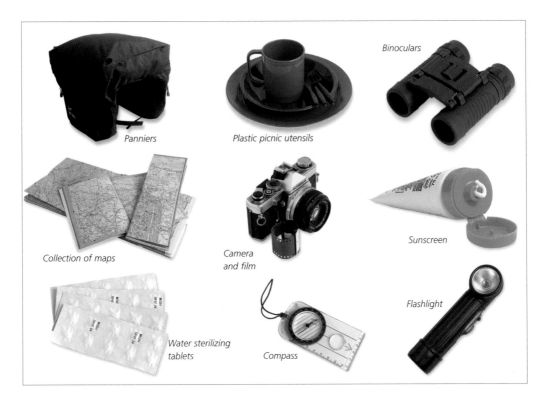

Panniers

Plastic picnic utensils

Binoculars

Collection of maps

Camera and film

Sunscreen

Water sterilizing tablets

Compass

Flashlight

Above: A selection of equipment that would be useful when touring includes panniers to fit on a bike, plastic picnic utensils, a pair of binoculars, a collection of maps to cover the area, a camera and film, a sunscreen of SPF25, water sterilizing tablets, a compass as an aid to navigation and a waterproof flashlight.

every day, it's best to bring plastic bags to put inside your panniers, to keep the contents dry. A raincoat will repel all but the heaviest rainstorms and keep your cycling clothes dry.

If all your kit is damp, and there is no prospect of a dry day's cycling, try to include an extra long stop at a friendly roadside café. While you enjoy a warming hot chocolate and cake, ask permission to hang your wet kit on a radiator or chair. The psychological boost of warming up and having dry kit to change into will make the difference between an enjoyable trip and the holiday from hell.

Touring checklist

Equipment	Day trip	Weekend away	Week-long tour	Expedition
Rear panniers	-	Y	Y	Y
Front panniers	-	-	(Y)	Y
Cycling shoes	Y	Y	Y	Y
Cycling clothes	Y	Y(2)	Y(2)	Y(2-3)
Raincoat	(Y)	(Y)	Y	Y
Spare tubes	Y	Y	Y	Y
Allen keys	Y	Y	Y	Y
Chain breaker	Y	Y	Y	Y
Spare spoke, cables and brake blocks	-	-	-	Y
Sleeping bag	-	(Y)	(Y)	Y
Tent	-	(Y)	(Y)	Y
Roll mat	-	(Y)	(Y)	Y
Cooking equipment	-	-	(Y)	Y
Plate, cup and utensils	-	-	(Y)	Y
Map	Y	Y	Y	Y
Money	Y	Y	Y	Y
Torch	-	-	(Y)	Y
Book	-	-	Y	Y

Above: It may be useful to copy this list and tick off items as you gather them together before packing your panniers.

Planning a Tour

For some cycle tourists, half the fun of a good cycling tour is in the planning. If you take some time and effort before you leave to make sure that your bike and equipment are in good order and that you have everything you need, the tour is likely to run without hitches.

It is fun to design an itinerary using maps and guidebooks. You don't have to carve a route in stone and adhere to it religiously – you may be tired one day, or you may want to stay an extra day – but if you have a plan of your route, your tour is likely to be rewarding.

The morning of your departure is not the time to organize your cycling holiday. The first decision should be made days, weeks or even months in advance – namely, where to go. There may be a particular area whose scenery you are attracted to, or a place you want to visit for cultural reasons. You might want to go to a quiet area away

Below: Spectacular scenery is one of the many joys of cycle touring.

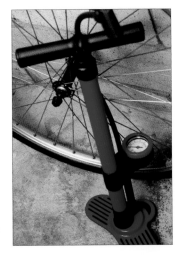

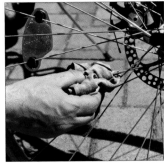

Above: A well maintained bike is essential: breakdowns can ruin a bike tour if you are miles from help.
Left: Before leaving for a tour of any distance, do pump up your tyres.

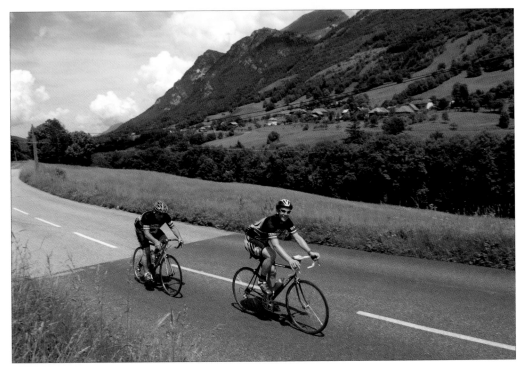

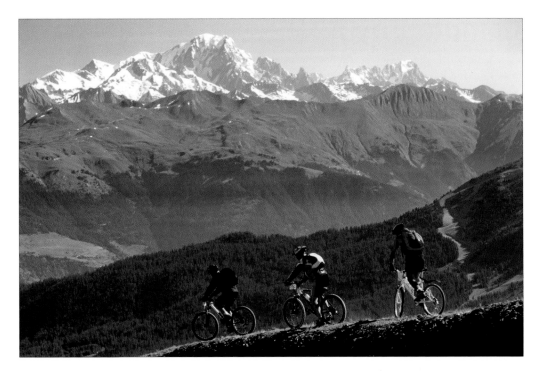

from the beaten track, or a region that is popular with tourists. Flat or mountainous? At home or abroad? The main thing to realize is that within limits, you are free to go cycle touring almost anywhere in the world.

Know your route

Once you have decided where you are going, you should buy a detailed road map of the area. If you are planning to stay in hotels, can you guarantee that the next town is close enough to reach in one day's cycling? You should plan your route using your map and according to your ability to cover the distance, with the emphasis on quiet roads and scenic routes. If you are capable of riding 65km (40 miles) a day, don't plan to stay in a hotel that is 95km (60 miles) from the last one. If you want to ride 160km (100 miles) every day, make sure to plan your accommodation accordingly.

If you are cycling in a mountainous area, gradients and altitudes are sometimes indicated on maps. Chevrons on the road indicate that the road is

going uphill, and in high mountain ranges such as the Alps or the Rockies, hills can go on for many miles. Ensure that your gearing is low enough for you to pedal with all your equipment in tow.

Most importantly, be flexible. If you are more tired than you anticipated, stop at the next town and stay there. You are free to do whatever you want.

Preparing for the tour

Your bike should be in perfect running order before you leave. Mechanical failure could stop your tour right where it happens, so look after your bike and give it a service before your departure. After the service, take it out for a ride to test that it is running well. If you are camping, it pays to double-check that none of the tent poles have gone missing or are damaged. Erect the tent in your garden, then pack it immediately and put it into your panniers. The day before you leave, wash and dry all the clothes you are taking with you, and pack them into your bags, along with all your other equipment. You are now set for the journey of a lifetime.

Above: Touring doesn't have to follow roads – with mountain bikes it is possible to strike out across country. Many countries have trails for bikes, but it is always best to check first.

---

10 steps to a successful tour

1. Decide which region you are going to cycle in.

2. Plan your route, including daily distances and stopping points.

3. If you are travelling farther afield, you may need a visa. Check for any restrictions or requirements for taking your bike on to trains, ferries or aeroplanes.

4. Plan accommodation, book if necessary.

5. Clean your bike, ensure it is running well, test brakes and gears, pump up tyres.

6. Make a list of equipment to take.

7. Check that the tent has all poles and fittings. Put it up to make sure it is in good working order.

8. Wash your clothes.

9. Get new batteries for lights.

10. Pack your panniers.

Enjoy the ride!

Camping by Bike

Cycle touring is a great way to enjoy an independent holiday. When you add camping into the equation, it becomes the ultimate in self-sufficiency. There is no need to worry about finding accommodation or a suitable place to eat supper.

Modern tents are lightweight, very easy to erect and pack down to take up very little space. You can buy single-person tents that are big enough to fit one person in a sleeping bag, and they weigh less than 1 kilogram (2 pounds). Modern synthetic sleeping bags are warm and light.

Camping does make a cycle tour more challenging. A roll mat on a hard surface is not as comfortable as a hotel bed. Nor is it as warm. If it rains, your tent is waterproof, but every time you go in and out with wet clothes on, everything becomes a little damper. Sleep might not be as deep as it would be in a bed, so you will be more tired, an important consideration when you are cycling a long distance the next day.

On the plus side, you are closer to nature when camping. If you are pitching wild, rather than staying at an organized campsite, the sense of escapism is hard to equal. Away from towns that are crowded with tourists and traffic, you can discover solitude, peace and tranquillity.

It is easier to plan your route around campsites, which allow you to pitch your tent in their grounds. This costs money, but not much, and if the idea of a week without human contact intimidates you, campsites are far more sociable.

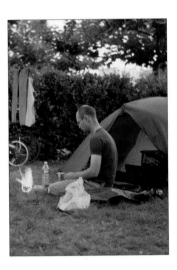

Right: When camping, stay organized and keep the campsite tidy.
Below: Camping by bike doesn't have to be a solitary pursuit.

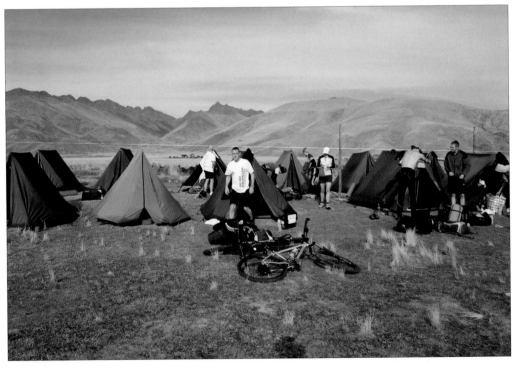

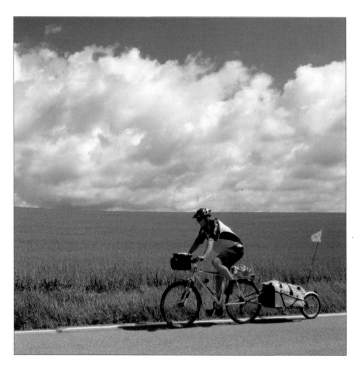

> **Dos and don'ts of camping**
> **Do...**
> - Seek permission to camp at a site if it is wild
> - Pitch camp before sunset
> - Tidy up after yourself, leaving the site exactly as you found it
> - Keep your kit organized
> - Leave early from a wild site
> - Bury toilet paper
> - Dry your tent before packing it – condensation makes it damp
> - Remember to buy food en route, so that you have something to eat in the evening
>
> **Don't...**
> - Leave litter
> - Pitch your tent in a field where there are animals or crops
> - Leave fires smouldering
> - Drink water from rivers without boiling it
> - Leave your bike unlocked, even if you think nobody is around

Left: A trailer can help take the strain.

Before you even get to the campsite, you should have planned your evening meal. Many campsites serve food, but you shouldn't rely on that unless you've checked in advance. If you are looking to save money, or are not at an official campsite, you have to provide your own food. Buy it en route, so you don't have to carry it all day. This means that when you arrive at your campsite, you don't have to go on last-minute shopping trips.

Making camp

As you have practised pitching your tent before your trip, it should present no trouble once you are on the road. If you have had to split the components of your tent between panniers, remember where everything is, and have it ready so that you are not missing the tent pegs just as your tent is about to blow away.

Roll your ground mat out, put your sleeping bag into the tent, stow the panniers, and your bed is ready for the night. Usually this can be done in less than 15 minutes, leaving you plenty of time to relax. If there is more than one of you, share the work out. One person

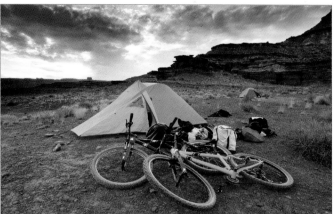

could pitch the tent, while the other starts to prepare and cook dinner. Dinner can be heated on portable stoves available from camping shops. The most convenient ones use gas cartridges, and it is important to carry a refill for longer trips. After your meal, clean all your equipment and keep it somewhere dry. In the morning, pack your things away, and be sure to dry the inside of your

Above: Camping wild can be an enjoyable experience – but be careful to always leave sites as you found them.

tent with a dry cloth – it will have got damp from condensation and will become musty if packed away when damp. If you are camping wild, try to remove all evidence that you were ever there, especially litter.

Touring in Northern Europe

Cycling is a popular activity in the UK and northern Europe, especially in the low-lying countries of the north – Belgium and the Netherlands. The flat terrain makes it especially easy and relaxing to get around and just enjoy the scenery.

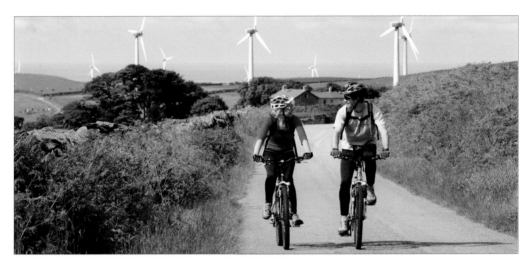

The United Kingdom is generally good for cycling tours, apart from the crowded south-east, where traffic congestion spills on to even the country roads. Luckily, outside this area, and the industrial Midlands, there are areas of quiet countryside and even wilderness. Scotland is sparsely populated and extremely hilly, even mountainous, and would be suitable for a camping

A mini tour of Devon, UK			
Day	**Route**	**Distance**	**Highlights**
Day 1	Exeter–Tavistock	48km/30 miles	Quiet roads through the wilderness of Dartmoor
Day 2	Tavistock–Barnstaple	105km/65 miles	Lydford gorge and waterfall
Day 3	Barnstaple–Minehead	80km/50 miles	Exmoor forest and moor
Day 4	Minehead–Exeter	80km/50 miles	The view from Exmoor over the Bristol channel

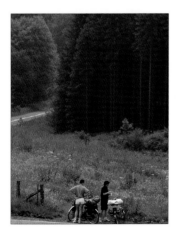

expedition. The farther into the Highlands you go, the more wild the terrain. North Wales is similar, with quiet roads and spectacular scenery. The Pennines, Lake District, Peak District and North Yorkshire Moors in the north of England are perfect cycling terrain. Devon and Cornwall are good cycling country, while in between all these areas are stretches of picturesque countryside waiting to be explored.

Planning a tour in the United Kingdom can spoil you for choice. Choose an area, buy a map and find the

Left: Touring cyclists pause to admire the view at Noirefontaine, Belgium.

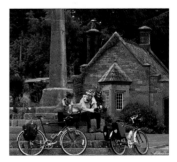

Above: With cycle touring you can stop for a break whenever you feel like it.
Top: When you are touring on a bicycle, head for smaller, quieter roads.

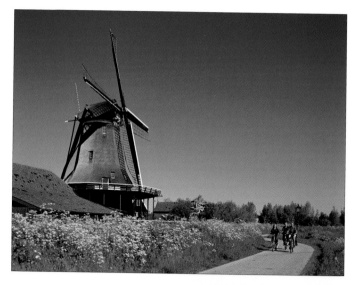

extensive network of cycle paths. Most main roads also have bike lanes running parallel, which in some cases are mandatory to use, but are safe and smooth. If you are embarking on your first cycle tour, and are worried about your fitness levels, the Netherlands and Belgium are perfect – the terrain is flat, and the towns are fairly close together, so that some days you can reduce the mileage between stops. Northern Germany and France are also ideal countries for novice and intermediate cycle tourists.

Left: The unmistakable scenery of the Netherlands, one of the most cycle-friendly countries in the world.
Below: Most cities are not ideal for cycle touring, but Amsterdam should be on everyone's cycle tour itinerary.

many ancient minor roads leading between villages and towns. Take a history book, too – hidden away in unpredictable nooks and crannies you can sometimes stumble on cultural and historical treasures.

In mainland Europe, cycling is a part of everyday life, which makes cycle touring much easier. A cycling tour in northern Europe offers more in the way of cultural variety than possibly anywhere else in the world. From Belgium, it would be possible to cover four more countries – Luxembourg, France, the Netherlands and Germany – in just a few days, each with a distinctive culture and landscape. The Netherlands and Belgium, especially, are geared to cycle touring, with an

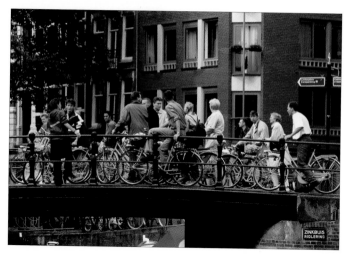

Cycling in northern Europe

Country	Terrain	Language	Climate	Notes
Belgium	Flat/hilly	Flemish/French	Warm in summer	Wind and rain common. Towns are close together – makes it easy to find accommodation.
Denmark	Flat	Danish	Warm in summer	Denmark is renowned for being expensive.
France (north)	Flat	French	Hot in summer	Beautiful cycling country.
Germany	Flat/hilly	German	Hot in summer	Hotels are expensive, but camping is cheap and popular.
Holland	Flat	Dutch	Warm in summer	Very accommodating of cyclists.
Luxembourg	Hilly	Luxembourgeois/ French/German	Warm in summer	Good camping country, and lots of very quiet minor roads.
United Kingdom	Flat/hilly	English	Warm in summer, prone to rain	Many minor roads make for good cycling.

Touring in Europe's Mountains

Mountainous regions are a challenge for the bicycle tourist, but the hard work of getting to the top of a mountain pass is usually compensated for by the sense of achievement and by the glory of the view once you get to the higher peaks.

The mountainous areas of Europe are tough terrain for cycle tourists, but offer some of the most spectacular scenery in the world.

In the French Alps, the highest mountain passes crest at almost 3,000m (10,000ft) above sea level, with climbs of up to 30km (18 miles). With a fully laden touring bike, it takes a great deal of fitness, stamina and determination to reach the top.

The Italian Dolomites and Swiss Alps are equally as hard. In Spain, desert-like conditions make for a challenging ride. There are also some very tough mountainous routes in the Apennines, in Umbria.

Training

When planning a touring trip in the mountains, preparation is even more important than on other trips. If you are new or relatively new to cycling, or are a little rusty, it is a sensible idea to undergo some training to prepare for the tough climbs. Be realistic, not optimistic, when planning your route, so that you won't spend the entire trip wishing you were anywhere else but on your bike.

In fact, training will add a new dimension to your tour and add excitement to the build-up. By acknowledging that your tour is both a bike holiday and a physical challenge, the feeling of achievement at the end of a trip will be all the more fulfilling.

Plan your pit stops

During the planning phase of your trip, look for towns along the way where you will be able to refill your water bottles and buy food.

In the mountains, towns are generally farther apart, and forward planning will ensure that you don't run out of supplies. As you are expending more energy than usual cycling up hills

A tour of the Alps, France			
Day	**Route**	**Distance**	**Highlights**
Day 1	Grenoble–Gap	113km/70 miles	Souloise Gorges
Day 2	Gap–Briancon	120km/75 miles	Col d'Izoard
Day 3	Briancon–St Jean de Maurienne	80km/50 miles	Col du Galibier
Day 4	St Jean–Bourg St Maurice	129km/80 miles	Col de la Madeleine
Day 5	Bourg St Maurice–Chambery	113km/70 miles	Cormet de Roselend
Day 6	Chambery–Grenoble	80km/50 miles	Chartreuse Mountains

(although the descent down the other side is a little less strenuous) regular refuelling is important. Almost every corner offers a spot with a fantastic view to rest for a few minutes and have a bite to eat and a drink.

Although the weather in southern Europe is generally warm, the conditions high in the mountains can change quickly. About every 100m (320ft) of altitude gained results in 1°C (2°F) of temperature lost. A 2,500m (8,000ft) pass can be 15°C (30°F) degrees cooler than the valley floor.

Below: Cyclists touring on the Lofoten Islands in Norway enjoy quiet roads and wonderful scenery.

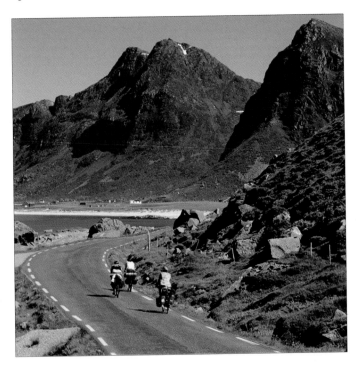

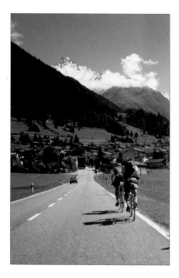

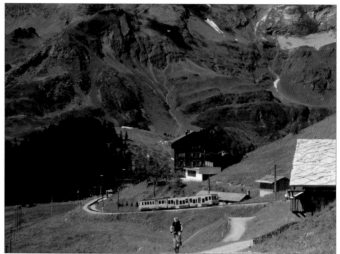

While climbing, you will be working very hard and sweating a great deal. As soon as you start descending, the air is cool and it is possible to catch a chill. Stop at the top to put on an extra layer to protect you from the cool air before you begin your descent. However, you've worked hard to get to the top so enjoy the descent and remember to brake carefully into the bends.

Above: Mountain passes such as that through Wengern Alp in Switzerland are a big challenge in cycle touring.
Above left: Two cyclists ride along a road through mountains in Switzerland.

Cycling in southern Europe

Country	Terrain	Language	Climate	Notes
France	Mountainous	French	Hot in summer	Well-surfaced roads through the Alps
Italy	Mountainous/hilly	Italian	Hot in summer	Beautiful cycling country
Portugal	Hilly	Portuguese	Very hot in summer	A high level of traffic accidents – be careful
Spain	Mountainous	Spanish	Very hot in summer	Long distances between towns
Switzerland	Mountainous	French/German/Italian	Warm in summer	Not many flat areas

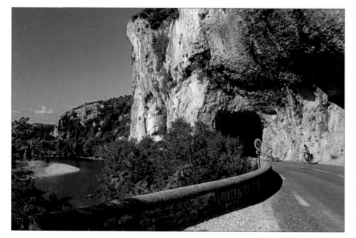

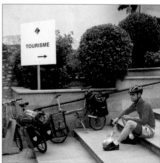

Above: Stop and take a break when you need to orientate yourself.
Left: When cycle touring in the Mediterranean, it can be very hot.

Touring in North America: West Coast and Midwest

Cycle touring is still in its infancy in North America, compared with Europe. On a typical day's touring in Europe, you will see tens if not hundreds of cycle tourists. However, North America has much to offer – fantastic scenery and a challenging terrain.

In North America, long distances between towns ensure that the primary means of getting around is the car. Bike touring is unusual. Why carry your equipment and luggage about on the back of a bike when you can carry far more in the trunk of a station wagon?

However, that attitude is gradually changing. Green issues are becoming more important, and Americans are becoming conscious of the low environmental impact of cycle touring.

Cycling is enjoying a boom in the States, thanks to public awareness of Lance Armstrong's seven Tour de France wins. It is now no longer a rarity to see bikes hooked on to the back of camper vans and motor homes so that when people set up camp, they can use their bikes to go and explore the surrounding area. It is only a small, logical step away from doing the whole trip on bikes.

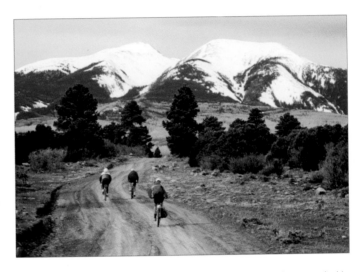

Below: A group of cyclists on mountain bikes set off on a touring trip around Kentucky, in the United States.

Above: Big sky, big landscapes and a big adventure – touring cross country in North America.

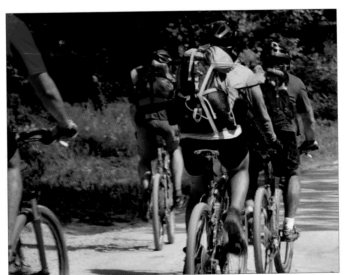

Where to go

The west of the United States is superb cycling terrain. Whether you like hot or cold weather, arid desert or humid forest, mountains or lowlands, densely populated areas with plenty of hotels and campsites or wilderness, you will find that the western states have it all.

One of the most popular areas for cyclists, and the most rewarding and enjoyable for cycle tourism, is California, where the climate is suitable for year-round cycling.

Central Los Angeles is no place for a bike, but even just an hour out of the city, the conditions are perfect – quiet roads, stunning scenery and varied terrain. Californians need not travel to France to cycle through vineyards, when there are vineyards on their own doorstep.

Farther up the Pacific coast, Oregon and Washington both offer good opportunities for cycle tourism, although they are cold and wet during winter.

Colorado has become a cyclists' Mecca – the Rocky Mountains are very tough to cycle in – while Montana and Wyoming are extremely challenging for wilderness expeditions.

The Midwest mountain states are generally hot in summer, and the terrain is very difficult, with long distances between towns. The planning for trips around these states should

Cycling in North America			
Region	**Terrain**	**Climate**	**Notes**
California	Hilly–mountainous	Hot	Coastal highway is a must. Go inland for hilly rides.
Canada (Rockies)	Mountainous	Cool	Wilderness, be prepared for long distances between towns.
Colorado	Mountainous–extreme	Cool	Sparsely populated, and altitude a challenge in the mountains.
Montana/Idaho	Mountainous	Cool	Long distances between towns, and challenging hills.
Oregon/Washington	Hilly	Temperate	Be prepared for wet conditions, but beautiful scenery.

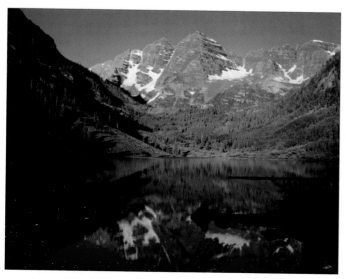

take into account that it will be necessary to carry more food and plenty of water. Self-sufficiency is vitally important, as you may find yourself a long distance from the next town and source of water. You may need to camp or sleep out if it's warm enough.

Left: Many Americans take short daily excursions, rather than embarking on a full cycle tour complete with luggage.
Below left: When cycle touring in North America, you can enjoy some truly amazing scenery.
Below: Always ensure that you carry plenty of equipment and supplies on a cycle tour when there are long distances between towns.

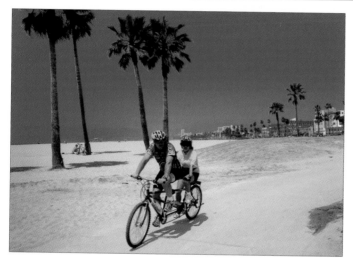

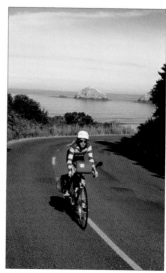

Touring in North America: East Coast

While the West Coast and Midwest are hard touring country, the eastern half
has a broader appeal. Parts of New England are remote, with tough cycling and
unpredictable weather, but the East Coast and the southern states offer an easier ride.

It is impossible to generalize about such a large geographical area, but the variety of terrain around the East Coast of North America is such that the cycle tourist will be able to find something that suits his or her level. There are diverse touring experiences available, with something to appeal to everyone, ranging from deserts, plains and mountain ranges to woods. An added attraction are the roads, which are well maintained just about everywhere. There are many parks which extend for miles and which are well organized with extensive services for people who are bicycle touring. To make it perfect for the cyclist, cycle lanes abound in many states and provinces, and there are also special bicycle trails.

Bicycle touring is also made easier in North America because there are so many campgrounds that are ideal for cyclists, which are either run privately or by the government.

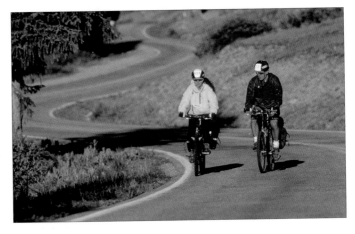

Flat terrain

The easiest cycling is to be found in Florida, which is very flat, with almost imperceptible undulations inland. When the highest point in the state is only 105m (345ft) above sea level, even novice cycle tourists can be confident that there will be no hills they can't manage. Although parts of the state are densely populated, it is easy to avoid the crowded areas. The weather will be the biggest challenge to a cycle tour – while winter temperatures are pleasant and temperate, the summer is scorchingly hot and prone to frequent thunderstorms.

When you plan your cycle tour holiday, always research the typical weather patterns for the time of year in which you are planning to travel.

Mountainous terrain

If you are looking for more challenging terrain, it is well worth considering planning a bicycle tour through the Appalachian Mountains. The mountains

Above: Some of the roads on the east coast are empty, which is ideal for touring. Below: When cycling in a hot area, particularly in summer, you'll need to take plenty of water.

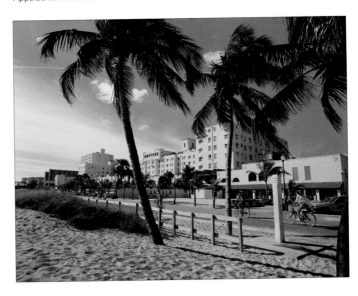

run for more than 1,600km (1,000 miles) from Alabama, which is in the southern United States, all the way to Newfoundland in Canada.

The Appalachians are a middle-mountain range – the roads are approximately half the altitude of a typical Alpine or Rocky Mountain pass.

The Blue Ridge Mountains in Virginia are ideal cycling country for the cycle tourist who has ambitions for a challenging tour, but who does not want to endure the extreme physical exertion of a route through a high mountain range. The roads in Virginia are quiet and rolling, with forests to shelter you from the midday sun. In high summer, Virginia is humid, but apart from this time, and winter, the weather is perfect for cycle tourism.

New England

A popular destination for cycle tourists in the United States is New England – the quiet backroads, moderate terrain, attractive scenery, temperate climate and the friendliness of the people make for good cycling country. You can choose between forested areas, farmland and New England villages. Summer and the famous New England Fall, when the foliage is at its resplendent best, are good times of year to explore.

Where to go?

With such a wide choice of destinations in North America, it can be difficult to make a decision – you may feel you want to go everywhere! The best starting point is to look at yourself and your touring companions. Ask yourself what you want to experience, and assess your ability to cover long distances or hard terrain. Factor in whether you want to ride through woods, towns or farming country, and if mountainous or flat terrain is preferred. This approach may seem coldly scientific, but your tour is much more likely to be a fun, rewarding experience.

Right: This tranquil road, which is perfect for cycle touring, goes through beautiful pastures in the Great Smoky Mountains National Park in Tennessee.

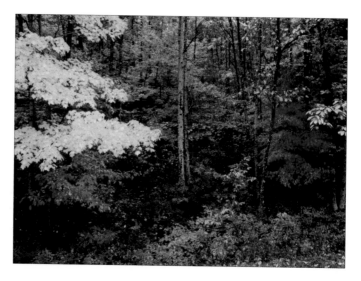

Above: Touring through New England is a great experience; it is fantastic cycling country and the scenery in the fall is particularly breathtaking.

Cycling in North America

Region	Terrain	Climate	Notes
New England	Hilly–challenging	Temperate	Very enjoyable cycling with a range of difficulties
Southern States	Flat–hilly	Hot	More densely populated and be prepared for hot temperatures
Virginia	Hilly	Temperate	Perfect cycling country, in Blue Ridge Mountains

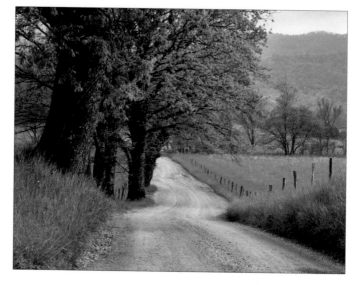

Touring Farther Afield

Africa, Asia and South America are a good challenge for the more experienced cyclist. They present more difficulties than Europe and North America, but, with a little foresight and packing the appropriate equipment, the result can be a holiday to remember.

A great deal of the enjoyment and challenge of cycle touring comes from the self-sufficiency involved in completing a tour. Whether you have ridden for two short days between hotels or three weeks in the Alps, the sense of achievement comes from having relied on your own horsepower to get from the start to the finish.

For an even more challenging cycle-touring experience, Africa, Asia and South America are as tough as it gets. The climate is hotter, the roads are less well maintained and the distances between towns are potentially huge.

Right: Cycle touring can be your passport to scenery like this.
Below: Conditions can be challenging when touring in remote areas – be prepared and plan carefully.

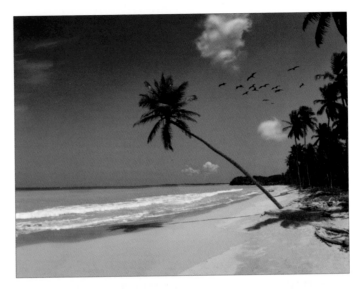

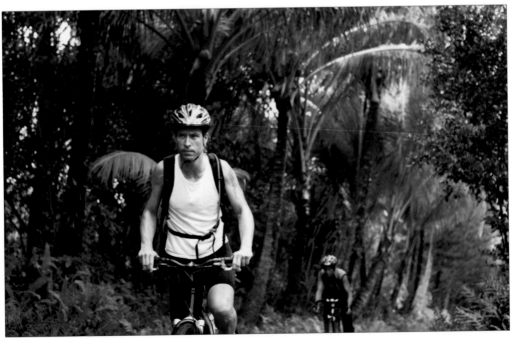

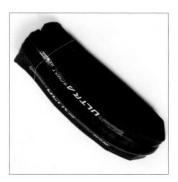

Above: Should you have a puncture en route, carrying a spare tyre is essential.

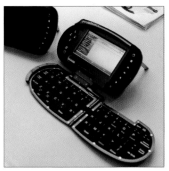

Above: A GPS phone is useful to help with navigation.

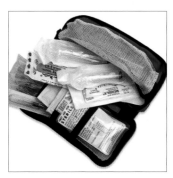

Above: Always take first aid supplies when touring off the beaten track.

You don't just have to be self-sufficient in terms of covering the distance, you have to take into account that you may need to carry more food and equipment. If your maps are inaccurate, you may even have to navigate yourself in order to get to your destination.

Remote areas

It is important to plan for every eventuality when organizing a cycling expedition to Africa, Asia or South America, from picking your destination, through making contingencies for mechanical failure, to researching the geography, roads and local people. Parts of south-east Asia have extremely busy roads, with the occasional erratic driver, but escape from the built-up areas and you will experience friendly hospitality from the people you meet.

A cycling tour in northern India should take into account the monsoon season, and the extreme terrain of the Himalayas. Avoid cycle touring during the monsoon – touring in pouring rain and extremely high humidity is no fun.

Touring in the Himalayas, or Andes, is a different proposition from the Alps. The roads suffer from weather damage in the freezing winter, and from land-slides, so surfaces are unpredictable and difficult to ride on. The altitude is higher than the Alps, with the highest road pass in the Himalayas, the Karakoram Highway, tops out at almost 5km (3 miles) – the thinner air makes exertion extremely tough. The roads can climb for around 50km (31 miles), so good

physical fitness is essential. In the southern half of India, the heat is not ideal for touring, but the terrain is less mountainous. In any country, assumptions about the weather can make or break your cycling holiday – find out the typical rainfall, humidity and temperature of the month you are visiting.

Cycle touring in China is also varied. Avoid industrial areas and the arid west – there's plenty to see elsewhere. Beijing is less cycle-friendly than it used to be, but once you are out of the city, avoid the expressways and keep to old minor roads.

Africa, on the other hand, offers wild, hot and challenging terrain. The roads range from good to non-existent. And South America is a continent of contrasts

for cycle tourists. The Andes are extremely challenging, while the wide open spaces of Brazil and Argentina make a more leisurely tour possible.

One more note – touring in Australia is fairly straightforward when keeping to the more densely populated coastal areas. But crossing the centre needs careful planning. Water stops are few · and far between, and the weather is extremely hot. Self sufficiency is the key to all cycle touring, but especially in conditions like these.

Be prepared

Self-sufficiency is important for both you and your bike when cycle touring off the beaten track. If there is a problem, you cannot ride to a town and buy a replacement part. You have to carry a few more tools and replacement parts to deal with any mechanical failure. If there are long distances between towns or stops, carry your own food and water, plus water purification tablets in case you have to use a local source.

Respect local culture

In some regions, the locals are not used to seeing western tourists, let alone a group of them on bikes. In most parts of the world, hospitality to strangers is a common trait, and you can find yourself being treated like a celebrity for the duration of your stay. However, it is important to respect local traditions. If local people have their legs and arms covered, cycle tourists should be aware of the impact of cycling into town in shorts and a teeshirt. It is rare, but the locals may take exception to westerners, in their eyes, dressing immodestly or behaving disrespectfully. Common sense is the best way to decide how to behave. A friendly and generous manner will get you a long way with most of the world's people.

Extra equipment for touring

As well as all the general equipment you will need for touring, planning for certain eventualities involves carrying more equipment. It is worth taking the following items, the extra weight will be well worth it: GPS phone, first-aid kit, water purification tablets, freewheel remover, lubricants, spare tyres, various dried foods and/or canned foods.

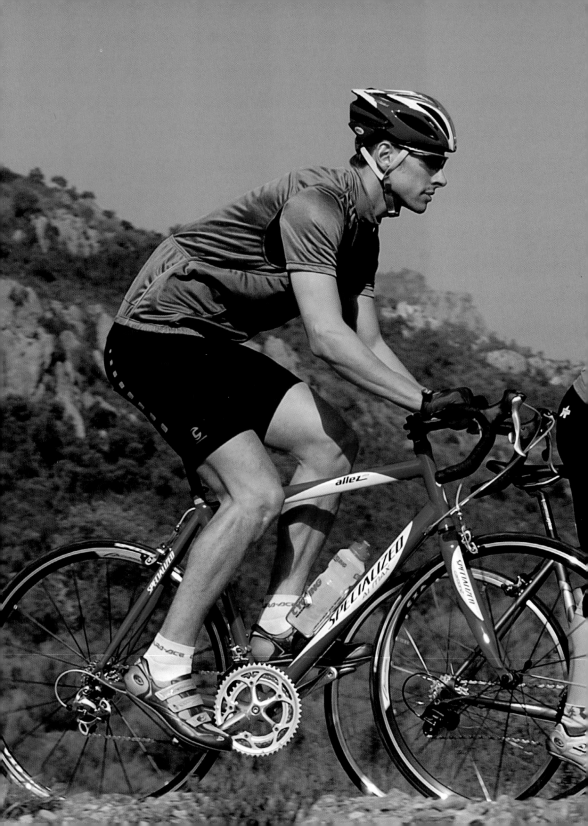

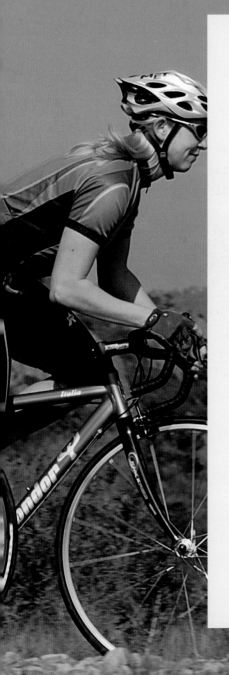

FAST RIDING

Riding bikes is practical and fun, and that is reason enough to ride. Regular riders will notice that cycling makes positive changes in their body. The more, and harder, they ride, the fitter they become. They start to challenge themselves with longer rides and a regular training schedule designed to move on to greater levels of fitness. There are many opportunities to challenge bike riders such as sportives and trail rides. Because of all the benefits, cycling is rapidly growing in popularity.

Left: Greater fitness levels make serious riding fun.

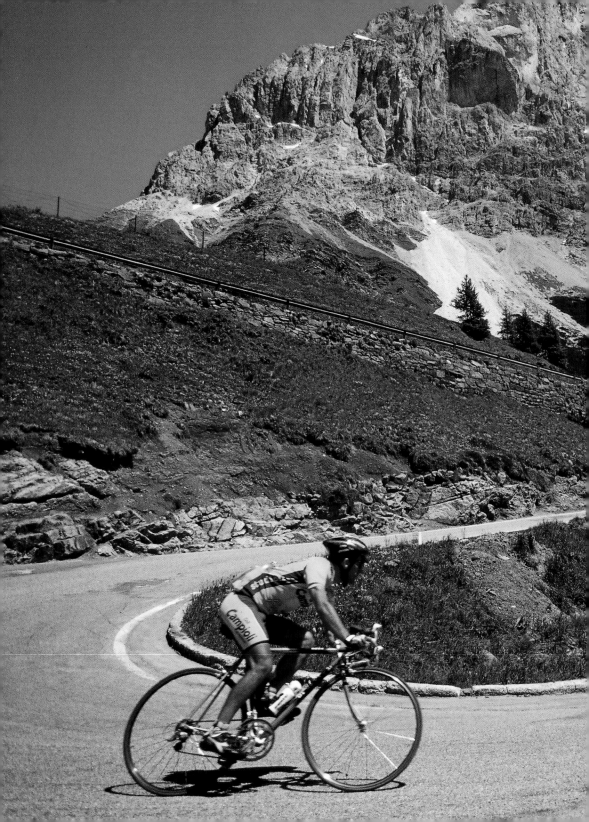

SPORTIVES

Sportive rides are the perfect compromise between leisure riding and all-out racing. Sportives have elements of both, and the best thing about them is that you can choose how seriously, or not, to take the event. Sportives are billed as personal challenge rides. They usually take place over long, but not impossible distances, sometimes taking in famous climbs, or arduous terrain – they are challenge rides, after all. Many also offer shorter distance rides to complement the main event, which means they are more inclusive.

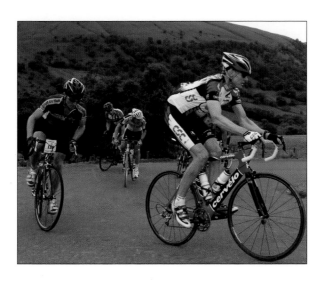

Above: A group of riders take part in a sportive ride.
Left: Sportive rides often take place in mountainous areas.

The Sportive Bicycle

A sportive bike can provide a similar performance to a racing bike. It is so similar, in fact, that most people who participate in both road races and sportives find that they can use the same bike without noticing any particular disadvantage.

Sportive bikes need to be reliable, light, fast, efficient and comfortable. They look very similar to racing bikes, with narrow slick tyres and drop handlebars. The only difference with a real high-end racing bike will be more relaxed geometry in the frame, which will make for a more comfortable ride over a long distance. A racing frame will be extremely rigid, so that little power is wasted in frame flex, while a sportive bike needn't be so rigid. However, in their speed and weight, they have far more in common with a racing bike than with a touring bike, for which comfort is everything.

Events

Sportives tend to range from 25km (15.5 miles) for a short distance event complementing another ride, to between 170 and 200km (105–125 miles) for the longest events. They often take a big loop into isolated terrain. It is important

Below: Sportive bikes need a good range of gears, and the compact chainset has become a popular choice because it offers the required flexibility.

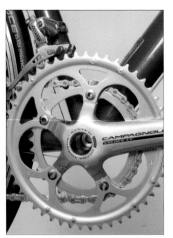

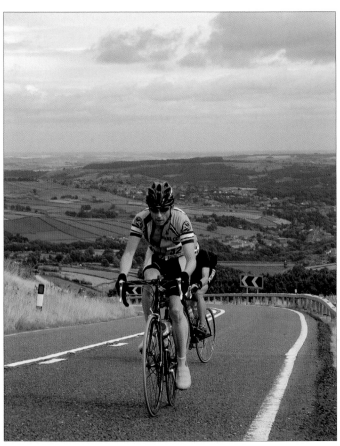

Above: A typical sportive bike is lightweight so that riding up steep hills becomes easier, but it is also comfortable for riding long distances.

that the bike is well-maintained so it won't let you down at a critical time.

Although there are sportives in all regions, from flat to mountainous, many take place in the Alps and northern Italy, where the routes take in large climbs. Popular British sportives are also very hilly, so a lightweight bike could help to make the difference between a gold and silver award.

Go for comfort

The length of most sportive events means that comfort is important. While a stiff, lightweight racing bike is the fastest option, don't sacrifice comfort for speed. If you do, you will ride the first two hours faster, then slow down for the second half of the event, as the discomfort increases. All except specialized racing bikes are suitable for sportive events.

The debate about frame materials continues, and there is no simple answer. The best material for one person may not be the most suitable for another. If you can afford a carbon fibre or aluminium frame, these will get you round the course the fastest. These frames are unlikely to last for a lifetime, however, while a good quality steel frame will last forever, well maintained.

After choosing which frame to use, the next most important decision involves gearing.

Racing bikes are designed for high speed events, and come with 52–42 or 52–39 chainrings, and 12–21 or 12–23 blocks on the back. For flatter sportive events, these might be sufficient but it is worth considering getting a compact chainset, with 50–34 rings, for riding in the hills. For self-sufficiency, make sure you can carry two water bottles, a pump, and a saddlebag or panniers containing spare tubes and tools.

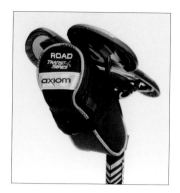

Right: Fit a saddlebag with spare inner tubes and tyre levers.

Anatomy of a sportive bike

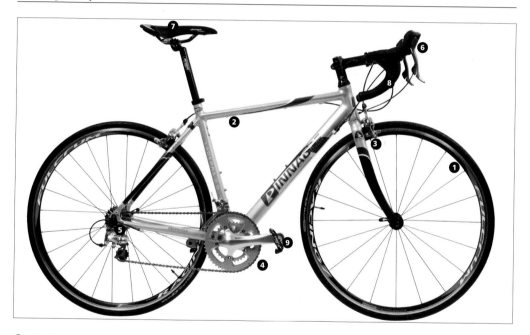

❶ Wheels: Size 700 x 23C with 28 or 32 spokes to save weight, narrow-section rims for aerodynamics, slick tyres for lower rolling resistance.
❷ Frame: Can be steel, or more modern lightweight materials such as carbon fibre or aluminium. Geometry is less relaxed than a touring bike, and similar to that of a racing bike, for a faster, more responsive ride.
❸ Brakes: Lightweight good quality calliper brakes. Models such as the Campagnolo Chorus and Shimano

Ultegra are popular, with very good performance.
❹ Chainrings: Compact chainsets, with a smaller inner ring, are becoming very popular with sportive riders. Fifty teeth on the bigger ring and 34 on the smaller is a good combination. Or possibly a racing set, with 52–42 toothed rings. Some people put a triple chainring on their sportive bikes, especially in mountainous events.
❺ Sprockets: Ten-speed freewheel, with a 12–25 block. For very steep

and long hills, depending on the chainring size, it might be advisable to fit a 27-tooth sprocket.
❻ Gear changers: Combined with the brake levers to save weight and for accessibility while riding.
❼ Saddle: Comfortable but narrow.
❽ Handlebars: Drop handlebars offer a range of positions. Riders can be aerodynamic on descents, and sit up for ease of breathing on the climbs.
❾ Pedals: Lightweight clipless pedals for shoes to attach to directly.

Clothing for Sportives

Sportive riding is a summer sport, so clothing needs to be lightweight, breathable, comfortable and aerodynamic. Modern fabrics are perfect in that they keep the body cool if necessary and also can act as insulation in cold weather.

One of the most important items of clothing for summer riding is a pair of Lycra racing shorts with a synthetic padded insert. For long rides on a fairly hard and narrow saddle, comfort is paramount. Ordinary cycling shorts are fine, but many racers wear bib shorts, which have straps stretched over the shoulders. Bib shorts fit snugly, and can be a more comfortable option over long distances.

Cold conditions

On chilly days, it is also worth covering the knees to protect them from the cold – longer shorts are available, but a better solution is to get some detachable knee warmers that extend from the thigh, inside your shorts, down to below the knee. If it warms up, you have the advantage that you can take them off.

A base layer is a good idea, even on hot days. Base layer garments wick sweat away from your body. In mountainous events, it can get quite chilly when descending, especially at altitude, and if you are covered in sweat this can be a problem. The lightest base layers have plenty of ventilation – some are string-vest style, which help keep you cool on hot days.

Wear an ordinary cycling top over your base layer. This should not be too baggy, otherwise it will catch the wind and slow you down. On the other hand, don't squeeze into a top that is a size too small either – find a comfortable snug-fitting breathable cycling top.

Like knees, arms can get chilly on cool days or on long descents. If it looks like being a cold day in the saddle, wear some detachable arm warmers. These will add a crucial layer of insulation, and

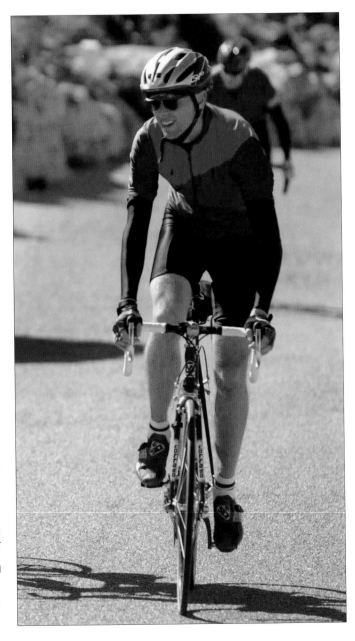

Right: For a sportive, lightweight, breathable clothing will make the event more comfortable.

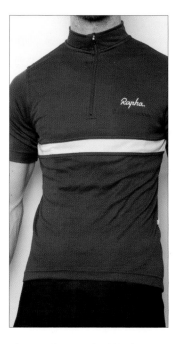

Above: Cycling tops should be fairly tight-fitting and snug, but should still feel comfortable.

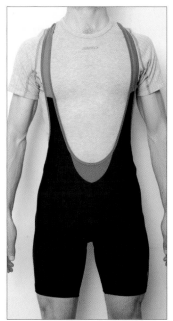

Above: Padded bib shorts over an insulating base layer are comfortable and aerodynamic.

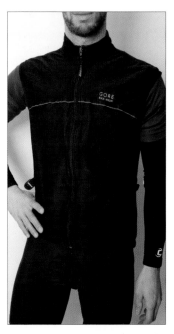

Above: In cooler conditions, a gilet and arm warmers add an extra layer.

pack down compactly if the day warms up. On cool days, also consider a gilet, which is a sleeveless zip-up top to insulate the body.

Footwear

Shoes should be stiff-soled, with attachments for shoeplates, which clip into the pedals. The stiff soles ensure that your feet do not bend around the pedals and so stop you wasting energy, and stop the feet becoming sore. Your shoeplates should use the same system as your pedals. Most shoes can accommodate all the main industry standard systems. When choosing shoes for size, be aware that your feet expand in the heat, so if they are tight when you buy them, they will be tighter when you are some distance into an event. You don't need to buy excessively loose shoes, but do buy for comfort. Shoes with Velcro fastenings are the most popular: they are easy to put on and take off, and can be loosened temporarily if your feet get uncomfortable.

Headgear

Most sportive organizers insist that you wear a helmet. It should pass all the safety standards (as should all helmets sold). The helmet should fit snugly and not move when the head is shaken about, and should also be well ventilated. Replace your helmet every two years, and at once if it suffers an impact (even if no damage is visible).

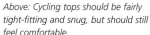

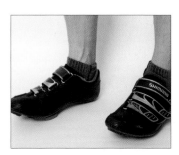

Above: Road cycling shoes are stiff-soled for better power transmission, and fastened with Velcro.

Sportive wear
Cycling shoes: Stiff-soled for efficiency
Cycling socks: Insulated
Cycling bib shorts: Padded
Knee warmers: Optional, for cooler days
Base layer: To wick away sweat
Cycling top: Lightweight and breathable
Arm warmers: Optional, for cooler days
Gilet: Optional, for cooler days

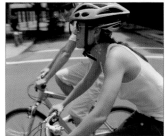

Above: If you are going to wear a helmet for a few hours in hot weather, comfort and coolness are important.

Setting Goals

Before entering a long-distance sportive, it is sensible to attempt to achieve the necessary level of fitness first. If you are an experienced participant in other sports, your fitness should transfer easily to cycling.

Your sportive riding experience will be more positive if you use it as a long-term goal, with a sensible build-up and a commitment to do your best.

Before entering an event, you need to assess two things – current ability and potential ability. You can then set your long-term goal and, with that in mind, decide how much training you are going to need to do to fulfil your potential.

If you are starting from zero, with little exercise in the last few years, the first thing you need to do is go to see a doctor for a medical check. Once you have the all-clear to begin your exercise regime, build up slowly and get used to riding the bike and accustom yourself to the physical exertion. It is realistic to set a goal of entering a shorter sportive within a few months, but try to think in terms of using shorter events and the time between them as stepping stones to a longer event a year down the line.

Commit yourself

You will get the most out of yourself and the sport if you work on the principle of building up to a certain

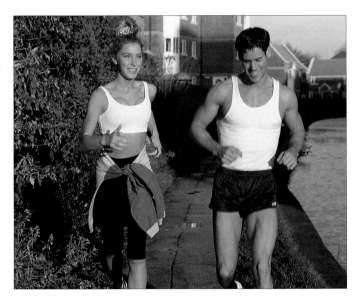

level, consolidating your fitness, then using that as a foundation upon which to build your step-up to the next level. In other words, make the bike into a lifestyle choice, and commit to

Above: Running provides good base fitness and lower-body workouts that are beneficial for cyclists.

improving yourself continuously. You will be amazed at how far you can make yourself go in this way. Over a few years, you could be riding 50km events in your first season, 100km events in your second, and full-length 170km sportives in your third. Along the way you will reduce body fat levels, become more toned, massively increase your energy levels, and achieve some incredible goals. If you are new to cycling, but are fit and have kept up an interest in other sports, it is realistic to set higher goals, but you must still be aware that it will take time for your body to adapt to the new stresses you are placing on it. With an adaptation period, and a sensible build-up, it is realistic to envisage riding a 100km event within three to six months of starting out, while

What should your goals be?	
Cyclist	**Non-cyclist**
Achievements attainable for a racing cyclist:	Achievements attainable for a regular sports player:
In 3 months: full-length sportive, silver standard	In 3 months: 100km sportive
In 6 months: full-length sportive, silver standard	In 6 months: full-length sportive
In 1 year: full-length sportive, gold standard	In 1 year: full-length sportive, silver standard
Long-term goal: Finish in top 20 of a big sportive	Long-term goal: gold standard in a full-length sportive
Commuting leisure cyclist	**Sedentary individuals**
In 3 months: 50km sportive	In 3 months: 50km sportive
In 6 months: 100km sportive	In 6 months: 50km sportive, at a faster pace
In 1 year: full-length sportive	In 1 year: 100km sportive
Long-term goal: silver standard in a long sportive	Long-term goal: full-length sportive

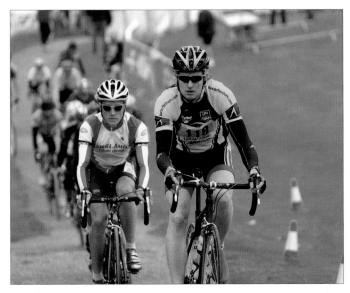

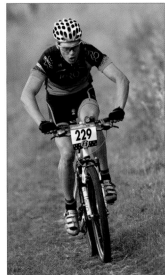

Above: After an organized training build-up, you are ready to enter your first sportive.

keeping an eye on setting a longer term goal of a full-length sportive within a year.

If you have ridden your bike regularly as a commuter or leisure cyclist, the adaptation should be straightforward, since your body is used to spending time in the saddle. The challenging part will be twofold – you need to get used to riding long distances, and you also need to get used to riding a little faster. The

easiest adaptation comes from racing cyclists who want a less time-intensive and stressful goal than road racing. Most amateur racing events are under 100km, so it takes a little extra time to get used to the longer distances. If the body is already used to cycling training, just alter the workouts a little.

Of course, most people fall somewhere in between all these categories. They also react differently to training – some become fitter very quickly, others take time to adapt. Some enter a marathon event such as the Tour de France's Etape du Tour,

Above: Mountain bike enduro events are a good target for riders who are aiming to increase their fitness.

which is a 180km ride through some of the most challenging mountain roads in cycling, with only a few months to train. The important thing is to always be aware of the signals your body is sending out.

Below left: Swimming helps to achieve stamina, strength and suppleness.
Below: Athletes who play sports such as tennis will build fitness quickly.

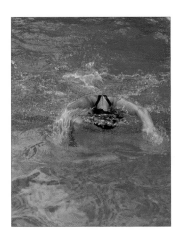

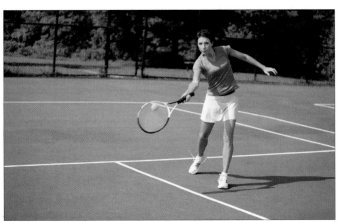

What to Expect in a Sportive

There are hundreds, if not thousands, of sportive events organized around the world, and each one is different. Some are very flat, while others include multiple climbs of 30km (18 miles). Some start with 5,000 riders or more; others attract 100 competitors.

Although a good foundation of base fitness in cycling will help you to get round any sportive fairly easily, training needs to be geared to the specific event you have entered. Before entering, try to find out as much information about the route as you can. Most events have internet sites, with downloadable maps and profiles of all the routes.

The profile is the most important part. It will show all the climbs and descents. Sometimes the scale can be misleading, so check the altitude scale on the left-hand side of the profile. Most sportive events have one, two or three signature climbs, which will be the main challenges of the day, and your success will depend largely on how well you pace yourself on these climbs.

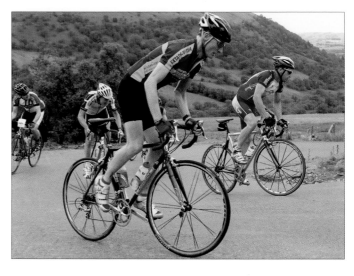

The ups and downs of racing

If an event includes a long climb, your training and preparation need to take this into account. A 15km (9 mile) climb places severe stresses on the body, and if your training rides all took place on flat roads, your body will be less able to deal with the challenge. Make sure that your training includes climbing. If you live in a flat area, consider going on a training camp in a hilly or mountainous area. If you have a good level of base fitness, a week spent in the mountains will allow your body to adapt to the rhythm and

techniques of long climbs. Not all events take place in the high mountains; there may be many shorter climbs, of between 3 and 7km (2 and 4 miles) in length. None are very hard in themselves, but the repetition makes each subsequent climb harder than the last. These are easier to train for – just try and replicate the number and length of climbs in your long training rides.

The downhill and flat sections are just as important – look at the profile to see where they are. A long descent is a

Above: Hilly sportives will test your fitness to its limits – success in these events depends on your long-term training technique.

good time to recuperate, so it might be worth trying a little harder on the climb in the knowledge that you have plenty of time to recover from the effort. Alternatively, some climbs lead you on to a plateau, or to the base of another climb – you'll need to be aware of the shorter recuperation time involved.

Steep terrain

Profiles can be misleading. Organizers concentrate on including the major climbs, but they may just draw a flat line between them. In reality, these flat sections may be a series of rolling climbs, with steep sections that sap your strength. Be prepared for this eventuality.

Left: The Etape du Tour follows the same route as a mountainous stage of the Tour de France and attracts thousands of entrants.

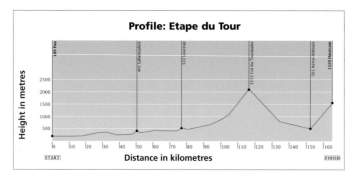

Profile: Etape du Tour

Height in metres

2500
2000
1500
1000
500

189 Pau | 401 Labaumalete | 521 Loucrup | 2115 Col du Tourmalet | 501 Ayros-Arbouix | 1520 Hautcam

|0 |10 |20 |30 |40 |50 |60 |70 |80 |90 |100 |110 |120 |130 |140 |150 |160

START   **Distance in kilometres**   FINISH

On the day

Most events start in the morning, so, depending on how far you live from the ride, it might be better to arrive the day before.

When you arrive, set up your bike so it is ready for the event. Pump up the tyres, make sure the components are clean and working well, double-check that the saddle and handlebars are in the correct position, and test the gears and brakes.

If you have had a long drive, your legs will be a little stiff, so it's a good idea to test the bike out on a short and easy ride. This is not the time for training – just a 30-minute easy ride to get your bike and body ready for the next day. Bring a spare set of kit for this ride, so you don't get your event clothes dirty or sweaty. Sometimes it is possible to sign on the day before, and you should do this if possible, so you can get your race number on the bike and avoid queues on the morning of the event.

The evening before, wrap your food and pack it into your pockets, prepare your drinks, eat a large dinner and get a good night's sleep. On the morning of the event, get up in plenty of time to eat a reasonable breakfast and get to the start. In larger events you will be directed to a pen according to race number, but in all cases, the earlier you arrive, the closer to the front you will be. If you want to win the event and you start at the back, you'll have several hundreds or thousands of riders to pass. Help yourself by getting there in good time. You are now ready to go.

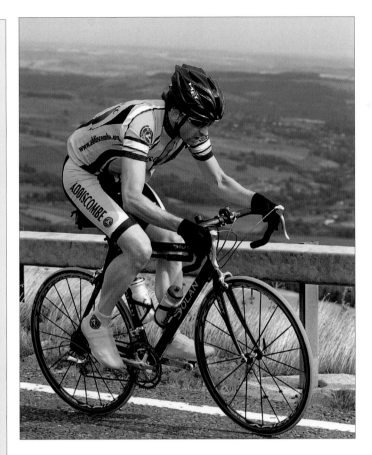

Above: Riding consistently well in a hilly sportive depends on fitness and determination – but the effort will be worth it.

Below: The Gran Fondo Pinarello is one of the biggest and most famous sportive events in Italy – its mountainous profile makes it a serious physical challenge.

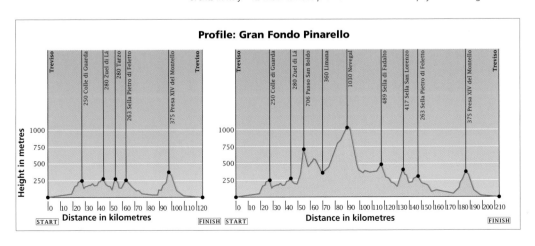

Profile: Gran Fondo Pinarello

Pacing and Gearing in a Sportive

Riding a sportive is not about pedalling like fury as soon as the gun goes off. Strategy and tactics and a thorough awareness of your own capabilities are more likely to get you to the finishing line with the chance of a good result.

A sportive is a race, so you naturally want to get around the course as fast as you can. But this does not involve putting your head down and riding hard from the gun. By riding intelligently, spreading out your effort and concentrating on riding as efficiently as you are able, you will achieve the best possible result.

Pacing

To succeed at pacing, you must look at the profile, have an awareness of your own ability and knowledge of the conditions on the day and be flexible in case of surprises. Preparation helps here – set your bike up correctly, with the right gears, and train for the challenges of your specific event. The best way to maintain a pace you know you can handle is by using a pulse monitor during training and the event. The effort you are making when cycling is reflected in a higher pulse as your heart works harder to transport blood to the muscles. Training with a heart monitor is covered on page 155, but the main point to remember is that you can only sprint for a limited period, whereas a steady, controlled effort can be sustained for longer.

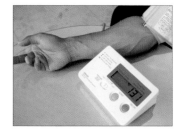

Above: A digital machine measures the pulse and blood pressure.
Below: Riding steadily over long distances will get you to the finish faster.

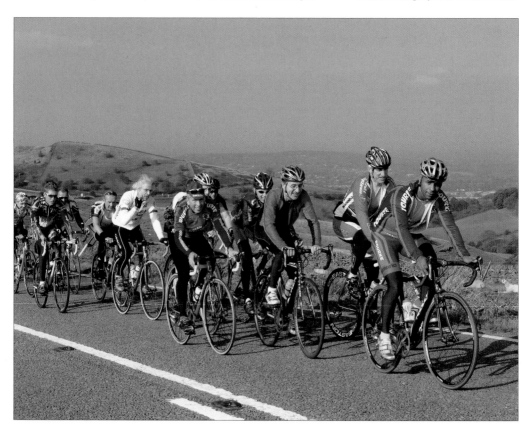

This is not a foolproof way of looking at it, since other factors, such as refuelling, previous efforts and even general tiredness also have a big effect on fatigue levels. However, by using a pulse monitor as a guide, you can maintain a sustainable level of effort. The more experience you gain in training and riding sportives, the more you will understand the way your body in particular reacts to the effort.

When no other factors are taken into consideration, it is theoretically ideal to maintain the same pulse rate and level of effort all the way through an event, but it is more realistic to anticipate changes of pace according to circumstances and the way you feel.

The golden rule, especially for inexperienced riders, is not to go too hard at any time. Accumulated fatigue can mount very badly if you go too hard early on. One good way of avoiding fatigue is to train yourself to spin the pedals faster in a lower gear. Different riders' bodies work efficiently at different pedalling rates, but according to sports doctors, pedalling a large gear slowly places greater stress on the muscles, which tire quickly, and pedalling a small gear fast places greater stress on the cardiovascular system while saving the muscles. Train yourself to turn the pedals at 90 revolutions per minute, and your body will become more efficient at handling the effort.

Gearing

For a mountainous sportive, it is a good idea to be conservative in your choice of gears. Fatigue builds up insidiously on long climbs, and if you are feeling weary, and already in your bottom gear, you can lose a lot of time.

Racing bikes tend to use 52 and 42 rings on the front, and 12–21 or 12–23 at the back. This is good for the fast and intense pace of a short race. However, for a sportive and for riders who are less fit, there is little point in trying to ride the same gears as a racer.

To provide lower gears, you can either fit larger sprockets to the rear wheel, or smaller chainrings at the front. If you change the block at the back to a 12–27, the difference between gears is

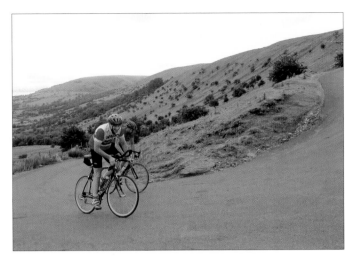

large, so that it is very difficult to find the right gear on a climb. You may be over- or under-geared, with no chance of finding the right rhythm.

The alternative is to fit a compact chainset. These have become popular with sportive riders in the last few years. These typically have 50- and 34-tooth rings, and combined with a 12–25 block at the rear, should bail you out of all but the very worst situations. More importantly, they also allow you to spin a lower gear and save energy.

Right: A compact chainset gives flexible gearing in most situations and is invaluable for sportives with long climbs.

Above: On the steepest hills, it doesn't matter how strong you are – you'll need to fit a low gear in order to be able to pedal up.

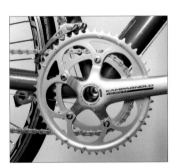

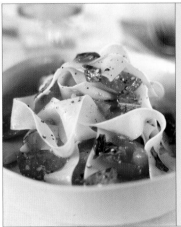

Maintaining energy levels

As sportives are long events, refuelling should be a vital part of your strategy. Start by eating a large meal with plenty of carbohydrates the evening before, followed by a substantial breakfast on the morning of the event. Carry some snacks that you can eat during the ride: try bananas, energy bars, dried fruit, sandwiches and anything that you find palatable during exercise. Drink plenty of water and energy drinks during the ride, especially on a hot day.

Left: Eating carbohydrates, such as pasta, produces more energy before a sportive event.

Climbing in a Sportive

Many sportive events include significant climbing. Organizers love climbs because they split the field up into manageable proportions, and riders love them for the challenge. With careful planning beforehand, you can turn the hills to your advantage.

Climbing hills on a bike is so difficult and energy intensive that by focusing your training and planning on going uphill as fast and as efficiently as possible, you can make a big difference to the success of your ride. That does not mean you can ignore other aspects of your cycling, but it is on the climbs that the most time can be lost – and gained.

Hill profiles
As part of the preparation for your sportive goal, check the profile to see how many significant climbs there are, and how difficult each one is. Some organizers even provide a detailed breakdown of the climbs, with average gradients for each kilometre ridden. This knowledge is a powerful weapon in your sportive-riding armoury – if you know that a 10km (6 mile) climb has 6 steady kilometres followed by 4 steep kilometres, you know not to overdo it in the early part of the climb and can

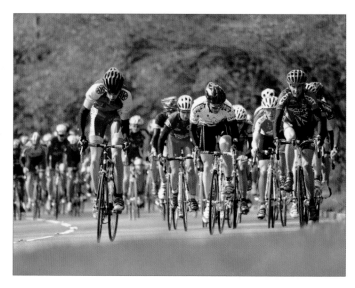

Above: When climbing in a group, follow your own pace to the top.

Below: Planning ahead and conserving energy when necessary is the best way to climb hills in a sportive event.

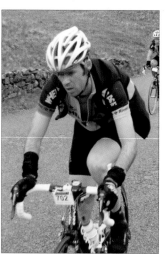

therefore save some energy for the difficult part. If the steep part comes at the bottom, it is a good idea to pace yourself carefully until the climb levels out a little, then go harder with the knowledge that it is not going to get any steeper.

Pace yourself
The frequency and positioning of the climbs will also make a big difference in your planning. The Auvergnate sportive, in France, has four significant climbs, crucially, two of them come right at the beginning. This is too early for heroics, so careful riders will pace themselves well on these two climbs.

Going hard right at the start of a sportive, especially uphill, might lead to an energy crash later. The Auvergnate's two hardest climbs come much later on – it is important to save energy for these two challenges.

Once you are on a climb, and you have an idea of the gradients, your fitness and your physical state, you can get on with tackling it as efficiently as possible.

Apart from physical strength and fitness, climbing well involves being able to focus and concentrate while relaxing. Relaxing sounds like the last thing you should do during such hard work, but while the legs turn, and the body provides an anchor for them to do so, the arms should be nice and relaxed, holding but not gripping the bars.

The right rhythm
Climbing is physically demanding: it hurts, and it can drain your resources incredibly quickly, but if you are able to remain focused and relaxed you can get into a good rhythm, which is what climbing is all about. This is easiest to establish on a steady climb, but it is still also possible on climbs that change in pitch every few hundred metres. Basically, the right rhythm is the one that

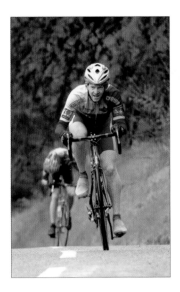

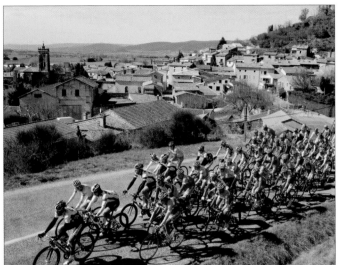

Above: On the steepest grades, reduce your speed accordingly – a constant effort up a hill is more efficient than a constant speed.

gets you to the top as fast as possible without going into the red zone (going too hard, then becoming very tired very quickly). The only way to really learn this is through experience. Use a pulse monitor if necessary, but it is better to learn to listen to the way your body feels so that your experience can tell you if you need to back off or go harder. This takes time but can be achieved.

Above: When making a long climb, pay constant attention to what your body is telling you and try to keep to your ideal rhythm.

Once you have established what feels like the right rhythm, sometimes it will take you all the way to the top. However, you must be focused enough to realize if you are going too fast or too slow, even if it is by a microscopically small degree. In this case, just try to alter your effort level a little, slightly up or down, and settle into the new rhythm.

On a climb that is constantly changing in pitch, you have to be able to maintain the same rhythm. This can be achieved by using the gears. Aim for the same pedal cadence and pulse rate by changing down on steeper sections, and changing up on shallower gradients.

Below: The profile of the climb at Mont Ventoux, in gradient percentages. The road to the summit has an average gradient of 7.6 per cent and is one of the most difficult and notorious climbs in the Tour de France.

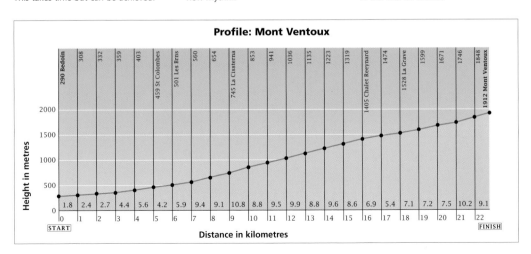

Riding a Sportive in a Group

On the start line of a sportive, you are sharing the road with up to several thousand other cyclists. It is unlikely that the group will ride round the entire course in one block, but by learning to ride in a smaller group, you can save a great deal of energy and time.

Cyclists riding in a group are faster than individuals riding on their own. The reason for this is that one of the biggest obstacles moving a bike forward is wind resistance. In a headwind, this resistance is made even worse, but it will have significantly less effect if someone is in front of you.

Efficient riding

By cycling behind another rider, it is estimated that you can save as much as 30 per cent of the effort he or she is making for the same speed.

What this means is that a group can work together efficiently and maintain a very high speed with less expenditure of energy. If a group of 12 riders spreads into a line and each takes a turn at the

front before moving to the back of the group, they will only spend a twelfth of the time riding into the wind, which is the hardest part. The rest of the time they are moving to the back of the group, which takes less energy, or sitting in the line sheltered behind another rider. In an hour, if everybody is sharing the workload equally, an individual will only have to spend 5 minutes on the front. That is a lot easier than riding into the wind on your own for an hour. The

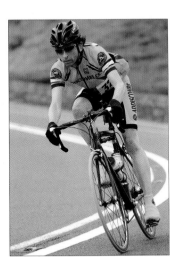

Right: Riding on your own is less energy-efficient than riding in a group.
Below: When you are riding a sportive in a group, share the work by taking turns at the front, where the air resistance is greatest.

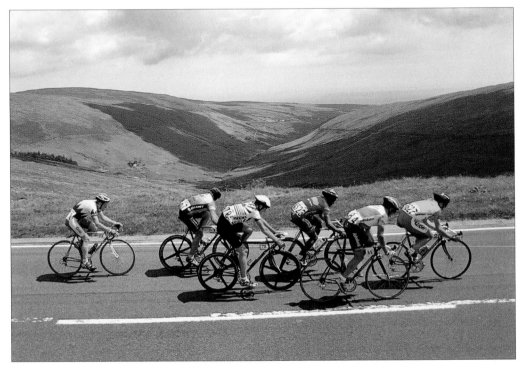

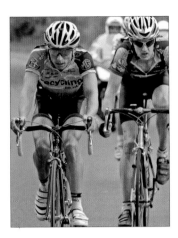

Above: Pace yourself and ride with others of similar ability, especially in a long sportive. Riders in a group who work out a formation will find that they can cut down their finishing time as well as increase their speed.

Tactical sportive riding

In the last few pages, we have emphasized that riding to your own pace is the best way of ensuring maximum performance and that going into the red zone can have a detrimental effect on energy levels later in the ride. (Going into the red zone is the equivalent of starting to sprint when out jogging.)

There are some occasions when other factors come into play. Imagine a situation where you are about 50m (165ft) from the back of a group near the top of a long hill, and riding at a rhythm which you know through experience is the right one to get to the top efficiently. You are better off riding at your own pace than trying to catch up faster riders. However, if they are only just ahead of you, it's worth chasing them down if there is a flat section after the descent.

By riding in a group, you will save energy in the long term and it will be worth the initial effort to catch them up for the effort you will save by sharing the workload.

If you are in the opposite situation, 100m (328ft) ahead of a small group of riders, it may be best to slow down and wait for them. If you are about to ride a long flat section, there is no point riding hard to hold them off – they will be riding far more efficiently than you, because they are sharing the workload. Instead, grab a bite to eat, sit up a little, stretch and wait for them. You will save a great deal of energy this way.

The guiding principle for sportives is: you are on your own on the climbs and descents, but co-operation with others on flat sections can make the difference between gold and silver awards.

technique of sharing the workload in the group is known as through-and-off, or drafting. It is not a simple case of riding in a straight line. Wind direction makes a difference, as do the relative abilities of the riders in the group. The wind is rarely a zero degree headwind blowing right into your face. More

often, with changes in road direction, it is a crosswind and comes from one side or another. The technique for riding in a crosswind still involves riding in a line, but riders also spread out laterally, with the first rider in the group on the side from which the wind is coming. The second rider sits behind him or her, and also to one side, with the following rider

taking a similar position and so on down the line. The front rider does his or her turn at the front, then goes back down the line to the back. And so on. This is an efficient way of riding, no matter how strong the wind, and if you join a strong group during a sportive, especially during the flat sections, it will make a difference to your finishing time.

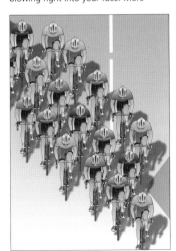

Above: When there is a crosswind, riders form a lateral formation for energy-efficient riding.

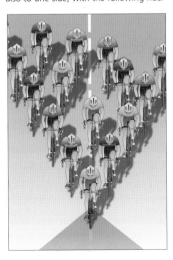

Above: When a group rides into a headwind, one rider takes the front position and others spread out behind.

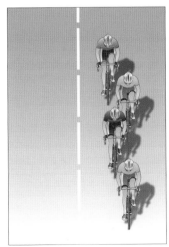

Above: In a smaller group, riders take it in turns to lead, while the others shelter behind the leader.

Descending in a Sportive

Some sportive organizers add to the cyclist's agony by finishing their events at the top of a hill. For all other events, what goes up must come down – for every mountain climbed, there is a descent waiting on the other side.

A lot of time can be lost on a descent. Nervousness about high speed and cornering can cause riders to overuse their brakes. They may also tense up, which makes it harder to flow through corners following the correct line.

Of course, the consequences of going out of control on a descent are far greater than on the flat or riding uphill. Speeds are much higher, so crashes are potentially far more dangerous.

By gaining confidence and relaxing, the descending involved in a sportive should be one of the most fun parts of the ride – and it hurts less than climbing.

Before you even start descending, the most important thing is to have trust in your bike. If it is well maintained, with sharp brakes, and correctly inflated, unworn tyres, you are reducing the chances of something going wrong. If your bike starts to rattle while you are going at 60kph (37mph) down a hill

because it has not been maintained, it is a problem. Second, you must have confidence in yourself and your ability to relax, focus and choose a line.

The shortest line

On a descent where the corners are not that sharp and you can see all the way through, just follow the shortest line down possible (without straying to the other side of the road). Allow your speed to rise to a point where you are totally confident of being able to handle it. If you find yourself starting to go faster than is comfortable, just feather the back brake to check, but not substantially reduce, your speed.

Your bike needs hardly any steering to get round these kinds of corners – shift your weight in the saddle, using your body to turn the bike, and just apply a little pressure to the handlebars to ease the bike through the turn. As

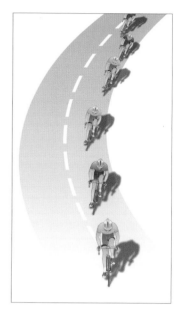

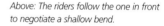

Above: The riders follow the one in front to negotiate a shallow bend.

your confidence rises, you will find yourself wanting to brake less. You will also relax, and start to lean your bike a little more as you round the corners. This is good, but don't relax to the detriment of your concentration – keep looking ahead for sharper corners or obstacles.

When descending, be aware of other competitors and road users and what is going on around you, and try to anticipate what others in front of you will do. If you are unhappy descending, drift to the back of your group so you can follow the other riders' lines through the bends. If somebody in front of you is going too slow, hang back until the right moment to go past them.

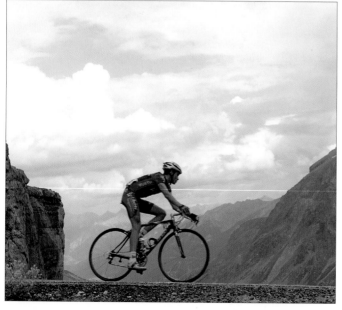

Left: When taking part in sportives in mountain areas, safe descent is vital.

Rounding a hairpin bend

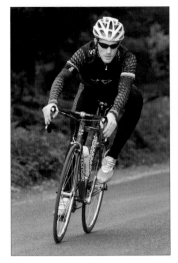

1 *Enter a bend from the wide angle.*

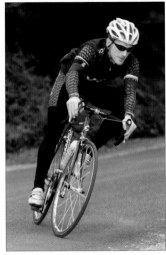

2 *Lean over and cut into the corner.*

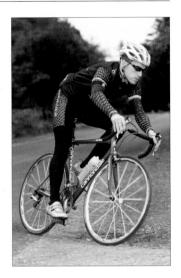

3 *Hit the apex with outer leg straight.*

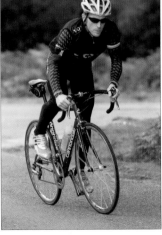

4 *Swing out again after the apex.*

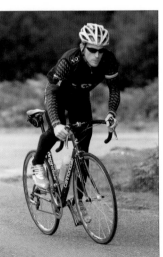

5 *Accelerate out of the bend.*

Hairpin bends

Descending becomes more complicated when the corners are sharper, as often happens in mountain regions. Engineers build roads with many hairpin bends, and getting around one of these losing as little speed as possible involves sound technique and steady nerves. As you approach a hairpin, you will probably be travelling quite fast. Keeping the same speed as you round the corner will result in a crash, so you have to check your speed. It is important to start and finish your braking before you start turning, or you risk your wheels locking and throwing you off the bike. The quickest way round is to enter wide, then lean your bike over and turn so that you pass close to the apex of the corner, then exit wide. Using the whole road is the way to maintain maximum speed, but if you cannot see through the corner, do not cross to the other side of the road as there may be oncoming traffic. If the way is clear, use a little more of the road, but safety should be your first concern.

As you turn, keep your inside leg up, point the knee towards the corner and put your weight on your outside leg, but don't be tempted to lean your whole body too far over. By keeping your head erect, you will hold your body upright enough to avoid toppling over. As you start to exit the curve, you can bring your inside knee back in, and you are ready to exit the corner.

By cornering on a hairpin bend, you have lost speed, and if you want to get to the bottom as quickly as possible, it will be necessary to accelerate hard once you are riding in a straight line again. With the gradient helping you, it won't be long before you are back up to full speed and ready to start braking for the next bend.

Applying Your Skills in a Sportive

Never go into an event without thoroughly researching the route. By doing your homework and analysing the distance and profile you can work out the best way for you to ride the race, and thus plan your training accordingly.

Riding a sportive successfully should be part of a long-term, goal-orientated strategy. The sense of satisfaction achieved by planning the build-up to an event, carrying out your training plan and riding the event successfully, is immense. If you surpass your expectations the sense of achievement is all the greater, and even if you are faced with unexpected challenges, dealing with them without panicking can also add satisfaction. Check out events well in advance in cycling magazines and websites.

Using the example of the Marmotte sportive in France, which takes in several Alpine climbs, a plan can be devised for the build-up, training and riding of the event to illustrate how these long-term goals can be achieved.

Research the profile and distance
Before starting the training and thinking about how to ride, you need to research the distance and profile of the event. In the case of the Marmotte, it is 174km

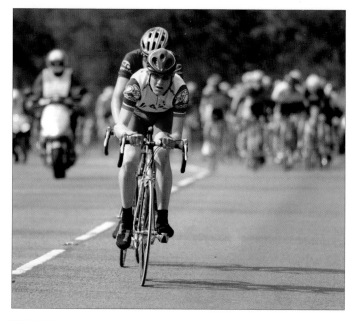

Above: Ride your target event at your own speed. Don't be pressured by anyone coming up behind you.

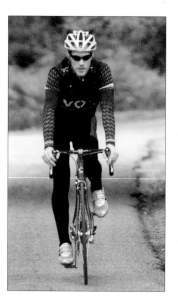

La Marmotte
Start Bourg d'Oisans, France.
Finish L'Alpe d'Huez.
Distance 174km/108 miles.
Number of significant climbs Four.
Total length of climbs 71km/44 miles.
Vertical height gain 5,000m/16,400ft.

(108 miles) long, which is above average. Your long training rides will have to be lengthened to prepare your body for the extra time in the saddle.

The profile of this event is intimidating. There are a few flat opening kilometres, followed by the long ascent of the Col de la Croix de Fer. The climb looks difficult – it is 27km (17 miles) long, averages a 5 per cent

Left: Train regularly in the months leading up to your target event. It will pay dividends during the competition.

gradient, and tops out at 2,068m (8,550ft) altitude. There is also a downhill section halfway up the climb, followed by a very steep upward incline. When riding, it will be important to pace yourself on the lower section to save some energy for later. Then you can rest on the descent before you reach the second section.

The descent of the Croix de Fer is nice and long – plenty of time to relax and save a bit of energy. It is followed by quite a long flat section to the foot of the next climb. During this part of the ride it is important to get into a group to save energy, and worth waiting for a group if there is none ahead of you.

The Col de la Télégraphe is the next climb – 12km (7.5 miles) long and less steep than the Croix de Fer, with less variation in gradient. It is important to establish a rhythm early on this climb, and make minor adjustments if you start to get tired or feel you are going too slow. The steepest part is at the top, so you might have to reduce speed in order to make the same effort for the final section of the race.

The descent of the Col de la Télégraphe is only a few kilometres long – not enough time to recover significantly, and with the 18km (11 miles) of the Col du Galibier approaching, it makes it all the more important to pace yourself sensibly on the Télégraphe.

The Galibier starts steadily, but gets steeper at the top. Pace yourself at the bottom, even if it feels like you are holding back. Then you will have more energy for the top half.

From the top of the Galibier, there are more than 40km (25 miles) of descent, which is an excellent opportunity to recuperate. This stretch takes you all the way to the foot of the final climb to L'Alpe d'Huez. There are 14km (8.5 miles) uphill to go, with the steepest section at the bottom. Pace yourself sensibly there, then establish a steady rhythm once the climb gets less steep.

Do the training
The training you need depends on whether your goal is to win the event, to achieve gold standard or silver

standard, or just to finish the event. You also need to tailor your training according to your experience and ability if you are to achieve your goal.

Whichever category you fit into, the training for the Marmotte needs to be extensive and regular.

Over a period of several months, you'll need to do at least one long ride each week, building up so that you can comfortably handle the distance. To prepare for the climbing, it will be necessary to practise riding uphill as much as possible. A great way of getting yourself into shape for a sportive is to ride another sportive. Why not find one about a month before the Marmotte to test your fitness and practise your pre-ride routine?

Ride the event
The Marmotte is long and hard, but with suitable preparation and training it should not hold any surprises for you.

The main thing to remember is to moderate your pace at the beginning of the route, especially during the first flat kilometres, where it is easy to get carried away and ride too hard.

Try to stay in a group for the flat sections, pace yourself carefully on the climbs and stay relaxed and focused for the descents.

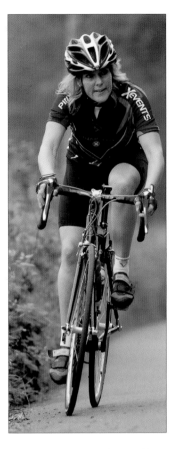

Below: The profile of the Marmotte shows that there are some very steep and difficult inclines to climb.

Above: Train hard over a few months before your chosen event. Practise on similar terrain, especially riding uphill.

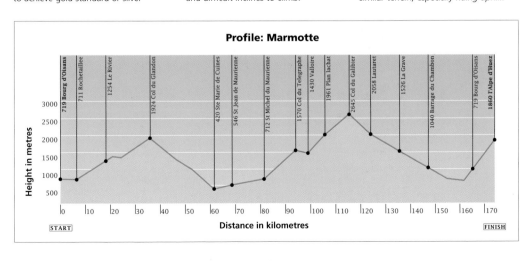

Profile: Marmotte

Great Sportives of the World: The Etape du Tour

The Etape du Tour is one of the most popular sportive events in the world. Each year, thousands of competitors ride a single stage of the Tour de France, during which they cross some of the most difficult mountains of the race.

The Tour de France is most renowned for its mountain stages. The fastest and fittest cyclists in the world compete with each other on the slopes of climbs such as the Col du Galibier, L'Alpe d'Huez and Mont Ventoux.

Since 1993, amateur cyclists and sportive riders have also been given the opportunity to compete on a Tour de France mountain stage in the Etape du Tour. Over the years, it has become a globally important sportive event, with 8,000 cyclists taking part.

More than 2,000 of these riders come from outside France. Most are from the United Kingdom and the United States, but some of the cyclists come from as far afield as Japan or New Zealand. The organizers of the Etape du Tour, who also organize the Tour de France, want

to make their event as spectacular as possible, and they often select one of the hardest stages of the actual race for the Etape route. With few exceptions, they favour stages from the Alps or the Pyrenees, involving the celebrated climbs of the race.

Because there are so many participants, the riders start in waves, counting around a thousand. Entry criteria are stringent, and there are cut-off points along the route – if you ride too slowly, you will be prevented from finishing the event. But while the rules are strict, the satisfaction to be gained from completing the Etape is immense, with the added bonus that you can compare your time with the professionals, who will ride the same course only days later.

A mark of how fit the actual Tour riders are is that the fastest Etape rider is often still an hour or so slower than the last-placed professional.

Tactics for the Etape

Unlike the Marmotte sportive, or the events in the following pages, the Etape follows a different route every year, which means that the preparation and tactics alter from event to event. The 2008 edition from Pau to Hautacam included a long, flat opening section, followed by two difficult climbs (the Col du Tourmalet and Hautacam), while the 2004 edition had a whole series of smaller climbs over the course of a long distance.

Meanwhile, the 2006 edition was one of the hardest in the history of the event, with three of the hardest climbs of the Tour de France – the Col d'Izoard, the Col du Lautaret and L'Alpe d'Huez – on the route.

On a route like that of the 2008 Etape, the biggest temptation would be to start too fast on the fast flat roads in the first half of the event. Pacing is even more important than usual when the end is harder than the start. The route also includes two smaller climbs early on – it's important to take obstacles like this easily, to prevent the build-up of fatigue. On the other hand, the first major climb, the Col du Tourmalet, is harder than the final climb. This means that it might be possible to make a bigger effort on this ascent, knowing that the final climb won't be as bad. However, the tactics for the 2007 event would

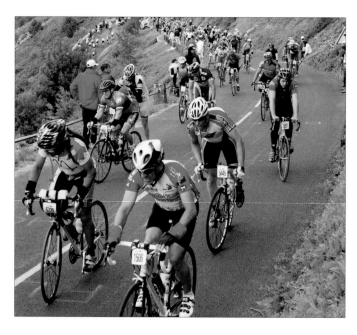

Left: The Etape du Tour is one of the most famous sportives in the world – it follows the same route as a Tour de France stage.

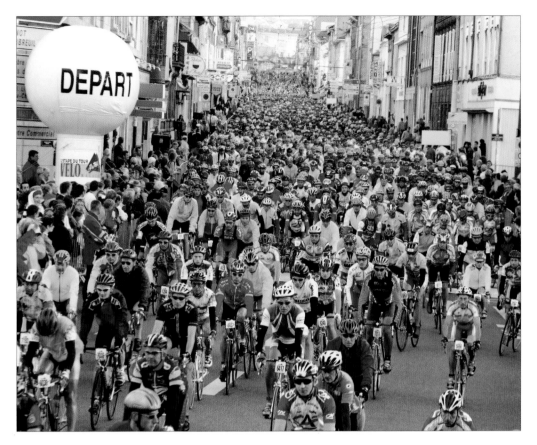

have been very similar to those of the Marmotte. With three major climbs en route, including an uphill finish, pacing needs to be steady and conservative.

In spite of its difficulty, or perhaps because of it, entries to the Etape are oversubscribed. Participants from outside France must enter through designated organizing companies, and provide a medical certificate. But if you are fit, and keen to emulate your heroes in the Tour de France, the Etape is one of the most rewarding sportives in the world.

Above: The huge popularity of the Etape du Tour is evident from this picture taken in 2004. The numbers have grown year on year, and as many as 8,000 riders from all over the world now take part. The route varies each year but it is always a difficult one.

The Etape du Tour in recent years					
Year	**Mountain range**	**Start**	**Finish**	**Distance**	**Climbs**
2008	Pyrenees	Pau	Hautacam	156km/97 miles	Col du Tourmalet, Hautacam
2007	Pyrenees	Foix	Loudenvielle	199km/124 miles	Col de Port, Col du Portet d'Aspet, Col de Mente, Col du Port de Balès, Col de Peyresourde
2006	Alps	Gap	L'Alpe d'Huez	193km120/ miles	Col d'Izoard, Col du Lautaret, L'Alpe d'Huez
2005	Pyrenees	Mourenx	Pau	179km/111 miles	Col d'Ichère, Col de Marie-Blanque, Col d'Aubisque
2004	Massif Central	Limoges	St Flour	239km/149 miles	Col de Néronne, Col du Pas de Peyrol, Col d'Entremont, Plomb du Cantal

Great Sportives of the World: Flanders and the Ventoux

The Tour of Flanders is one of the most famous professional bike races in the world. The climb of Mont Ventoux is among the best-known ascents in the Tour de France. It's possible to tackle both in the form of a sportive.

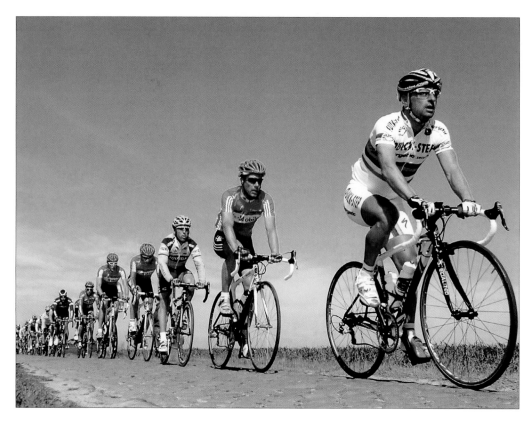

The Tour of Flanders and the Mont Ventoux sportives are a good challenge for ambitious amateur cyclists. Both cover the routes of well-known bike races, although they are very different in their challenge and character.

The Ventoux sportive is similar to the majority of this kind of event – it covers large climbs and is extremely arduous. The Tour of Flanders is different – because it takes place in Belgium, it therefore cannot include

Above: The Tour of Flanders attracts many amateur riders who want to follow in the tracks of their professional cycling heroes.

high mountain passes. But it still remains an extremely challenging and tough event.

The Tour of Flanders

Unlike the Tour de France, which is a stage race taking place over three weeks, the Tour of Flanders is a single-

day event. Flanders, in Belgium, is probably the most cycling-obsessed region in the world, and thousands of fans turn out to watch the race, which happens on the first Sunday of April.

While the Tour de France has its mountains, Flanders has its bergs – these are small but very steep climbs that range between 300m (984ft) and 3km (4 miles) in length, and often have a cobbled surface which makes riding them extremely difficult. Although the route alters slightly most years, there are always between 15 and 20 bergs, which are packed with fans on race day.

The day before the professional event, there is an amateur event over the same roads. The professional race is 270km (168 miles) long, which is an extremely tough proposition, even for fit amateurs, so the organizers also run a 140-km (87-mile) sportive.

Weather conditions are often difficult in Belgium in early April – the Tour of Flanders is traditionally run over flat roads which are extremely exposed to crosswinds. Rain and cold also make it a challenge. Tactically, to do well in the Tour of Flanders sportive, you must be skilled at riding in a group, to minimize the effect of the wind. If the wind is coming from ahead, ride directly behind the rider in front. But if the wind is coming from either side, move to one side of them, so that you are protected.

The climbs also take a special technique, especially in wet conditions. The cobbles are bumpy and slippery, and the steepness of the hills means that traction is easily lost. Usually on a steep hill, standing up on the pedals is the most efficient way to the top, but on slippery cobbles, stay seated, keeping your weight over the back wheel to stop wheelspins from happening. And ride in a low gear, to prevent stalling – the steepest of the climbs are around 25 per cent (one-in-four) gradient.

The Ventoux

The 'Giant of Provence', as Mont Ventoux is known, is one of the most arduous climbs regularly used in the Tour de France. It rises 1,912m (6,273ft) above sea level in Provence, and is all the more impressive for its isolation – it towers above the surrounding hills. Mont Ventoux gained infamy in the Tour de France when British cyclist Tom Simpson died of heatstroke, exacerbated by performance-enhancing drugs, on its slopes during the 1967 race. Ventoux is also famous for being one of the few mountain stages in the Tour de France that seven-times winner Lance Armstrong never managed to conquer.

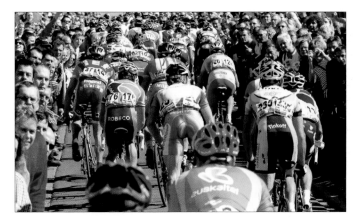

Above: The Tour of Flanders in 2007 attracted many spectators to watch the professionals ride by.

The Ventoux is a hard, steep climb, with a summit very exposed to wind and sun. There are three roads to the top. The Ventoux sportive is an annual event which takes place in the early summer. It starts and finishes in Beaumes-de-Venise, and is unusual in that the route crosses the climb twice – once from the hardest side, which starts in the town of Bedoin, and once from the easiest side, which starts to the east in Sault. The route includes hilly sections between the two main ascents, and a final 30km (18½ miles) with two significant climbs. The route is 170km (106 miles) long, so it is hard even for the fittest cyclists. This means that tactics for the Ventoux need to be carefully planned. The first 30km (18½ miles) are flat and fast – it is easy to go too hard here, so instead, find shelter in a group of riders and take it easy to the bottom of the first ascent of the Ventoux, which is the hardest part of the course. The climb from Bedoin to the summit of the Ventoux is consistently steep, and 23km (14 miles) long, which means that it takes most amateur cyclists at least an hour and a half to climb it. Too hard an effort here will result in fatigue later.

Right : The mountainous route of Mont Ventoux is so steep and long that even professional cyclists find it difficult.

The final 7km (4 miles) take riders above the treeline, where they are exposed to the hot sun on clear days, and often strong winds. The descent of the Ventoux is one of the fastest in any sportive in the world, but following it, there are 50km (31 miles) of rolling roads where it is easy to go too hard. On both the initial climb and this section, save a bit of energy for the final climb of the Ventoux, up from Sault. This climb is less steep than the approach from Bedoin, but fatigue makes it as hard, or harder than the first climb. And you still need to save energy for the final 30km (18½-mile) stretch to the finish.

If you wish to enter the Ventoux sportive, go to the event's website, at www.sportcommunication.com.

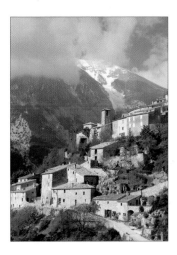

Great Sportives of the World: Cape Argus and Gran Fondo Gimondi

Two of the most popular sportive events in the world are the Cape Argus Cycle Tour and Gran Fondo Felice Gimondi. One takes place in South Africa, the other in Italy, and both are renowned for their dramatic scenery.

Sportives are not just a physical challenge. One of their main attractions is that they take place in spectacular locations, in the mountains, in often beautiful settings. Many events, including the two described here, are a perfect combination of leisure, enjoyment and challenge.

Cape Argus Cycle Tour

This event happens in March, and it is the biggest sportive in the world. Unusually, it takes place outside Europe, in South Africa, with a route that skirts the Cape Peninsula in Cape Town. The event, which started in 1978 with 525 cyclists, has now grown to attract 35,000 entrants who include elite international athletes at the front, covering the 100km (62-mile) route in under 2½ hours, through serious amateurs, to leisure cyclists looking for a personal challenge.

The biggest attraction of the Cape Argus Cycle Tour, aside from the privilege of sharing the road with the biggest group of cyclists in the world, is the breathtaking scenery along the South African coast. The press photographs of

Below: Cyclists climb Suikerbossie Hill in the annual Cape Argus Cycle Tour.

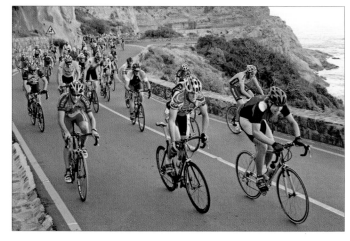

thousands of riders snaking along the coastal road of the peninsula, which is closed to traffic for the day, are so impressive that they attract great public interest in the sport of cycling.

The Cape Argus differs most from the traditional European sportives in the difficulty of the route. It's hilly, but by no means mountainous – the highest point of the event is under 200m (640ft) above sea level. This means that it is more

Above: The Cape Argus Cycle Tour is the world's largest individually timed race.

accessible to leisure cyclists. And at 100km (62 miles), it can be achieved by anyone who has done a little training.

There are five main hills, and many smaller rises along the route, which are steep, but are mainly under 4km (2½ miles) long. Entrants can thus ride in a different way than in the big mountain sportives of Europe. Along the flat roads of the coast, riding in a group will help enormously, by providing shelter from wind resistance. It's also possible to ride at a much more even speed, which makes judging overall pace much easier. Don't start too hard, but the route is not so difficult that you need to save yourself specially during the early stages.

Gran Fondo Felice Gimondi

While the Marmotte and Etape are very hard, events like the Gran Fondo Felice Gimondi are the perfect balance of physical challenge, and rideable terrain.

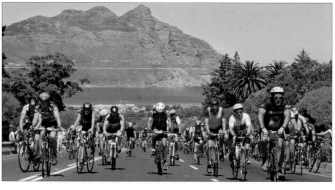

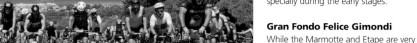

Climbs of the Gran Fondo Felice Gimondi				
Climb	Length	Altitude	Height gain	Average gradient
Colle dei Pasta	3.8km/2 miles	406m/1,340ft	140m/1,340ft	3.7%
Colle Gallo	7.5km/5 miles	763m/2,518ft	426m/1,405ft	5.7%
Selvino	11km/7 miles	960m/3,168ft	653m/2,155ft	5.6%
Forcella di Bura	20.4km/13 miles	766m/2,528ft	613m/2,023ft	4.5%
Forcella di Berbenno	4.5km/3 miles	663m/2,188ft	273m/901ft	5.3%
Costa Valle Imagna	9.5km/6 miles	1,014m/3,346ft	715m/2,360ft	6.6%

The Gimondi, which starts and finishes in the cycling-crazy town of Bergamo in Italy, has six significant climbs, the highest of which is about 1,000m (3,200ft) in altitude. Rather than the steep 25km (15½-mile) slogs of the Alps, these are much smaller climbs, which offer a reasonable challenge without being too tough. At 163km (101 miles), the distance is about average for a big international sportive.

The Gimondi is an interesting study in how to ride a sportive. The climbs vary in difficulty. The Forcella di Bura, which is the fourth climb of the day, is over 20km (12 miles) long, but only has an average gradient of 4.5 per cent, whereas the Costa Valle Imagna, the final climb of the day, is less than half the distance at 9.5km (6 miles), but is much steeper at 6.6 per cent. Each climb demands a different effort, and

it is important in this event not to ride too fast on the early climbs. The Colle dei Pasta, which is the first climb, is more of a warm-up for the later climbs, but the second and third hills, the Colle Gallo and Selvino, are increasingly longer.

The final climb is the hardest, which means that pacing is very important – there are five chances to go too hard earlier in the ride, and it is usually better to resist the temptation and reserve plenty of energy for the end.

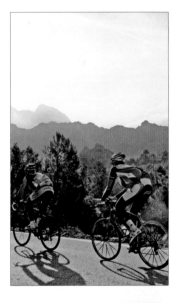

Right: Two riders cycle home after taking part in a sportive event.
Below: The Gran Fondo Felice Gimondi is a major sportive event, named in honour of Felice Gimondi, a notable professional racing cyclist in the 1960s. He won three Grand Tours, one of only four cyclists to do so.

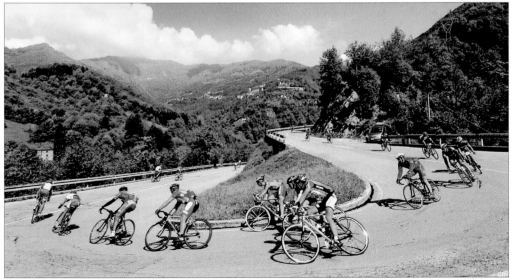

Great Rides of the World: The Great Races

You don't have to enter a sportive event to experience the great races of the world. Sometimes, it is enough to go and just ride them as a one-day event. All you need is a map, a bike and no small amount of energy and enthusiasm.

At the Etape du Tour, you can ride a stage of the Tour de France. The Marmotte, Gran Fondo Felice Gimondi and Ventoux sportives all offer the chance to compete against thousands of other cyclists on some famous cycling routes. But it's also possible to just go and ride the routes of some of the great races without having to enter a sportive. Road racing takes place on roads which are open to the public for the other 364 days of the year, and it's possible to ride any of them.

Milan–San Remo

Known as the 'Sprinters–Classic', the route of Milan–San Remo is mainly flat, along the northern Mediterranean coast of Italy. As a result, sprinters, who are generally big, strong, heavy riders who are less good at climbing hills, dominate the race history. The best part to ride is the final 100km

Below: The champion, Eddy Merckx, won the prestigious Milan–San Remo seven times.

(60 miles) of the race, or more if you are fit enough. The route is a pleasant ride, with only a few hills to deal with. The most difficult are the 6km (4-mile) Cipressa and 4km (2.5-mile) Poggio, in the final 30km (18.5 miles) before the finish, but they are well-surfaced and steady.

Milan–San Remo
Where to stay San Remo.
The ride Savona–San Remo (110km/68 miles).
Climbs Capo Mele, Capo Berta, Cipressa, Poggio (max altitude 240m/780ft).
Other rides in the area Head inland from the coast to explore the quiet hills.

Paris–Roubaix

Most cycling events get their difficulty from hills. However, Paris–Roubaix is one of the flattest races in the professional cycling calendar. It gets its toughness from several sections of cobbled farm track, which have bumpy and unpredictable surfaces and are extremely

---

Paris–Roubaix
Where to stay Valenciennes.
The ride Valenciennes–Roubaix (110km/68 miles).
Climbs No significant ones.
Other rides in the area Cross over the Belgian border to explore the Chimay.

---

difficult to ride on. The best preparation for riding on the cobbles is to modify your bike so it will absorb as much of the shock as possible. You will need thicker tyres, and stronger wheels if possible. Professional cyclists put two layers of bar tape on, to make gripping the handlebars easier.

When riding the cobbles, maintaining speed is very difficult, but crucial if you are to avoid getting knocked off your line. Stay relaxed and vigilant and try to look a few metres ahead at all times,

Below: The roads of the Paris–Roubaix race are as challenging and difficult as any mountain pass.

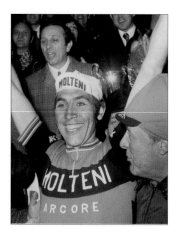

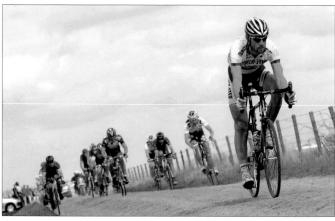

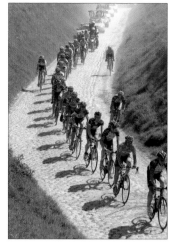

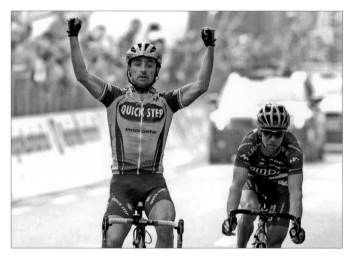

*Above: The cobbled track in the Paris–
Roubaix event is very hard to ride on.*

*Above: Italy's Paolo Bettini is a former
winner of the Tour of Lombardy.*

so you can spot any large cobbles that
jut upwards. This kind of surface takes a
lot of getting used to.

Liège–Bastogne–Liège

A more traditional cycling challenge is
Liège–Bastogne–Liège – its difficulty
comes from a succession of long and
steep climbs winding through the forests
of the Ardennes in Belgium. The race
starts from Liège, and heads down to
the turning point at Bastogne. It's a
good idea to pick it up from here – the
hills are almost exclusively in the second
half of the race. None of the climbs are

longer than a few kilometres. But their
steepness and repetitive nature sap the
energy from the legs. One good idea is
to fit a compact chainset, so that you
have a wide selection of low gears.

> **Liège–Bastogne–Liège**
> **Where to stay** Bastogne.
> **The ride** Bastogne–Ans (150km/93 miles).
> **Climbs** Many, including the Côte de Stockeu,
> Haute-Levée, Redoute and Sprimont.
> **Other rides in the area** Head west to
> Huy to ride the famous Mur climb, which
> features in the Flèche Wallonne race.

Tour of Lombardy

The climbs of the Tour of Lombardy, in
Italy, are in some of the most beautiful
cycling country in the world. They are
long, moderately steep, and offer a
good physical challenge. The route
circles Lake Como, and covers 260km
(162 miles). Even missing the first part of
the race and riding from Como involves
220km (137 miles) of hilly riding – it's
probably best to divide it into two
halves, and stop over in Parlasco, on the
west side of the lake.

Approach these climbs like mountain
roads – it's important to establish an
early and good rhythm, because if you
go too hard too soon, you will suffer in
the final kilometres. The most famous
climb of the Tour of Lombardy is the
Madonna del Ghisallo, with a chapel at
the top, filled with cycling memorabilia.

*Left: The peloton starts in Liège for the
Liège–Bastogne–Liège challenge ride.*

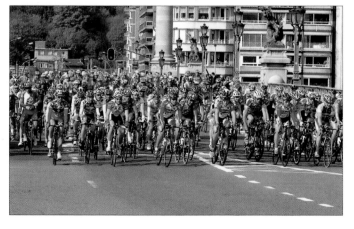

> **Tour of Lombardy**
> **Where to stay** Como.
> **The ride** Como–Como (220km/136 miles).
> **Climbs** Parlasco, Colle di Balisio,
> Madonna del Ghisallo, Civiglio, San Fermo
> di Battaglia.
> **Other rides in the area** The hills around
> Lake Como are some of the best for
> cycling in the world.

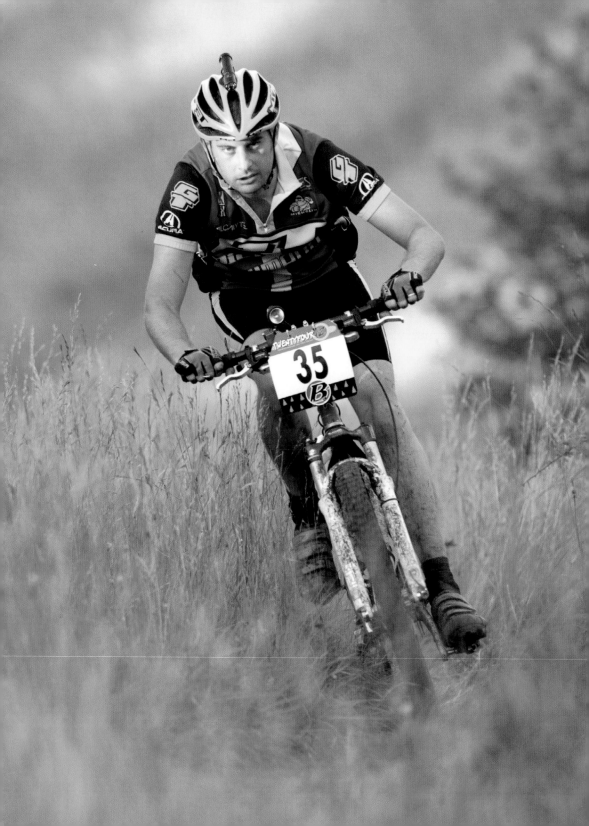

MOUNTAIN BIKING

Mountain biking is one of the most beneficial
and fun exercise regimes you can follow. While
road riders have to share the road with traffic, on a
mountain bike you are generally in splendid isolation, in
beautiful surroundings, on challenging terrain.
It doesn't even matter if it rains. While bad weather
can be demoralizing for other forms of cycling, wet
weather is all part of the fun of mud-plugging (off-road
riding). There are many different disciplines to try out
on a mountain bike, from trail riding and downhill
riding to freeriding.

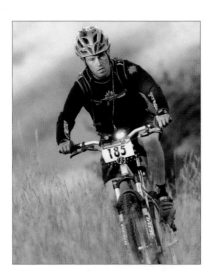

Above: Riding off-road is one of the pleasures of mountain biking.
Left: Mountain biking through a forest on a rocky road will help to improve your fitness,
while being extremely enjoyable.

Choosing a Mountain Bike

With such a wide range of off-road bikes available, it can be hard to choose what type to buy, let alone a specific model. When buying a bike your needs, budget and ambitions all have to be taken into consideration.

Before taking the plunge to buy a bike, you have to decide whether you want a specific bike for a specific task, or a more versatile model to allow you to explore more than one branch of off-road cycling.

Specific bikes are easy to decide on. If you want to ride trials, only a trials bike will do – the specification is so exact and developed that a normal mountain bike will be unable to meet performance needs. You really need a downhill bike for cycling down hills properly. It is possible to ride down some courses on a hardtail bike with suspension forks, but

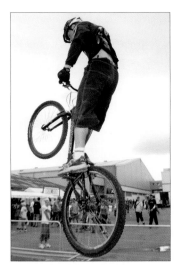

Right: For trials riding, you'll need a specialized bike.
Below: A full-suspension mountain bike is suitable for heavy-duty off-road riding.

you will have to keep your speed so low to cope with the bumping and shock that it will detract from the fun.

If you decide that you are going to ride off-road, then you need a more general bike, and this is where the massive choice starts to get confusing. You might be more specific, and decide that you want to race cross-country, but then you have to choose between hardtail and full suspension, V-brakes or disc brakes, even between eight- and nine-speed freewheels.

For those who just want to enjoy the occasional bit of trail riding, a hardtail bike with V-brakes and suspension forks will probably return the maximum benefit. A bike like this is versatile enough to be ridden on the trails and make it a rewarding experience, but it is

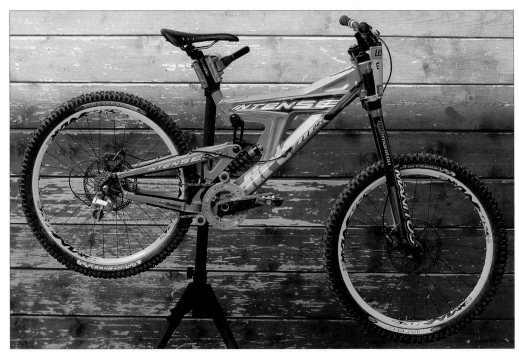

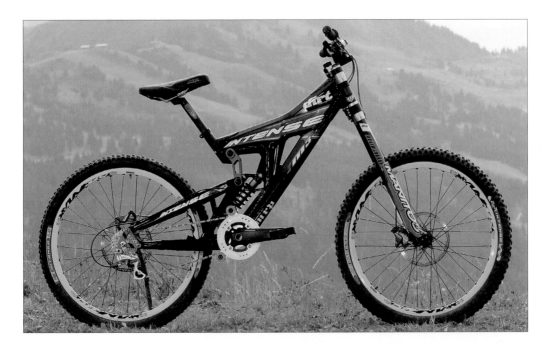

Above: A downhill bike is designed for one purpose only – it's too heavy to ride back up a steep slope.

not so specialized that it can be used only for this purpose. There is also the advantage that it can be used as a runaround urban bike and fulfil that function perfectly well.

If you are going to take the sport more seriously and hit the trails on a regular basis, perhaps embarking on longer challenge rides, your equipment needs to be a bit more specialized.

There is no easy answer to the hardtail versus full suspension debate – the topic has been debated for years. All you can do is make your own decision, based on what you think you will get out of each type of bike.

If you are light and good at climbing, you might consider going for the full suspension – the extra weight will slow you down on the hills, but as you climb fast, you can afford to slow yourself down marginally. On the other hand, when it comes to bowling down the other side of the hill, the full suspension will allow you to maximize your speed and efficiency. Likewise, an occasional

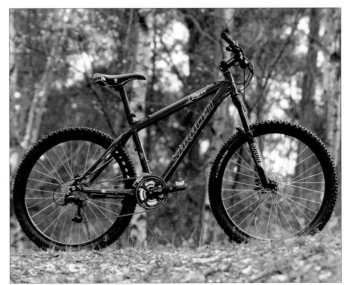

rider who prefers a bit of light trail riding on a warm day might not need to install disc brakes, when V-brakes will do just as well. If you are planning to go out in all weathers throughout the year, disc brakes are probably the right option. The most important thing is to

Above: Hardtail mountain bikes are good for off-road riding, and are more efficient for all-purpose riding.

work out which bike will give you the most enjoyment and let you cycle effectively.

The Hardtail Bike

Hardtail mountain bikes are light and fast and handle precisely, and they are excellent for speed and efficient climbing. The front suspension provides comfort and control of the bike and the fat tyres allow smooth riding on roads.

A basic mountain bike, either with suspension or regular forks and a normal aluminium frame, is known as a hardtail. Although full-suspension bikes are currently popular for their greater shock absorbency in bumpy conditions, a traditional hardtail can still be the best bike for basic cross-country and trail riding. They are lighter than full-suspension models. They also have the advantage that, combined with slick tyres, they make a far better road bike. When buying a mountain bike, it is easy

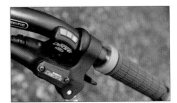

Right: Gear shifters are located on the handlebars for quick changing.

Anatomy of a hardtail bike

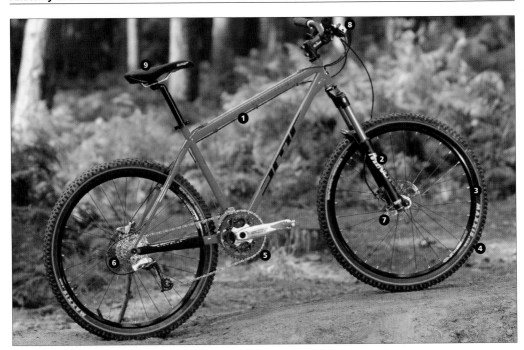

1 Frame: Aluminium frame, compact, but with plenty of clearance for fat tyres. Skinny seatstays absorb much more impact.

2 Fork: Suspension fork for shock absorption and a more comfortable ride on rough and bumpy surfaces. Most forks can be adjusted for shock absorbency, depending on the type of terrain.

3 Wheels: 32-spoked wheels, with 26in rims, which are smaller than those on a road bike. Width can be 1.5–3in.

4 Tyres: Thick and knobbly for extra grip on loose surfaces.

5 Chainrings: Triple chainrings offer more possible gears.

6 Sprockets: Eight or nine, depending on preference and model.

Much wider spread, to give very low gear options for steep hills.

7 Brakes: V-Brakes for greater stopping capacity than regular callipers. Disc brakes are becoming more popular for their efficiency in all weathers.

8 Gear shifters: Integrated into brake system for ease of access.

9 Saddle: Comfortable, supportive saddle, good for rough terrain.

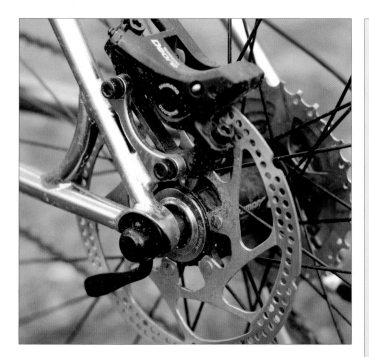

to be impressed by the sophisticated technology of full-suspension designs, but depending on your needs, hardtail mountain bikes are resilient and reliable. Hardtails are more sensitive to accelerations, giving a more responsive ride, which purists and traditionalists prefer. For general fitness riding and enjoying getting out on the trails, a basic hardtail model with eight-speed freewheel and V-brakes is a good choice.

Frames and components
The majority of hardtail frames are aluminium, and they are compact and low. A long seatpin, small frame and 26in wheels, which are smaller than road wheels, keep the rider's weight low to the ground. This makes the bike more controllable at low speeds, either going up steep hills, or dealing with highly technical sections. Riders often have to jump off their bikes, and a low top tube makes this easier.

The triple chainset, with chainrings with 42, 32 and 22 teeth, plus an eight-speed freewheel is a good combination for riding your mountain bike over a

Above: Disc brakes are powerful enough to check speed even on loose surfaces and down steep hills.

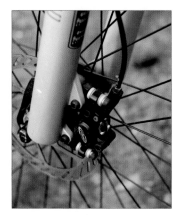

variety of terrains. On very steep hills, which you can often encounter on a trail ride, the inner chainring should be able to deal with the gradient.

Brakes can be either disc or the traditional V-brakes, depending on what you want to get from your riding. Disc brakes perform better in bad

Trials bike
Trials bikes are an offshoot of mountain bikes used for jumps and riding over obstacles, either artificial or natural. Riders keep their feet up, and ride, hop and jump from obstacle to obstacle, balancing on the super-fat tyres even when the bike is not moving.

A trials bike has a very short seat tube, which enables the body to move over the bike and perform a jump called a sidehop, in which the bike jumps both up and laterally. The frame is very stiff and responsive, with no need for energy-absorbing suspension. Riders gain control from a wider set of flat handlebars, which give more leverage.

Wheels are usually 26in, with fat tyres at low pressure to grip surfaces. A single small chainring, usually fitted with a guard to protect it from damage when it hits an obstacle, is combined with a seven-, eight- or nine-speed freewheel. Brakes need to be very strong – many riders choose hydraulic systems, which lose less power than a traditional cable. Some riders don't even use a saddle on their trials bike – the jumps are all executed standing up.

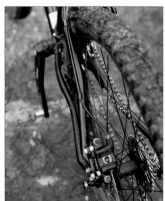

Above left: Suspension forks and disc brakes help control your bike.
Above: Chunky tyres are necessary for off-road riding, to aid grip.

conditions, and overall, offer more stopping power. V-brakes are simpler and lighter.

Full-suspension Cross-country and Downhill Bikes

In recent years, the technology of full-suspension frames has improved significantly. For trail riding, the full-suspension bike gives a much more comfortable ride, which is especially important when riding long distances.

Bumps and shocks tire and bruise the body – riding a full-suspension bike can reduce these shocks and make the experience of trail riding positive and even more enjoyable.

Full-suspension bike
There is no doubt that riding a full-suspension bike down hills is easier than on a hardtail, on which all the bumps you ride over are transmitted straight to your saddle area. The suspension irons out the lumps and bumps, giving a faster, more comfortable ride.

The payoff for the extra comfort, however, is reduced speed and extra weight. Full suspension adds a few kilograms to the weight of your bike, because of the extra tubing and machinery involved in the suspension system. Every time you ride up a hill, you will be carrying more weight than a

Below: Full-suspension frames make for a less harsh ride over bumpy ground.

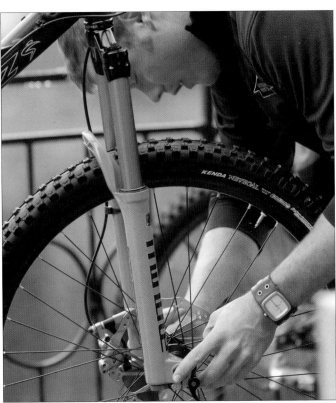

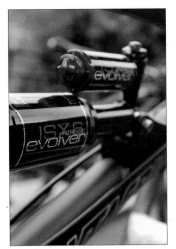

Above: Keep your mountain bike clean and well maintained – riding off-road in poor conditions can wear down components very quickly.

traditional hardtail, and the efforts quickly mount up and can tire you out. However, the more technical the terrain, the more the full-suspension bike comes into its own. So over the course of a long ride, including uphills, downhills and technical sections, the full suspension will probably have a net benefit effect on the speed of your ride.

Downhill mountain bike
With most other types of mountain bike, riders always have to compromise between speed and comfort. The downhill mountain bike is designed purely to absorb bumps and shocks. Downhill mountain biking has its roots right back in the origins of the sport. The first mountain bikers were the Californians who rode general-purpose

bikes down Repack Hill in the 1970s, and the tradition has continued to the present day, when the downhill is a major event in the World Cup series, attracting huge crowds with spectacular races. Downhill cycling is a time trial from the top of a hill to the bottom, with bends, jumps and steep straights on which riders can reach massive speeds, sometimes over 95kph (60mph). The downhill bike, more than any other, relies on strong suspension with a great deal of travel (amount of give in a suspension system) to absorb the shocks at speed. It also needs to be manoeuvrable – courses often include sharp bermed (high-sided) corners and narrow sections that demand great control, even at speed.

Frames are full suspension, with lots of travel and large springs to absorb the impact of bumps that are hit at 80kph (50mph). The fork suspension travel is enormous, since it is the front wheel that takes the brunt of the hits. Controlling speed effectively means that disc brakes are the only real option, as they have a larger braking surface than regular mountain bike V-brakes. The chain is kept in place with a retainer, and the chainring is protected.

The riding position on a downhill bike is not over-streamlined, in spite of the fact that aerodynamics are important. The saddle is kept low, to keep the rider's weight close to the ground and the bike stable.

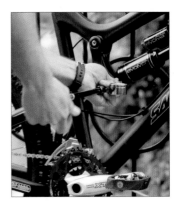

Above: The travel on full-suspension bikes can be altered depending on the terrain you expect to encounter.

Anatomy of a full-suspension cross-country bike

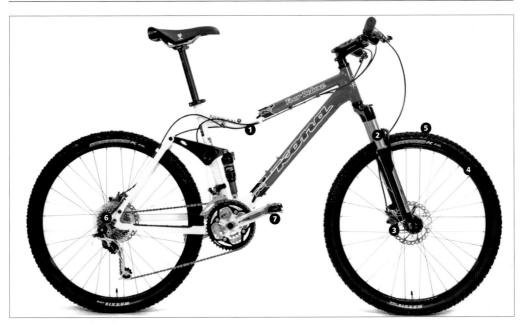

❶ Full-suspension frame: Provides greater shock absorbency, and greater control and traction in rough terrain.
❷ Suspension fork: Takes all the impact where the bike feels it most – at the front wheel.
❸ Brakes: Disc brakes are essential for better stopping power at speed and

for cycling in poor conditions such as mud and water, bumpy surfaces and rocky roads.
❹ Wheels: Rims are 26in with 32 spokes for lightness and strength. Width is 1.9 or 2.1in, for the right balance between grip and rolling resistance.

❺ Tyres: Thick knobbly tyres grip the ground in rough terrain.
❻ Gears: Nine-speed freewheel, combined with a triple chainring with 22, 32 and 42 teeth.
❼ Pedals: Reversible clipless pedals so that the shoe can clip into either side of the pedal.

Clothing and Equipment

The varied conditions experienced when out mountain biking mean it is a sensible idea to wear specialized clothing that will minimize discomfort. Comfort is a priority as well as protection from the cold and wet.

In the summer, clothing is simple. A pair of shorts, plus a base layer for your top, and a loose cycling jersey are the most comfortable option. Some mountain bikers wear skin-tight Lycra road-racing shorts, while others prefer the look of baggy shorts, but be careful of catching them on your saddle as you stand up on the pedals. Jerseys do not need to be as tight fitting as those of road riders, since speeds are lower and aerodynamics less important. A loose-fitting jersey will help keep you cool.

Gloves are essential. No one is immune from crashing, and you will need to protect your hands and fingers if you stack your bike. Full-fingered gloves are advisable for off-roading.

Helmets, too, are just as important for off-road riding as they are on the road. If you come off, you could be seriously injured if your head hits a rock or tree roots.

If you are not planning on having to put your feet down, you can use stiffer-soled shoes similar to those of road cyclists. However, most mountain bikers will want the kind of shoe that clips into your pedals, but is also comfortable and

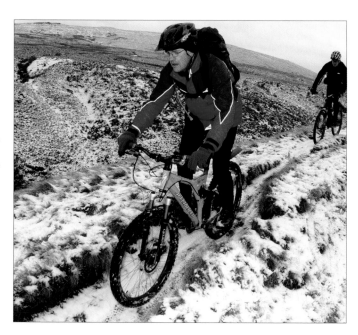

Above: Extreme conditions make it necessary to wrap up warm.

flexible for walking. For steep sections of trail you may need to dismount and walk, and it helps to have some grip.

In winter it is important to dress well because of the wet conditions. Depending on how mild or cold it is, you may need a windproof and waterproof jacket. Even if it is not raining, water can still spray up off your companions' wheels. Long leggings will keep your legs warm and shoe covers will protect your feet from the elements. A warmer pair of gloves and a hat are also useful. Even when the sun is not shining, it is a sensible precaution to wear goggles to protect your eyes.

Left: A lightweight waterproof jacket will protect you from the rain.
Right: Keeping feet warm is important.

Mountain bike tyres pick up mud and stones and sometimes they can be flicked up into the face of the rider behind.

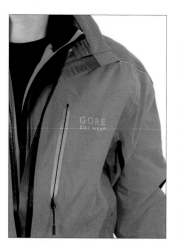

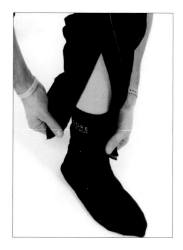

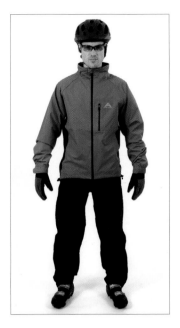

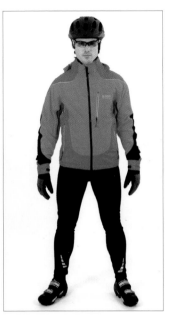

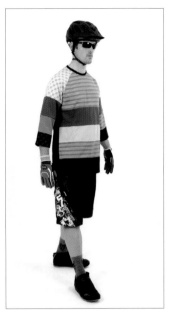

Above: Baggy winter clothing is warm and practical for off-road riding.

Above: If speed is important to you, Lycra leggings are more aerodynamic.

Above: In summer, shorts and a long-sleeved top will protect you from scratches.

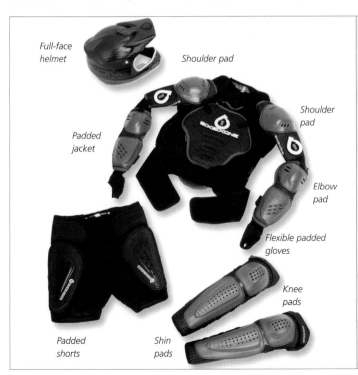

Full-face helmet

Shoulder pad

Shoulder pad

Padded jacket

Elbow pad

Flexible padded gloves

Knee pads

Padded shorts

Shin pads

Downhill body armour

Downhill racers need serious protection for their bodies, in case of a crash.

On your head, you need a full-face helmet. It is not enough just to wear an ordinary hard shell helmet – these do not protect the face. A comfortable and effective full-face helmet will protect the whole of your head, as well as the back of your neck. Cover your eyes with goggles that fit inside the opening of the helmet.

Body armour will protect your arms, legs and body. Parts of your anatomy tend to hit the ground more than others and these parts have extra-hard shell protection. The knees and shins have a hard shell, as do the shoulders, elbows, wrists and chest. Downhill crashes tend to cause injuries from skidding along the ground, Full body armour, however is specifically designed to minimize this damage.

Padded downhill gloves are flexible, to allow you to control the brakes and steering without loss of sensitivity, while for your feet, protective shoes with thick soles help when you put your feet down in the corners.

Trail Riding Skills: What to Expect

Riding a mountain bike along a trail is exhilarating and fun, but it also requires concentration and a good skills base. By practising your technique, you can make your off-road riding a much more rewarding experience.

The very best mountain bikers rarely bounce along bumpy trails, they glide and flow. This is the riding style you should aim for – relaxed, efficient and comfortable. By shifting your weight around subtly, finding the right line and letting the bike do some of the hard work, you can start to ride with more economy.

Each different kind of surface demands a slightly different approach, but there are some general rules and techniques to apply to your riding that can help you improve. These involve keeping momentum, absorbing shocks and keeping your weight back.

On rough surfaces, it can seem as if the bike is fighting you and trying its best to stop. These surfaces can cause inexperienced riders to lose speed, and the slower you go over or through an obstacle, the harder it becomes to deal with. So try to maintain momentum into, through and out of especially

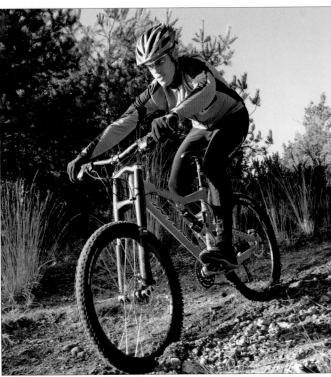

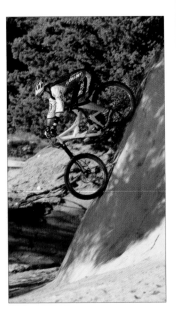

rough patches. Try not to hit obstacles at maximum speed, but keep a positive pedalling action and pick your way through trying to lose as little speed as possible. Losing speed means using more energy to keep going.

Shocks

Absorbing shocks is an important part of maintaining momentum. When you hit a loose surface or technical section, sometimes the reaction is to try too hard to control the bike, which makes your body tense and stiff. Relaxed arms and legs are natural shock absorbers, and if

Left: On extreme descents, keep your weight back as far as possible.

Above: When descending, keep your weight over the rear wheel for traction and balance, while at the same time lightly braking.

you can absorb the bumps, your progress will be smoother.

Lastly, your bike will react better to the terrain if more of your weight is over the back wheel. If you hold your weight too far forward, steering is compromised on rough terrain. Putting your weight over the back wheel increases traction while pedalling and will give you more control over your speed. Your front wheel should be free to manoeuvre, but should not be so loosely held that it bounces around.

Muddy conditions

The more sticky the mud is, the lower the gear you will need. Sit well back and maintain traction. Pick your line and try to stick to it, keeping your weight off the front wheel so that if it starts to get stuck you can easily pull it out before it sinks and pitches you off. You should be able to ride over the rocks, but hitting them at a bad angle knocks the front wheel out of alignment, affecting momentum and steering, so plan ahead

to follow a line that avoids bigger stones. The ride is bumpy, so stand up and bend your arms; the arms and legs act as shock absorbers. In most off-road situations, spinning a low gear is better than pushing a large gear, but in rocky terrain, a larger gear is better to try to maintain speed and momentum. If you are deflected into a new line by bigger rocks, follow that new line. When you steer, use your body and hips to help to change line.

Riding over roots

Roots are present on many off-road trails. In wet weather they usually become slick, and if you hit them at the wrong angle, you can take your bike out from under you, even if you have fitted rugged tyres. The way to tackle roots is to hop the front wheel over them, avoiding wet roots if possible, then use the back wheel to generate speed to pass over them in a straight line, at a right angle to the root.

Dealing with mud and rocks

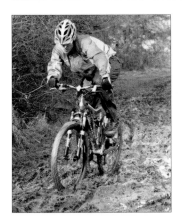

Mud *Put the bike into low gear. Pick a line and try to stick to it.*

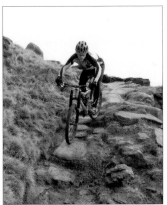

Rocks 1 *Follow a line and plan ahead to avoid large stones.*

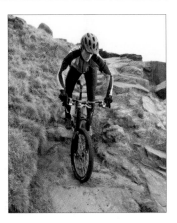

Rocks 2 *Stand up in the saddle so that the legs and arms absorb the shock.*

Dealing with roots

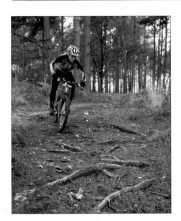

1 *Approach the roots and plan a path through them.*

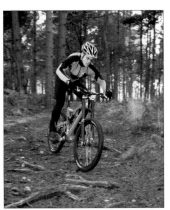

2 *Hop the front wheel over the roots. Beware of wet, slippery roots.*

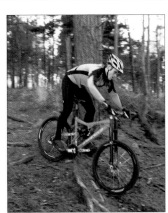

3 *Pass over the roots at a right angle to the direction of growth.*

Trail Riding Skills: Choosing a Line

Riding in a straight line is easy but the challenge of mountain biking involves the unpredictable nature of the trails. Being able to pick your line, anticipate problems and corner fast and safely are important skills.

When riding, it is natural to look just ahead of the front wheel, so that you can deal with problems as they arise. But looking farther ahead is far more efficient – that way, you can avoid problems before they happen, rather than have to deal with them.

Look ahead

Pick your line well in advance. When you can see a rough patch approaching, look for a suitable entrance point, a good line through, and a possible exit. That way, you have already ridden the section in your mind before you actually get to it on the bike and will be prepared for each stage. Sometimes you may have to change your tactics if your original line turns out to have a hidden obstacle, but that is all part of the fun and challenge of mountain biking.

Looking ahead can help with gear selection, too. If you get caught out by a sudden steep rise it is easy to stall, but if you have changed down already in preparation for a climb, you will be ready to ride all the way up.

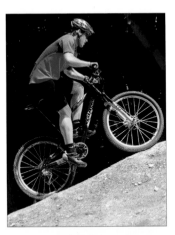

Right: Even when pedalling uphill out of the saddle, it's still important to concentrate on controlled steering to get you safely up.
Below: Allow your bike to steer for you by following the natural line of the trail.

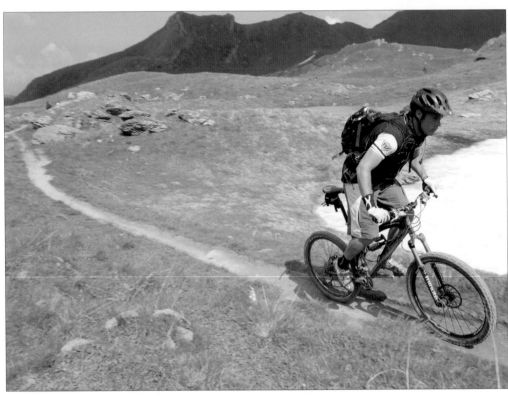

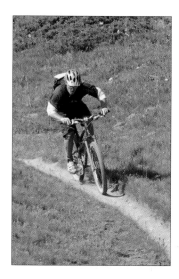

Above: Be prepared to take action if you come to a sudden corner on a singletrack.

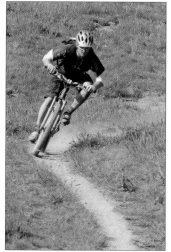

Above: Use your upper body to help steer your bike, leaning into the turns to aid traction.

straight line – you'll be constantly turning and changing your line during the course of a ride.

Cornering involves three phases – the approach, the turn and the exit.

In the approach, use your brakes to moderate your speed. The aim is to enter the corner as fast as possible without the risk of overshooting. As you enter the corner, lean your body over to counteract the centrifugal force, and stay seated. This allows you to push down on your outside leg while bending your inside leg away from the bike for extra balance. Keep your weight centred over the bike, spreading it equally between the front and back wheel to maintain grip.

Once you are past the apex, your aim is to accelerate out of the corner. As soon as you have rounded the bend and can see your exit point, start to pedal.

On a smooth corner with a banked surface, your speed can be high all the way through. Be prepared to slow down more for gravelly surfaces, adverse cambers and other obstacles.

Singletrack

Riding singletrack is one of the most rewarding off-road cycling experiences you can have – it tests your reflexes, fitness and bike handling.

Singletrack is just that – a one-lane mountain bike trail wide enough for one bike at a time. It twists and turns unpredictably, and has all the variety of surfaces that off-road riding has to offer. Often they come unexpectedly –

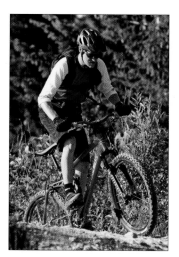

you may dive out of a sharp corner only to discover a large rock under your front wheel or find yourself up to your hub in mud. Riding singletrack is a matter of ducking and diving around the corners and being able to deal with obstacles that come when you least expect them. Singletrack demands a much more erratic speed than larger trails. You will very often have to brake sharply for corners, then accelerate out of them. The aim is still to maintain flow, but within the bounds the singletrack imposes on you.

To control speed in twisting sections, use the back brake, and manoeuvre the bike using both body weight and turning the handlebars. Use the front brake for sharper stopping. You'll need to change gear often as the speed alters. Because of the need to accelerate, it is better to spin a lower gear and anticipate changes down so that you are ready to speed up again.

Cornering

An important skill in mountain biking is cornering quickly and safely. There are very few trails that travel in a totally

Left: Always try to anticipate what is coming up when riding at speed.

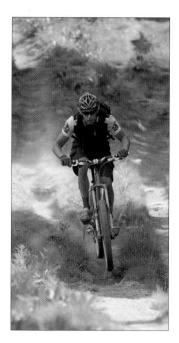

Above: Accelerate out of tricky situations to prevent getting stuck in a rut.

Trail Riding Skills: Descending

Descending is theoretically the easiest thing about trail riding on a mountain bike. Gravity pulls you downward, and all you do is control the bike by keeping your weight back. Then just relax, steer, brake a little and enjoy the ride. But it takes skill, too.

Your main priority when descending is safety. On shallow descents this is straightforward – keep a laid-back position, and use the brakes when you need to. Look well ahead and plan your line. If the surface gets bumpy and you have a hardtail bike, stand up on the pedals to let your legs act as shock absorbers.

Steep descents involve a little more care. You need to be aware of your centre of gravity, and be more focused on the movement of the bike underneath you. Your line should be the shortest one, surface permitting, so cut corners tightly.

Keep your weight back when descending – too much weight above the front wheel can move your centre of gravity far enough forward that you become unstable. The steeper the descent, the farther back you need to sit. Once it becomes really steep, you can hang off the back of the saddle with

Right: Keep weight back when descending to prevent tipping over forwards.
Below: When descending, use your arms and legs to support your body weight.

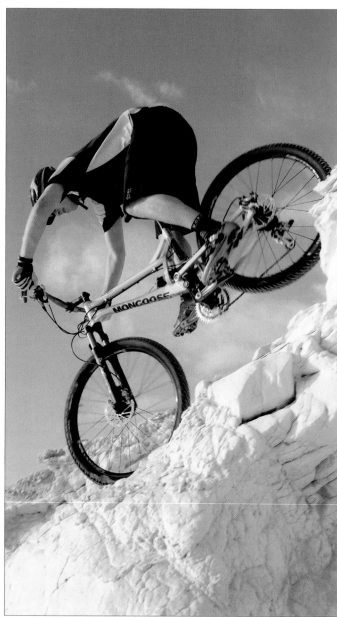

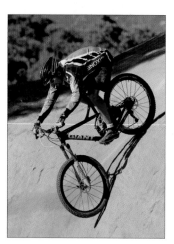

*Right: Keeping your weight above your
back wheel helps maintain traction and
allows you to react to obstacles.*

your bottom above the rear wheel. In
this position, your centre of gravity is still
low enough to keep you stable, but pay
attention to your steering.

Finding a way down

Steering on the descents is easier if you
shift your weight and lean rather than
turn the handlebars. This is all part of
being relaxed and letting the bike do the
work of finding its own way down.

On a slippery or loose surface,
descending becomes more complicated.
Overusing the brakes can result in a
crash, so the best technique is to
moderate your speed before you hit the
gravel. Unless there is particular difficulty
ahead, don't brake on a loose surface,
but if you have to, keep your weight
well back, your centre of gravity low,
and feather the brakes so that you
regain control.

Drop-offs

On some off-road descents, mountain
bikers can encounter drop-offs, which
are vertical drops in the path or trail.
Some are so small that you might
not even notice them, but others
are quite dramatic and take a lot of
practice before you can deal with
them confidently. To ride a drop-off,
you don't need to be riding fast, but
it helps if you are riding positively
and confidently. Do not use your
brakes once you are committed
to the move.

On the approach, move the bike into
a straight line and put your weight
slightly over the rear wheel. As the front
wheel goes over the edge, pull your
handlebars up, bending your arms, and
stay back over the rear wheel. Your rear
wheel should hit the edge, and your
momentum should cause both wheels to
land together at the bottom of the
drop-off. Your bent arms will take some
of the shock of landing.

During the final approach, look
at where you intend to land and plan
your exit strategy so that you don't
lose momentum.

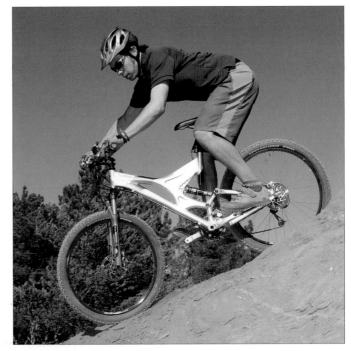

Drop-offs

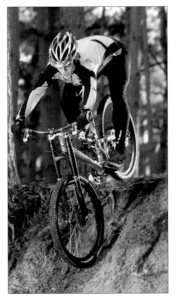

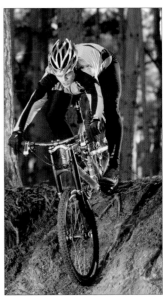

1 *Put your weight over the rear wheel
and pull up the handlebars.*

2 *Look ahead and decide where you are
going to land.*

Trail Riding Skills: Climbing

Climbing is an unavoidable, and difficult, part of trail riding. It is part of the huge variety of terrain you can come across, even on just a single ride, and being able to do it effectively will make your ride a more positive experience.

The steepness of a hill dictates how you tackle it on a mountain bike. On a shallow incline, it is just a case of sitting comfortably, with your body stretched out as you ride to the top. On steep climbs, or climbs with loose surfaces, technique plays a significant part in getting up.

Relaxation is also important. Instead of bunching up your entire body and holding the handlebars in a death-grip, concentrate on breathing evenly, open out your chest a bit, and hold the bars firmly, towards the outside. If you have bar-end attachments, use those to stretch yourself out a bit.

Maintain traction

When the surface of the climb is loose, keeping traction is the biggest challenge. A wheelspin can slow your progress almost to a halt, so to ensure it

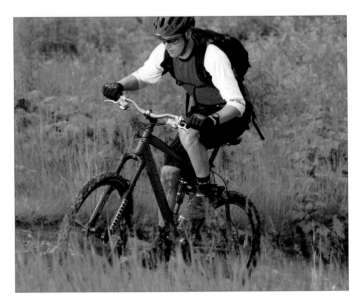

Above: When climbing steady gradients off-road, stay in the saddle and sit back, spinning a low gear.

doesn't happen, sit back and keep your weight over the back wheel. At the same time, to keep your centre of gravity low and increase traction in both wheels, stretch out so that your body is almost parallel to the top tube.

Loose surfaces can also affect your bike when you are standing up and pedalling up a hill. If you sway your bike from side to side, as sometimes feels natural, you run the risk of it slipping out from underneath you. Try instead to move your body from side to side, keeping the bike upright beneath you.

On a very steep climb, with your weight back, it is possible for the front wheel to come off the ground and cause you to lose momentum. On a steeper climb, move your weight forward a little, consciously maintaining traction in the rear wheel.

Golden rules of climbing

1 Stay in the saddle

Climbing is all about establishing a rhythm, and the easiest way to do this is to relax and focus, and stay in the saddle. Grip the bars firmly but not tightly, settle your weight where it feels comfortable and effective, and climb with good rhythm. Save standing up for where you have to accelerate, or stretch out your legs.

2 Bend forward, stretch yourself out, keep your weight back

When climbing, rear-wheel traction is everything. Keep your weight back over the rear wheel to prevent it slipping, but stretch forward with your upper body to get a lower centre of gravity. This will also help traction.

3 Use a low gear

It is less tiring to your muscles to spin a low gear fast than try to turn a big gear over. By staying in a low gear you will have more energy later on. Also, changes in gradient can slow you down – if you are already pedalling slowly you run the risk of stalling.

4 Change the numbers

You can climb faster without even having to go out riding. Climbing effectively is all about power-to-weight ratios. So spend some time and effort, and money if necessary, on losing weight, both you and your bike. Then do some specific hill-climbing training to boost your power. Your climbing will improve out of all recognition.

5 Take the easiest line

The easiest line is not necessarily the shortest one. Corners are often much steeper on the inside than on the outside. The extra distance on a shallow gradient can be less tiring than the short distance up the inside with a steep gradient.

Climbing

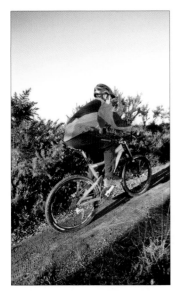

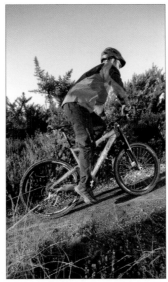

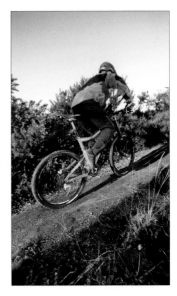

Sit down *Most of your climbing should be done sitting down, with the weight over the back wheel for traction.*

Weight back *If necessary, stand on the pedals on steeper gradients, but keep the weight back.*

Side to side *When climbing, move from side to side. Keep the bike straight, to prevent it slipping out beneath you.*

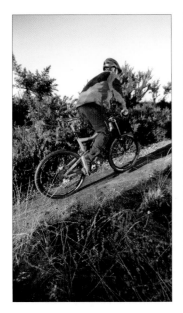

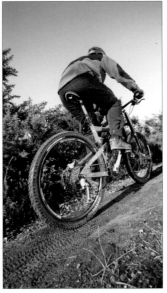

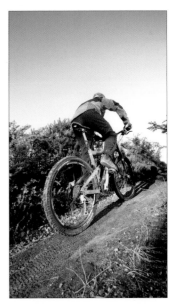

Stand up *Standing up on the pedals stretches the legs, helps combat tiredness and gives a little extra acceleration.*

Weight forward *On the steepest climbs, move your weight forward a little for traction with the rear wheel.*

Keep going *Maintain your speed and effort to the top of the climb to prevent stalling.*

Downhill Racing

Taking part in a downhill race is not as easy as just sitting back and freewheeling while the bike does all the work. It is a serious athletic challenge, and all mountain bikers should have a go at it – it is fast, exhilarating and fun.

On the face of it, downhill riding looks like the easy option for mountain bikers. Dressed from head to toe in protective body armour, riders plummet down steep paths on bikes that look more like motorbikes. If they want to go down again, they catch the ski-lift back up to the top. This isn't simply laziness; downhill mountain bikes are so engineered that they weigh a great deal more than normal bikes, and riding back up would be very difficult.

Downhill riding takes a cool head, nerve, co-ordination and skill. It also takes physical strength – on well-designed courses riders rarely freewheel. Instead, shallower gradients and sharp corners require fast riding and acceleration to maintain velocity.

Your first few downhill runs should be more about gaining confidence and getting used to the way a downhill bike handles. Get used to the brakes and acceleration, and then ride a bit harder. Preparation on a downhill run is essential, and it's worth walking the course to inspect it before you ride. By getting a mental picture of the right line to take, and where to brake, when it

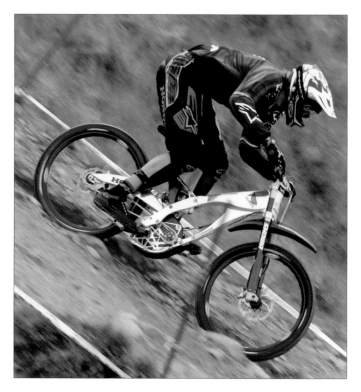

does happen it will be more natural. Actually riding the correct line is a matter of experience and anticipation. By looking well ahead of your front wheel, you will be in a position to choose the right line.

Corners and jumps

The start of a downhill ride is an important part of the whole descent. The margins of victory in competitive downhilling are often very small, and the difference can be made in the initial acceleration. A powerful sprint out of

Left: Full protective body armour is absolutely essential for anyone taking part in downhill racing.

Above: Riders can reach incredible speeds on the steepest gradients in downhill events.

the starting blocks will give your ride physical momentum. It is also a statement of intent – by starting as fast as you mean to go on you can give yourself a psychological boost. Once you are into the ride, you can deal with the sections as they come.

Most corners have berms, which help you to maintain your line through them. When you approach a bermed corner, brake before you start to turn, then hit the berm on the top half. Lean over and shift your body weight on to your outside pedal, which should be down,

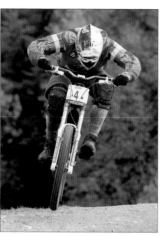

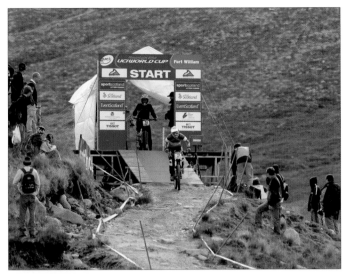

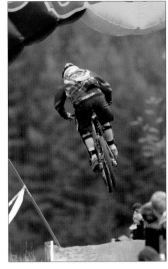

and following the line should be straightforward. Follow these steps and your cornering will be a lot faster and better controlled.

Some corners don't have berms, and the best technique is to use your lower leg in the corner for balance. Riders come round some corners so fast that their bike is almost horizontal, with their leg skidding around on the floor to keep them upright, and to help the bike around the corner before getting it upright again. Use longer, straight

Above: At the start of a downhill race, acceleration is all-important, and riders sprint out of the gate.

sections to build up speed, but be careful of your exit – if you fly too fast into a technical section, you can crash. Some sections will be quite flat, and it's important to try and sprint through these, in order to maintain your speed.

At certain sections, there are small jumps. Hit these jumps with your wheels straight, lift the front wheel up, closely

Above: Hitting a ramp at speed means riders can jump. It's vitally important that the bike is straight for landing.

followed by the back wheel, and be careful to land straight. Look ahead while you are making the jump, so that the exit from your landing is as safe and speedy as possible.

The most important and useful skill to develop, along with your confidence, is your ability to let yourself and the bike flow down the hill. Your reactions to the course have to be fast and fully committed.

Left: Cornering at speed on a berm.
Below: During flat sections, the rider holds speed by pedalling hard and maintaining an aerodynamic tuck.

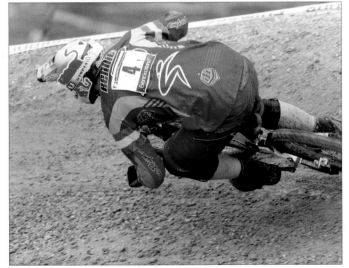

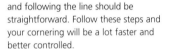

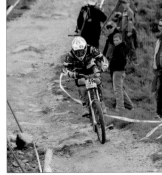

Freeriding

A recent development in mountain biking is freeriding, which is perhaps the ultimate expression of the sport. It is an improvisatory way of combining cross-country riding, downhill riding, trails and trick riding.

The inspiration for freeriding initially came from snowboarders. Freeriding in snowboarding takes place off-piste, away from the beaten track; mountain bike freeriders do the same. Sometimes freeriding involves building jumps and narrow wooden walkways to ride on. Often it is a case of finding your own trail and using logs and rocks.

The definition of freeriding by the sport's originators in British Columbia is that there is no definition.

There is an element of downhill riding, but freeriding also involves riding through more technical terrain. While downhill riding involves getting from A to B as quickly as possible, freeriding means getting from A to B in as stylish and innovative a way as possible.

Freeriding has provided cycling with some of its most photogenic moments since its development at the turn of the century. Freeriders have sought out steeper drops to ride off, and they build ever larger jumps. The original freeride trails incorporated narrow walkways 3m (10ft) in the air. These days the walkways are 12m (40ft) off the ground.

A freeriding bike is very like a downhill bike. The frame is heavy duty with full suspension, although as it often

Right: Freeriders build their own obstacles, putting narrow walkways up to 12m (40ft) off the ground.
Below: Huge jumps are an integral part of freeriding, with the best riders finding ever larger drops to ride.

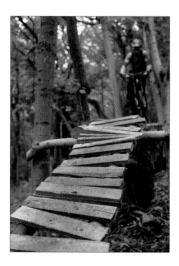

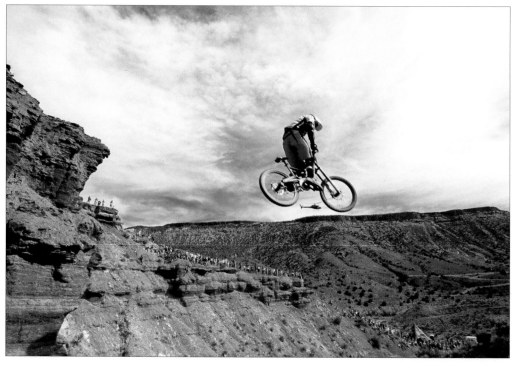

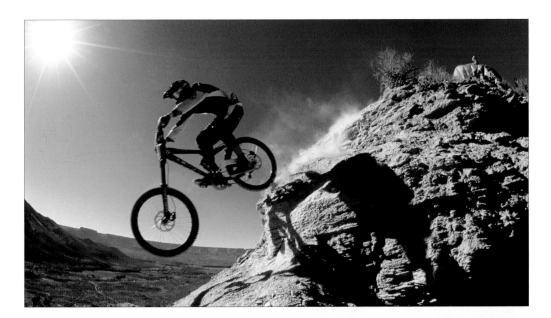

Above: Freeriding bikes have full suspension, with enough travel in the front forks to absorb impact off jumps.

has to be ridden up hills and for longer distances, it is not as bulky. Its wheelbase is shorter and the head tube is steeper, which gives more control when performing jumps.

Special bike features
The long travel suspension forks have been retained from downhill bikes – freeriding involves dropping off obstacles and jumps, and the shock of

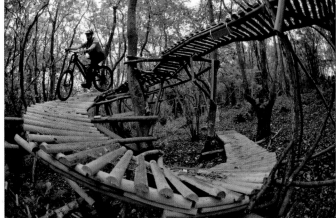

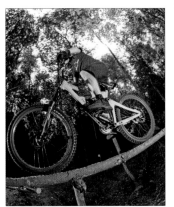

landing needs to be taken in the forks. Disc brakes with a large braking surface also survived from downhill bikes – landing off a 3m (10ft) cliff involves a fair amount of acceleration, and speed might need to be checked very quickly.

Unlike a downhill bike, however, the freeride bike has a triple chainset and therefore a larger range of gears. The

Left: Freeriding courses often incorporate narrow log beams, which test the riders' balance to the limits.

Above: There is no limit to the complexity of freeriding courses.

greater variety of terrain expected to be encountered by a freerider also requires the gears to deal with it.

Freeriding involves elements from many mountain bike disciplines: the trick-riding abilities of the trials rider, the reflexes and nerve of the downhill rider, the physical strength and urge to explore shared by all trail riders, and the competitive instincts of the racer.

Mountain Biking: Branching Out

Mountain biking isn't just about trail riding and cross-country. There are a multitude of other racing and riding disciplines that are challenging and fun, including bicycle four-cross, slalom, trials and dirt-jump riding.

Mountain biking is primarily about having fun, and there are a variety of disciplines outside cross-country riding. Four-cross and slalom are action-filled races over short distances including jumps, berms and downhills. Trials riding is more technical – it's all about hops, jumps and tackling obstacles. Dirt-jump riding is an underground scene with the emphasis on style and expression.

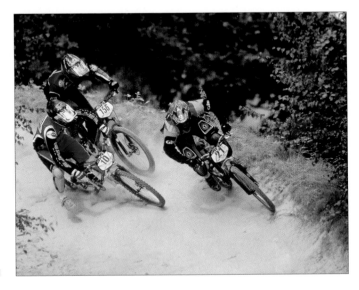

Four-cross

At a bicycle four-cross event, four riders start at the same time, and race to the bottom. Bikes are full suspension, with short seat tubes and low saddles like a trials bike, and crashes are common. Riders need nerves of steel and great technical ability to ride down a steep section of hill with jumps and corners, elbow-to-elbow with other riders. Speed alone might not be enough – races are often decided by the jumps, and course designers keep the suspense alive to the finishing line by incorporating as many unpredictable elements as possible.

Slalom

A type of racing that involves two riders going head-to-head on two near-identical but separate courses down a hill is

Above: Bicycle four-cross is a fast and furious race on specially designed courses, with four riders going elbow-to-elbow in a downhill dash to the line.

'slalom'. Originally, it was simply erecting the poles in a field and letting the riders go, but it evolved into an organized part of the sport. The course became more technical, with jumps and berms between the slalom poles. With the development of the 'dual' slalom, in which riders start separately, until their lanes merge, there was more conflict. Once you have established a lead in an event like the slalom, it is easy to keep it, so a typical race sees aggressive fighting to reach the merged lanes in first place.

Trials

Another form of mountain biking, trials, entails performing tricks and jumps over a series of obstacles. In trial biking

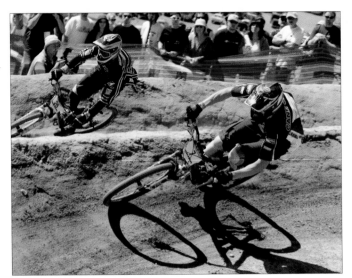

Left: In a slalom race the bikes ride down separate but identical courses.

Trials riding: jump

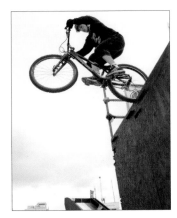

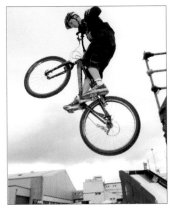

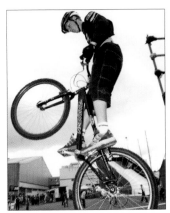

1 *A rider starts to jump off the top of an obstacle.*

2 *In mid-air, the rider positions his bike to effect a good landing.*

3 *The rider is not allowed to put his feet on the ground.*

competitions, riders have to negotiate a set course without putting their feet down, or allowing any part of their bike apart from the tyres to touch the obstacle. If they do, they are penalized. There is also a time limit, and when riders exceed it, they gain a penalty point for every 15 seconds taken over the limit.

Below: Four-cross courses can incorporate jumps taken at great speed to try to gain an advantage over rivals.

Trials riding takes great skill and balance – riders can use their strong brakes and soft, grippy tyres to balance on their rear wheel and hop on to obstacles up to 1.5m (5ft) in the air.

Dirt-jump

One of the more underground areas in the sport is dirt-jump mountain biking. While other riders go off in search of obstacles, part of the process of dirt-jumping is building your own. This has

led to clashes between dirt-jumpers and landowners who have recently discovered that there is an unapproved dirt-jumping track on their land. Like freeriders, dirt-jumpers insist that their sport is not about competition but free expression. The aim is not to be the fastest, or the highest, or even to be able to perform the best tricks, but simply to execute a jump in a way that feels natural and expressive to the individual rider.

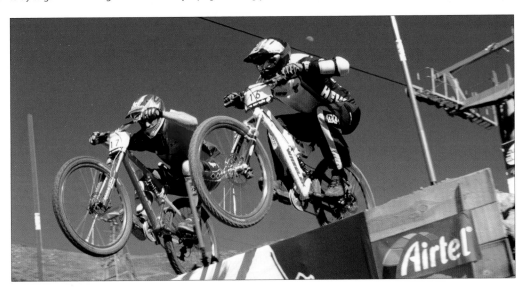

Great Mountain Bike Rides in Canada: North Shore and Whistler

North Shore, in British Columbia, is one of the world's major centres for mountain biking. Initially it was a well-kept local secret, based around Mount Seymour, Mount Fromme and Cypress Mountain. Whistler has hundreds of mountain bike trails.

The North Shore is endowed with challenging trails for singletrack riding, while Whistler has trails for every ability.

North Shore

Now regarded as the home of freeriding, North Shore, with its jumps, ramps and elevated trails offers some of

Below: British Columbia is a major area for cross-country mountain bikers.

	British Columbia Bike Race		
Stage	**Start**	**Finish**	**Distance**
One	Victoria	Cowichan Lake District	112km/70 miles
Two	Cowichan Lake District	Port Alberni	115km/72 miles
Three	Port Alberni	Comox Valley	83km/52 miles
Four	Comox Valley	Sechelt	60km/37 miles
Five	Sechelt	Gibsons	55km/34miles
Six	Squamish	Whistler	75km/47 miles
Seven	Whistler	Whistler	25km/16 miles

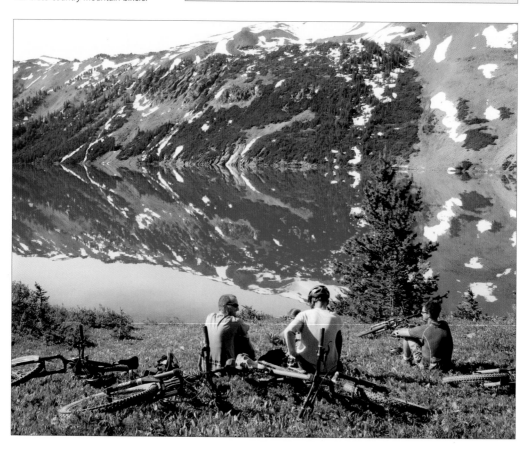

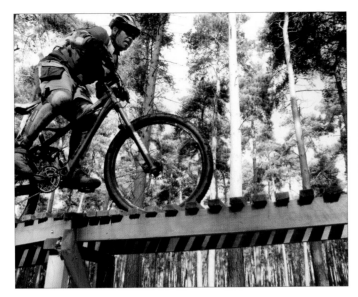

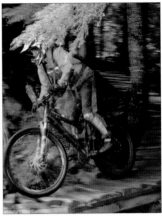

Above: Although there are well-marked trails, many riders choose their own.
Left: The North Shore area was where freeriding developed.

the best and most varied mountain biking in the world and it is legendary in the sport. There are many watercourses and forests with huge trees, and because there are creeks and fallen timber, narrow, high bridges have been built that are often used as launch ramps. The trails at Mount Fromme are easy to explore, although riders are expected to stick to a few rules regarding the trails, other users and the environment. Exploration is in keeping with local traditions – just arrive and see what happens.

Whistler

One of the biggest cross-country trail locations in the world, Whistler has hundreds of kilometres of trails, based at three locations in the area. One of the most famous rides in Canada is the seven-day British Columbia Bike Race, from Victoria to Whistler. Each day involves around 4 to 8 hours riding and a daily distance of 50–100km (31–62 miles). There are seven stages of the ride and the climbing can be exacting. Mud can make the route hazardous. If you have prepared and are in fair shape, you will have a good riding experience.

Right: The cross-country riding in British Columbia is challenging, but the views make the effort worth it.

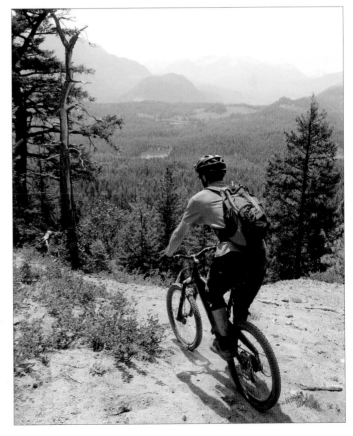

Great Mountain Bike Rides in the USA: Moab, Utah

Moab, in the south-eastern corner of Utah, is one of the best places for mountain biking in the world, with mile upon mile of trail of every description. Every mountain biker should go there at least once.

The most famous trail in Moab is Slick Rock, a 15.5km (9.6-mile) loop of sandstone rock. While it gains its name from the difficulty of riding horses on the hard stone, for mountain bikers there are few better surfaces to ride on. The sandstone offers unbelievable traction. The original trail is marked out with white paint. The terrain is steep and hard, and set in a Moon-like landscape. While it is short compared to many off-road loops, the demanding technical nature of the course is such that it can take hours to complete.

What makes Slick Rock such a natural place for mountain bikers is that it couldn't have been better designed as a technical mountain bike course. The trail incorporates natural bowls, some with steep sides, which are ideal places to experiment with tricks, jumps, drop-offs and more extreme riding. There are none of the restrictions that define most trails – on a singletrack course you have no choice but to follow the path. On Slick Rock, going off-piste and improvising your own way down is part of the experience.

The other main off-road trail in Moab is the Porcupine Rim Trail, which is less famous than Slick Rock, but has a better reputation among Utah's mountain bike aficionados. It is a 33km (20.5-mile) trail that finishes in Moab and consists of extended stretches of broken rocky singletrack. It is known for the 915m (3,000ft), 18km (11-mile) descent from the top of the first climb all the way

Below: The arid sandstone area of Moab, Utah, is one of the biggest mountain biking challenges in the world.

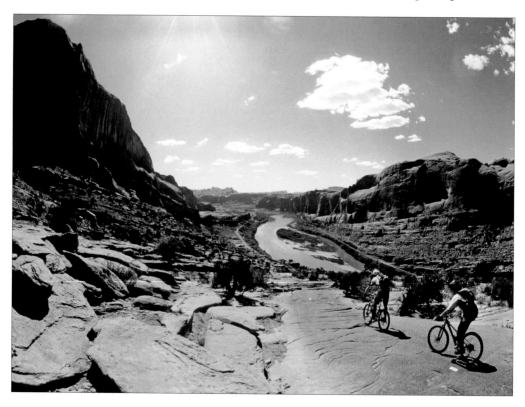

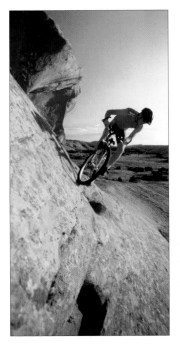

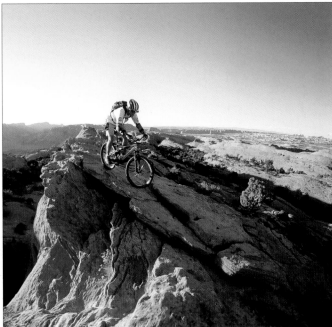

down to the Colorado River. In Moab there are also dozens of short trails, long trails, hard trails and beginners' trails. One trail, farther from Moab, the White Rim, is based on a 160km (100-mile) loop in the Canyonlands National Park. This ride takes two or three days, and you need camping equipment.

Above left: Although this looks as if it would be extremely difficult, Moab sandstone has superb traction, making technical manoeuvres like this possible. Above: The trails in Moab are highly demanding and technical – riders often have to improvise their way out of difficult situations.

Below left: The desert around Moab is wide open, with plenty of opportunities for easier, less technical riding. Below: With the changing scenery and riding like this, it is no surprise that Moab is now considered to be one of the top worldwide mountain biking destinations.

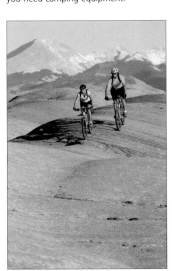

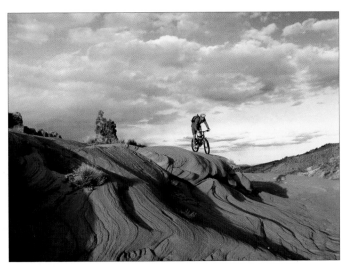

Great Mountain Bike Rides in Europe

The mountain ranges of Europe are natural playgrounds for the off-road enthusiast. For cross-country and downhill riders, the French Alps and Pyrenees are among the most desirable destinations in the world for off-road riding.

Mountain biking has become a major summer sport in the Alps. Those in the tourism industry have realized that ski resorts can be used by mountain bikers during the summer, and in some areas have made great efforts to design attractive destinations for off-road riding.

Rides in France

In the French Alps, Morzine has become a Mecca for downhill riders with four of the best downhill tracks in the world within a few kilometres of the town. The Les Gets course is used for the World Cup event, while the Super Morzine is one of the longest downhill tracks in Europe. There are many trails for riders of all abilities, ranging from steep and difficult

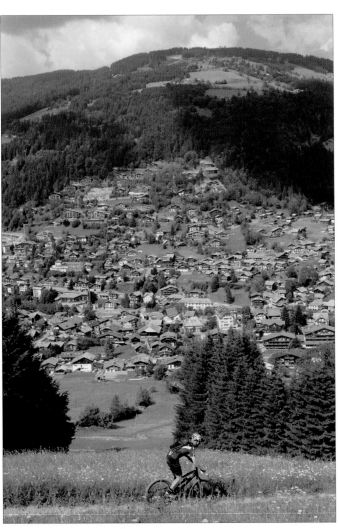

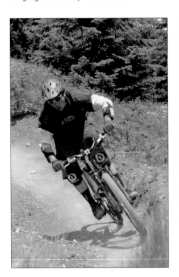

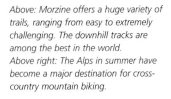

Above: Morzine offers a huge variety of trails, ranging from easy to extremely challenging. The downhill tracks are among the best in the world.
Above right: The Alps in summer have become a major destination for cross-country mountain biking.

downhills at the top of mountains to easy cross-country trips.

Morzine is also a centre for cross-country riding, with popular local routes into the mountains. The Col de Cou is a steep climb which rises 400m (1,312ft) from bottom to top with a 1,000m (3,280ft) descent to reward the effort of making the top. Morzine has more than 400km (250 miles) of bike-specific tracks for mountain bikers, but the most interesting proposition for experts is the 110km (68-mile) Portes de Soleil route.

Many of the cross-country rides can also incorporate chairlifts to take out some extended uphill grinds, although for some this is all part of the fun. And whether you pick an easy trail or a serious downhill run, there is fantastic scenery to enjoy.

As well as Morzine, Chamonix, in the shadow of Mont Blanc, has developed many mountain bike trails.

Rides in Spain

Spain has an advantage for mountain bikers, especially in the south, in its good all-year-round weather. The Sierra Nevada mountain range has some of the highest mountain biking in Europe, while the Alpujarras in Andalucía has been described as a cross-country paradise for aficionados.

The Pyrenees are following close behind the Alps as a destination for mountain bikers. The Valle de Tena is located in the western Pyrenees, right on the French border, with a good network of trails, and no restrictions on routing. The Val d'Aran has abundant cross-country trails, and you can create longer routes by including road links.

The Picos de Europa, which is based around Potes, is one of the world's best mountain bike destinations, with challenging trail rides and many long descents.

Top right: The terrain makes mountain biking in Spain a challenging experience.
Right: Many European mountain biking centres have extensive singletrack trails.
Below: Mountain biking in Europe benefits from clement weather all year.

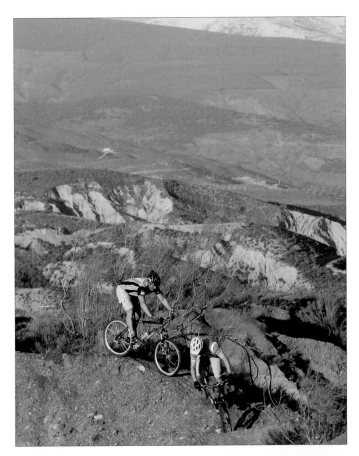

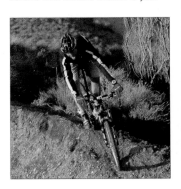

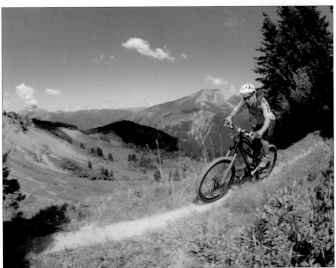

Great Mountain Bike Rides in the UK

There are many fantastic rides in the UK; among the most notable are the trails in the South Downs, Wales and the innovative 7stanes in Scotland, which links seven mountain bike centres in the south of Scotland by a variety of trails.

Although spectacular mountain bike rides in the UK are numerous, a handful stand out. For a long ride, the South Downs Way is unbeatable. Wales is crisscrossed with trails and there are mountain bike centres to help along the route. Scotland, however, is acknowledged as having the most diverse and difficult rides.

South Downs Way

The first national trail in the UK to be designated a long-distance bridleway, the South Downs Way has become a challenge for mountain bikers. It starts in Winchester and follows the South Downs all the way to the coast at Eastbourne. The total length, from end to end, is 160km (100 miles), with 4,150m (13,600ft) of ascent and

descent. The highest point is Ditchling Beacon, at 248m (814ft) altitude. The ride is seen as a serious challenge not for the toughness of its terrain, but its distance. It has become a challenge to ride the entire length in a day, although most people tend to split it into two days.

Rides in Wales

Established as the main area for British mountain biking, Wales has hundreds of miles of purpose-built singletrack and trails shared between the biggest centres at Coed y Brenin forest and the Afan

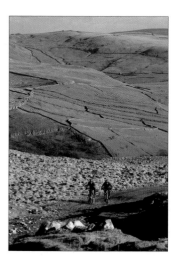

Right: Empty moorland in Derbyshire is ideal for cross-country mountain biking. Below: This route on the South Downs Way can be tackled in one or two days.

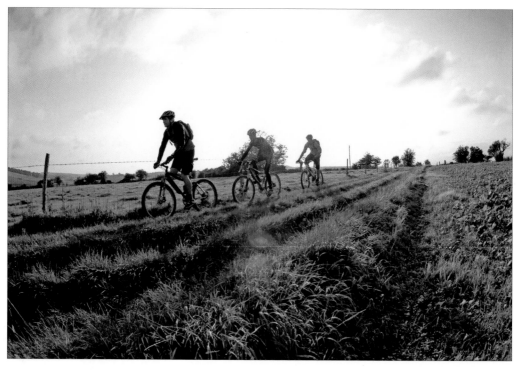

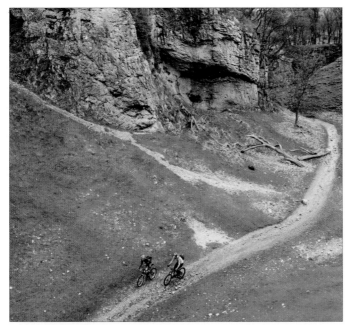

Forest Park. Purpose-built mountain bike centres are a good way of enjoying the sport without the risk of cycling on private land or getting lost. Afan Forest has a network of trails, including the original 22km (13.6-mile) Penhydd trail, which is a suitable distance for ambitious novices and intermediate riders. For more experienced riders, trails such as the Skyline Trail, at 46km (28.5 miles) in length and with 2,000m (6,500ft) of vertical gain, are a substantial challenge.

Rides in Scotland

Mountain bikers in the UK find that Scotland has the most varied and challenging terrain. The low population and mountainous landscape are perfect for long rides and expeditions. Biking centres have sprung up over the last few years, such as the 7stanes network. Trails range from 400m (1,310ft) in length to the 58km (36-mile) Glentrool ride. Fort William has become popular since hosting the World Cup mountain biking events.

Above left: Even in a densely populated country like Britain, there are still some wide-open spaces to explore.
Left: The UK has some of the best and most extensive singletrack riding.

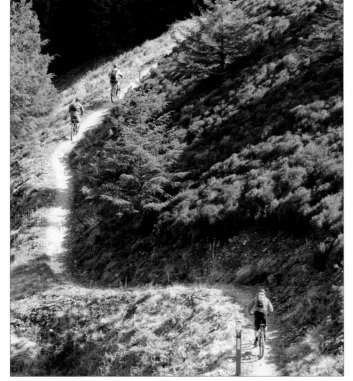

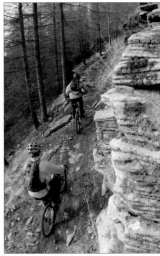

Above: Riders tackle a challenging cross-country mountain biking trail in Afan Forest in Wales.

Great Mountain Bike Rides: Multi-day Events Around the World

For the ultimate mountain biking challenge, many riders are signing up to multi-day events in the great mountain ranges. The TransAlp, TransRockies and Cape Epic Challenges give riders a chance to test themselves against the toughest terrain in the world.

For more experienced riders, multi-day events are increasingly popular. The TransAlp, the TransRockies and the Cape Epic, all with great climbs, are three of the most demanding.

The TransAlp Challenge

An eight-day challenge ride across the Alps, the TransAlp climbs a series of high passes in daily stages ranging between 50 and 100km (30–60 miles). It has run every year since 1998, starting in Mittenwald in Germany and finishing in Riva del Garda in Italy. The routes are a combination of off-road tracks, gravel paths and asphalted surfaces. Some days involve a height gain of over 3,000m (9,842ft). It is an extremely arduous race, one of the most difficult mountain bike events in the world. Riders have to be fit and follow an advanced training schedule to prepare. Such is the popularity of the TransAlp that more than 500 teams take part every year.

2008 Route TransAlp Challenge Ride				
Stage	Start	Finish	Distance	Altitude gain
1	Füssen	Imst	80km/50 miles	1,962m/6,437ft
2	Imst	Ischgl	76km/47 miles	3,171m/10,403ft
3	Ischgl	Scoul	75km/47 miles	2,547m/8,356ft
4	Scoul	Livigno	77km/48 miles	2,621m/8,599ft
5	Livigno	Naturns	122km/76 miles	2,909m/9,544ft
6	Naturns	Kaltern	97km/60 miles	3,930m/12,894ft
7	Kaltern	Andalo	74km/46 miles	3,071m/10,075ft
8	Andalo	Riva	62km/39 miles	1,480m/4,856ft

2008 Route TransRockies Challenge Ride				
Stage	Start	Finish	Distance	Altitude gain
1	Panorama	K2 Ranch	52km/32 miles	2,478m/8,177ft
2	K2 Ranch	Nipika Resort	74km/46 miles	3,813m/12,582ft
3	Nipika Resort	Nipika Resort	44km/27 miles	1,514m/4,996ft
4	Nipika Resort	Whiteswan Lake	110km/68 miles	2,567m/8,471ft
5	Whiteswan Lake	Elkford	89km/55 miles	2,147m/7,085ft
6	Elkford	Crowsnest Pass	102km/63 miles	2,998m/9,893ft
7	Crowsnest Pass	Fernie	79km/49 miles	2,101m/6,933ft

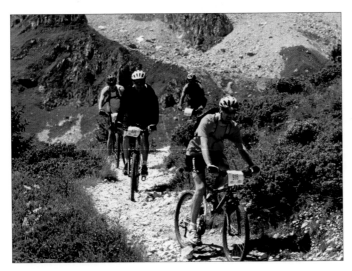

The TransRockies Challenge

The success of the TransAlp Challenge led to its format being copied around the world, with the Canadian TransRockies Challenge starting up in 2002. The route is still developing, but it can be extremely punishing, and the weather can be variable. Like the TransAlp, the TransRockies is split into daily stages, covering 600km (372 miles) in seven days and climbing a total of 12,000m (39,000ft), a little below the TransAlp, but still a very hard challenge.

The short history of the TransRockies gives a perfect illustration of the unpredictable nature of this kind of event – in 2003 forest fires forced the

Left: Riders negotiate the TransAlp, one of the most difficult bike events.

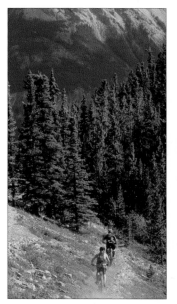

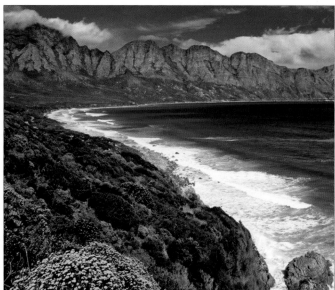

Above: Mountain bikers tackle a scree trail in the Rocky Mountains.
Above right: The route of the Cape Epic is entirely off-road and goes along rugged tracks, through the beautiful scenery around the Cape.

2008 Route Cape Epic Challenge Ride				
Stage	Start	Finish	Distance	Altitude gain
Prologue	Pezula	Pezula	17km/11 miles	310m/1,020ft
1	Knysna	Saarsveld	123km/76 miles	3,091m/10,141ft
2	Saarsveld	Calitzdorp	137km/85 miles	2,518m/8,261ft
3	Calitzdorp	Riversdale	133km/83 miles	2,340m/7,677ft
4	Riversdale	Swellendam	121km/75 miles	2,620m/8,596ft
5	Swellendam	Bredaarsdorp	146km/91 miles	1,819m/5,968ft
6	Bredaarsdorp	Hermanus	130km/81 miles	2,095m/6,873ft
7	Hermanus	Grabouw	91km/57 miles	1,985m/6,512ft
8	Grabouw	Lourensford	68km/42 miles	1,760m/5,774ft

organizers into a swift re-routing exercise at very short notice, while the 2004 event was hampered by heavy rain.

The Cape Epic Challenge
The first event in the South African Cape Epic Challenge, in 2004, attracted more than 500 riders for the 800km (500-mile) route, and within two years it had doubled in size to 1,000 riders and increased its length to 921km (572 miles). Every year it starts in Knysna Waterfront and finishes in Lourensford Wine Estate. The total climb for the eight-day 2007 event was 15,045m (49,360ft), comparable to the TransAlp.

Preparation
Taking part in multi-day events like the TransAlp, TransRockies and Cape Epic is not to be undertaken lightly, because 100km (62 miles) is a long way to ride off-road on a single day, let alone on

several days. To get the most out of the experience, it is necessary to be honest and realistic about your own capacities, and to train hard over a long period to prepare for the event. Try following or adapting some of the training programmes in this book to prepare yourself, and take part in some shorter events to make sure that your body can take the longer distances and repeated efforts of a multi-day event.

Right: Many challenging mountain bike races go through spectacular, mountainous terrain, such as this one at Mount Hood, Oregon.

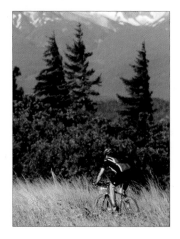

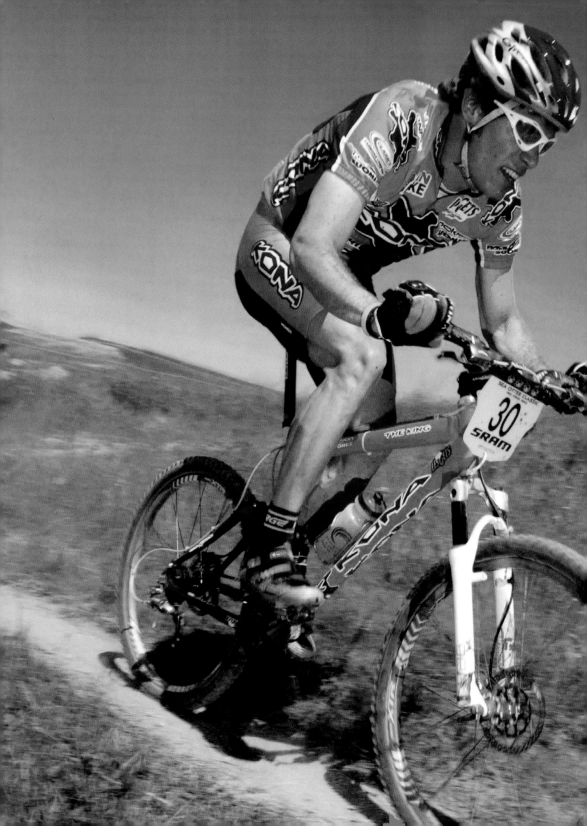

RACING

For some people, racing is the purest expression of bicycle riding. The bicycle was invented to be an efficient machine, and nowhere is this more important than in a bike race, when man and machine strive to be the fastest and best. No sooner had the bike been invented than people began to wonder how fast they could be pedalled and who could pedal them the fastest. As technology improved, other branches of bike racing evolved. With the advent of mountain bikes has come off-road racing. Track racing is one of the centrepieces of the Olympic Games. Racing demands specific skills, and the next section explains how to develop them.

Left: Bike racing on- or off-road takes dedication and determination.

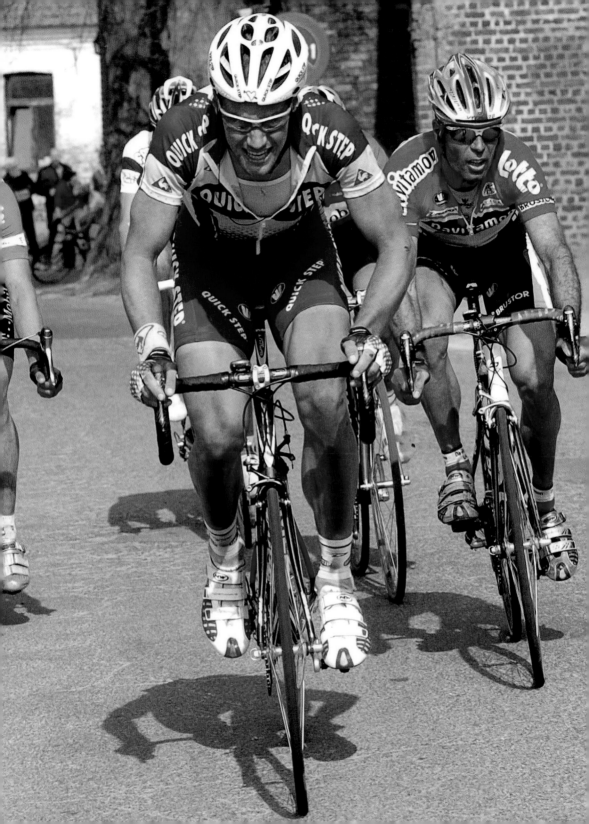

ROAD RACING

The thrill of the road race has few equals in modern
sport. As part of a multi-coloured pack, riders fly up hills
before swooping down the other side, and cruise at
great speeds for miles before unleashing a fearsome
dash for the line. Finishing a road race takes more
than great speed and stamina. A number of riding skills
are needed to survive in a road race – how to climb,
how to descend, how to infiltrate a breakaway,
how to outsprint your rivals, and how to use team
tactics to your advantage.

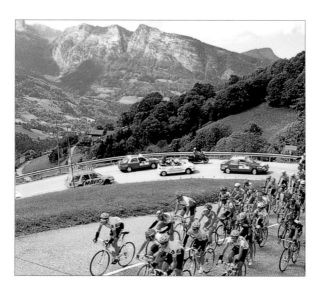

Above: Road racers round a sharp bend in a mountainous race.
Left: Professional bike racers are among the fittest athletes on the planet.

The Road-racing Bicycle

Road-racing bikes are sleek, lightweight and fast. Ergonomic and aerodynamic principles are used in design so that everything possible is honed to a minimum, in order for the rider to be able to generate more speed.

Each element in a racing bike has been designed to be lightweight so that the rider can achieve maximum speed and responsive handling.

Frames

Carbon fibre or aluminium are used to make frames, or even a combination of the two, in which the main triangle of the frame is stiff aluminium, while the forks and seat stays are carbon fibre, to absorb some of the road shock. Frame tubes are wider than traditional steel bikes because aluminium is so much lighter than steel. Larger diameter tubes are stiffer, but even though more material is used in their construction, they are still much lighter than a comparative steel frame.

Right: A lightweight front mech (mechanism) on a racing bicycle.

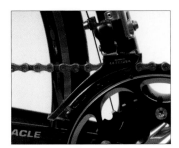

Anatomy of a racing bike

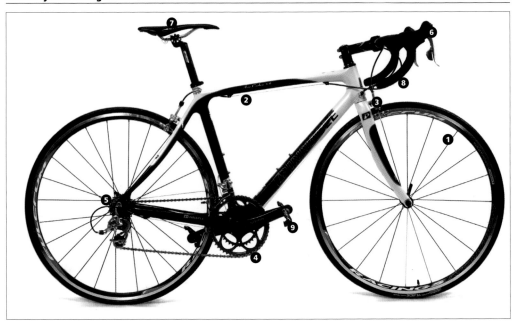

1 Wheels: size 700x20c, with 24 spokes and slick, lightweight tyres. Having a narrow section is much more aerodynamic.
2 Frame: Carbon fibre or aluminium, with compact design and sloping top tube.
3 Brakes: High performance dual pivot calliper. Carbon fibre brake levers to save weight.

4 Chainrings: 53–42, attached to hollow bottom bracket axle and hollow cranks to save weight.
5 Sprockets: 10-speed freewheel with 12–21 block.
6 Gear changers: Brake levers also function as gear changers when they provide instant gear-changing ability.

7 Saddle: Narrow and hard, with titanium seat rails to save weight.
8 Handlebars: Dropped carbon fibre handlebars with ergonomically designed tubes for more comfortable and effective riding.
9 Pedals: Lightweight pedals with special bindings for shoeplates to clip into.

The modern trend is for sloping top tubes and compact frames, which are smaller than traditional frames. A compact frame is stronger, because the tubes are shorter. They also allow frame manufacturers to make frames in fewer sizes, with most compact frames coming in three different sizes. Individual riders can tailor their position with precision using seatpins, stem, cranks and handlebars. Clearances between wheels and frame are reduced to almost nothing, and the profile of the bike is as narrow as possible, for better aerodynamics.

Specifications of wheels

Wheels are narrow – 700x20c, with 24 spokes, or fewer for the front wheel, depending on the model and spoke pattern. Tyres are slick and lightweight, with little or no tread – with such a small area of the tyre on the road at any one time, this actually offers the best grip. The fastest tyres used to be one-piece tubulars, which were extremely lightweight and glued to the wheel. However, the performance of traditional tyres, with a wire-on outer layer and inner tube, is now similar to tubular tyres. Wire-on tyres are easier to mend.

Components

Gearing in a racing bike is higher than the bikes that have been covered so far – road-racing bikes need to travel at high speeds, and the pace is rarely slow enough in a road race to justify using very low gears. Even on climbs, the riders try to go up so fast that their bottom gear doesn't need to be super-low. A typical racing bike has 52 or 53–42-tooth chainrings on the front, although this can be adapted to 53–44 if the course is less hilly, or 53–39 if it is especially hilly. At the back, a typical block would be 12–21 or 12–23, depending upon the type of terrain. Professional sprinters use an 11-tooth sprocket, but you should be very fit and strong before you attempt to turn over such a large gear. Brakes are lightweight and high performance.

Road-racing bikes feel very stiff, with all effort going into moving the bike forward. Most road races are

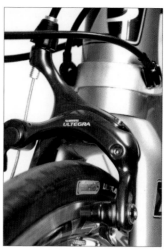

Above: Brake levers on a racing bike combine brakes and gear-changing functions at the same place.

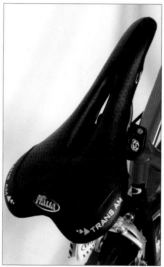

Above: Brakes on a racing bike are light, but strong, making it easy to control your speed on a fast descent.

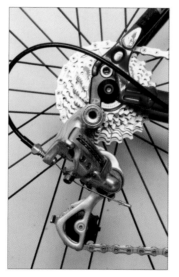

Above: Modern racing bikes have as many as 11 sprockets on the rear wheel, giving a total of 22 gears so that riders can travel at high speeds.

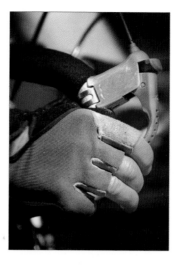

Above: Racing saddles are narrow, for improved aerodynamics. Choose a saddle that is comfortable for you by testing as many as possible.

shorter distance events, taking between 1 and 3 hours to complete, so that for this distance it is possible to sacrifice a little comfort for stiffness and responsiveness.

Tour de France riders, however, can sometimes spend as much as 6 hours at a time on a racing bike so for the long distances they ride, comfort is of paramount importance.

Choosing a Racing Bike

Which racing bike are you going to buy? You will probably want a bike that is light, fast and responsive but your choice should depend on your current ability, your potential ability, your ambitions and the depth of your wallet.

By choosing to buy a good quality racing bike, you are already demonstrating that you are serious about riding fast and racing. To help achieve your maximum potential, the better the bike you buy, the faster you will ride.

As a rule of thumb, you should always buy the best possible equipment that you can afford, without getting into the mindset that you cannot ride fast without it. By focusing too much on equipment you run the risk of relying too hard on it. Instead of working overtime to afford a titanium seatpin bolt, you might end up going faster by investing that time in training more effectively.

Matching components
It is important to buy a bike with a matching level of componentry and frame. If you spend all your budget on a professional level frame, and only have

Right: Buy the racing bike that best suits your needs and level.
Below: Carbon fibre is one of the lightest and strongest materials for making racing frames.

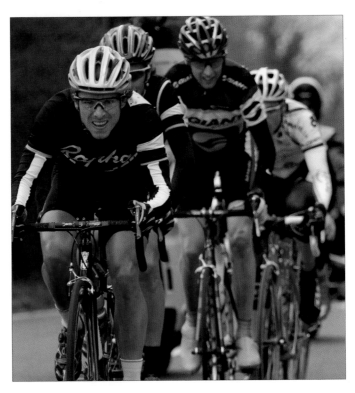

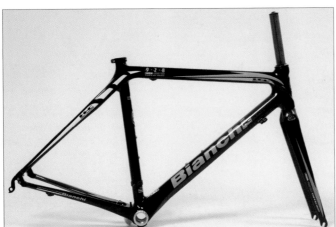

Carbon fibre or aluminium?
Bicycle technology has reached a point where there is so much choice that nearly everybody can find a racing frame that suits his or her needs and abilities perfectly. Deciding between carbon fibre and aluminium can, however, prove to be a difficult choice. Both are light, corrosion resistant and strong. Both give a stiff, responsive ride. The best way to choose is to test ride a model made in each material and see which you prefer.

Some people believe that a full-carbon frame tends towards a harsh ride. A good compromise is an aluminium frame that has carbon forks and seat stays.

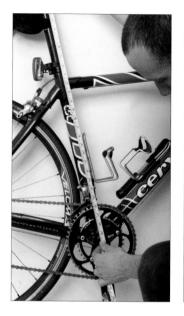

Positioning

With compact frames available in three different sizes, it is easy to judge which suits you. What is more important is to set up a comfortable and efficient riding position.

The two most important measurements are saddle height and reach.

There are several ways to determine the correct saddle height. Former Tour de France winner Greg Lemond recommends multiplying the distance between your crotch and the floor by 0.833. To do this, stand with your feet flat on the floor at the same distance apart as they would be on your bike, and keep your legs straight. Have a friend measure the distance for you.

Multiply this length by 0.833, and you have the correct figure for the distance between the centre of the bottom bracket and the saddle.

Your handlebars should be about 3cm (1¼in) below the level of your saddle. For greater aerodynamics, your handlebars can be a little lower, but this will come at the sacrifice of comfort.

When sitting on the saddle and holding the drops, your nose should be about 2cm (¾in) behind the horizontal part of the handlebar.

You can make micro-adjustments in your position, which will give you a more comfortable and efficient riding experience. When your pedals are at the same height, the front of your forward knee should be vertically above the central line of the axle of your pedal. Move your saddle back or forward a little to ensure that this is the case. If you have to do this, you may have to tweak your saddle height and stem, to ensure that all the angles are correct.

If you have long thighs, or a longer upper body, all this has to be taken into account when choosing your frame and setting up position.

enough left for a cheap groupset (the brakes, gears and drivetrain), there will be a compromise in performance.

For high-level racing, most riders choose between Shimano and Campagnolo groupsets. Shimano Dura Ace and Campagnolo Record are the

Above: Check that the distance from the saddle to the pedals is correct for you.
Right: When setting up your bike, make sure that the reach is set at the correct distance for your size.

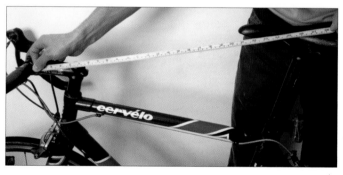

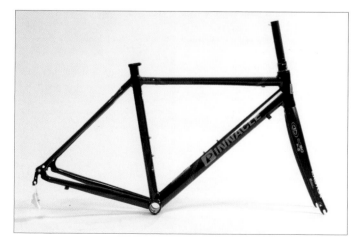

top range, and are highly engineered and reliable. As with choosing between carbon fibre and aluminium frames, the performance of both is so good that selecting one over the other is a matter of preference. The gear-changing system is different, and Campaganolo offers a more definite 'click' in between gears.

Wheels should have hubs compatible with the gearing system, and light, good quality rims. Advances in design, materials and spoke patterns ensure that there is a wide choice. For top level racing, a deep-section carbon rim is the best, but these are very expensive.

Left: An aluminium road and mountain bike frame is preferred by some riders.

Road-racing Skills: Breaking Away

Winning road races isn't easy. You share the start line with 150 other riders, who all want to win. Some are great climbers and others are great bunch sprinters. In a hilly race, if you are a good climber or a sprinter, you should make the most of these skills.

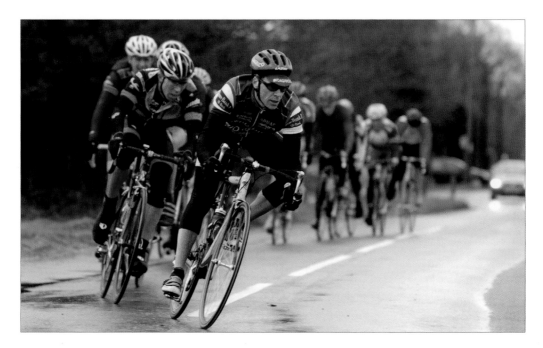

If you do not excel at sprinting or climbing, try to get into a breakaway. It's a rare road race in which the entire field rides round and waits for a group to sprint together (the bunch sprint). Attacks often go from the gun, and it takes special circumstances for the attack to be the right one.

Leading the charge

Attacking is energy-consuming. It is better to attack once, successfully, than four times unsuccessfully. The energy consumed in four unsuccessful attacks could make you miss the fifth, which is the one that disappears up the road. On the other hand, it might take those four attacks to succeed – the bunch may tire of chasing you down and let you go. Each race is different in this respect. But don't ever attack just for the sake of it. Choose your moment.

The best times to go are when the bunch slows down, either due to a corner, a hill, the fact that another group has just been chased down, or simply because the riders at the front stop riding hard. When you notice this happen, go as hard as you can. You may escape on your own, you may be followed by a small group in counterattack, or you may get chased down. After a few minutes, turn around and see which of these has happened. If you are on your own, but can see a small group working together to catch you 20 seconds behind, while the bunch is at a minute farther back, you are better off waiting for the small group to catch you. The short-term sacrifice of a handful of seconds is worth the long-

Right: The joy of victory – get it right and the win is yours.

Above: In a race, getting into the right breakaway is a crucial tactical skill.

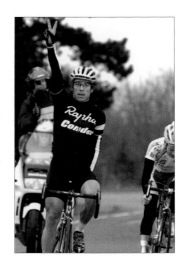

term gain of being in the breakaway group and getting farther from the bunch than you could on your own. Be careful of who joins you, however. If the best sprinter in the race has made the bridge, there is little point in working well together – you might want to sit up and wait for the bunch to catch you. It may be a waste of energy, but so is towing a superior sprinter to the line, unless you are confident you can drop them before the finishing straight.

If you see somebody else attacking, your reaction must be fast. Every moment of hesitation means that there is a bigger gap to cross. When you see the telltale sign of a rider lifting themselves out of the saddle, try and make it a reflex to do exactly the same and put yourself right in their slipstream.

Individual riders often get away, but the most common breakaway is a small group, of between three and ten riders. Initially, these groups tend to work hard together to ensure that they are building a healthy lead over the pack.

You also need to know what the bunch are doing behind you. If they start chasing harder, it is worth marshalling the group to ride especially hard for 10–15km (6–9 miles). It's harder work, but if you can keep the gap at a constant level the bunch may become demoralized and back off. You will be more tired, but when the bunch slows, you can too.

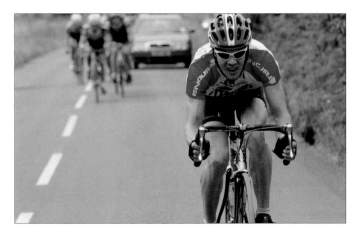

Playing the field

Once groups have a minute or two of lead, riders work together, either by putting the lead at risk, or letting one or more riders do less work than the others. These riders will be fresher at the finish. There may be two riders from one team in the group. It may be your team. If there's a good sprinter in the group, you will need to get rid of them before the end. If you have superior numbers from your team, you can start to dictate things. If you or your team-mate is a good sprinter, it's worth the other rider sacrificing their chances in order to chase down attacks, lead the group at a fast pace to prevent attacks, and to do more of the work in order for the

Above: Solo breakaways are the hardest way to win, but the most spectacular.

sprinter to stay fresher. Or you can take turns in attacking, forcing the other riders to chase you down. If you attack enough times between you, it's a matter of time before an attack is successful.

Up against these tactics, you have to ride cleverly. If you are isolated you will have fewer opportunities to make an effort, but when you do, make sure it is the successful move. If another rider is pulling their team-mate to a sprint victory, make sure they are doing all the work and tiring themselves out, then launch a surprise attack near the finish. When two team-mates are attacking in turn, allow others to chase them down the first time at least. When the second or third attack happens, react at once, get into their slipstream and wait. If you are away, you now have a 50 per cent chance of winning. If you get chased down, go with the counterattack from the other team-mate.

In a breakaway situation, your main aims are working hard to ensure the break stays away, then using as little energy as possible when the tactical games start. Relax, watch your breakaway companions, and make your race-winning effort at just the right moment.

Left: Share the work with your breakaway companions, but be careful to watch them all the time.

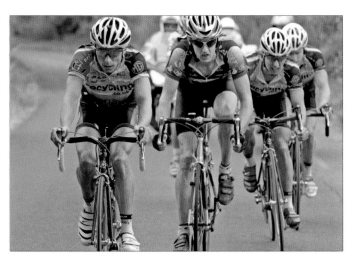

Road-racing Skills: Climbing

Climbing is the hardest part of bike racing. Even good climbers suffer when they ride uphill, while for bad climbers, hills can be the difference between winning and losing a race. It is important to know how to climb.

A strategically placed hill can blow a race apart, so you need to know how to deal with them in a race.

Some people are born climbers. They are generally light, skinny and small, with a large power-to-weight ratio. For these lucky people, hills are where they can really put pressure on the rest of the field. If they also have good technique and tactical sense, they are very hard to deal with in a race.

Others don't climb so well. Larger, heavier riders have more weight to carry up the hills. Others find it difficult to react to changes in pace on uphills. However, even poor climbers can greatly improve their performance by using the best tactics in each situation.

In a race, whether you are a good climber or bad climber, it is important to be at the front when the climb starts. Poor climbers hope that by doing this, they can slip back through the bunch, and still be in contact as the race passes over the top. If these riders start the hill at the back, that is where they will stay. Good climbers need to follow the same tactic, so that they are in position to

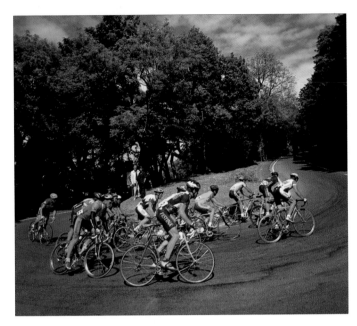

dictate the race or react to others trying to do so. It can take several kilometres of racing to get to the front in time for the bottom, so be prepared.

Hitting your stride

On a long climb, cadence and rhythm are important. Pushing a big gear slowly is an expensive way of riding, and increases the chances that you will tire before the top. The best way of riding is to train yourself to ride in a much lower gear. This gives your legs greater 'snap' when making or reacting to an attack.

Breathing is difficult when climbing, so when climbing sitting down, try and sit more upright, holding the tops of the handlebars, thereby opening up the chest. Sometimes, when the speed

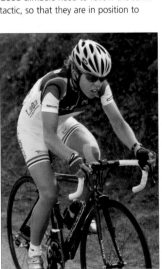

Left: Climbing in a race can be intense and painful – always maintain focus, as this rider is doing here.

Above: The easiest way around a hairpin bend is towards the middle of the road. Follow this line and you could save crucial energy for later on.

increases, or just to stay on top of the gear, you will need to stand up. A good climber can vary their position and rhythm between seated and standing climbing – train yourself to do this so that when you need to do it in a race you are ready.

The best line to follow through the corners on a climb is not necessarily the shortest one. Road corners are often much steeper on the inside than the outside, which could force you to work harder than you need to to maintain your speed. The most advantageous way is halfway between the two sides of the road, unless the corner is really steep, in which case it might be more efficient to move out farther. The important thing is

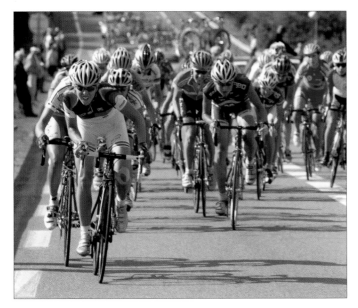

Left: If you are a good climber, attacking uphill can put dangerous rivals out of contention.

If they increase the pace slowly, go with it. It is going to hurt, but you will be maintaining a rhythm, which is more straightforward than responding to varying pace. If they attack suddenly, don't attempt to follow them, as you would an attack on the flat. Remain calm, and slowly increase the pace. Unless they are in super shape, an attack by a climber will be followed by a deceleration. Accelerate slowly to the point where you can bring them back. By catching them, you can make them doubt their ability to get away. If a climber is varying the pace, try to ignore them and ride at your own rhythm.

When climbing gets really painful, it can help to use mental techniques to master the pain. Counting to 10 over and over again will help you focus through the pain. If the climb is a long

to conserve as much energy as possible, and spinning through the less steep part of a corner enables you to do this.

What is necessary while climbing, for good and bad climbers alike, is having the self-knowledge to know your limits and how you react to riding at certain speeds, and to be able to focus through periods of great discomfort. Train yourself in both of these, and your climbing will improve.

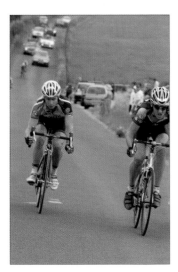

Tactics for a good climber

The best climbers use three methods to make life exceedingly miserable for everybody else in a race. The first is the most straightforward and involves going to the front and gradually accelerating until they are riding as fast as they can. Hanging on to them in this kind of situation is difficult.

The second is by attacking hard, and quickly accelerating away. The third method is, perversely, slowing down. Climbers can deal with changes in rhythm much better than non-climbers can, and by slowing things down they are making the other riders vulnerable to attacks.

If you are a good climber, practise all these methods and try to use them to your advantage.

Tactics for a bad climber

Bad climbers will have to come up with ways of dealing with the methods employed by good climbers to put them to the back of a race. By training hard and being confident of your tactics you may be able to neutralize the climbers.

Left: If you get attacked on a climb, respond, and it may help to discourage further attacks.

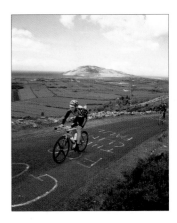

Above: On long, steady climbs, stay as relaxed and focused as possible and hold your pace.

one, focus on getting to the next bend. Break the climb into smaller sections, which are mentally easier to deal with.

Bad climbers are especially vulnerable on races with hilltop finishes. There is no way you can hope to compete with a good climber here. Instead, you should work on getting into a break, giving you a head start.

Road-racing Skills: Cornering and Descending

Taking a corner fast, either on the flat or riding downhill, takes skill, balance and confidence. Deficiencies in any of these areas can lead to a rider being dropped. All these skills are easy to work on, and can be used to advantage in a race.

Your bike can only lean over through a corner so far before one of two things happens. Either your pedal will scrape the floor (if you are pedalling), with dire consequences, or your tyres' traction will be lost, which would be equally catastrophic. On a gravelly surface, this can happen at a very slight angle.

Dealing with a corner in a bike race involves three phases. First comes the approach, during which you adjust your speed to the level necessary to go through the corner. Next is the apex, which is the sharpest part of the corner. And finally there is the exit, which is where you can accelerate out again.

Cornering

In a bunch, the first rider will choose the racing line around the corner, generally swinging out in the approach, then turning their wheel and passing close to the apex. Finally they will swing out again as they accelerate away. If the bunch is strung out in a single line, follow the rider ahead, using the same line, trying to lose as little speed as possible. Do not attempt to overtake on the inside, where you are vulnerable to crashing and also disrupting the flow of the line of riders. By cutting up the inside, you are effectively moving into the racing line of other riders as they cut into the apex, which will make you unpopular. If riders are bunched up, follow close to the racing line and adjust your speed to match the riders around you.

When going around the apex, keep the outside leg down, and lean your bike, while keeping your head upright, to maintain the maximum speed possible. The idea is to cut from the outside of the road to the inside through the apex, then swing wide again once you have passed it. As soon as your bike

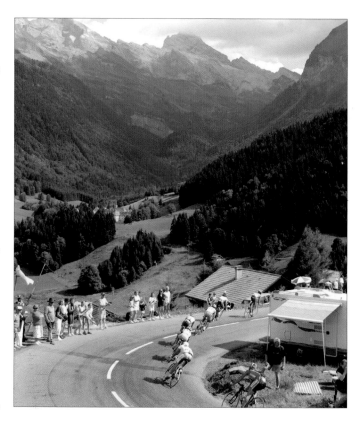

stops swinging wide, you have entered the exit phase and are ready to start pedalling again.

In a race, you can make others work harder through corners by getting to the front, keeping the speed high, and then accelerating hard out of the corner. This has the effect of stretching out the bunch, and riders have to work hard to close gaps that have opened up. Repeat this a few times, and your rivals may not have the energy to chase an attack.

Above: Descending fast and safely is an essential skill in bike racing – getting the racing line right is crucial.

Some bike races are flat, but most include hills for the sake of variety and to add a challenge. Going up the hill is not the only challenge – bunches race fast down the other side, and this is where the less confident descenders get found out.

If your race is taking place on open roads, your first priority should always be safety in the case of meeting cars or other

Cornering on the flat

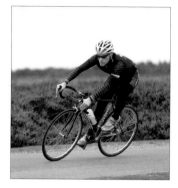

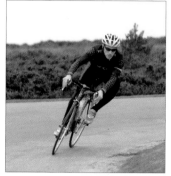

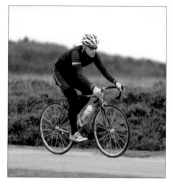

Approach *During the approach, adjust your speed to go around the corner.*

Apex *The sharpest part of the corner is the apex. Lean into it as you go around.*

Exit *The exit is the final part of the corner where you begin accelerating out.*

traffic. Stay on the correct side of the road in case there is a car around a blind corner. The same warning applies for training rides.

Descending

The first rule of descending is to keep your head up, look ahead and anticipate what is going to happen in front of you. Unless you are leading the bunch, you may have to react to the movements of other riders.

Effective descending means having a comfortable and aerodynamic position on the bike. Always hold the drops of your handlebars, with one or two fingers on the brake levers, so you can react fast to obstacles. Keep your centre of gravity low,

for better balance and aerodynamics. If you can see a long way ahead, you can go into a tuck position, with your hands on the tops of the handlebars and your chin almost touching your wrists. Use your legs as shock absorbers by putting more of your weight on the pedals and sitting on the tip of your saddle.

It is important to corner well going downhill. Slow down before you hit a corner, to a speed that will allow you to go around the bend without crashing. If you are in a bunch, don't make sudden movements if you want to change your position, but do signal your intentions clearly in case somebody in turn is trying to get around you.

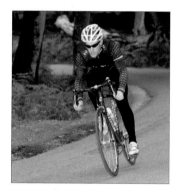

Above: To enter a bend, swing wide, then cut in to the apex of the curve.

Cornering on a descent

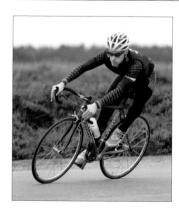

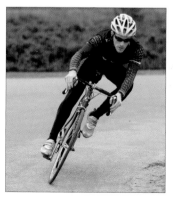

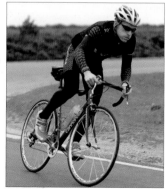

Approach *To begin, swing wide, and accelerate towards the corner.*

Apex *Follow a natural line, stay relaxed and look forward with head up.*

Exit *Start pedalling as you hit the exit with the bike starting to straighten.*

Road-racing Skills: Sprinting

Sprinters win far more bike races than any other kind of bike rider. They have the advantage of being able to wait until the finishing line is in sight and then unleashing their primary weapon. Various tactics can be employed to win the day.

Field sprinting demands nerve, speed, strength, determination and timing. When a rider has all of these attributes, he or she is very difficult to beat.

Sprinting, at a basic level, involves riding as fast as possible over a short distance, but there is more than one way of doing this.

Some sprints are won by a rider jumping to the front early in the race and holding their speed all the way to the line. Others are won by a rider getting into the slipstream of the rider who has made the early jump, taking advantage of the wind protection offered by their rival, then overtaking them in the final 50m (164ft).

Strength or speed?

Some riders rely on sheer brute strength in their sprint. If they can turn a bigger gear than anybody else, they can go the fastest. These riders favour a long,

drawn-out sprint. Riders at the opposite end of the sprinting scale rely on leg speed. They don't need to use as high a gear as the power sprinters, but instead turn a smaller gear faster. The advantage of this method is that their acceleration is far quicker, enabling them to speed away from other riders very quickly.

In a race, the preparation for a sprint starts as far as 20km (12.5 miles) from the finishing line. If you want to be involved in the sprint you need to make sure you are riding near the front well before the finish. Take time to move up the bunch, staying out of the wind as much as possible. Ideally, you will have a team-mate or two to help you do this.

In the Tour de France, the sprinters' teams maintain a very high speed at the front of the bunch for the final 10km (6 miles), to discourage breakaways from spoiling their leader's chance of a win. In smaller races, the run-in tends to be

more of a free-for-all. Stay near the front without going into the lead, so you can watch the way the race is developing.

Jockeying for position

With 3km (1.8 miles) to go, the real manoeuvring starts. Riding behind another rider saves energy, so the sprinters bump and barge each other to defend their position behind another rider. If there is a strong sprinter in the field, other riders keep close to their wheel, following them in the sprint and jumping around them to steal the win. There is only one place on his wheel, even if four or five riders are fighting for it.

As the race enters the final 500m (1,640ft), the riders start to fan across the road as the sprint is launched. Although every sprint is different, you should be aiming to start your final sprint with about 200m (656ft) to go. Try to stay on another sprinter's wheel until this point. Accelerate hard at this point and spend the next 50m (164ft) building up to speed. Then try to hold your top speed all the way to the finishing line.

Phases of sprinting

Acceleration and speed maintenance are the two phases of sprinting. Acceleration has to be a sudden increase in speed to reach top speed as fast as possible, to get around riders in front of you, and to shake off riders who are on your wheel. If gear selection is too high, it will take too long to accelerate; too low, and you will not be able to reach top speed. Terrain and wind direction must be taken into consideration. Grip the drops of the handlebars firmly, stand up on the pedals and jump as hard as you

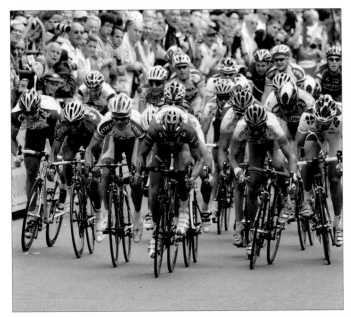

Left: Bike races are often decided with a fast and furious bunch sprint. Good tactics make all the difference in a sprint.

How to sprint

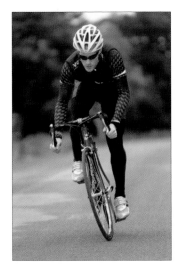

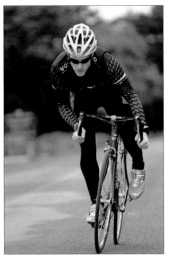

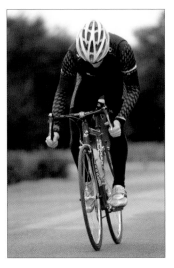

1 *To sprint, jump hard, holding the handlebars firmly.*

2 *Push down with one leg; pull up handlebars with the opposite hand.*

3 *When your reach maximum speed, maintain it as long as you can.*

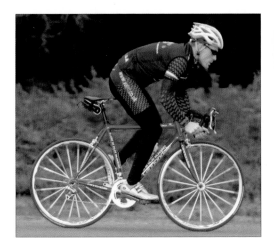

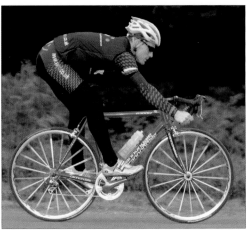

4 *Bend your arms. Use the upper body to best effect.*

5 *Extend arms and legs to push the bike over the line.*

can, putting as much force through the pedal stroke as you can, again and again. Use your upper body and each arm in turn to pull the handlebars up as you push down on the pedal with the opposite foot. Initially your acceleration will be slow, but as momentum builds up, you can get towards your top speed.

Finishing the sprint

Once you hit top speed, your aim is to maintain it to the finishing line. If you start to slow, other riders who have timed their sprint better will come past you. Keep your eyes forward, ignore other riders, and maintain a straight line to the finishing line to avoid obstructing other riders, for which you can be disqualified.

It is also the shortest distance. Don't slow in the final metres, even if you think you have won, but pedal hard through the finishing line, with the final strong thrust of the pedals coinciding with straightening your arms to 'push' your bike ahead. This is called 'throwing' the bike, and it can be the crucial skill that gains you victory.

Road-racing Skills: Strategies and Teamwork

It is often said that cycling is a team sport for individuals, and it is true that only one rider can win the race. However, that victory may well be partly due to the sacrifice and hard work of the rider's team-mates.

Getting into the right position in a race involves thorough pre-race planning, and clever decision-making during a race. Team tactics must be well thought out and flexible enough to allow unpredictable events to be dealt with.

Before the race

The most important part of preparation for a race is to train properly for the weeks and months leading up to it. Turning up at a race unfit is a waste of your time. If the race is an important one, ease off your training in the run-up to it, so that you are in tip-top condition on the morning of the event.

Well before the race, you should research its route. Knowledge of the roads you are racing on is a huge advantage. If the race is local, you can train on the route, get used to the corners, decide which gears you need to use, find out where the course might be exposed to crosswinds, and notice subtle variations in the gradient of the finishing straight. All of this information is a powerful tool in riding a good race.

Knowing that there is a hill might not be good enough. You need to know if it is steep at the bottom, or steep at the top. Is there a descent straight away, or does it emerge on to a plateau, which will be windy and could split the bunch up even more than the climb? Is there a sharp corner just at the bottom of the climb? If so, going around it in first position will enable you to accelerate and gain distance on your rivals, who will have to work hard to chase you down. Does your race finish on a hill,

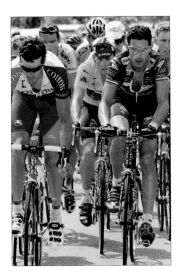

Above: Lance Armstrong was helped to seven Tour de France wins by his US Postal and Discovery Channel teams.

and if so, who is your team's best climber? Is there a sharp corner 400m (1,312ft) before the finishing line? No detail is too small to help in your preparation. By knowing the course, you can also train specifically for its challenges, which will stand you in good physical stead.

Know your enemy

The course is one area that you should research well before the race; another is your rivals. They want to win the race as badly as you do, and they have their own plans for doing so. Good climbers need to be neutralized during the flat part of the course. Good sprinters need

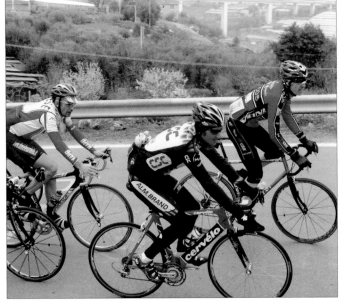

Left: Researching the route and working out strategies with team-mates ahead of the race can give a team an advantage.

to be kept to the back in the hills. If there is a particularly strong team taking part, rather than trying to beat them single-handedly, it might be better to apply the old saying, 'if you can't beat them, join them.'

Try to get into breaks with their riders and work with them, which effectively makes them, and the riders they have in the bunch, your temporary team-mates. You can work out how to beat them once you have carved up the race between you.

Lastly, look at the weather forecast the day before the race and bring the correct riding clothes for the conditions.

During the race

You should have formulated 'Plan A' before the race. This might involve getting a specific rider in your team away in an early attack on the first climb of the race. Or it could involve waiting for the finishing sprint.

Because these plans are fairly inflexible, and could be compromised by the actions of other riders in the race, you also have to react well to the prevailing circumstances. You might designate one or two riders who are under instructions to make sure that at least one of them is in every early break. This takes the pressure off the rest of your team to chase breaks down.

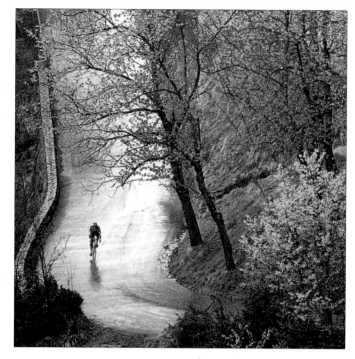

If you find yourself with a team-mate farther up the road in a break, your job is twofold. First, there is no need to expend energy in chasing down the break – you can leave this to others. Second, you should be vigilant for counterattacks, which might put your

Above: If you are a strong climber, use hills to get ahead during a race.

escaped team-mate in a weaker position. If counterattacks happen, it's worth trying to get another team-mate into them. If the tables are turned and your team has missed the break, it will be your responsibility, along with other teams who missed the break, to chase it down. If this is the case, don't use the whole team to ride as hard as possible on the front, or you will all be burned out by the finish. Instead, try and share the work with another team, using just a couple of riders to up the pace gradually and eat into the break's lead.

Apart from these strategies, the main aim of the race is to expend as little energy as possible so that you are still strong at the end. Stay close behind other riders as much as is practical. Don't panic as events unfold, but react to them calmly.

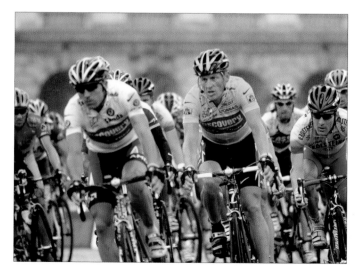

Left: By sheltering their leader (in the middle) from the wind, team-mates help him to save vital energy in a race.

Road-racing Skills: Time Trialling

The ability to time trial is one of the most important skills in cycling. Being able to ride fast and maintain a fast pace is a necessity not only in time trialling but also in road racing, when you are in an escape, or when chasing down a break.

Time trialling involves riding at a steady and consistent rate. The aim is never to ride so fast that you are unable to maintain your pace, and not to slow down – a feat which requires concentration, nerve, resistance to pain, endurance and strength.

Some riders are naturally better at time trialling than others. It is also a trainable skill. By working hard on your body position and endurance, and practising a lot, you can bring about improvements in your time-trialling results.

Time trials can be individual races, or part of a stage race. In the latter, you can afford to lose a little time if you know you can gain time in another stage. In an individual race, the fastest man or woman wins. It involves getting up to speed quickly and steadily, then maintaining the effort until the finish.

Your starting effort in a time trial should not be the same as an attack in a road race, or a jump in a sprint. Instead, accelerate gradually so that you don't overwork your muscles. At the same time, don't relax too much at this point – you need to be at cruising speed sooner rather than later.

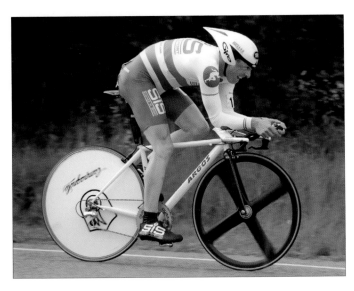

Pacing yourself

Finding out what pace you can sustain over a long time trial involves training with a pulse monitor and working out

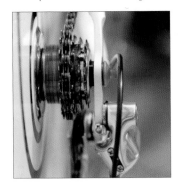

the percentage of your maximum heart rate you can ride at without becoming exhausted. This takes experimentation. Maintaining this pace should not be a comfortable process. During a time trial, your body will be in a great deal of pain, and you need to focus through this and be confident that you can maintain the same level of effort.

Riding at the same pace during a race is often made difficult by corners, hills and weather conditions. Some riders make the mistake of trying to maintain speed up hills and into a headwind; the extra effort will make them collapse later. The effort should be the constant, not the speed. There is no need to panic if it feels like you are riding slowly – your rivals will be doing the same. As with road races, knowing the course will

Left: Time-trial bikes need fewer gears than road bikes, especially on the flat.
Right: Time-trial bikes handle less well than road bikes, so you have to take care to avoid crashes.

Top: Good time trialling requires an aerodynamic position, good equipment and the ability to endure pain.

assist in planning your race. If you have paced yourself correctly, you should be feeling weary in the second half of the course. This is the time to hold your nerve and focus. If possible add a little extra effort, without crossing into the red zone, ensuring that by the finishing line you are at your peak output.

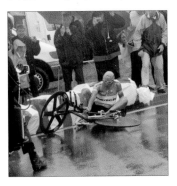

Time-trialling bikes

Road-racing bikes and time-trialling bikes are different. Aerodynamics are important for time-trialling bikes, since the speed will be greater than in other kinds of race. The bike is narrow, and puts the rider in a position in which the arms are ahead of the body, the back and head are as low as possible, while still letting the legs turn at maximum capacity.

Frames are stiffer than for bikes for road-racing. The greater distances in road racing mean that stiffness has to be balanced against comfort. Time trials tend to be shorter and comfort is not so important. By making the frame stiffer, less power is lost by the frame flexing, resulting in a faster ride.

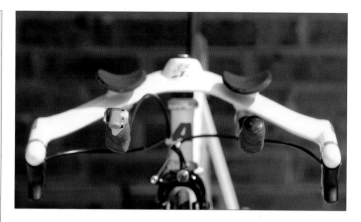

Above: Time-trialling handlebars are arranged so that they put the arms and body into an aerodynamic tuck, with the head and back in a low position.

Anatomy of a time-trial bike

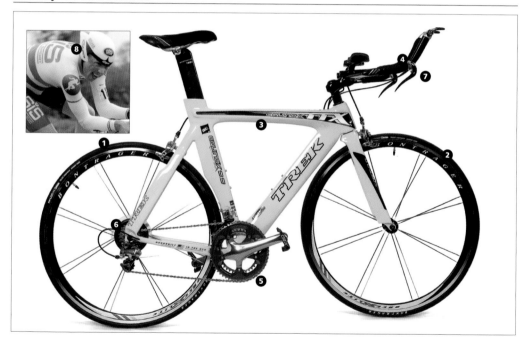

❶ Rear wheel: Solid disc wheels are more aerodynamic than spoked wheels.
❷ Front wheel: Deep rims cut down on the length of the spokes, which are flat, to reduce drag.
❸ Frame: Moulded carbon fibre frame with flatter tubes. Extremely stiff, at the expense of long-distance comfort.

❹ Handlebars: Special low-profile 'tri-bars' allow the rider to rest on their elbows with the arms stretched out ahead, giving a far more aerodynamic profile.
❺ Chainrings: 53–44 or even less discrepancy in size, unless the bike is to be used on a very hilly course.

❻ Sprockets: 8- or 9-speed freewheel with 12–19 or 12–21 block.
❼ Gear-changers: These are mounted on the end of the tri-bars for ease of access.
❽ Clothing: One-piece tight-fitting skinsuits and profiled helmets catch less wind than regular cycling clothing.

Racing Skills: Triathlon

Triathlons involve sandwiching a bike race between a swim and a run. For many cyclists, they are an extra challenge that also contribute to greater all-round fitness. The training discipline for a triathlon is very similar to that for cycling.

Triathlons are almost a pure endurance sport, in which judgement of pace and resistance to fatigue are the most important skills. The three sports are difficult enough on their own, but together they form a unique challenge.

When cyclists start triathlon training, the greatest challenge is forcing the body to work with different muscle groups. When making the transition, it is recommended that you spend a few months just getting used to swimming and running without going into any structured training routines.

Once your body is used to working in these different ways, it is a good idea to work with a swimming coach, who will improve your technique. The typical swim for an Olympic-distance triathlon is 1,500m (approximately 1 mile) – bad technique over this distance will slow you down and tire you out, and good cycling may not be enough to compensate. Better technique will greatly improve your swimming times.

If you are an experienced cyclist going into triathlons, work on maintaining your cycling economy and fitness – this

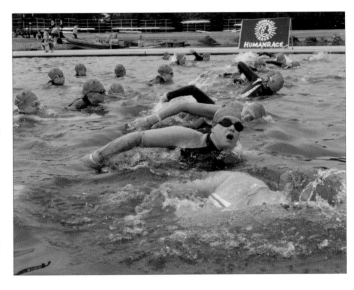

Above: Triathlons often begin with a massed start swim in which positioning is a crucial factor.
Below: Experienced cyclists have an advantage over their competitors in the bike leg of a triathlon.

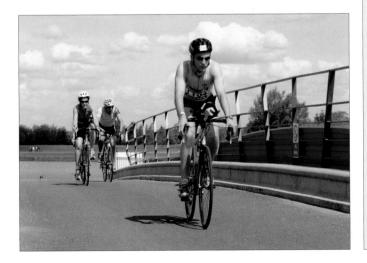

Triathlon bike

At first glance, a typical triathlon bike looks very similar to a time-trial bike. However, the special nature of the exertion in the course of a triathlon means that the athletes have some needs not shared by time triallists.

First, the position of a triathlete is not as low down as a time triallist. The saddle should remain at the optimum height for maximum performance, but the handlebars should be raised so that the position is not so extreme. The bike section of a triathlon is followed by a run, which puts strain on the hamstrings. If the triathlete uses a low position, he or she risks injury during the run.

Second, there are two water bottles carried on the frame. The athlete will not have had a chance to rehydrate during the swimming leg. The bike is a good time to refuel and ensure consumption of enough energy to get through the run. Both bottles will probably be necessary.

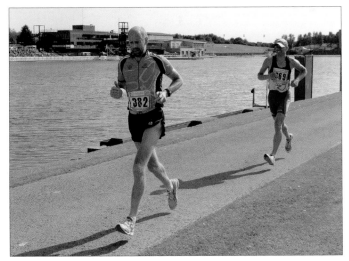

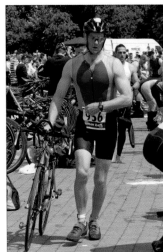

is the part of the race in which you will have an advantage over swimmers who are starting the bike stage ahead of you.

The running stage is an unusual kind of exertion. Although running training is absolutely necessary, you also need to train yourself to run after a long bike ride. Your body is tired by now and this will slow down your running, so, as well as swimming, cycling and running training, you also need to incorporate what are known as 'brick' sessions into your training routine. These involve a training session linking two of the disciplines, most often cycling and running. A typical brick session might involve a 30-minute warm-up followed by 10-minute sets alternating between the bike (on a stationary trainer, unless you have an exact training route) and running. Cycle at 75 to 80 per cent of MHR for 10 minutes, then run at the same intensity for 10 minutes. Then repeat, before warming down. These sessions are essential if you are to achieve your potential in a triathlon.

Quick changes

The other challenge facing triathletes is to 'transition' as quickly and efficiently as possible between the three stages.

Right: Save time in the transition zone by having your equipment prepared exactly as you want it.

Above: The run leg of a triathlon is extremely arduous because of the fatigue after the swim and bike legs.

This is complicated by the fact that competitors often wear a wetsuit for the swim (if it is in cold, open water), and need to change shoes for both the cycle and the run. Organization and relaxed focus is necessary to do this as quickly as possible. When you leave the water, start to unzip your wetsuit as you jog towards the bike pen. Take your wetsuit off carefully but fast, so your feet don't get caught, then run with your bike

Above: During the transition time, take the opportunity to refocus on the next discipline.

(with shoes attached to pedals) out of the bike pen to the start of the bike leg. Mount the bike and put your feet into your shoes as you move off.

For the next transition, take your feet out of your shoes at the end of the ride and dismount the bike, running to the pen. Get your running shoes on as quickly as possible, and you are set. Transitions are an easy process, but rushing can add minutes to your finish time.

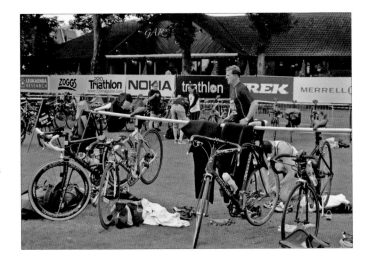

Great Road Races: The Tour de France

The Tour de France is the greatest race in cycling history. Because it is the first and oldest of the Grand Tours, with the best slot on the cycling calendar in mid-July and terrain perfectly suited to bike racing, it captures the imagination of the cycling world each summer.

The Tour is a stage race. The approximately 3,000km (1,865-mile) route is divided into daily stages, generally between 150 and 250km (93–155 miles), with time trials on some days. The riders start each stage together, and their accumulated time is added into the general classification.

Yellow jersey

The leader of the general classification wears a yellow jersey. There is also a points classification, for the rider who consistently gets the best stage placings, and a red and white dotted jersey for the best climber, known as the King of the Mountains. The yellow jersey is that colour because the original sponsoring newspaper, *L'Auto*, was printed on yellow paper. In the early years of the race it was pointed out that nobody knew who was winning the race, and the tradition of handing them a yellow jersey at the end of each stage was born.

Test of strength

The race is extremely arduous, with only two rest days during the three weeks. The route is different every year and in recent times has followed a clockwise direction one year and the next year, an anticlockwise direction.

The race always spends five or six days in the high mountains, crossing the Alps and Pyrenees. Riders can lose huge amounts of time in these stages, and many are forced to pull out.

In some years, when the organizers want to make the event particularly tough, the race goes into the Massif Central mountain range in central France for a day or two. The race has a different start – known as 'Le Grand Départ' – every year, but always finishes with a well deserved celebration stage on the Champs Elysées in Paris.

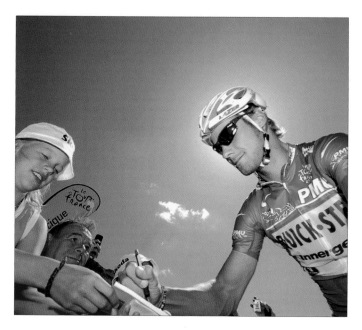

Above: Fans flock to the Tour de France in their thousands every summer, hoping for a glimpse of their cycling heroes.

1952

The most impressive Tours are the closest ones, and those that are dominated by a single rider. The year 1952 saw an Italian climber at the peak of his powers, with his rivals simply unable to keep up with him.

Fausto Coppi probably would have won whatever the route in 1952, but the organizers blessed him with a mountainous route including the first ever summit finishes – three of them, at Puy de Dôme, Alpe d'Huez and Sestrières. He won each of these stages, as well as a long time trial early in the race. Journalists, with very little to write about in the way of a close race (second-placed Stan Ockers was at least 28 minutes behind, which

was a massive margin), waxed lyrical about Coppi's win, seeing it as nothing short of legendary.

Below: Fausto Coppi was one of the first heroes of the modern era, winning the Tour de France three times in the 1950s.

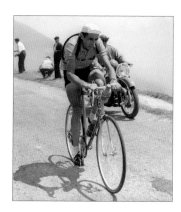

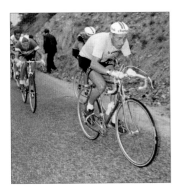

Above: Frenchman Jacques Anquetil, who was the first man to win the Tour de France five times.

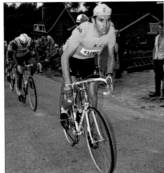

Above: Eddy Merckx, who won five Tours in dominant style during the 1960s and 1970s.

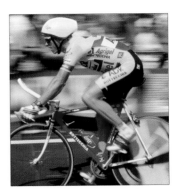

Above: Greg Lemond time trials his way to victory in the 1989 Tour de France, the closest race ever.

1964

In 1964, the race was a battle between two Frenchmen – four-times winner Jacques Anquetil and his great rival Raymond Poulidor. Anquetil was the more successful on the bike, while Poulidor was more popular with fans.

In 1964, Poulidor came very close to toppling Anquetil. On the climb of the Puy de Dôme, the two rode side by side, elbows clashing, weaving up the road as they fought to win. Unbeknown to Poulidor, Anquetil was feeling terrible, but he bluffed his way up, fighting the agony to stay with Poulidor. Poulidor only realized too late that Anquetil was vulnerable and he attacked with sufficient time to drop Anquetil, but not enough to take the yellow jersey, which Anquetil eventually won by 55 seconds.

1969

As in 1952, 1969 saw a single rider dominate the race. His name was Eddy Merckx, and he was about to take the first of his five Tour de France victories. His nickname was the 'Cannibal', which referred to his voracious appetite for winning races and destroying the opposition. In 1969 the 24-year-old Belgian was unrivalled. He took the yellow jersey as the race entered the Alps in the first week, and held it to the finish. He took a brilliant solo victory on the 17th stage in the Pyrenees, attacking early and spending the day on his own at the front. He won by almost 20 minutes.

1989

This was simply the most dramatic race in Tour history. The excitement started when defending champion Pedro Delgado turned up late for the first stage and lost almost 3 minutes before he had began turning the pedals. The lead swung between Greg Lemond, on the comeback after a hunting accident, and two-times winner Laurent Fignon through the flat first week and the Pyrenees. Delgado began to claw his way back into contention.

In the Alps, Fignon looked the stronger, and two attacks on successive days put him 50 seconds into the lead with only a 30km time trial into Paris to go. Lemond beat him by 58 seconds, gaining the yellow jersey by 8 seconds.

2003

Lance Armstrong had dominated the race for four years previously, but in 2003 he almost failed. He was unable to stamp his authority on the race in his usual style, and although he wore the yellow jersey through the Alps and Pyrenees, his lead was slim, and he looked vulnerable to the attacks made by his rivals. He took a beating in a long time trial. On one day, one of his closest rivals, Joseba Beloki, fell off directly in front of Armstrong on a steep corner in the Alps. Armstrong was forced to take spectacular evasive action, and ended up riding across a field, jumping off his bike and carrying it back on to the road. In

the Pyrenees, his handlebar got caught on a spectator's bag strap, pulling him off his bike. He still managed to put in a race-winning attack farther up the road, defending a slim lead in the final time trial.

2008

The Tour in 2008 was one of the most tactical and closest ever. There were no outstanding favourites, and with only days left to race, there were still six riders within a minute of the lead, an unprecedented situation. In the Alps, in the last week, Spanish rider Carlos Sastre made an all-or-nothing attack on the Alpe d'Huez climb, and gained enough time to win the Tour.

Below: Lance Armstrong, the absolute record holder in the Tour, with seven wins.

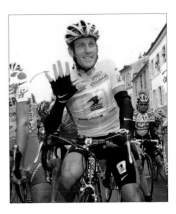

10 Best-ever Tour de France Riders

The Tour de France is one of the most important stage races for cycling aficionados. It is a tough race, taking around 23 days and covering more than 3,000 kilometres (1,865 miles). To be the best, riders need endurance and great physical strength.

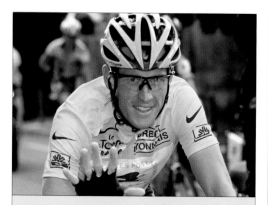

1) Lance Armstrong (USA)
TOUR WINS: SEVEN
Armstrong dominated the Tour de France between 1999 and 2005. He won seven on the trot, and in six of these he was unchallengeable. The exception was 2003, when he started tired, and struggled all the way to victory only 1 minute ahead of German rival Jan Ullrich.

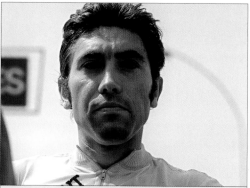

2) Eddy Merckx (Belgium)
TOUR WINS: FIVE
Merckx won five Tours between 1969 and 1974, as well as virtually every other race on the calendar. His insatiable appetite for succeeding ensured that he won more stages than any other rider and spent more days in the yellow jersey than anyone else.

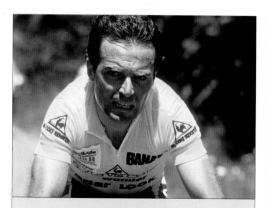

3) Bernard Hinault (France)
TOUR WINS: FIVE
The last indomitable French winner of the Tour de France took his fifth title in 1985. Hinault had an aggressive, confrontational style, in life as in racing, and didn't suffer fools gladly.

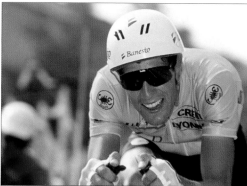

4) Miguel Indurain (Spain)
TOUR WINS: FIVE
Indurain was the first rider to win five successive Tours, between 1991 and 1995. He was an awesome time triallist, building a big lead in the individual tests, and hanging on to the best climbers in the mountains.

5) Jacques Anquetil (France)

TOUR WINS: FIVE

Anquetil was the first rider to win five Tours, taking his first in 1957, then another four between 1961 and 1964. His career was defined by his great rivalry with the more popular Raymond Poulidor, whose nickname 'the eternal second' revealed which of the two riders was faster on the bike.

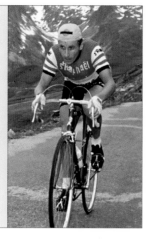

6) Greg Lemond (USA)

TOUR WINS: THREE

Lemond was the first American rider to win the Tour de France. His career was interrupted by a hunting accident in which he nearly lost his life. On recovering, he showed his ability in an amazing comeback, and stormed through to win the 1989 race by only 8 seconds, which was the closest race in history.

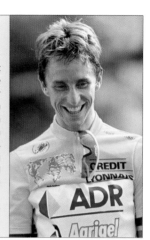

7) Louison Bobet (France)

TOUR WINS: THREE

Bobet won three successive Tours between 1951 and 1953, starting a golden age in French cycling. Including his wins, French riders won 11 out of 15 Tours, a record they have rarely approached since. His performance in the 1953 Tour was considered to be one of the finest ever because the conditions were so difficult.

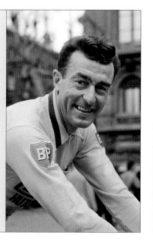

8) Philippe Thys (Belgium)

TOUR WINS: THREE

The first triple winner of the race, Thys would probably have won a lot more Tours if his career had not been interrupted by World War I. Although he started off as a cyclo-cross champion, he went on to win the Tour de France in 1913, 1914 and 1920. He won five stages in 1922 and two stages in the tour of 1924.

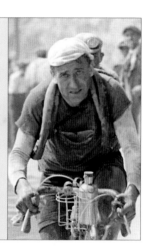

9) Fausto Coppi (Italy)

TOUR WINS: TWO

As with Thys, war took Coppi's best racing years from him and his racing career took place when travelling across borders was not particularly easy. He dominated the Tour in the mountains in a way rarely seen in the history of the race. His 1952 win has been described as the best Tour de France victory.

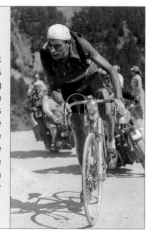

10) Laurent Fignon (France)

TOUR WINS: TWO

Fignon won the Tour at the age of 22 in 1983, and after thrashing Bernard Hinault the following year, it was expected that he would go on to win many more Tours. But plagued by injury, poor morale and a spate of bad luck, the rest of his career was blighted, and he missed out on winning in 1989 by just 8 seconds.

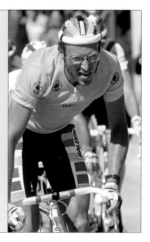

Great Road Races: The Giro d'Italia

The cycling season doesn't begin and end with the Tour de France. There are two other Grand Tours, the Tour of Italy and the Tour of Spain, as well as a whole host of stage races and one-day races from February through to October every year.

The Giro d'Italia, or Tour of Italy, is the first Grand Tour of the year, taking place in late May and early June. Like the Tour de France, it is three weeks long, and is contested in the same way, with daily stages and a general classification. The leader of the race wears a pink jersey, known as the 'maglia rosa', in the same way as the Tour de France leader wears a yellow jersey.

The race is as tough as the Tour de France, with stages in the Alps and Dolomite mountain ranges. In recent years, the Giro d'Italia organizers have tried to design ever-tougher mountain stages, to make it the hardest race in the world.

1949

Just like in the 1952 Tour de France, Fausto Coppi dominated the 1949 Giro with superb lone attacks in the mountains. His closest rival was Gino Bartali, who finished 24 minutes behind.

On a sporting level, it was a one-horse race, but the rivalry between Coppi and Bartali divided the nation. As Italy emerged from the chaos of World War II, it stood at a crossroads between the old ways, and the modern ways of the Western world. Bartali was a pious Catholic, who attracted the older, more conservative fans, while Coppi, divorced and conducting a public affair with another woman, represented the secular,

modern world. The fans played out the cultural war using Coppi and Bartali as symbols of their beliefs.

1987

The 1987 Giro d'Italia was possibly the most entertaining Grand Tour of them all, with a bitter feud raging at the heart of the race. Irishman Stephen Roche was the winner. He took the lead midway through the race, with an attack on a mountain stage. That might not have been a problem in itself, except that he was riding for an Italian team, in Italy,

Below: The Irish cyclist, Stephen Roche, who won the 1987 Giro d'Italia.

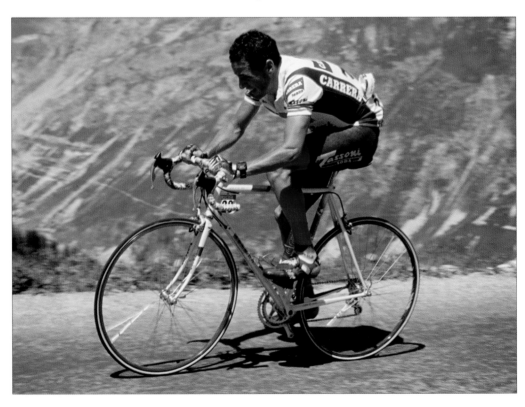

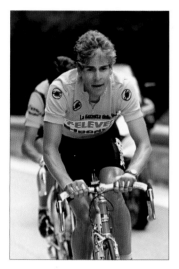

Above: Andy Hampsten, winner of the 1988 Giro d'Italia. He won the race in terrible conditions in the mountains.

and the rider he relieved of the pink jersey was his Italian team-mate Roberto Visentini. It caused a scandal.

Visentini spent the rest of the race conducting a war of words in the press with Roche, who could no longer rely on the support of his team-mates. The crowds by the roadside yelled abuse and threw missiles at Roche as he rode past, while Visentini tried to knock him off his bike. Roche prevailed and went on to win a historic triple in the same year – the Giro, the Tour and the World Championships.

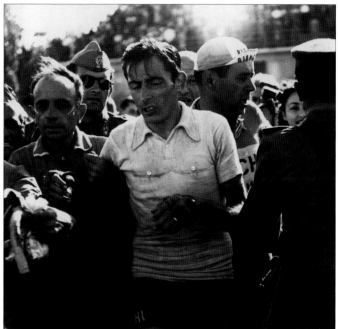

1988

After the drama of 1987, it was only a year before the next big drama in the race. On a mountain stage to Bormio, in the Dolomites, the weather took a turn for the worse. It was raining in the valleys, but the stage was going over the 2,600m (8,500ft) Gavia pass, where the rain turned to snow. In apocalyptic conditions, the organizers refused to stop the race, forcing riders to struggle up through

Above: Fausto Coppi, who became a hero for Italian fans by winning the Giro d'Italia five times in the 40s and 50s.

the blizzard, then, which was worse, ride down the other side. American Andy Hampsten and Dutchman Erik Breukink handled the conditions the best, putting almost 5 minutes between them and the next rider, and Hampsten went on to win the race.

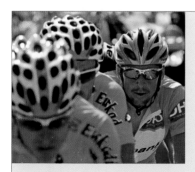

Above: The 18th stage of the Vuelta a España in 2007.

The Vuelta a España

The Tour of Spain, known as the Vuelta a España, is the third Grand Tour of the cycling season. It is not as big or brash as its counterparts in Italy and France, and suffered from a crisis in confidence when it was moved from May, when it used to attract good quality international stars, to September, towards the end of a long and tiring season. It is said that there are two kinds of riders at the Vuelta – those who want to win the race, and those who have been sent there as punishment. The Vuelta is a three-week stage race and the route changes each year but usually includes steep climbs. Nevertheless, it is still an important race. Spain emerged as a powerful cycling nation in the late 1980s and 1990s. Pedro Delgado and Miguel Indurain's Tour de France wins brought more fans to the Vuelta.

Nobody has ever dominated the Vuelta like Merckx dominated the Giro and Armstrong dominated the Tour – the record for victories is three by Swiss rider Tony Rominger between 1992 and 1994, and even Merckx only managed to win it once. Indurain famously never managed to win it, claiming it came at a time of the season when allergies affected his form.

Great Road Races: The Classics

As well as the Grand Tours, there are also many one-day races throughout the cycling year. The biggest and oldest are the five major Classics held at venues in Europe. The only other one-day race that comes close in terms of prestige is the World Championships.

For many riders and fans, the five Classics and the World Championship races are the ultimate prize – even more important than the Tour de France. For each Classic, there is an outstanding race or a rider that fought against all the odds to win. These races will never be forgotten.

Milan–San Remo

Known as 'La Primavera', Milan–San Remo happens as spring reaches northern Italy. It is a mainly flat race, which attracts the bunch sprinters, but two strategically placed hills near the finish always have the potential to stir things up. The most memorable race took place in 1983. This race has a fond place in the hearts of Italian cycling fans. The home favourite, Giuseppe Saronni, was the winner. He was wearing the rainbow jersey of world champion, which simultaneously heaped the pressure on to his shoulders, and made his victory all the more worthwhile. He attacked alone on the Poggio, the final climb into San Remo, and held off the bunch on the descent to the finish line.

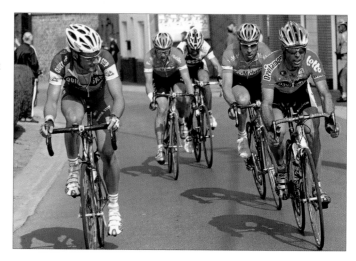

Tour of Flanders

The whole of Belgium stops what it is doing on the day of the Tour of Flanders. Belgian cycling fans are among the most passionate in the world, and if they get a home winner, the excitement is comparable with a national holiday.

The race includes several steep cobbled climbs, called 'bergs', and rutted, sometimes muddy tracks, where the atmosphere is second to none. The race is usually decided on the climbs.

Belgian cycling fell into something of a decline when Eddy Merckx retired in 1977. The country embarked on a fruitless search to replace their hero, whose ability and wins will probably never be equalled in the sport.

In 2005, however, a new national hero emerged in the form of sprinter Tom Boonen. He dominated the race, making his rivals look second-rate with a searing attack in the final 10km (6 miles).

Left: Andrei Tchmil wins the Paris–Roubaix, the best performance of modern times.
Right: Giuseppe Saronni, who won the unforgettable 1983 Milan–San Remo.

Above: Tom Boonen (left), the Belgian rider who won a famous Tour of Flanders in 2005.

Paris–Roubaix

Famous for the cobbled farm tracks that appear with increasing frequency in the second half of the race, Paris–Roubaix is a hard race to ride. The rough tracks turn the race into a war of attrition,

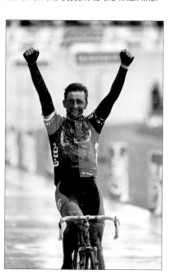

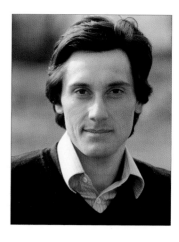

which only the strongest can survive. Riding on cobbles is hard enough – it is atrociously difficult even for the strongest professional cyclists. In 1994 persistent rain added to this difficulty, turning the roads into quagmires, covering the riders in thick mud and causing crash after crash. The formidable Russian Andrei Tchmil emerged from the chaos to take victory, riding away from the other favourites with 50km (31 miles) still to ride.

Liège–Bastogne–Liège

The oldest of the Classics is a hilly race in the Ardennes region of Belgium. It tends to attract the type of rider who is also a contender for the Tour de France – the constant climbing whittles down the field until only the strongest climbers are left.

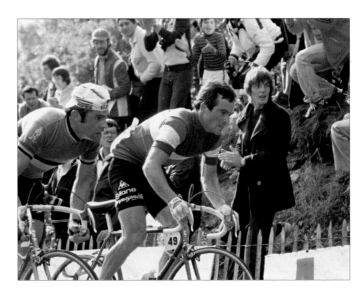

Above: Bernard Hinault en route to winning the 1980 World Championships in dominant style.

Lemond, and Irishman Sean Kelly, who would become one of the most prolific Classics winners of them all.

As the group sprinted towards the line, there was a blanket finish, with four riders flashing across the line. In first place was Kelly, only half a wheel ahead of Lemond.

The World Championships

Held at a different venue every year, the World Championships take place over a course based on laps of the same circuit. Unusually, riders compete for their country, rather than the professional trade teams they represent the rest of the year. The winner of the race is presented with a white jersey with rainbow stripes, which he has the right to wear in races for the next year.

In 1980 the course was more mountainous than it had ever been before, based at Sallanches in the French Alps. This coincided with French cyclist Bernard Hinault, a notoriously prickly character, coming back from injury, during which he had been written off by the media. He took his revenge by thrashing his rivals, attacking on the climb on each lap until he was on his own.

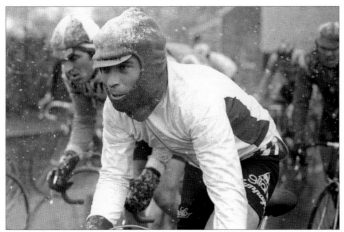

Above: Hinault, this time battling through arctic conditions at the 1980 Liège–Bastogne–Liège.

Frenchman Bernard Hinault won the 1980 Liège–Bastogne–Liège in a terrible blizzard that besieged the riders throughout the race and subsequently wiped out more than half of the field. As rider after rider abandoned the race, Hinault forged ahead on his own, finishing 9 minutes ahead of the next rider. The cold was so terrible that Hinault never regained the feeling in one of his fingers.

Tour of Lombardy

The 'race of the falling leaves' takes place in northern Italy at the end of the cycling season. The race winds through the scenic wooded hills surrounding Lake Como – the biggest climb, the Madonna del Ghisallo, is named after the chapel at the top. Cycling fans consider this to be the most beautiful race of the season.

A race as hard as the Tour of Lombardy is usually won by solo escapers, but in 1983, a group of 13 riders poured into the finishing straight, including recently crowned world champion Greg

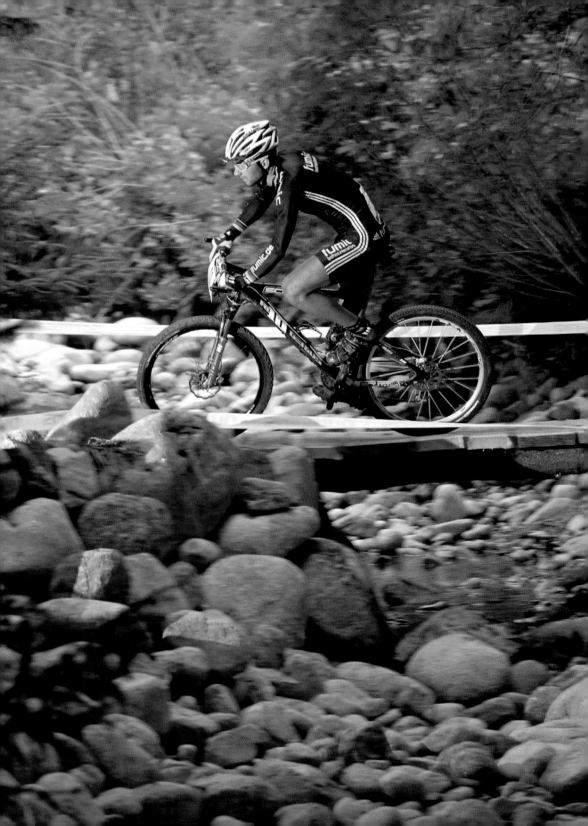

OFF-ROAD RACING

The next step up from riding off-road trails is racing along them. With the boom in mountain biking, off-road racing has grown along with the popularity of the bikes themselves. Mountain bike cross-country racing is now an Olympic sport, while thousands of people enter long-distance enduro races.

The sport of cyclo-cross, which developed along with the sport of road racing, has enjoyed a mini-boom on the back of mountain biking. As people discover the fun of racing mountain bikes, cyclo-cross gives them a different opportunity to race off-road.

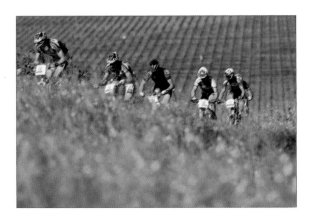

Above: Cross-country racing on mountain bikes has become more and more popular.
Left: Off-road racing is a tough but rewarding sport.

The Cross-country Race Bike

A good cross-country bike has to meet many requirements. Cross-country racing is technically demanding, testing physical strength and stamina and bike-handling ability across a wide variety of terrains.

In a cross-country race held on a small or medium-sized circuit, a rider can expect to encounter steep uphills, technical sections demanding occasional dismounting, twisty descents and long flat sections. Added to all that, the prevailing weather must also be taken into consideration. If it is raining, wet surfaces can completely change the

character of a circuit. What is perfectly acceptable to ride on in the dry might be a totally different proposition in poor weather or in muddy conditions.

There is a perfect cross-country bike for each course, but most people cannot keep a stable of mountain bikes, all set up differently, to take down when they are needed. Sometimes, a compromise is

necessary, in which case you should simply get a bike that you feel comfortable with and that suits you and your riding style.

Most cross-country courses include punishing technical sections that make great demands on both bike and rider, so it is also a good idea to emphasize reliability.

Anatomy of a cross-country race bike

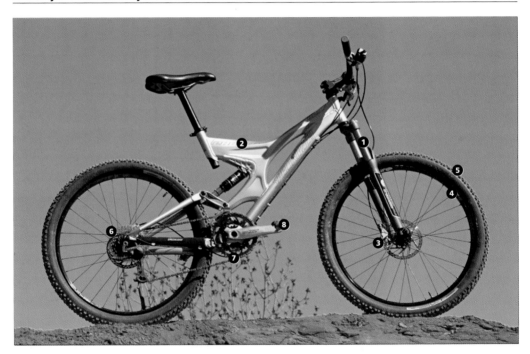

❶ Suspension fork: Medium or short travel or 'give' – some shock absorbency is needed.
❷ Full-suspension frame: Greater shock absorbency is needed for technical sections of the races. Some models can lock out the suspension system for better conditions and easier terrain.

❸ Brakes: V-brakes are the lightest, most efficient option, and they provide good stopping power.
❹ Wheels: 26in spoked wheels.
❺ Tyres: Knobbly tyres are good for maximum traction. If the course has less in the way of loose surface, such as stones, semi-slicks can be substituted instead.

❻ Gears: Nine-speed freewheel. Gear levers are integrated with brake levers.
❼ Chainset: Triple chainset for a wide range of gears – some technical and steep sections need very low gears to prevent stalling.
❽ Pedals: Clipless pedals to be used with off-road shoes. Shoeplates can clip into either side of the pedal.

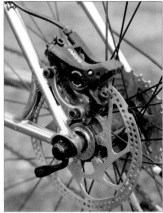

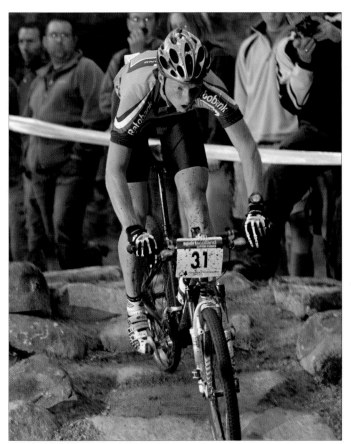

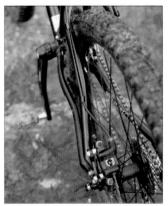

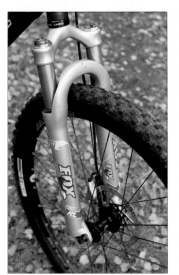

Choosing a cross-country bike

The first question is whether to go for hardtail or full suspension. The hardtail will be lighter uphill, but is much less comfortable and manoeuvrable down the other side. Until full-suspension bikes are made lighter, this choice will have to be made. With suspension, both at the forks and rear of the bike, travel is an important factor. For leisure riding, greater travel in the suspension gives a more comfortable ride. But racing riders want speed rather than comfort. Ideally there will be minimal travel in the forks and just enough travel in the rear to take the shock out of bumpy downhills.

Left: Suspension forks are needed for all but the easiest of cross-country courses, dampening the shock of hitting bumps, rocks and tree roots.

Top left: Many cross-country courses have technical sections that test riders' abilities to the limit.
Top: Powerful disc brakes help control speed.
Above: Thick, knobbly tyres are necessary for grip and traction.

Sizing is important. Cross-country racing bikes have a long top tube for aerodynamics and efficiency on long hills but a shorter bike is easier to pedal up short steep hills. Cross-country bikes use 26in wheels, with a width of between 1½ and 2in. The narrower the wheel, the lighter, but a 1.5in wheel will be a compromise between lightness and durability. Tyre pressures need to be higher, so rough terrain is hard to ride on. On a fast, dry course, less tread gives a more efficient ride.

Cross-country Race Skills

Cross-country races can be won on your ability to go up and down hills successfully. Practice can really pay off in this situation. If you cannot climb, you will find it difficult to win a cross-country race because most courses are hilly.

By training for climbs and riding them effectively, your chances of victory or a top-ten finish will be increased. Even if you are well behind the leaders, riding to your own potential is a satisfying experience. While most hills will probably be short, steep sprints, there will still be significant amounts of climbing in most courses.

As well as training, there are two things you can do to lighten the load and increase your climbing speed – losing weight yourself, and losing weight from your bike. At the same time, work on your climbing technique and you will see big improvements.

The longer top tube typical on racing cross-country bikes is an aid to climbing – it stretches your upper body out and gives you a lower centre of gravity. Bar-end attachments will get you even lower.

Depending on the steepness and the surface, move backward and forward on the bike to maintain traction. A steep

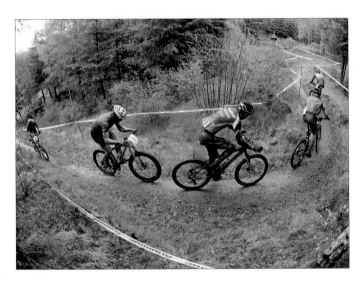

climb needs more weight forward, while you can stay back for a steady climb. It may sometimes be necessary to climb out of the saddle but this reduces traction in the back wheel, so you must judge whether the terrain is suitable. Climbing out of the saddle can be useful when a hill is very steep or if you are trying to get to the top ahead of another competitor before reaching a technical section you want to lead.

Descending and cornering

While cross-country races can be won on the uphill sections, they can equally be won or lost in the downhills. Descending fast is an essential part of cross-country racing – you will need to be able to relax and stay controlled.

If you have a full-suspension bike, your job is already easier – by taking some of the shock out of the bumps,

Left: On less technical descents, keep your weight back and stay in control of your bike.

Above: Be careful of letting gaps go during uphill sections, and always be on the lookout for overtaking chances.

the suspension will allow you to control your line and bike much better.

To ride down steep hills fast, you need to allow the bike to do some of the work while you stay supple and relaxed. Get your weight back – on some very steep hills, you need to be well over the back wheel, with your stomach touching the saddle. Check your speed by feathering the back brake, and pick your line well ahead.

In corners, depending on your speed, the angle of the track and how sharp the bend itself is, the correct technique is to use shifts in your weight, as well as steering, to get round. With more body weight over the front wheel, you can gain traction and control.

Many bends are banked, which helps in getting round them – moderate your speed before you hit the bend, lean the bike over, keep your head at 90 degrees

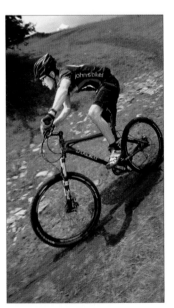

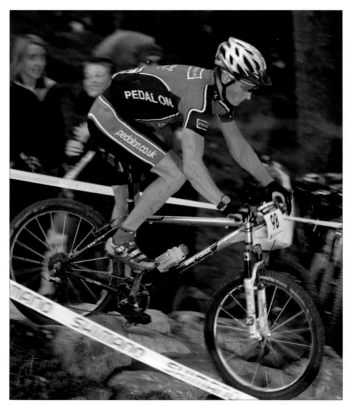

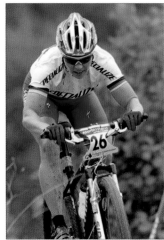

Above: During complicated sections, keep your fingers over the brakes in case of sudden obstacles.
Left: Tackle descents that have obstacles with care. Stay relaxed and balanced.

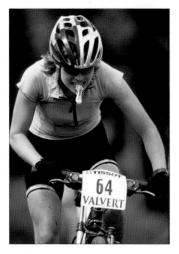

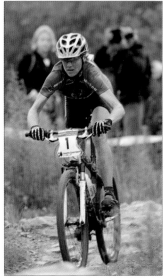

to the ground, steer as much as you need to and let the banking and centrifugal force do the rest.

Planning and fuelling
For longer races, it is not enough to simply turn up and ride. Since no external assistance is allowed in cross-country racing, you have to help yourself in the case of mechanical trouble. You are also responsible for making sure that you eat and drink enough to prevent yourself running out of energy.

It is your choice how much mechanical gear you take with you in a race, but if finishing is a priority, then you will need to carry spare tubes, tyre levers and a chain breaker. With these tools you can improvise a repair that will get you up and running again.

For race food, modern energy bars and gels are light and take up very little space – in a long race you need to eat at least one energy bar or gel an hour.

They can be carried tucked into a pocket. Drink plenty of fluid, depending on the weather: experience will tell you how much you need.

Above: Aim to control your line and your bike when riding down a bumpy or rocky descent.
Above left: In longer races, riders have to refuel on the go. It's a good idea to keep an energy gel tucked in the shorts for easy access.

Cross-country Race Strategies

The difficult terrain of cross-country events is such that technique and tactics throughout the race really count if you are to win. As with most cycle races, trying to have a plan for every eventuality is the best bet.

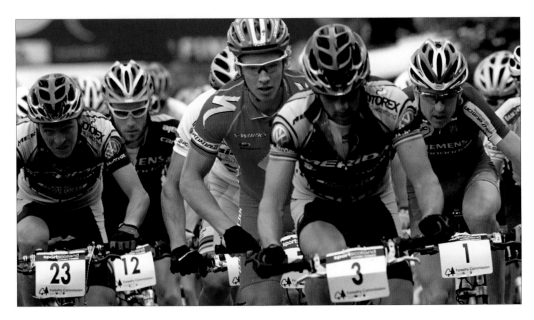

At the start of a cross-country race it is crucial to get to the front as soon as possible. Courses tend to narrow down to a singletrack fairly quickly, making overtaking very difficult. The more people get in front of you at the start, the harder it is to make any headway on the leaders. Some starts are organized by race number or seeding, with the best riders on the front row, and the others in lines behind them. Others are based on order of arrival.

There are two things that will affect your initial placing in a race – your grid position, and yourself. If you are on the front line, you will have a clear run at the first corner. If you are back on the third row, you'll be fighting for position.

A good start, in either position, will significantly help your chances. Before the start, warm up thoroughly – your legs have to be ready for an immediate big effort. A physical warm-up is not the only necessity – go through the first minutes of the race mentally, which will get you focused on what you need to do.

When the starting gun goes, get clipped in quickly and go as hard as you can to get to or stay at the front. The sprint for the first corner, or the first narrow section, is as important as the sprint for the finish line. You need to be strong and determined, and able to recover quickly from the effort.

Pacing

Cross-country races, even short ones, are extremely hard work. Uphill sections build up lactic acid in the muscles. The start puts you into oxygen debt. Long technical sections of singletrack force you to constantly brake and accelerate. Even supporting your body weight and absorbing the shocks on the downhill sections is very hard. Fitness is crucial, and so is the ability to pace yourself. Trying too hard in the first half of a race can leave you with no energy in the second

Above: Cross-country mountain bike races start with all the riders in a group.

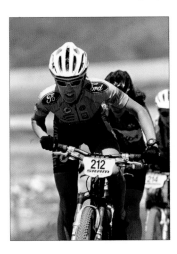

Above: Cross-country races involve consistent and intense efforts.

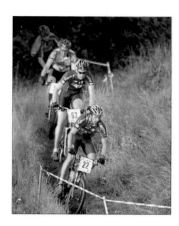

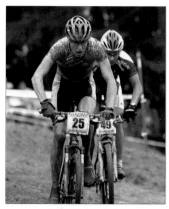

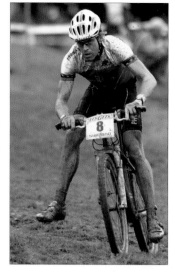

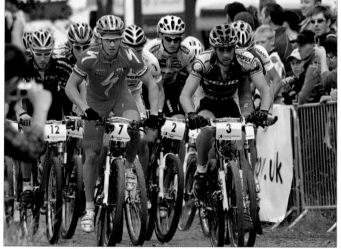

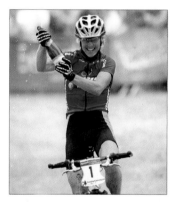

half but sitting back to save yourself for the second half will leave you well down the field, with stragglers blocking up the singletrack. Experience will tell you how hard you can go. But cross-country is not a time trial – it is a race against other people. Sometimes it is important to go harder or ease up. If you are a handful of seconds ahead of the rider behind and you know that there is a stretch of singletrack coming up, try to get there first. It's worth making the effort to stay ahead – they will find it difficult to get past once the singletrack starts, and you can recuperate there. If you are in second place, you know that a really hard dig for a few minutes will be worth it if you can get past.

Overtaking

Singletrack is great for technically skilful riders. During a singletrack section of a cross-country race, good bike handlers and trail riders come into their own.

On a singletrack, having the skills needed to overtake when you get stuck behind a slower rider is crucial. You could always wait until the next climb or wider track to overtake, but that might be several minutes away. Instead, you should press for a chance to overtake.

To overtake on singletrack takes acceleration and foresight. Follow your opponent's wheel, assuming he or she is on the racing line, and look past them for small gaps, or wider sections. Keep pressing, staying as close as possible,

Top left: Don't lose concentration during downhill sections.
Top middle: Always keep your eyes open for overtaking opportunities.
Top right: When you start to get tired, try to keep going and pace yourself.
Above left: The start of a race is a crucial time for getting into the best position.
Above: With luck, fitness and ability, comes victory.

so that when the opportunity presents itself you will be ready for it. When it comes, attack hard and try to surprise your opponent. If you can get your front wheel in front of theirs, you can dictate the racing line. The openings will be brief, but they are there to be taken.

Great Mountain Bike Races

The World Cup, the World Championships and the Olympics are big events for mountain bike competitors. Attracting the elite of international mountain bike riders, they are popular with tourists and also with aspiring riders.

In a notable series of mountain bike events that are scheduled around the world during the course of a year, four stand out.

The World Cup

In this event, riders win points in each round, which count towards an overall title at the end of the year in a variety of disciplines including cross-country, downhill and four-cross racing.

Events attract huge crowds, and the World Cup has evolved into the most important mountain biking competition in the world, after the Olympic Games. The various events have proved popular as tourist races – amateurs can ride on the same terrain and courses as their professional heroes.

Right: Ned Overend, a formidable and successful competitor in many mountain biking events.

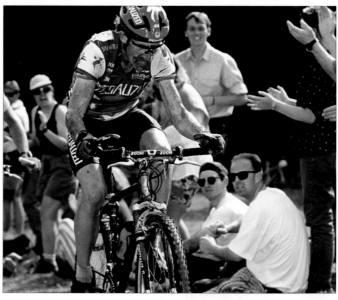

The World Championships

The mountain bike World Championships started in 1990 and are now a one-off event held annually in a different venue every year. Disciplines added from 1992 include cross-country, trials riding, downhill and four-cross. The blue riband event is the men's cross-country race, which was first run in 1990 and won by US mountain biking legend Ned Overend. Winners of the events receive a gold medal and are eligible to wear the rainbow jersey for similar events for a year.

The World Championships are arranged by nationality rather than by teams, and are usually held at the end of the mountain biking season.

The most successful rider at the World event has been Danishman Henrik Djernis, who won three world championships in 1992, 1993 and 1994. In recent years Julien Absalon also won a hat trick, between 2004 and 2006.

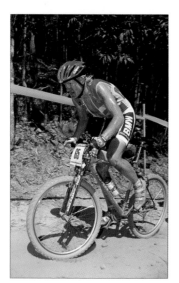

Above: The Dane, Henrik Djernis, has won countless races in his long career.

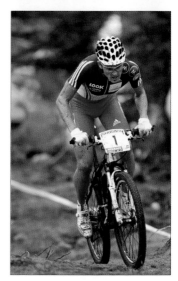

Above: French mountain biker Julien Absalon won the Olympics in 2004.

The Olympic Games

The cross-country race has been part of the Olympic Games since 1996, and is seen as the pinnacle of mountain biking competition. It is the only form of mountain biking discipline practised at the Summer Olympics, and the gold medal winners have gone down in history as legends of the sport.

The first Olympic cross-country race for men in Atlanta 1996 was won by Dutchman Bart Brentjens, while Italian Paola Pezzo took the women's race. The Americans hosted the event with expectations of victory, but the home of mountain biking came away with nothing except a bronze medal in the women's race. Their top finisher in the men's race was Tinker Juarez in 19th place. France has performed well since then, having taken two gold medals in the men's cross-country race. Miguel Martinez dominated the Sydney Olympic race in 2000, while Julien Absalon was the winner in Athens in 2004.

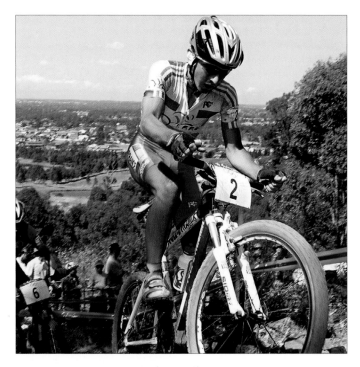

The Sea Otter Classic

One of the biggest off-road cycling festivals in the world is the Sea Otter Classic. The World Championships, the World Cup and Olympic Games have the official stamp of approval, while the Sea Otter Classic welcomes amateur racers as well as the top elites. Sea Otter takes place in Monterey, California, and hosts events such as dirt-jumping, slalom, cross-country, downhill and elite-level races as well as trials demonstrations. The Classic attracts more than 50,000 mountain biking enthusiasts, and spectators and riders alike enjoy one of the largest cycling events of the year.

Above: Miguel Martinez on his way to a gold medal in the 2000 Summer Olympics in Sydney.
Below: Bart Brentjens, who won bronze in the 2004 Summer Olympics.

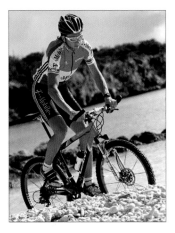

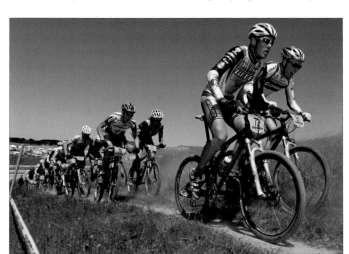

Left: The popular Sea Otter Classic in Monterey celebrates the sport of mountain biking with several events for all levels and all ages.

Cyclo-cross

The winter sport of cyclo-cross is the original off-road racing – it was around for years before mountain bikes came on to the scene. Cyclo-cross is very different from mountain biking; both take place off-road, but there the similarity ends.

A cyclo-cross bike looks more like a road bike than a mountain bike, with dropped handlebars and minimal extras. In a race, riders get off their bikes during steep sections and run with their bikes on their shoulders, sometimes for significant distances. Unlike mountain bike races, which are predicated on self-sufficiency, cyclo-cross races allow mechanical assistance. Riders often use two bikes in a race – one to ride, while the other is cleaned and prepared by a helper.

Obstacles along the way

Cyclo-cross races are short and sharp. They take place on a circuit, upon which the riders do enough laps for the race to last an hour. Like a mountain bike race, overtaking is difficult, with many circuits offering enough room for only one rider to pass. Circuits can incorporate muddy sections, wooded paths, sand, steep hills, cambered sections and occasionally even stretches of road. Tree roots and rocks have to be cycled over, jumped or riders simply have to dismount. Many organizers incorporate short sections of boarded jumps, about 30cm (12in) high, which have to be crossed on foot, although the 1989 world championships were won by Belgian Danny De Bie, who developed a technique of bunny-hopping the obstacles and staying on his bike while others wasted time dismounting, running and remounting. Depending on the time of year and weather, there may be obstacles such as water and ice. Coping with these challenges will improve your chances in a race.

Right: Weary cyclists carry their bikes during the Three Peaks cyclo-cross event in Yorkshire, England, which is one of the longest and toughest events in the world. It covers 61km (38 miles) over three of the highest hills in the country.

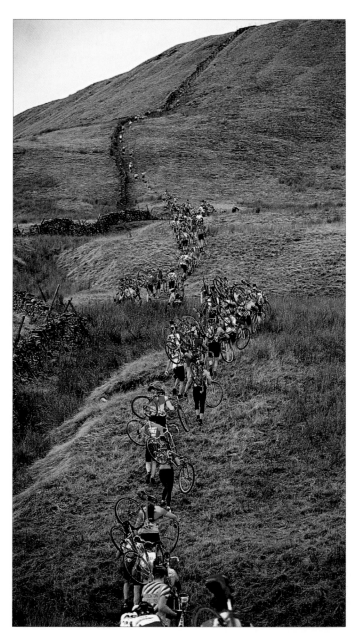

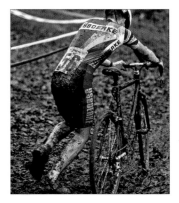

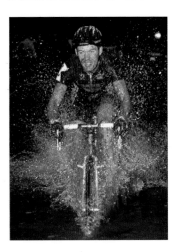

Mud

Cyclo-cross is referred to as 'mud-plugging', which describes the conditions encountered in a cyclo-cross race. After rain, the course becomes stickier and more slippery. Sticky mud gets into the tyre treads and the workings of your bike, adding to its weight and detracting significantly from its performance. A bike change every lap can help, but the mud soon builds up again, sapping your strength. Slippery mud comes with more rain. Keeping your balance is difficult, especially on cambered surfaces or around corners.

The main technique to use when riding in mud is to put the bike into a lower gear, and sit more upright, putting more weight on the pedals so that you are still sitting on the saddle but also letting your legs take the strain. This will give more traction. This takes a little weight off the handlebars, which results

in a more relaxed riding style, and it leads on to another technique that is easier to do than explain. It involves letting the bike take some decisions for you – don't force it to follow a certain line. In really atrocious conditions, let some pressure out of your tyres to give more traction in the mud.

Dry conditions

You can approach a dry cyclo-cross course very differently from a muddy one, and the going will be easier and faster. Depending on the surface of the course, it might be worth putting on tyres with less tread and inflating them to a higher pressure. You will not need to change bikes so often, or perhaps at all – plan for this, and your race strategy will be more effective.

Roots and bunny hops

To ride over roots, lift your front wheel over them and let your back wheel follow. This way you can maintain maximum traction and acceleration.

To clear bunny hops, lift the front wheel first, pulling your arms up. Then, immediately pull up and backwards with your legs to get the back wheel over the obstacle. If they are too high, the only way is to jump off and run over them.

Ice and snow

The hardest surface of all to deal with is ice – the slightest deviation in your line, or on the surface, can have you off your

Left: Riders have to get off and run when bunny hops are too high to jump.

Above left: On muddy ground, riding becomes less efficient – sometimes it is faster to get off and run.
Above: When the weather is dry, races are much faster.
Below: Cyclo-crossers should be prepared for all kinds of conditions.

bike very quickly. Being able to avoid crashing on an icy course is a big advantage. The technique for riding on ice is to turn a big gear and sit low, to keep your centre of gravity nearer the ground. Fatter tyres, at a lower pressure, help to maintain grip.

Snow can be similar to mud and clogs up the workings of the bike, especially the brakes and the sprockets. For this you will need tyres with a deeper tread on the rear wheel and a file tread on the front.

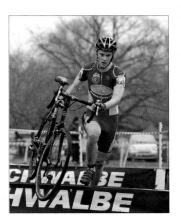

The Cyclo-cross Bike

Cyclo-cross is a winter sport, so bikes are subject to constant abuse from rain, mud, sand and grit. Mud and dirt builds up in the crannies of the frame, in the brakes and in the gears, so to get a good performance from your bike, maintenance is essential.

Cyclo-cross bikes may look like road racing bikes, but they have a number of modifications that make them ideal for off-road racing. Bikes for cyclo-cross need to be as light as possible so that they are easier to carry. On a technical course, with steep hills, the riders will spend a great deal of time running with their bikes on their shoulders, and every extra gram counts. Comfort is a consideration, although most cyclo-cross events tend to be short at around an hour, so it is not as important as it would be with a mountain bike or a sportive bike.

Choosing a cyclo-cross bike
Cyclo-cross frames tend to be about 1cm (½in) shorter along the top tube than an equivalent road bike for the same rider. Aerodynamics are not as important, so riders sit more upright, with higher handlebars, and brake levers positioned higher up, giving a shorter position. Frame geometry differs – a shallower seat angle, and a moved-back saddle pushes the rider back so that their weight is farther over the rear wheel. This helps steering and control and adds traction over rough terrain.

Anatomy of a cyclo-cross bike

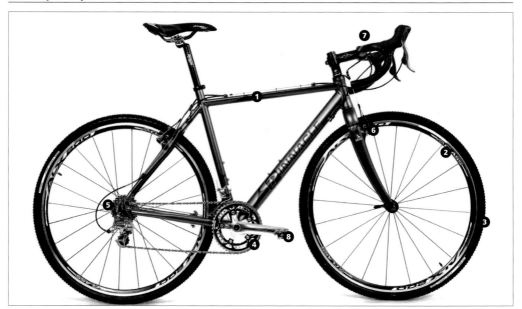

❶ **Frame:** Lightweight for easier carrying, with large clearances to avoid mud build-up.
❷ **Wheels:** Lightweight, for easier carrying. Mud builds up on spokes, so modern wheels have fewer of them. V-shaped rims are easier to clean. Size is usually 700x28C, but larger or smaller wheels can be used according to conditions.
❸ **Tyres:** Fat and knobbly for extra traction on loose surfaces. Pressures are lower than for road tyres, which also helps traction.
❹ **Chainset:** Single, double or triple chainrings, according to terrain. A triple offers more gears, but weighs more. Generally, double is most popular, using 39–48. Cranks are marginally longer than a typical road bike.
❺ **Sprockets:** Nine-speed freewheel with 13–26 sprockets.

❻ **Brakes:** Cantilever brakes avoid mud build-up. Brake levers incorporate gear levers for accessibility. Some riders ride with an extra pair of brakes on the top, with separate cables to the brakes.
❼ **Handlebars:** High handlebars for an upright position, with dropped ends, for use when accelerating.
❽ **Pedals:** Clipless pedals to be combined with an off-road shoe.

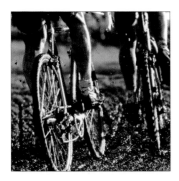

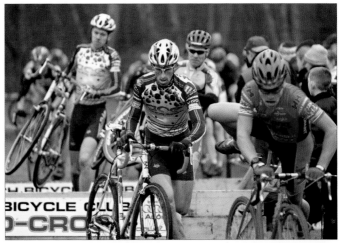

Above: Cyclo-cross bikes have to be set up to deal with clogging mud.
Right: Riders in cyclo-cross events need to be prepared to spend a lot of time running with their bike.

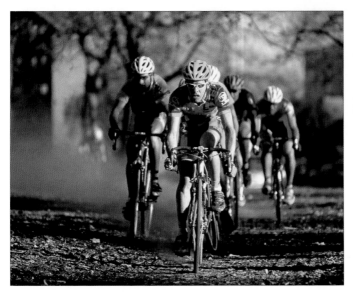

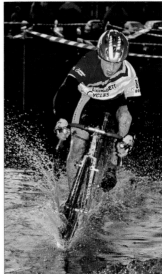

The clearances on a cyclo-cross frame are large, with no bridge between the chainstays, and the fittings are designed to take cantilever brakes. These have separate calliper arms attached to pivot points on the frame and forks, joined by a central cable that runs to the brake levers. The advantage of cantilever brakes is that they do not clog up with mud.

Wheels need to be lightweight. Carbon composite wheels can be used, which have fewer spokes and are very easy to clean. On these wheels, the braking surface is aluminium, for better performance. Carbon wheels are an expensive option, however, and a set of lightweight spoked wheels will also offer good performance. Deep, V-shaped rims are less likely to clog up around the spokes, and are easier to clean.

Tyres need good traction. Cyclo-cross tyres are knobbly to prevent slipping.

It is possible to ride cyclo-cross races with single, double or triple chainrings, according to the terrain. A single chainring saves weight, but there will be

Above left: Cyclo-cross bikes are similar to road bikes, but note the thicker tyres and cantilever brakes.
Above right: Stay upright when riding through challenging or technical sections.

fewer gears. Doubles are the best option generally, using a 39–48 combination, with 13–26 sprockets at the back. In very steep terrain, a triple might be necessary, but it is often easier to get off and run up steep hills because of the rough ground.

Cyclo-cross Skills

Racing cyclo-cross requires a wider set of skills than racing on the road. Accidents apart, road racers mount once and dismount once, before and after a race. Cyclo-crossers may do this 50 times or more in the course of a race so it's an important skill to perfect.

Running with the bike on your shoulder will be quicker than riding in many situations. You should learn to dismount and mount in relaxed, confident movements, making them part of the forward progress of your bike.

When and how to dismount

The reasons for dismounting are a steep hill, or an obstacle that you cannot jump the bike over or ride around. On a steep hill, first try riding out of the saddle with your weight back to maintain traction. If the hill is too steep, dismount from the bike. In the approach to the dismount, ride in an upright position, with your hands on the brake hoods. Unclip your right foot and swing it over the back of the saddle, and grab the top tube with your right hand as you jump off. Unclip the left foot. With the bike still moving, start running as your feet hit the ground, and lift your bike on to your shoulder. If the hill you are about to ride up is rideable at the bottom, don't

Dismounting from your bike

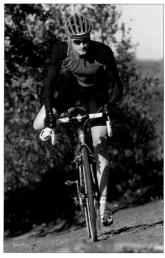

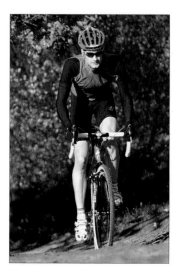

1 Approach a dismount with your hands on the brake hoods.

2 Unclip your right foot and start to swing your leg over the saddle.

Handling on slippery hills

Cyclo-cross climbs are short and steep, and the fastest way up when they are rideable is to ride out of the saddle with your hands on the brake hoods. But the muddier the ground, the harder it is to gain traction. When it is especially slippery, stay out of the saddle, but try to put your weight back over your rear wheel to prevent it from slipping, and ride in as straight a line as possible.

Descending is straightforward – hold the drops, and relax, with your weight set back to keep traction, and staying out of the saddle so you can use your legs as shock absorbers. If you feel the bike slipping, or you can see an especially difficult section coming up, unclip one foot from the pedal and touch it to the ground for balance.

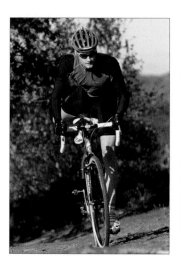

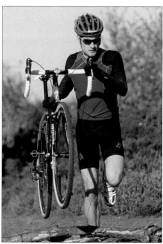

3 Unclip your left foot and jump from the bike.

4 Lift your bike on to the shoulder or, if you are tall, hold the frame.

dismount until then. Try not to grind to a halt, but swing your right leg over, keeping both hands on the brake levers. Jump off, push the bike along the ground to maintain momentum, then pick the bike up. Running with a bike unbalances your natural rhythm and weighs you down. Carry the bike with the top tube on your right shoulder, with the wheel turned inward. Taller riders may find it more comfortable to hold the head tube with one arm, and the handlebars with the other. Shorter riders hook their arm under the down tube, and hold on to the drop of the handlebar. Most running sections are short, so concentrate on strong running.

How to remount

Once you have cleared the obstacle, remount. Grab the top tube with your right hand, and put the bike on the ground. Push forward to get moving again, at the same speed as you are running. Put both hands on the brake hoods and jump back into the saddle, with your right leg over the back wheel. Once you are on the saddle, look down to the pedals, and clip both feet in.

Climbing

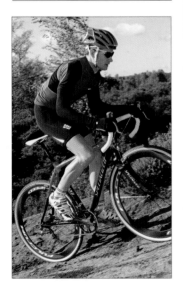

Climbing *When climbing, keep your weight back over the rear wheel.*

How to run with your bike

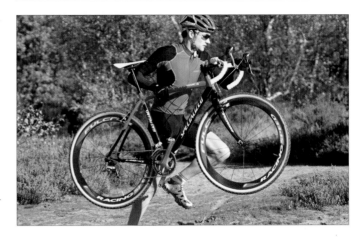

Running *Lift the bike on to your shoulder, or if you are tall, hold it by the frame. Look ahead to where you are going and stay upright, relaxed and balanced.*

Remounting your bike

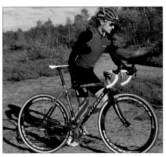

1 *Put your bike on the ground while you are still running.*

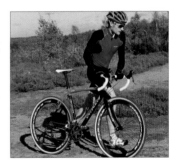

2 *Place your hands on both handlebars before remounting.*

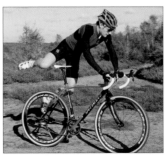

3 *Jump back on, swinging your right leg over the saddle.*

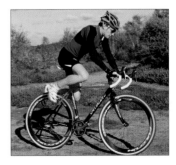

4 *Land in the saddle as you clip in with your left foot.*

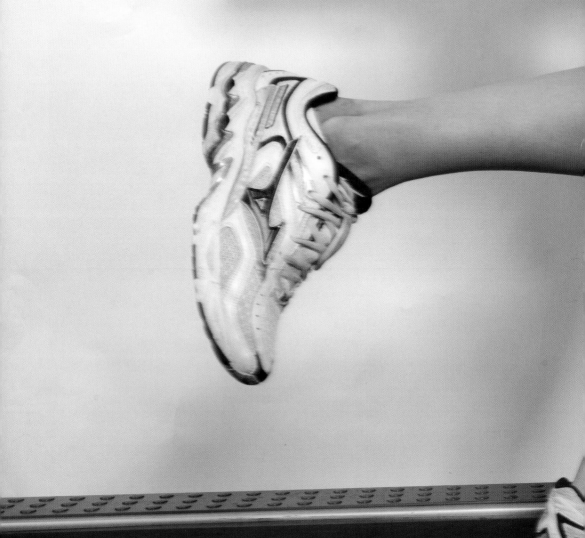
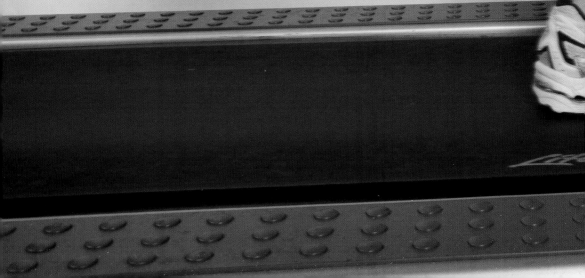

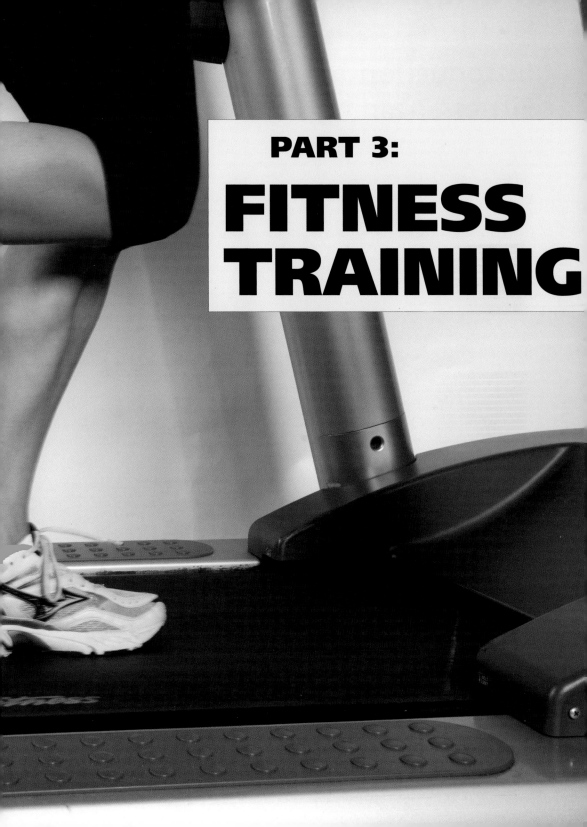

PART 3:
FITNESS TRAINING

Introduction to Fitness Training

Going to the gym and jumping on the treadmill will not necessarily give you the results you want from your exercise regime. There are so many different exercises that you can do, some of them far more beneficial than others, and it is important to find a training plan that works for you.

Before you begin, decide what it is you want from your exercise routine. Advice on body types, health measurements and fitness tests will help you to identify the areas which you might need to work on, and how you can build a programme around these.

This section will give you an understanding of which exercises will help you to achieve your goals, with detailed descriptions of how and when to do them so that you can be confident that you are performing them correctly. To achieve fast, effective, long-lasting results you will need variation in your training. Each exercise lists the muscles used so that you can determine which part of your body is being used, giving you the chance to change your work-outs and challenge your body to promote better results.

There is always something that you can do. Even if you are injured, there are exercises that will help you to recover. The following pages provide you with basic knowledge to help with diagnosing injury, understanding the recovery process and preventing the injury from recurring.

Fitness and exercise are not just about sweating in the gym. Core stability and flexibility training are just as important to prevent injury and give you the strength to train harder, push big weights, run marathons or cope with the demands of everyday life.

Similarly, nutrition is also a vital part of any fitness regime. Everything you eat has some effect on you – your food can turn to fat or energize you; it can help you to improve your fitness level, recover from injury, change your body shape and alter your self-image. This section provides you with an understanding of the effect that different foods have, the optimum nutrition combination for what you hope to achieve, and the best time to eat and drink.

Regular exercising and a healthy diet will not only help you to gain physical fitness, providing a big boost to your self-esteem; you will also have increased energy, and benefit from a more active and positive outlook.

Right: There are no short cuts to getting fit, but it is much easier if you have the right information about appropriate training.

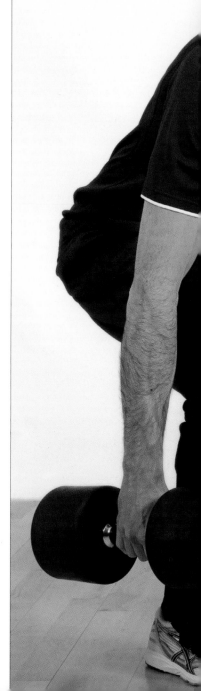

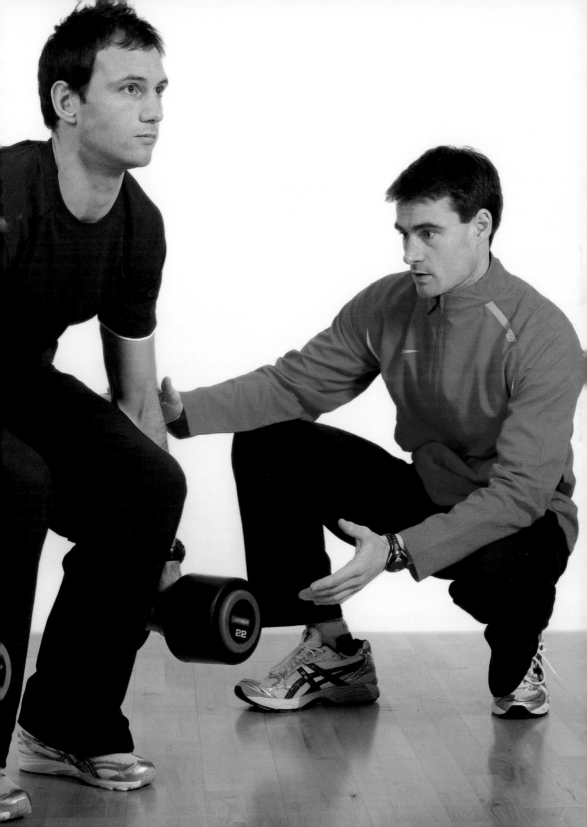

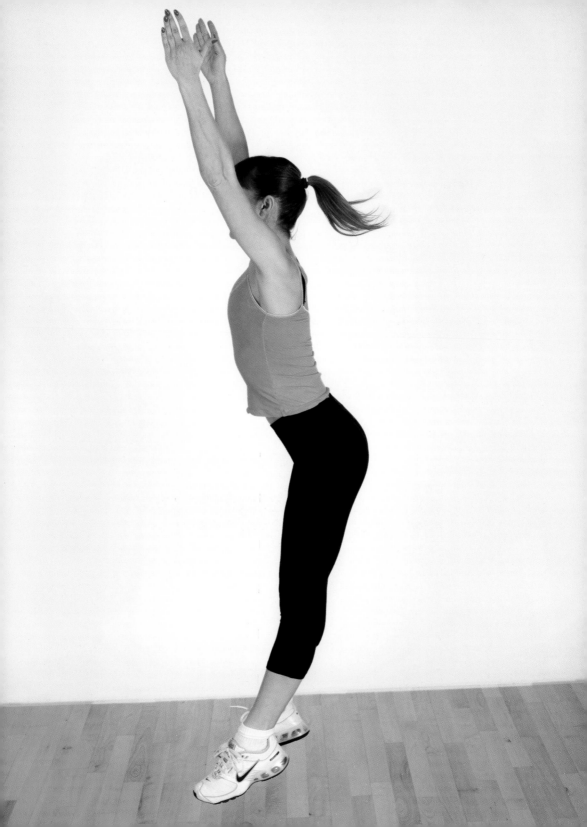

GETTING STARTED

Before you begin your journey to a fitter lifestyle, this chapter outlines a realistic approach to a successful fitness training programme, including accurately assessing your starting point, setting achievable goals, taking and analysing body measurements, performing fitness tests to measure your progress, keeping a training diary, and determining which exercises are best for you. Armed with this new knowledge, you will come to appreciate why you are not intended to live a sedentary lifestyle, and commit to making health and exercise priorities in your life.

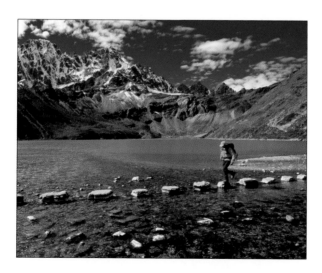

Above: Whatever your fitness goals may be, you will certainly enjoy achieving them.
Left: Fitness training will help you discover more about yourself.

Three Steps to Fitness

We are bombarded today, on one hand, by news items stressing the importance of a healthy lifestyle, and on the other by pictures of glamorous celebrities. Can you ever look that good? Yes, but not by wishing for it – it takes determination, motivation and knowledge.

As everyone knows – or should – there is no such thing as overnight success in any walk of life, and certainly not in the area of health and fitness. Unfortunately, we live in a culture of conflicting messages that do nothing to nourish our wellbeing. On the one hand, it is impossible to escape media images of thin, toned, buffed and sculpted role models of quite out-of-reach physical perfection. On the other, advertising and the food industry pump fat-filled, sugar-coated, carbohydrate-rich food at us from every direction. Consequently, we

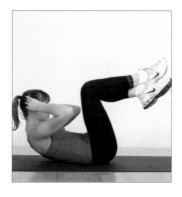

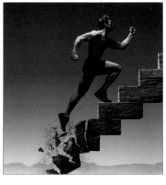

Below: Hours of training steps up all the systems in your body and helps you to run faster.

Above: You don't need to be in the gym for this type of floor exercise; you can easily do it at home.

Above: The buzz you get from being supremely fit will help you continue your fitness regime.

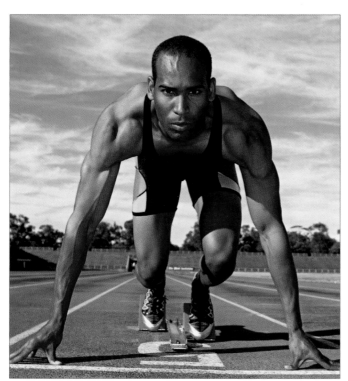

have become an unfit society in thrall to endless aspiration, and sold on the promise of nips, tucks, jabs, instant gratification and quick fixes. Quite simply, becoming fit and healthy – safely, effectively and in the long term – does not and will not happen quickly. You will, however, get real results if you follow this three-step plan:

Determination Look at other areas of your life in which determination has been a force for change, such as passing exams, bringing up your children in the best way possible, getting a better job or making more money. Transfer some of this determination to the job of making yourself fit and healthy.

Motivation Have a goal in mind, such as running a half-marathon, fitting into a wedding dress or simply getting up the stairs without being out of breath.

Fitness can't be bought
Simply paying a monthly subscription to a gym is not enough to help you get fitter. You can buy many things in life, but fitness involves regular, hard work.

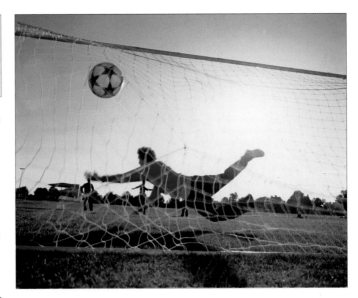

Use this chapter to determine your goals by analysing all aspects of your life and making a note of your strengths and weaknesses. Once you have set your goals, keep visualizing how great you will feel once you have achieved them. This is something you are doing for yourself and no one else. Family and friends can try to motivate you but until you actually want to do it for yourself, it won't work. After all, no one is asking them to make sacrifices – you are the one who has to change your lifestyle and do the physical training.

Knowledge Gather as much knowledge as possible to plan your new personal training plan. It is not possible to get results without understanding how your

Below: If you want to succeed in your aims quickly, get help and advice from professionals in the field.

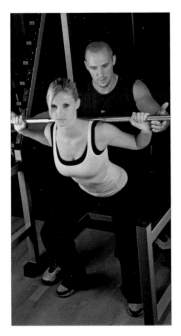

body works and what type of training will be best for you. Be aware, though, that a little knowledge can be a bad thing. For example, the suggestion that resistance training will make you gain weight is a myth. The truth is that resistance training will make you gain lean muscle mass, which will have a positive effect on your metabolism and therefore make you lose fat.

Knowing what to eat, and when to eat it, is also essential. Without good nutrition, you won't have the energy to train, recover from training or see the benefits of your training. There are no short cuts or quick fixes – your nutrition plan will require preparation to make it practical for you to stick with it every day.

Know yourself

Once you have the basic knowledge, you can apply the correct training to achieve your goals. In some ways you have far more knowledge of yourself than a gym instructor because they have only known you for a matter of hours, whereas you have known yourself since the day you were born. You know how determined you can be and what your motivation is. You know what you enjoy and what you dislike. You can be honest with yourself about how you look and

Above: Just a little extra fitness can mean the difference between winning and losing.

how you want to look. You know how much energy you have and how much more energy you would like to have. Your exercise plan has to suit you and no one else.

Plan ahead

Be practical and think ahead. For example, if you are travelling for business or on holiday, plan your training to be harder in the week before and after you are away. Don't use the time away as an excuse – there is always some kind of training you can do, whether it's going for a run or doing exercises in your hotel room. Keep your goal in sight and remember that consistency is the key to achieving it.

No excuses

There are two types of people who want to get fit: those who think about results and those who think of excuses. If you look for excuses, you are setting yourself up to fail. If you focus on achieving results, you will win. From the moment you pick up this book, the excuses stop and you set yourself on the path to success – to fitness and health.

A Lifestyle that Works for Your Body

One of the main reasons for a general lack of fitness in developed societies is that so many people lead sedentary lifestyles, and abuse their bodies daily through poor diet and other bad habits. The simple fact is – we are not designed for the way we live.

Compare your lifestyle with that of someone who lived approximately 10,000 years ago. When people lived as hunter-gatherers, constantly on the move looking for food, they led very active lives.

From hunter-gatherers to channel-flickers

Today, many people lead an unhealthy desk-bound, sofa-lounging, channel-flicking lifestyle, their longest walk being to the car and back. It's time to take stock of the fact that although we live in post-industrial, urban environments, our bodies have not evolved to keep pace with the demands of life in this developed world. We are still built to live as our ancestors did, many thousands of years ago. Unfortunately, that's causing us a lot of problems. Take control of your lifestyle before it's too late.

Below: If children are encouraged to try a sport when they are young, it will stand them in good stead later on.

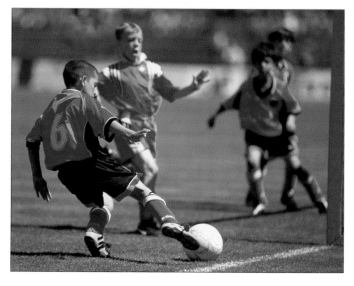

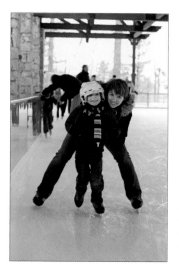

Life expectancy and lifestyle

There is a direct correlation between life expectancy and lifestyle. A person who drinks excessive amounts of alcohol, smokes, eats unhealthily and lives a sedentary lifestyle will have a shorter life expectancy than someone who looks after their body and takes regular exercise. However, it is not just about the length of your life. Quality of life is just as important, and if you don't take care of yourself, your life will not only be shorter, it may well be unpleasant too.

Most disturbing of all, there is ample evidence that these bad habits are starting earlier and earlier in life. Little to no exercise or outdoor games, endless hours sat in front of computer games and a diet high in sugar and saturated fat have triggered escalating and alarming rates of obesity and related illnesses among children. The net result will be, if left unchecked, a generation of children likely to live shorter lives than their parents.

Above: Children thrive on fresh air and exercise; limit the time spent playing computer games indoors.

Our healthy ancestors

We know people lived relatively healthily 10,000 years ago because there are people still living the same lifestyle in some areas of the world today – the last 84 tribes of hunter-gatherers in the world, who can be found in Australia, Africa and South America. Fit with lean muscular physiques, these people continue to live very active and healthy lives, and experience markedly lower levels of diseases such as cancer and heart disease.

This much we know

People in the developed world cannot go back in time, but they can get an understanding of what they should do to find a balance in their lifestyle, in order to stay healthy. We know that exercise makes you fitter, boosting your immune system and protecting you from

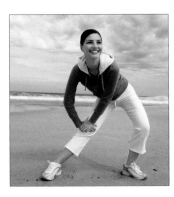

Above: Sea air and exercise is a great combination for a healthy and happy way of life.

disease. We know that some exercise each day will counteract the negative effects of sitting at a desk all day staring at a computer screen, and will give you the get-up-and-go to have fun with family and friends. We know that eating certain foods will give you energy and make you look good and feel good. Let's take this knowledge and put it to good use so that we can all live longer and happier lives.

Below: Your body is not designed to sit in a car all day. Try to change your mode of transport to include walking.

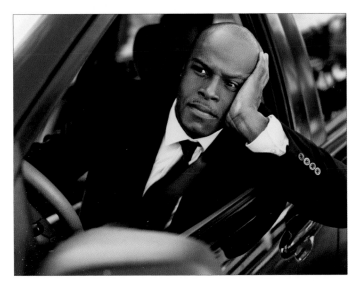

The perils of modern-day life

There are many aspects of modern life that are intrinsically bad for our physical and mental wellbeing. From the daily grind of office life to the stresses and strains of travel and the junk food that we consume, living in a developed country has a downside.

Desk-bound injuries Sitting still in front of a computer all day long, and doing no exercise, contributes to back and neck problems. Physiotherapists and osteopaths owe most of their income to this fact. Correct exercise would prevent all of these problems – problems that didn't exist generations ago. We didn't need core-stability exercises to avoid such aches and pains, because working the land made these muscles strong.

Mental exhaustion We are not designed to work long hours and feel stressed about hitting deadlines. The body is designed to hunt and gather, then rest and build strength for the next day. Having to retain huge amounts of information can be exhausting; it leaves you feeling too mentally tired to do any exercise. Of course, taking exercise will provide you with the energy to continue to hit targets and deadlines at work, and enable you to work long hours.

Travel woes We were not intended to travel in planes or for any great length of time by other means of transport.

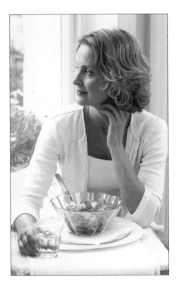

Above: Fast food is fine occasionally, but it is good to be aware of your body's nutritional needs and eat healthily.

Travelling through time zones, especially at altitude in a short space of time, can be very tiring, and of course there are the additional negative effects of sitting still for hours.

Junk food and booze We are not designed to eat convenience foods, which are often full of sugar that will affect your energy levels and body weight. Alcohol is viewed as a natural accompaniment to food, but even modest amounts of alcohol can lead to a number of illnesses and damage to some of the major organs of the body. Even if food is 'natural', the nutritional content may only be a fraction of what it was many years ago. In many areas, the land has been over-farmed and saturated with chemicals, which leaves crops tainted with an unhealthy chemical residue.

Labour-saving, life-shortening We were not designed to use labour-saving devices. We were designed to use our hands and the materials from the land to build shelters and weapons to catch animals and provide food. Today, there is a gadget or machine for almost everything, which simply encourages us to become lazier still.

The Importance of Exercise

Regular exercise leaves you full of vitality and a get-up-and-go attitude. People who do physical training regularly already know that if they skip a few days they start to feel tired and lethargic, which is how many people feel who never exercise.

The right exercise and nutrition can dramatically reduce the risk of many common illnesses and diseases, including cardiovascular disease, various cancers and type II diabetes:

Heart disease Exercising three to four times a week and eating healthily have a positive effect on your heart. Exercise also lowers cholesterol levels and blood pressure, which considerably reduces the chances of suffering a heart attack.

Osteoporosis Regular weight-bearing exercise helps to build bone tissue and prevent age-related bone-density loss.

Cancer Exercise reduces the risk of some cancers. Two ovarian hormones that are linked to breast cancer, estradiol and progesterone, are reduced by exercise. Studies have shown that regular exercise can help prevent breast cancer by up to 60 per cent. Several studies also show that obese people who live sedentary lives are at increased risk of endometrial, colon, gall bladder, prostate and kidney cancers.

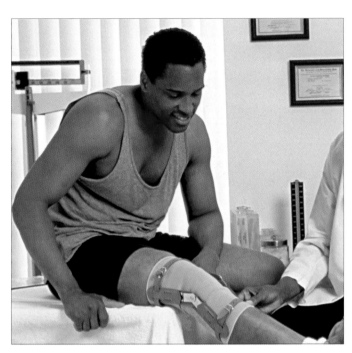

Above: Sporting injuries should always be assessed by a professional.

Below: If you attempt to practise a healthy lifestyle, you are less likely to worry about the doctor's findings.

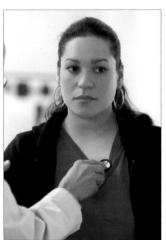

Type II diabetes Regular exercise will dramatically reduce the risk of developing type II diabetes. A weight increase of 5–10kg/11–22lb doubles the risk of developing type II diabetes. More than 80 per cent of people with type II diabetes are overweight or obese, which is why it is also referred to sometimes as 'diabesity'.

Joint and back pain These common ailments can be reduced with the correct physical training, which will build muscle and increase flexibility and core stability.

Obesity A combination of cardiovascular and strength training will increase the metabolism and improve the body's capacity to burn calories. This helps to

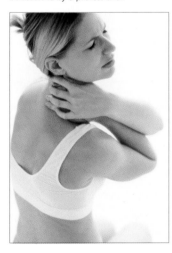

Right: Regular physical exercise can greatly reduce unpleasant neck pain and headaches.

reduce the risk of developing one of the many obesity-related diseases as well as increasing wellbeing.

Psychological health The symptoms of depression and anxiety can be reduced by regular exercise. Stress is part of everyday life but exercise can equip you to cope with it. Exercise will give you greater endurance to tackle daily tasks, improve your sleep, increase your energy and give you an improved body shape, which will improve your self-esteem.

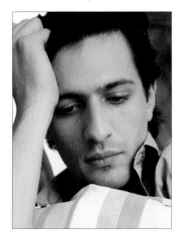

Above: Lack of exercise can have the effect of making you feel lethargic and demotivated.

Below: Fruits are a healthy alternative to sugary or fatty snacks.

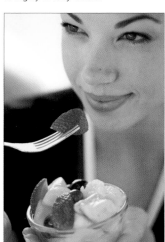

General health Regular exercise has many health benefits. It can boost some vital processes in the body, such as stimulating your digestion, liver function and your glycogen system (stored glucose, mainly in the muscles and the liver). Exercise will lead to an improved immune system, it can revitalize and enhance your sex life, and may well add some years to your life. Strength training has the ability to tone, build and improve the speed of muscle contraction and reaction time through the development of strong neuromuscular pathways. You will also become more agile and benefit in many ways from improved co-ordination and balance.

Don't put it off

Fear is one of the biggest factors in motivating exercise. If you were to stand in a line of 100 people waiting for a heart attack, where in the queue would you be? If you are near the front, then fear will probably be the motivating factor that drives you to a healthier lifestyle, but why should it be this way? Be healthy before you get to the fear stage. Most importantly, respect your body – it's the only one you've got – and aim to feel good on the inside and the outside by exercising regularly.

Below: Regular strength, flexibility and core-stability training can help to prevent back pain.

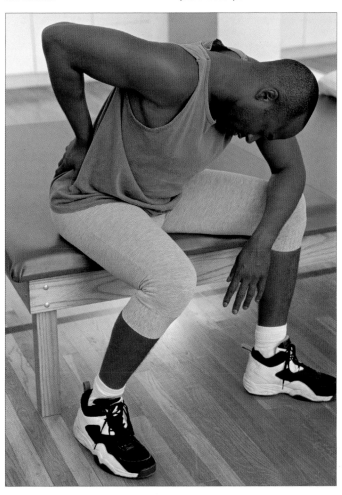

Setting Your Goals

Before you start to exercise, you must be clear about what it is you want to achieve. Do you want to run a marathon, lose weight or gain muscle? These are all big goals and in order to achieve them, you need to prepare both your body and your mind.

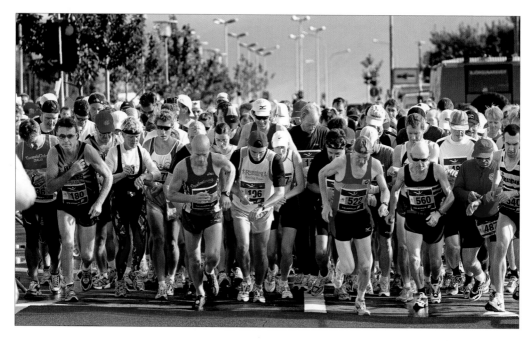

Begin by setting out smaller goals. For example, if you want to run a marathon in six months' time, set yourself deadlines, such as being able to run 10km/6.2 miles after the first two months of training, and 20km/12.4 miles after three months. A gradual improvement in stamina and ability will help you to focus on the big goal.

There are also other factors to take into consideration, such as what it will be like to run among so many other athletes. Research the marathon course and talk to people who have run it previously so that you are familiar with its organization and structure. Consider the equipment you intend to use, your fluid intake and tactics for the big event. Running a half-marathon is an excellent way to get first-hand marathon experience. Plan when to change your training shoes in order to get the best

out of them, but do not turn up on the start line with shoes that are worn out or brand new shoes that may give you injuries or blisters. Read around the subject of injury so that you can identify early signs of injury immediately.

If you want to lose weight, follow a six-week plan that incorporates a low GI diet and exercise. So that you can monitor your weight loss and progress, keep a training diary.

When you want to gain muscle, plan your training sessions carefully, enlisting the help of a personal trainer if necessary. They will be able to help with the appropriate type of exercises for specific muscles.

Make your own goal wheel
It is important to focus on other factors in your life that will have an effect on your goal. For example, if you want to

Above: Even if you don't succeed immediately, there is nothing wrong with setting long-term goals.

lose weight, you will struggle if you have low self-esteem, suffer from lack of sleep and work too hard to do any exercise. Use a goal wheel to help you change your lifestyle and keep achieving. The goal wheel is similar to the wheel of a bicycle. The wheel has an outer rim, a hub in the centre and spokes running between the rim and the hub. Each of these spokes represents a different factor in your life. Because people's lives are very different, you can make the spokes represent whatever you like.

An example would be spokes for physical exercise, social life, nutrition, sleep, family, work, injury and psychology. Each spoke has a score

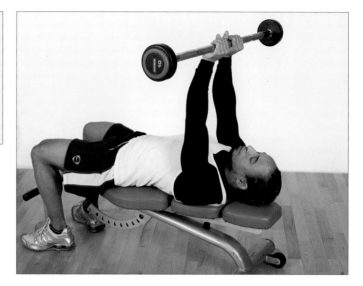

on it going from ten at the hub to zero at the rim. You personalize your wheel by putting a cross on each spoke. For example, if you take little or no physical exercise, you would put a cross close to the rim of the physical exercise spoke. If your exercise routine is going well and you really enjoy it, mark a cross close to the hub.

Once you have put a cross on each spoke, join the crosses up. It is highly likely that you will have a jagged pattern within the wheel. Some crosses will be close to the hub and others will be farther away. Every spoke that has a cross close to the rim of the wheel represents the lifestyle factor that you need to work on. It is important to

remember that all the factors are related. For example, your psychology score may be low if you never take any exercise and your nutrition is poor. If you spend all your time working and socializing and especially if this involves a lot of drinking alcohol, you won't be able to run a marathon successfully.

Above: Always keep in mind the goals you have set yourself; this should help you stick to the training.

There simply won't be enough time to train adequately, and if you try to take part, it could result in feelings of depression and even physical injury.

Below: Getting weighed weekly will help you assess the progress you are making in your training plan.

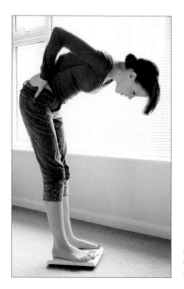

Goal wheel

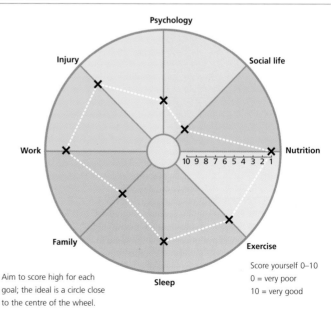

Aim to score high for each goal; the ideal is a circle close to the centre of the wheel.

Score yourself 0–10
0 = very poor
10 = very good

Training Diary

Keeping a training diary will help you to achieve your goals and stay motivated. Make the diary realistic and useful. Don't cram it with information that will become irrelevant later on in training – only note facts that motivate you and help you to track your progress.

A diary can help to re-motivate you as you look back through all the other fitness improvements you have made.

When losing weight you may find that over the first six weeks of training you lose 10kg/22lb but then you don't lose any in the seventh week, which can lessen your motivation. However, it's not just the weight loss that matters; for example, if you have been walking in an effort to accelerate your weight loss, and could only walk for 1.6km/1 mile in your first week, but can now manage 4.8km/3 miles, this progress will motivate you to keep going.

If you are training for a marathon, keep a diary of all your training, including details such as whether your training is road or off-road running, the time of day, your nutrition and hours of sleep. This way, if you do suffer from any problems, such as an overuse injury, a coach or physician will be able to use your diary to see when the problems may have started and may be able to determine what caused them. Noting what you eat will help you determine which foods work best for your performance and recovery.

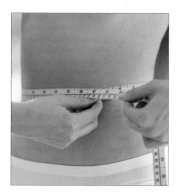

Above: By taking your measurements, you can work out that you have lost fat and are more toned than before.

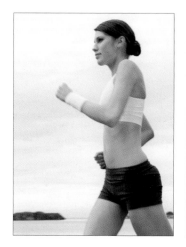

Above: If you step up your walking, note the details in your diary, to allow you to assess your progress better.

How to keep your training diary
You should record details of your training, the goals you want to achieve and an assessment of your training to date. Include test results, nutrition information and body measurements.
Daily records Record the following information in your diary every day:
• The physical training you intend to do against the actual physical training that took place, marked out of ten.
• Hours of sleep the previous night.
• Resting heart rate, taken first thing in the morning.
• Any injury or signs of fatigue.
• All food and fluid intake, including what time you ate or drank.

Also note what you did on rest days, as your activity on these days will have a significant effect on your performance. For example, if you stayed up late on a rest day, or drank alcohol on two rest days before a big competition, your performance will suffer and when you check the diary you will know why.

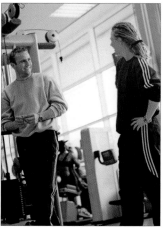

Above: Your training needs to work the way you want it to. You can discuss your progress with an instructor at the gym.

Big goals and small goals At the front of your diary list the goals you want to achieve, and when you want to achieve them by. For example, if you weigh 70kg/154lb on 1 January and you want to lose 10.8kg/24lb over six months, or 1.8kg/4lb per month, mark your desired weight – your small goal – on the appropriate page for each month; so on the page for 1 February, you would note that you want to weigh 68kg/150lb, and on the page for 1 March, you would note that you want to weigh 66kg/146lb, and so on.

Weekly assessment At the end of each week assess how your training has gone. Note the average score you have given to your training and how you felt each day. Look back over your nutrition for the week and mark down any changes you want to make. Assess your fluid intake for the week and check that you are drinking enough. Add up the total number of hours you have been

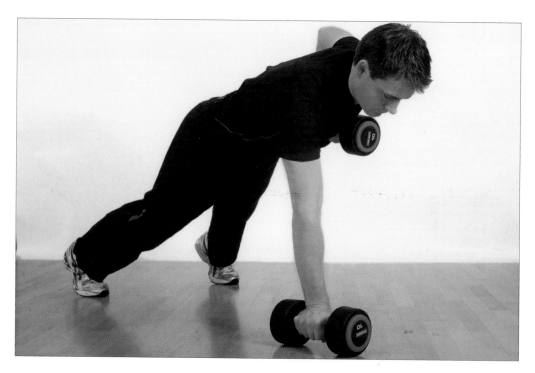

Below left: Note any injury; what you were doing and for how long. It may help you alter your training plan.

Below middle: An accurately filled-in training diary can prove to be an invaluable asset at a later date.

Below right: Keep a record of the hours that you sleep to get an insight into your sleeping patterns.

training and compare it with the week before. Make a note of measurements such as body fat, weight and Body Mass Index (BMI).

Weekly review If the overview of your week is not positive, consider where you may have gone wrong and note the changes that you intend to make in order to get more from your training. These changes might involve a different combination of exercises, taking more

Above: Even if your goal seems daunting at times, try to meet the challenge and stay on track.

rest days or working harder to achieve intensity levels in certain sessions. Look back at the goals you have set yourself, written at the front of the diary, and make changes to the small goals – adding new ones and ticking off the ones that you have achieved.

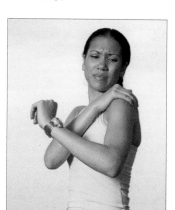

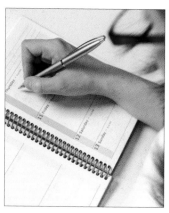

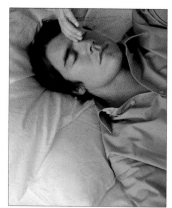

Body Type

We are all born with a body type, some naturally physically stronger than others.
However, with the right exercise and nutrition, we can become stronger and fitter,
change our type and fine-tune our strengths for specific sports and physical activities.

Your body type will have a direct influence on your sporting performance. For example, if you are a gymnast or Tour de France cyclist, being lightweight is a priority. However, if you take part in contact sports or weightlifting, you need to be heavy enough to hold your ground in the scrum or have the muscle power and strength to lift weights.

American psychologist W.H. Sheldon (1898–1977) developed a system in the 1940s that recognized three body types: endomorph, mesomorph and ectomorph. Most people share many, but not all, of the features of one of these body types.

Endomorphs

People with this body shape carry the most body mass of all three types. They are pear-shaped and often overweight. Endomorphs are likely to have the most sedentary lifestyles of all of the body types. They are not good at endurance activities, but if they have strong enough muscles, they can lift weights and use their own weight to provide power. Consequently, disciplines such as javelin and hammer throwing naturally suit them. People of this body type have a high Body Mass Index (BMI) and are at a greater risk of poor health than any other body type.

Mesomorphs

The most athletic and muscular-looking of the three body types, mesomorphs find it easy to compete in most sports and are able to build lean muscle, lose and gain weight fast, and maintain low body fat. They are stronger and fitter than other body types and will be good at adapting their body to cardiovascular and strength-training exercises. Mesomorphs are at less risk of health problems than any other body type. Mesomorphs can train harder than any other body type but need to watch their diet to make sure they are getting the correct fuel for their activity; they can get away with eating unhealthy food much of the time, but it won't provide them with the fuel for activity or aid their recovery after exercise.

Ectomorphs

These are the most fragile of the body types. They are thin in appearance and struggle to gain weight. Their low level of body fat makes them more susceptible to health problems. However, they are the best body type for endurance activities such as running marathons or cycling long distances. With the correct training, ectomorphs can have very high power-to-weight ratios, making them fast over long distances and good at climbing hills, for example.

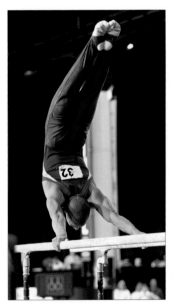

Left: Some people are more flexible than others, but this degree of flexibility requires more than just genetics.

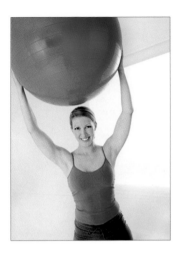

Above: Try a regime to change your body shape and, as a result, you will be happier with the way you look.

Making the changes

You may be an endomorph now but this doesn't mean you have to stay that way. The right exercise and food will change your body shape and decrease the risk of health problems. If you want to have a more athletic figure, you will need to follow a plan that involves burning as many calories as possible, while eating healthily, using the glycaemic index as a guideline in order to balance your blood sugar levels and prevent you from depositing fat. You will need to exercise three to four times a week,

A combined approach

To change your body type, you will need to adjust your training and your nutrition. One without the other will never get you the desired result. Once you have changed the way you look, you will need to continue working hard to maintain your new body shape.

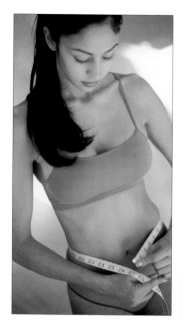

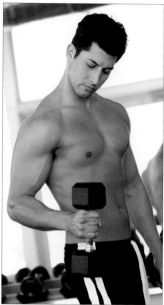

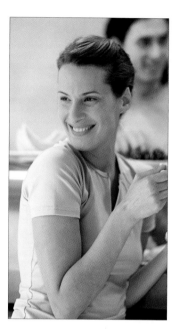

Above: Ectomorphs are naturally thin and have a low level of body fat. They often find it hard to gain weight.

Above: Mesomorphs are the fittest, with more lean muscle and low body fat. They easily lose and gain weight.

Above: Endomorphs have the largest body mass and may be overweight. They often have a sedentary lifestyle.

incorporating: cardiovascular training to burn calories and build a better and more efficient aerobic system (which in turn will allow you to burn yet more calories); and resistance training to build muscle and increase your metabolism.

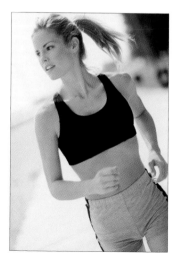

Endomorph to mesomorph If you are an endomorph, the chances are that you constantly struggle to motivate yourself to eat healthily and exercise. To make the necessary changes, you will need to alter your habits. Focus on reducing your calorie intake and increasing cardiovascular fitness and resistance training to increase your metabolism and lose weight. As you feel the benefits and increase your energy levels, you should see results more quickly, which will, in turn, reinforce your motivation.
Ectomorph to mesomorph You will need to consume more calories to feed your muscles and help them grow. At the same time you need to reduce your cardiovascular training time and focus more on resistance training, which will help you to build muscle.
Mesomorph to endomorph This is the easiest transformation and one that, unfortunately, usually happens quite by

Left: If you eat a healthy diet and exercise appropriately, you will be able to alter your body image.

accident. People who were athletic in their youth but have less time for exercise as they grow older, and perhaps have a sedentary job, are likely to change body type in this way. The bottom line is that if you consume more calories than you expend, then an endomorph you will become.
Mesomorph to ectomorph If you have bulky muscles, you may want to change shape, but this is hard to do. It requires you to lose muscle, not just fat. You can try to lose muscle by reducing your calorie intake so that you have to burn up muscle and use it as an energy source. Add long-distance endurance running or cycling, but avoid resistance training, as this will build muscle.

Altering your body type
Expect changes to your body shape to take time. Don't be discouraged by this. Keep the end goal in sight and stay motivated. If your body type changes too quickly, you will not be able to sustain the transformation.

Body Measurements

There are many different ways of measuring your body on a regular basis and assessing your progress. As you see your body shape gradually but definitely changing, it will help to give you the motivation you need to keep training.

The weighing scales are one of the oldest but most effective ways of recording your weight. Always use the same scales to weigh yourself at the same time of the day, on the same day of the week. Place the scales in the same place on a hard floor each time to get a true measure. If your goal is to lose weight, only weigh yourself once a week to give yourself a chance to see the weight decrease. Weighing yourself first thing in the morning will reduce the chance of the measure being affected by what you have eaten, as you probably won't have eaten anything for at least 8 hours. However, dehydration after a heavy night of drinking alcohol can make you seem lighter on the scales, so don't be fooled by this.

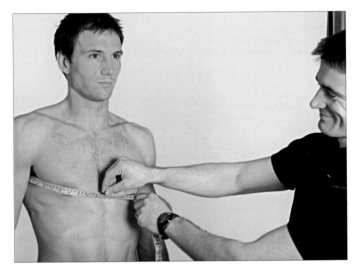

Above: Using a tape measure is an accurate indicator that your fitness regime is working well.

Measuring tape
A measuring tape is another useful way of monitoring your progress. Take measurements once a week at the same time as weighing yourself. Measure several different areas of the body each week. Breathe normally and don't suck your belly in when you measure.

Below: Scales don't always tell the whole story. You may have changed shape, but muscle is heavier than fat.

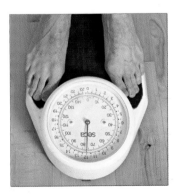

If the scales don't show a change in weight, the measuring tape might be your saviour. If your measurements are reducing, you know you are going in the right direction, even if you haven't lost weight. This change in shape and weight may be a result of more training, as muscle weighs more than fat – in fact, the same volume of muscle weighs nearly twice as much as the same volume of fat.

Use your body measurements to create your long- and short-term goals, but remember to be realistic. If you are trying to lose weight and your waist measures 102cm/40in, set a goal to lose 1cm/½in every two weeks until you reach your end goal of a 81cm/32in waist. If you are trying to gain muscle and change body shape, and your chest is 97cm/38in, set targets of a 2.5cm/1in increase in size until you reach your goal.

How to measure yourself

Chest: measure around the body, in line with the nipples.

Waist: measure around the body, in line with the belly button.

Hips: measure around the widest part of the hips.

Thighs: measure around the leg 15cm/6in up from the top of the knee.

Calves: measure around the mid-point of the lower leg.

Biceps: measure around the mid-point of the upper arm (decide whether you want to do this with the muscle tensed or with a straight arm, and use the same method of measurement each time so that you will be able to record any differences accurately).

Shoulders: measure from the middle of the side of one shoulder across the back to the middle of the side of the other shoulder.

Neck: measure around the mid-point of the neck.

Photographs and mirrors

One of the best ways to measure your progress is to look in the mirror and assess what you see. Obviously, you will not be able to remember what you see from one week to the next, so take photographs to compare the difference. This is especially important if you are trying to lose weight, change body shape or put on muscle mass. You can also use the mirror to assess your muscle definition if you are trying to put on muscle and look leaner. If you use a tape measure to measure your biceps, and the measurements don't change from week six to eight but the mirror and photograps show a distinct change in appearance, you will be instantly motivated to continue training. If you have been working on your running technique for your next 10km/6.2-mile race or marathon, run in front of the mirror or use photographs or a camcorder to see the difference in your technique.

Using a mirror for most weight-training exercises, especially with free weights, is essential. You need constantly to check whether you are using the right technique. Many people use weights that are too heavy for them and so fail to work the correct muscles, because the

Below: By regularly examining your body in a mirror, you will notice any areas that look different.

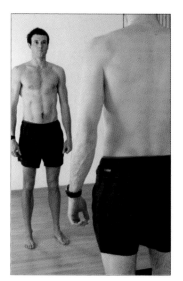

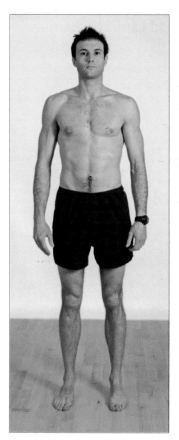

Above: If you have photographs taken at intervals, you will easily be able to see any bodily changes.

weight forces them to use other parts of their body instead of isolating the muscles they really want to work.

Clothes that fit

How your clothes fit is one of the best measures of your progress. The scales and the tape measure may at times suggest that your body has not changed at all, but if you go down a dress, trouser or shirt size, you will be inspired to continue training – it clearly is working. Clothes can tell you more than any measuring tape; for example, it is hard to use a measuring tape to measure the size of the buttocks but if your trousers feel looser, then obviously you have become thinner – in that area

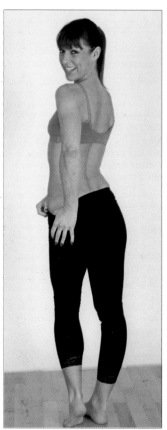

Above: How your clothes fit is a good indicator of losing body fat. After weight loss, they feel much looser.

at least. Buy clothes that you want to fit into in the future, and use this as a small goal on the path to achieving your goal.

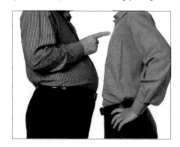

Above: If you are prepared to put in the required effort, you will achieve the results you want.

Measuring Body Fat

If you are trying to gain weight in the form of muscle, and you are eating more and taking supplements, measuring body fat regularly will help you to see whether you are gaining muscle or fat, and keep you on track to reach your goals.

As already stated at the beginning of this book, fad diets simply don't work. Many of them, in fact, can result in a higher percentage of body fat because a diet that leads to fast results often causes you to lose just as much muscle as fat. This reduction in muscle means that your metabolism will be lower, and as a result you will put on more fat, especially after the diet has come to an end – which, invariably, it will.

If your weight on the scales is the same as before you started the diet, but your body fat has dropped from 15 to 10 per cent, you will know that you have gained a considerable amount of muscle.

Below: Don't be discouraged if you are not losing weight quickly; slow and steady ensures it stays off.

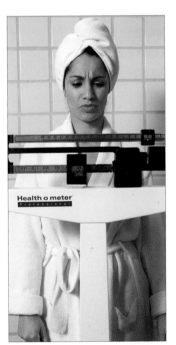

Health o meter
Professional

Body fat table			
Once you have calculated your body fat, compare your percentage with the figures on this table. You should try to stay within these boundaries – having some fat is essential for regulating the body's temperature and protecting vital organs.			
Age	**up to 30 years old**	**30–50 years old**	**50+ years old**
Female	14–21 per cent	15–21 per cent	16–25 per cent
Male	9–15 per cent	11–17 per cent	12–19 per cent

How to measure body fat

There are several different ways to measure body fat. The most accurate is hydrostatic weighing, which works by submerging the subject in a tank and measuring the water that is displaced. It is one of the most reliable tests, as factors such as how much fluid has been drunk in the last hour will not affect the results. However, you are unlikely to have a suitable tank at home and you won't find one at many sports clubs either. Instead, you are more likely to encounter body-fat scales and callipers.

A set of body-fat measuring scales will give you a rough estimate of your body fat. A low level electrical current is passed through the body and the impedance (opposition to the flow of current) is measured. The result is used with your weight and other factors to give you a body fat percentage. However, your body's impedance level can be affected by the amount of water in your body, any recent exercise and your skin temperature. If you are going to use body-fat scales to measure body fat don't eat or drink for at least 3 hours before measuring and avoid exercise for 12 hours before measuring.

Using body-fat callipers is more accurate if the same person does the measuring each time; the same amount of skin is pinched; the same side of the body is measured (usually the right-hand side); and the same equation is used to calculate body fat. If you repeat the same test in a month's time, and your fat

percentage has gone down, you know your training plan is working. There are a few rules you should stick to:
• The same person should measure you every time.
• Measure at the same time of day.

Below: This woman is having her fat measured in a hydrostatic weighing pool, which is a very accurate method.

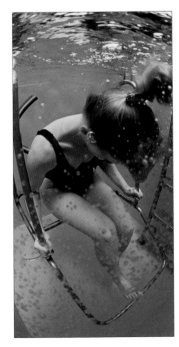

Body fat by sport

Average body-fat percentage for athletes.

Sport	male	female
Baseball	12–15	12–18
Basketball	6–12	20–27
Football	9–19	15–30
Cross-country running	5–12	12–18
Tennis	12–16	16–24
Triathlon	5–12	10–15

• Avoid drinking and eating for at least 3 hours before measurement.
• Avoid exercise for at least 12 hours before measuring.
• Hold the skin fold between the thumb and the index finger.
• Apply the callipers at a depth equal to the thickness of the fold.
• Repeat the measurement three times and take an average, so that you get an accurate reading.
• Add the readings for the different areas of the body together and use the equations that follow.

Instead of converting your skin-fold measurements into an actual body-fat reading, you could just add up your skin-fold measurements and use this to determine whether you are losing or gaining fat. If you want to focus on one area, such as losing weight from your stomach, then simply take one skin-fold measure from your abdomen using the following method. With a thumb and finger, pick up a skin fold with two thicknesses of skin and subcutaneous fat. Grip the skin with the callipers 1cm/½in from the fingers, at a depth the same thickness as the skin fold.

Measurements

Remember that muscle weighs more than fat so if the reading on the scales doesn't change don't feel defeatist. To check if you are losing fat, take body measurements using a tape measure, measure your skin folds with callipers and use your mirror to see the changes. Use your scales only twice a week unless you are an athlete in training.

How to calculate body-fat percentage

Specially calibrated callipers that grip the skin and fat are used for the measurement; three readings are taken at each site and an average is used for the calculation of body fat.

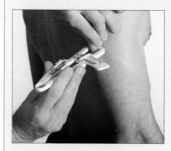

Triceps: *the back of the arm located halfway between the shoulder and the elbow. Measure vertically.*

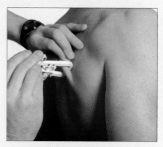

Sub scapular: *situated just below the shoulder blade. Measure at a 45-degree angle.*

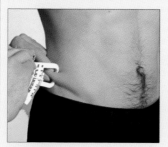

Supraspinale: *on the side of the abdomen just below the line of the belly button. Measure horizontally.*

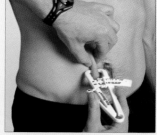

Abdominal area: *this is just beside the belly button. Measure the fat vertically.*

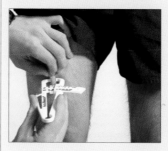

Thigh: *at the midpoint of the front of the thigh. Measure vertically.*

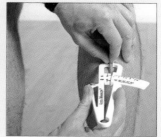

Calf: *taken at the back of the largest part of the calf. Measure vertically.*

Calculate your body-fat percentage using an equation such as this:

Equation for males: percentage body fat = (0.1051 x sum of triceps, sub scapular, supraspinale, abdominal, thigh and calf) + 2.585

Equation for females: percentage body fat = (0.1545 x sum of triceps, sub scapular, supraspinale, abdominal, thigh and calf) + 3.580

Yuhasz, M.S., *Physical Fitness Manual*, University of Western Ontario, 1974

Body Mass Index and Health Measurements

While the Body Mass Index is generally a useful way to assess whether your body mass is obese, overweight, normal or underweight, it is not always a straightforward measure, depending on who you are. It pays, therefore, to understand it in some detail.

Body Mass Index (BMI) is a measure of a person's weight scaled according to their height (see box 'Measuring your BMI'). This parameter is a useful tool for monitoring your progress in health and fitness. However, it is not accurate in all cases. For example, power athletes may have the same BMI score as an overweight person, even though they are carrying no fat. The reason for this is that the BMI does not account for the amount of lean muscle the athlete is carrying. Likewise, many endurance athletes have a BMI score indicating that they are underweight, even though they are actually a healthy weight. In older people, BMI

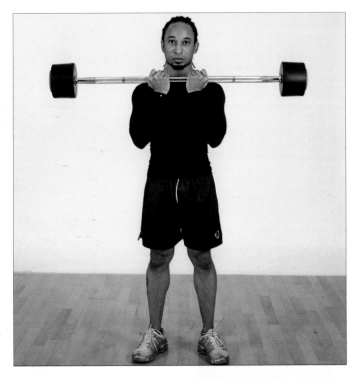

Measuring your BMI

Use the following methods to find your BMI:

Metric
BMI = body mass in kilograms/divided by height x height in meters

Example:
A 1.78m tall person, weighing 79.83kg would have a BMI of 25:
79.83kg/(1.78 x 1.78)
= 79.83/3.16
= 25

Imperial
BMI = body mass in pounds/divided by height x height in inches multiplied by 703

Example:
A 5ft 10in (70in) tall person, weighing 176lb would have a BMI of 25:
176lb/(70 x 70) x 703
= 176/4,900 x 703
= 25

Above: Muscular people may have a higher BMI. This does not, however, mean that they are unhealthy.

Right: Long-distance runners who are lightweight will generally have a low BMI.

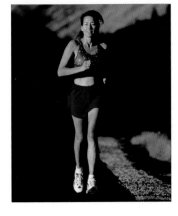

readings may be of little use, as they will not take into account loss of muscle mass. Neither can the BMI be an accurate measure for children or breastfeeding mothers. However, those exceptions aside, the BMI provides a good basic guideline to follow for the general population.

How to measure your waist-to-hip ratio

Take your waist measurement by measuring round your body at the midpoint between the bottom of your waist and hips. Measure your hips by measuring around your body where your buttocks stick out the most. Divide your waist measurement by your hip measurement. For example, a 81cm/32in waist and 102cm/40in hip would be calculated as a waist-to-hip ratio of 0.8. This ratio is reasonable for a man but is the upper limit for a woman.

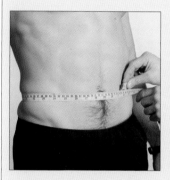

Above: To measure your waist, hold the tape measure between the lower part of the waist and the hips.

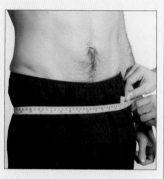

Above: The hips are measured by holding the tape measure at the widest place.

Blood pressure

If your blood pressure is higher than 140/100, you should consult a doctor before you start any exercise routine. It is easy to measure blood pressure yourself with a blood pressure monitor that you can buy from larger pharmacies. It is best to take the test before you have done any exercise that day, as that may affect the result. However, if you have already exercised, then make sure that you rest for at least 30 minutes before you take a reading.

Cholesterol

Your doctor can check your cholesterol level by a simple blood test. The result is reported in millimoles per litre (mmol/l) or milligrams per decilitre (mg/dl). A cholesterol level of 5 mmol/l/200mg/dl or less is desirable, 5 to 6 is borderline, and above 6 puts you at a high risk of a heart attack. In the UK, 75 per cent of adults aged over 40 have a level higher than 5, and 54 per cent of heart attacks are linked with levels of over 5.

Waist-to-hip ratio

Other body measurements are also useful for monitoring health. Simply measuring your waist and hips, then calculating your waist-to-hip ratio, can be just as effective as the BMI measurement for highlighting health risk factors, especially for heart disease

Below: There is no need to visit the doctor to take your blood pressure; you can easily measure it yourself.

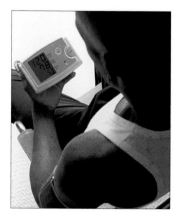

and type II diabetes, as it has been proven that people who carry excess fat around their middle are more at risk of these illnesses.

The risk of health problems has been found to increase if a man has a waist measurement of over 102cm/40in, or a woman has a waist measurement of more than 89cm/35in. A waist-to-hip ratio of more than 1 for men and 0.8 for women is highly detrimental to your health. At this point, the risk of heart disease, hypertension and type II diabetes is dramatically increased.

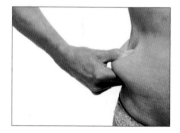

Above: The amount you can firmly pinch indicates extra weight and also the state of your wellbeing.

BMI and health risks

Studies show that the BMI score is linked to health risk factors. Compare your score with those on the chart below. If your health risk is high or very high, you should consult a doctor and start taking exercise and eating sensibly immediately.

BMI score	Classification	Health risk
Less than 18.5	underweight	moderate
18.5–24.9	normal	very low
25–29.9	overweight	low
30–34.9	obese class 1	moderate
35–39.9	obese class 2	high
Above 40	extreme obesity	very high

Cardiovascular Fitness Tests

It is essential when following a training programme that you test your cardiovascular fitness, and there are a number of ways you can do this. It is equally important that the test you choose is appropriate to the sport you will be doing.

Tests vary depending on the sport and the first step when testing your cardiovascular fitness is selecting the right test for you and your sport. If you are a sprinter, you need to set yourself tests on the track covering the distances, or similar distances, that you will be running in competition. Testing yourself over 5km/3 miles will be of little use to you.

If you are a cyclist, test your fitness with a 8km/5-mile or 16km/10-mile time trial over a familiar route – one that you can use in the future for comparison.

For invasion sports such as basketball or netball, test yourself by running different lengths of the court and timing

Measuring up
When testing your fitness, use a treadmill or run on an athletics track so that you can easily measure your distance.

The VO2 max table fitness assessment

Female

Age	Very poor	Poor	Fair	Good	Excellent	Superior
13–19	<25	25–30.9	31–34.9	35–38.9	39–41.9	>41.9
20–29	<23.6	23.6–28.9	29–32.9	33–36.9	37–41	>41
30–39	<22.8	22.8–26.9	27–31.4	31.5–35.6	35.7–40	>40
40–49	<21	21–24.4	24.5–28.9	29–32.8	32.9–36.9	>36.9
50–59	<20.2	20.2–22.7	22.8–26.9	27–31.4	31.5–35.7	>35.7
60+	<17.5	17.7–20.1	20.2–24.4	24.5–30.2	30.3–31.4	>31.4

Male

Age	Very poor	Poor	Fair	Good	Excellent	Superior
13–19	<35–36	36–38	38.4–45.1	45.2–50.9	51.0–55.9	>55.9
20–29	<33.0	33.0–36.4	36.5–42.4	42.5–46.4	46.5–52.4	>52.4
30–39	<31.5	31.5–35.4	35.5–40.9	41.0–44.0	45.0–49.4	>49.4
40–49	<30.2	30.2–33.5	33.6–38.9	39.0–43.7	43.8–48.0	>48.0
50–59	<26.1	26.1–30.9	31.0–35.7	35.8–40.9	41.0–45.3	>45.3
60+	<20.5	20.5–26.0	26.1–32.2	32.3–36.4	36.5–44.2	>44.2

Cooper, K.H., *The Physical Fitness Specialist Certification Manual*, The Cooper Institute for Aerobics Research, Dallas, Texas, 1968

Below: Sprinting demands a fast delivery of oxygen to your muscles. This is known as 'aerobic exercise'.

Below: If you enter a triathlon, you need to ensure that you do regular cardiovascular training.

Below: Games require a fast, efficient cardiovascular system to enable rapid recovery between points.

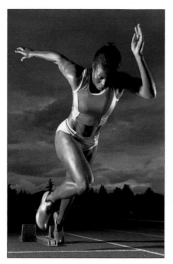

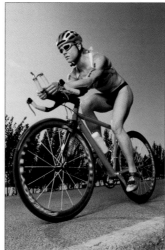

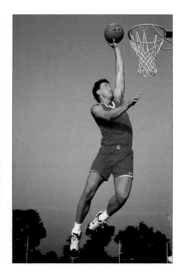

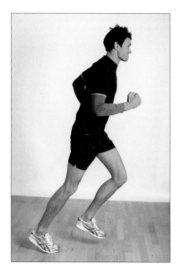

Above: If you have a high level of fitness attempt the Cooper 12-minute run test, in which you run or walk for 12 minutes.

yourself. Try starting at the back of the court and running to the halfway mark and back five times, and then running to the far end of the court and back five times and getting an overall time.

For rowing, set a distance such as 2,000m/2,187yd and time yourself. Then test yourself again in the future to check for fitness improvements.

There are three useful measurements that test either aerobic fitness or the cardiovascular system: the VO2 max, the Cooper 12-minute run and the Harvard step test.

VO2 max The VO2 max test measures the maximum volume of oxygen (O₂) that an athlete can use during intense exercise. The test is suitable for elite athletes who are able to push

themselves hard without risk of injury or other health problems. It is also one of the best measures of cardiovascular fitness because it shows you how efficient your body is at utilizing oxygen and represents your maximum aerobic capacity. It is expressed as ml/kg/min (millilitres of oxygen per kilogram of body weight per minute).

The most accurate way to test VO2 max is to exercise to failure (when you reach the point that you simply cannot push your body any further) and use laboratory techniques to work out the exact amount of oxygen you are able to utilize by measuring the air that you exhale. However, there is a simple test you can do to predict your VO2 max without using specialist equipment, and which does not involve exercising to complete failure:

The Cooper 12-minute run Like the VO2 max, this test is also suitable for elite athletes used to pushing themselves hard. It measures the body's ability to use oxygen while running. Run or walk as far as possible in 12 minutes, then measure the distance in metres/yards to predict your VO2 max. Use the following formula to calculate your estimated VO2 max in ml/kg/min (milligrams of oxygen/ kilogram body weight/minute):

Miles: VO2 max=35.97 x miles - 11.29
Kilometers: VO2 max=22.4 x km - 11.3

An endurance athlete, such as a marathon runner would generally have a high VO2 of around 70ml/kg/min, an average level would be 35 and a poor level is 25 or below.

The Harvard step test Anyone who wants to get fit can use the Harvard step test, which monitors the cardiovascular system. This is a basic test that involves stepping up on to a 40–50cm/16–20in high gym bench once every 2 seconds for 5 minutes and recording your heart rate. Note your heart rate 1 minute after finishing the test (HR1), again after 2 minutes (HR2) and, finally, again after 3 minutes (HR3). Use the following calculation to assess the state of your fitness:

The Harvard step test results

>90	excellent
80–89	good
65–79	above average
55–64	below average
<55	poor

McArdle, W.D. et al, *Physiology: Energy, Nutrition and Human Performance,* 1991.

Fitness level = 30,000/2 x (HR1 + HR2 + HR3). For example, 30,000/2 x (120 + 100 + 80) = 50.

A high level of 80 or 90 is good, indicating a healthy cardiovascular system, while 50 or below is poor. Before you attempt any form of cardiovascular test for the first time, you should consult your doctor. Always have somebody with you during the test.

Below: The Harvard step test is a way of noting your heart rate to assess your state of fitness.

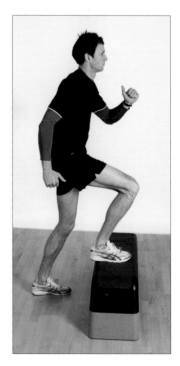

Strength Tests

When devising a training plan – and before you actually embark on it – it is important to find out how strong you are. Otherwise, you could quickly overreach yourself and do yourself an injury. When measuring your strength, use a test that best suits you and your specific goals.

The test that you choose should be determined by the goal you have in mind. If you want bigger arms, then use bicep and tricep exercises to generate a test that will assess your performance on the way to achieving your goals.

To recover from a knee operation using exercise to build strength in your quadriceps, use a leg extension test to assess the strength in your quadriceps and monitor your rehabilitation programme.

If you want stronger, wider shoulders, do shoulder presses in order to assess shoulder strength.

Below: Test your body for strength on the areas that you most want to work out.

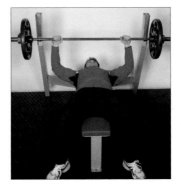

Above: The bench press test is a method for assessing the strength of the pectorals and shoulders.

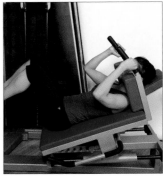

Above: You can easily find out how strong your legs are by using the leg press.

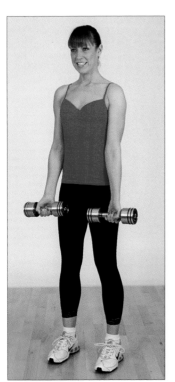

To assess hamstring strength (muscles at the back of the thigh), use a hamstring curl machine.

For upper-back strength, do chin-ups and add weights, wearing a weights belt to test your strength.

Take precautions

Before you do any strength test for the first time, consult your doctor. If you are testing to find your one repetition maximum (ORM), make sure to have a training partner to help you when your muscles tire. Use supports and foot rests on exercise machines when you start to fail on a weight. Struggling to lift a weight that is too heavy for you is one of the most common causes of injuries.

One Repetition Maximum test

This is the gold standard of strength tests. Most ORM tests involve the bench press and leg press, as these two exercises involve the majority of the large muscles in the upper and lower body. Follow this procedure to find your ORM:

1 Warm up for three sets using a weight you can lift for at least ten repetitions.
2 Add 5–10 per cent to the weight and complete three repetitions.
3 Add a further 5–10 per cent to the weight and try to complete three repetitions.
4 Continue to add 5–10 per cent to the weight until you can only do one repetition (ORM).

Strength assessment					
Bench press	Poor	Fair	Good	Very good	Excellent
Male	0.6	0.8	1.0	1.2	1.4
Female	0.3	0.4	0.5	0.6	0.7
Leg press					
Male	1.4	1.8	2.0	2.4	2.8
Female	1.2	1.4	1.8	2.0	2.2

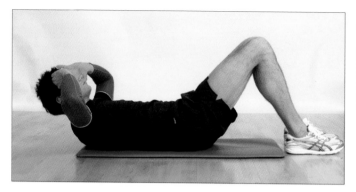

Good technique

Achieving a good score on these tests is not necessarily attributed to strength alone. As your body gradually gets used to the technique, you will start to see an improvement in your scores.

Left: The sit-up test lifts the head and shoulders up. It measures the strength of the abdominal muscles and hip flexor muscles. The more sit-ups you can do in 1 minute, the stronger your muscles.

Once you have found your ORM for the bench press and leg press, divide the weight you have achieved by your body weight to get a score. This is the calculation if your ORM for the bench press is 100kg/220lb:

100kg/220lb (ORM bench press)/
80kg/176lb (body weight) = 1.25

A good result for a male would be more than 1.4; a poor result is less than 0.6.

Strength endurance test

You can easily do this test at home. It involves doing as many sit-ups and press-ups as possible in 1 minute. Because women do not have the same upper-body strength as men, women can do the press-ups with their knees on the floor. Use the scores in the table to assess your strength endurance.

Using the strength tests

Anyone can adapt the strength tests to their chosen sport. For example, if you are a cyclist, use the leg press to find your ORM. For the strength endurance test, see how many step-ups or squats you can do in 1 minute. If you want to build a bigger, stronger chest, do an ORM test using the bench press, and for strength endurance, do as many press-ups as you can manage in 1 minute. Repeat every four to six weeks to monitor your progress.

Right: For the female press-up test, the knees balance on the floor.

Above right: The male technique for a press-up test lifts the body off the floor.

Strength endurance assessment					
Sit-ups	**Poor**	**Fair**	**Good**	**Very good**	**Excellent**
Male	20	30	40	50	60
Female	10	20	30	40	50
Press-ups					
Male	10	20	30	40	50
Female	10	20	30	40	50

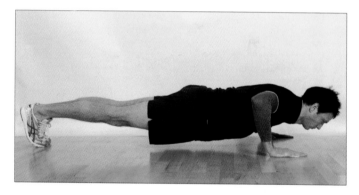

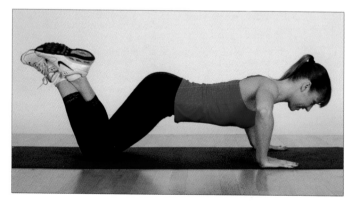

Equipment for Cardiovascular Training

Before you use cardiovascular equipment, in the gym or at home, you need to take into account a number of important factors. These include, location, space, value, safety, hygiene, familiarity with the controls and, most of all, using machinery that 'fits' you.

Whether you decide to train at home or in a public gym, the location and its surroundings are very important. The place you choose for your training must be somewhere that you really want to go. It must be somewhere to look forward to, especially if you are going to train after a long day's work. If you are going to join a public gym, there are a number of factors to consider.

Gym conditions

Always check the level of instruction on offer at the gym. Find out whether the instructors are qualified, and to what level. Find out how much help is on offer. If you have not used a gym before, you will need all the help you can get to set up machinery and feel safe with what you are doing. There also needs to

Below: Understanding the equipment will make your workout more enjoyable and useful.

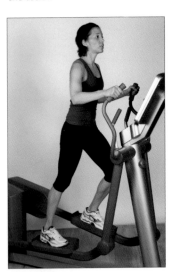

be plenty of natural light or, failing that, good-quality artificial lighting and ventilation to keep you supplied with plentiful fresh air. Air-conditioning will help to cool you down, but it may lead to greater dehydration, especially during cardiovascular exercise, so take care to carry a drinks bottle with you at all times.

Spend some time at the gym before you join and study closely what it is like at different times of the day. It may be very quiet on your first visit at 10 a.m., but it may be packed with people waiting to use the machines at 6 p.m. – the very time you are most likely to want to train, if you have a regular job. Make sure, too, that the machines are kept in good order and are hygienic.

The machines that you will be using for cardiovascular training include treadmills, exercise bikes, cross-trainers, rowing machines, steppers, trampolines and vibration plates.

Measuring up and splashing out

You may not feel like using the gym close to you; a gym environment is not ideal for everyone, in which case, you should consider training at home, but check carefully the amount of space you have, and the access, before ordering any unnecessary gym equipment. For cross-trainers and treadmills, you will need considerable ceiling height. Buying cardiovascular equipment can be very expensive. It doesn't have be the most state-of-the-art to be useful to you but, generally, the more costly it is, the more functional and robust it will be. If you want to work out using smooth machinery with lots of built-in cardiovascular programmes, then spend more money. Many manufacturers describe

> **Practise first**
> Make sure you make yourself familiar with the motion of any machine you are going to use, along with all the buttons that you will need for your workout. For example, if you are on the treadmill, practise adjusting the speed before you embark on an interval training session. Also, check that you know where the stop button is and practise walking on the treadmill before you run on it for the first time.

their cardiovascular equipment as being for 'domestic use' or 'commercial use'. The commercial use equipment will be more expensive, but it will last longer because it is designed for continual heavy use in a public gym.

Below: The heart-rate monitor is worn around the chest, over the heart. A reading can be seen on the wrist device.

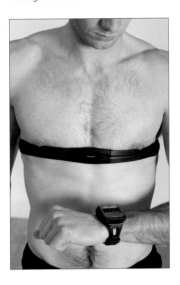

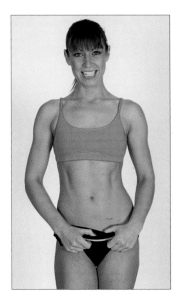

Above: It is essential to wear a supportive sports bra when doing vigorous training.

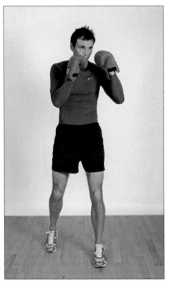

Above: Always check your equipment for safety. For hygiene, wear only your own boxing gloves.

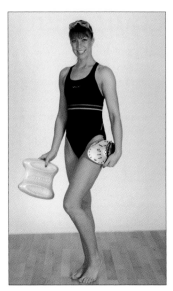

Above: Swimming aids such as floats and pull buoys will help to improve your technique.

From treadmills to rowing machines, the choice of cardiovascular equipment is endless. If you can afford it and have the space, have at least two pieces of cardiovascular equipment so that you can vary your exercise routine. There should be a number of programmes to stop you getting bored. Also, keep in mind that treadmills have different maximum speeds and levels of incline. Rowers use different pulley mechanisms, while cross-trainers vary in size and motion. Some stationary bikes are more adjustable than others. Try out the equipment before you buy and make sure the machine is right for you.

Heart-rate monitor

Constantly use a heart-rate monitor to analyse your training efforts. Most good heart-rate monitors allow you to set zones for your desired level of intensity. You can buy more expensive versions that allow you to download the data to your PC and copy the workout data into a diary, if you wish. However, being able to view your heart rate easily during your training session is the most important factor. Make sure that your

---

Divert and motivate

Distractions when you are doing cardiovascular exercise are good. Use an MP3 player or watch television to turn your routine into a pleasant experience and make the time go faster. Knowing that you can watch a favourite TV programme may motivate you to get to the gym.

---

heart-rate monitor is coded so that it only picks up a signal from you and not your training partner's signal.

Clothing

For running, rowing or other similar cardiovascular exercise, wear loose-fitting, lightweight, breathable clothing. Always wear good footwear with plenty of support and cushioning. Females should wear good-quality supportive tops to prevent them feeling uncomfortable or self-conscious in front of others.

For boxing, it is essential to always have the correct protective pads and gloves. For hygiene reasons, always try to use your own gloves in a public gym. If you do have to use other

people's gloves, remember to wash your hands thoroughly afterward. Remove all your jewellery and watches to prevent injuries.

For swimming, wear a well-fitted swimming costume that is supportive but will allow you to move with maximum efficiency through the water. Use pull buoys and floats to help you improve your swimming technique. Choose goggles that attach firmly to your face with suction before you've even put the strap around your head. This is the sign of a good fit; wearing loose goggles when swimming are next to useless; they will allow water to get into your eyes, and will only interfere with the smooth timing, enjoyment and effectiveness of your session.

Suitable equipment

If you are training outdoors, always take a pack with the necessary clothing, including waterproof outerwear, and sun cream, when appropriate. Also, remember to take with you a water bottle, other drinks and snacks.

Equipment for Strength Training

With both free weights and machines, expensive equipment, though preferable, is by no means necessary. It is much more important that you combine different pieces of equipment for maximum effect – and know how to use them correctly and safely.

You don't need to spend lots of money on strength-training equipment, but if money is no obstacle, then having expensive, well-built equipment may well help to motivate you to exercise. This equipment is normally the easiest to adjust to suit your personal needs; it will offer a greater range of movements and require less maintenance.

You can choose between using free weights, body weight or machine weights, such as weight-training benches, squat stands, single stations and multi-gyms. Or, you can use a combination of all three for the best workouts. No single piece of equipment is better than any other piece. The most important factor is how you use the equipment. If used correctly, you will benefit from it; if used incorrectly, you may do yourself more harm than good.

Below: In a gym, dumbbells are stored on a convenient rack according to their size.

Use of free weights

Free weights such as dumbbells or barbells require you to recruit more muscle mass to provide balance and stability, unlike machines, which simply require you to push a weight in one direction. Free weights demand that you control the weight in all directions.

Free weights

Free weights involve barbells or dumbbells.
Barbells These are long, straight bars with weight plates attached at each end. Some gyms have a variety of barbells, with the plates permanently fixed to the bar. Sometimes, the plates can be removed so that you can adjust the barbell size and weight. If you intend using adjustable barbells, make sure that you use the safety collars on each end to retain the weights.
Dumbbells These are short bars with weighted plates on each end. The plates

may be fixed or removable, depending on the size of the weights area. Most gyms have a variety of dumbbells with permanently fixed plates.

If you want to use equipment at home, free weights are a good option compared with machines. Machines take up a lot of room and may give you the option of working only one or two different exercises – unless you've bought a multi-gym (a unit with lots of exercise stations coming off it). By contrast, free weights take up very little room and can be used for a variety of exercises.

Weight machines

Machines with multiple weight stacks give you an easily adjustable weight. You simply adjust the weights stack with a connecting pin that runs through the middle of the weight you want to select.

Below: This weights bench is adjustable to most sizes but it is best to check first that it is suitable for you.

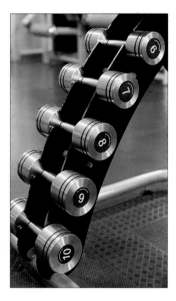

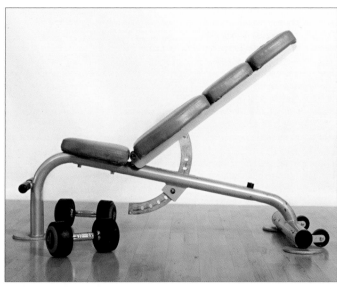

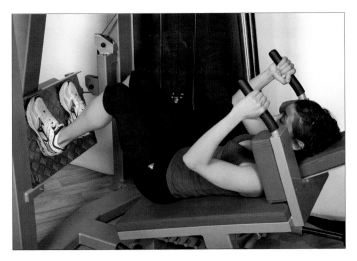

Above: Before exercising, adjust the machine to fit you correctly. If it does not feel comfortable, do not use it.

Machines are often seen as safer because you cannot drop the weights on the floor or lose your balance, or even control of the weight, and injure yourself. Be warned: machines can sometimes be designed in such a way that they do not 'fit' you very well. Setting up machines in the correct position for you takes experience and, possibly, some assistance from a qualified instructor. You could unknowingly put yourself in a position that will cause muscle or joint pain. For example, sitting on a chest-press machine with the handles set too high will force your shoulders to do all of the work, not your chest. Some machines are designed as 'one size fits all', but they do not always live up to their billing. If you are particularly short or tall, you need to ask yourself whether a

particular machine is going to be best for you. How can you tell? Quite simply, if it feels wrong or awkward when you try to use it, use free weights instead.

Make sure that you are completely familiar with the safety aspects of each machine that you will be using before you start training on it. For example, if you are going to use a leg-press machine, before you release the weight and start bending your legs back toward your body, be clear about what you need to do in case you fatigue and you cannot straighten your legs again. Always check to see whether there is any kind of safety mechanism to stop your legs being crushed.

Body weight

If you are in a restricted space, or have a limited budget, then simply use your body weight – it's highly effective. Even top bodybuilders use exercises such as press-ups and lunges. To make these exercises effective, make sure that you are using the correct technique to isolate the muscles you want to work and avoid injury. Using just your body weight in warm-up exercises is also a great way to stimulate the muscles you intend to work using free weights or machines, giving you a better workout all round.

Getting started

If you do join a gym, you are most likely to be shown how to use the machines for your strength training. But if you find

you are mainly using machines in your workouts, take time to vary your exercise and introduce exercises that involve just your body weight and free weights. That way, you always have a familiar exercise programme when you are staying away from home and have limited or no access to a gym.

For weight-training, wear comfortable clothing that allows you the full range of movement. Clothing that fits close to your skin will enable you to see if the correct muscles are working. Always wear a number of layers to make it easy to adjust to changes in the temperature you are working in, and to keep your muscles warm.

Below: You can easily assess your position and ensure good technique by looking in a full-length mirror.

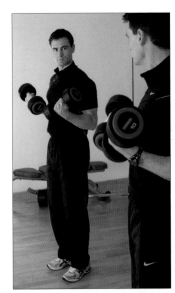

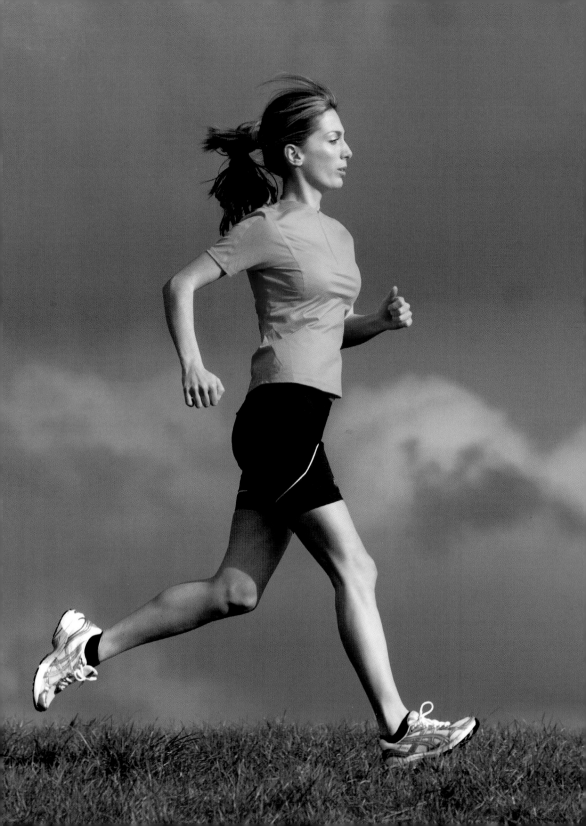

CARDIOVASCULAR TRAINING

Any form of exercise that raises your heartbeat is cardiovascular, whether it is walking to the shops or swimming a long distance. What matters is finding the exercise that suits you best and slowly building up your level of intensity in order to achieve your goals. At the outset, you do not need to suffer to feel the benefits. However, to challenge your body, make it fun and get the best results, include variety in your training, and keep a record of your exercise to monitor your progress and stay motivated.

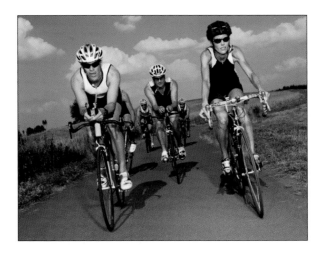

Above: Training in groups can make fitness fun.
Left: Running can be enjoyable, as well as helping you to achieve fitness.

The Benefits of Cardiovascular Exercise

Whether you are planning to run a marathon, take part in a triathlon or simply improve your general health and fitness to deal better with everyday demands, cardiovascular training has the added advantage of promoting your wellbeing.

Cardiovascular exercise has a beneficial effect on the body. It will promote weight loss and enable your heart and lungs to work more efficiently and become stronger. It will help to increase bone density, reduce stress and decrease the risk of heart disease and some cancers, particularly colon, prostrate and breast cancer. Regular cardiovascular exercise relieves depression, increases your level of confidence, improves your sleep patterns and gives you more energy to combat challenges at home and at work. It can help to lower cholesterol, triglyceride (fat in the bloodstream and fat tissue) and blood pressure levels. Glucose tolerance (how your body breaks down blood sugar) and insulin sensitivity (how well the insulin in the body controls blood sugar levels) will also improve. For athletic performance, the more cardiovascular exercise you do, the faster your heart rate will recover, and metabolize glucose to give your muscles the energy they need.

Below: The cardiovascular system consists of the heart and a closed system of arteries, veins and capillaries. Because the heart and lungs are made from muscular tissue, they need to be trained, just like other muscles.

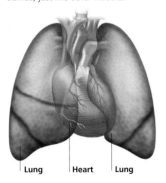

| Lung | Heart | Lung |

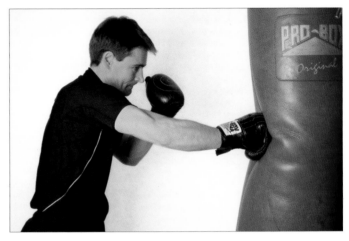

Appropriate exercises

Different exercises will benefit different people, depending on their fitness level and injuries. For example, a big muscular person will benefit more from rowing, in which there is no impact and they can use a large amount of muscle mass. Running, however, involves constant impact and is more likely to cause injury. It relies on the legs to carry the weight and doesn't use the upper-body muscles.

Losing weight

• To achieve weight loss and maintain your new lower weight, you must combine cardiovascular training with resistance training, because resistance training will increase your muscle metabolism and help you to burn more calories.

• To lose weight, do exercises that use greater muscle mass. The rowing machine and the cross-trainer work both your upper and lower body and will burn more calories compared to other cardiovascular exercises.

Above: Boxing provides a complete workout for your cardiovascular and endurance systems.

Enjoy yourself Choose a cardiovascular activity that you enjoy, so that you'll want to do more of it. If you dread going to the gym, try training with a partner, perhaps competing side by side on a bike or doing some boxercise. Use music to distract yourself from the exercise, especially if you are exercising at low intensity to burn fat. To motivate yourself before a training session, think about how great you will feel after you have completed a good cardiovascular session – energized, fresh and stress free.

Challenge yourself If you run for 5km/ 3 miles on the treadmill every other day, your body will soon get used to this exercise, and the lack of challenge will result in fewer calories being burnt and only a small improvement to your fitness level. Rather than doing the same exercise at the same level of intensity, combine different exercises and levels of intensity all the time to give your body new

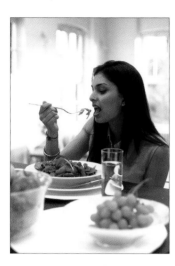

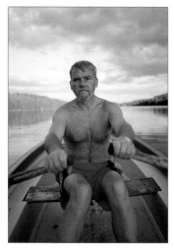

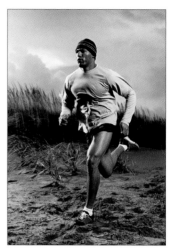

Above: Eat a healthy, nutritious diet to prepare for and recover from cardiovascular workouts.

Above: Rowing trains your cardiovascular system without the impact of running.

Above: Make running a more challenging experience by trying out different surfaces and terrains.

challenges. For example, run for about 3 minutes at a steady pace, then accelerate and hold a fast pace for the fourth minute, before returning to a steady pace. When out walking, adjust

Below: Weights alone will not benefit your cardiovascular system – you need a mixture of different types of exercise.

your training route to include more hills to challenge your body and increase your heart rate, thereby making you work harder to achieve fitness.

When to train
Everybody has a preferred time of day to train. If you train first thing in the morning before eating, you will burn

straight into your fat stores as your glycogen stores (stored glucose, mainly in the muscles and liver), which you usually use in the first 20 minutes of exercise, will have depleted overnight. If you follow resistance training with cardiovascular training, you will also burn straight into fat stores. This may seem like a more efficient way of burning fat but be careful – you may start to feel dizzy and you may even pass out if your glycogen levels are low. Training will increase your energy level, so you may want to train during your lunch break so that you have greater energy for the afternoon's work.

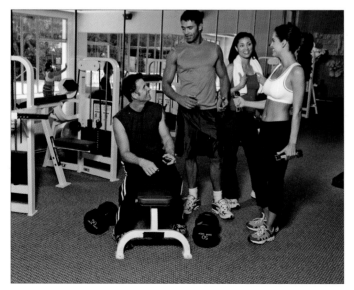

Training tips
• To start burning fat, your exercise regime should last for at least 20 minutes.
• To feel the maximum benefits of cardiovascular exercise, you should train at least three times a week at between 60 and 90 per cent of your maximum heart rate.
• Elite athletes need to train at between 75 and 95 per cent of their maximum heart rate if they want to make significant fitness improvements.

Cardiovascular Energy Expenditure

When estimating the number of calories you will burn in an exercise session, you need to take into account duration, speed and intensity of exercise, along with your body type and the muscle requirement of each exercise.

The longer you exercise, the more calories you will burn. If you are unfit, you should exercise at a lower intensity so that you can exercise for longer before fatigue sets in. For example, if you are trying to run for the first time, begin by alternating 1 minute of jogging with 3 minutes of walking, then repeating for as long as possible. If you attempt to jog continuously, the chances are that you will last less

Below: Boxing is extremely demanding, and around just 3 minutes of hard boxing can seem a very long time.

than 10 minutes. By alternating walking and jogging, you may be able to last for up to 1 hour.

Speed of exercise
The faster the exercise, the more calories you burn. Going faster will force your body to work harder, and muscle cells to contract faster. You have to burn more calories to maintain a fast work rate.

Intensity level
The greater the intensity of the exercise, the higher the number of calories you will burn. Intense exercise will not only

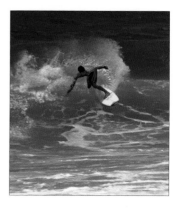

Above: If you constantly paddle out, catch a wave and surf in again, you will burn more calories.

burn calories during exercise, it will also make you burn more calories after the exercise has stopped. Interval training and sprinting will have this afterburn effect because your muscles need energy to recover, which in turn burns more calories.

Body type
Mesomorphs are naturally leaner and possess more metabolically active muscle cells. This means that they will have a higher metabolic rate, even at rest, and will, therefore, burn a greater number of calories, further helping them to stay lean.

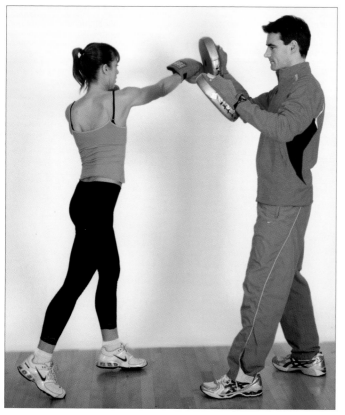

Appropriate nutrition
If you are quite lean already, make sure that your food intake is sufficient to keep up with your exercise demands. If it is not, you may be forced to break down muscle to provide energy. In the long term, this means less muscle mass and, therefore, a reduced potential for burning calories.

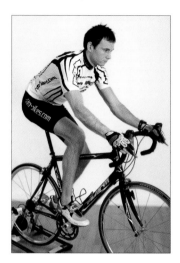

Above: Cycling at speed uses up a lot of calories and they continue to burn even after the exercise has stopped.

The heavier a person is, the more calories he or she is likely to burn during exercise because they have got more weight to move around. For example, the energy required for a runner who weighs 63kg/140lb is far less than the energy needed for a runner who weighs 90kg/200lb, or almost twice as much. The lighter runner burns off fewer calories.

Below: For someone of average weight, baseball burns up around 350 calories in 1 hour.

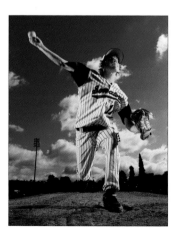

Muscle use

There is a simple equation to keep in mind when it comes to exercise and calorie burn. Exercises that involve using greater amounts of muscle will burn more calories. For example, a training session on the rowing machine will burn more calories than a similar session on a static bike because rowing uses both your upper and lower body. However, cycling, when riding at speed, may burn up a lot of calories, even though it uses only your leg muscles. Competitive sports require high-speed running or sprinting and can burn off hundreds of calories in an hour.

Calorie burn by exercise

The following list shows an estimate of how many calories you can expect to burn in 1 hour of constant exercise, depending on your body weight, and the speed you are going at, for a variety of popular sports and activities.

Exercise	59kg/130lb	70kg/155lb	86kg/190lb
Aerobics, general	354	422	518
Aerobics, high impact	413	493	604
American football	593	783	866
Baseball	295	352	431
Basketball	472	563	690
Cycling <16kph/10mph	236	281	345
Cycling >32kph/20mph	944	1,126	1380
Cycling, mountain bike	502	598	733
Boxercise	531	633	776
Rowing, racing	708	844	1035
Rowing, leisure	17	211	259
Dancing, fast	325	387	474
Dancing, slow	177	211	259
Football	531	633	776
Golf	236	281	345
Handball	472	563	690
Hockey	472	563	690
Horse riding	236	281	345
Ice hockey	340	485	592
Rugby	590	704	863
Running 16kph/10mph	944	1,126	1,380
Running 13kph/8mph	796	950	1,165
Running 10kph/6mph	590	704	863
Ice-skating	413	493	604
Skateboarding	340	495	604
Skiing, cross-country	826	985	1,208
Skiing, downhill	354	422	518
Skiing, water	354	422	518
Squash	708	844	1,035
Surfing	177	211	259
Swimming, fast	590	704	863
Swimming, leisure	354	422	518
Tennis, singles	472	563	690
Tennis, doubles	354	422	518
Volleyball	472	563	690
Walking 6kph/4mph	236	281	345
Walking 5kph/3mph	207	246	302
Walking 3kph/2mph	148	176	216
Weightlifting	354	422	518

Heart Rate

The heart circulates oxygenated blood from your lungs to the working muscles. Using a heart-rate monitor will help to monitor the stresses you are putting on your heart and will reduce the risk of injury and overtraining.

Your heart rate is measured in beats per minute (bpm). You can measure your heart rate by using the pulse on your wrist or neck and counting the number of pulses in 6 seconds and then multiplying it by ten. However, the best way to monitor your heart rate is to use a heart-rate monitor. It's easy to use: simply place the strap around your torso just underneath the top of your chest or bra line. The best time to measure resting heart rate (RHR) is first thing in the morning when you wake up – before the stresses of the day, eating and exercise can affect the reading. For an average reading, take your RHR every day for three days.

Heart rate can be used as a measure of how fit you are. The sooner your heart rate returns to its resting value after exercise – 55bpm for example – the fitter you are. It is worth monitoring your average heart rate (AHR) throughout similar exercise sessions to compare your fitness levels and keep you motivated. For example, if you regularly do a 4.8km/3-mile cycle ride in 15 minutes and your AHR reading is 155bpm, and you do the same bike ride a month later, in the same time, and your heart rate averages 145bpm, you know you are getting fitter.

Maximum heart rate

The maximum number of times your heart can contract in a minute is called the maximum heart rate (MHR). This is the best indicator to use to work out the intensity levels of your training. There are two methods to determine your MHR: the first involves increasing the intensity of exercises, step by step, over the space of 10–20 minutes until you reach total exhaustion. For example, ride the exercise bike at 16kph/10mph and increase the speed by 1.6kph/1mph every minute until you can't go any farther. You should not try this test unless you have a doctor with you, in case you have cardiac problems. The second method uses the following formula: MHR = 220 - your age.

Heart rate and health

You can use your heart rate to monitor your health and prevent yourself overtraining. If your RHR is five to ten beats higher than normal, this

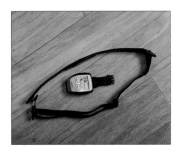

Above: The strap of a heart-rate monitor, worn around the chest, sends information to the wrist monitor.

indicates that you may be coming down with an illness. You should, therefore, consider adjusting your training or taking a rest before you do any more damage. If your heart rate will not increase to the values you normally see when you are doing high-intensity

Below: The heart rate can easily be calculated by feeling for, and taking, your pulse.

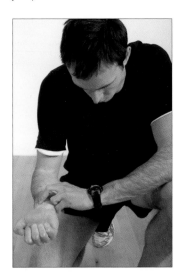

HRZ

To train safely and effectively, you need to establish your correct heart rate zone (HRZ) for the various training levels. To do this, you first need to calculate your heart resting rate (HRR), using this formula:

HRR = maximum heart rate (MHR) – resting heart rate (RHR)

Calculating HRR

220bpm (MHR) – 60bpm (RHR) = 160bpm (HRR)

Your HRZ can be set using percentages of your HRR, using this formula:

HRZ = (HRR x percentage level of intensity) + RHR

Use the formula to work out your heart rate zone (HRZ) for all your training levels of intensity. Most heart-rate monitors will have a facility to set training zones. The watch will flash or make a noise if you go above or below the appropriate zone.

Calculating HRZ (Level 3 high intensity)

75–90 per cent (160 HRR x 75 per cent) + 60 RHR = 180bpm (bottom of L3) HRZ;

(160 HRR x 90 per cent) + 60 RHR = 204bpm HRZ (top of L3 HRZ).

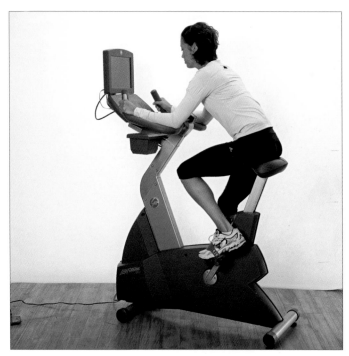

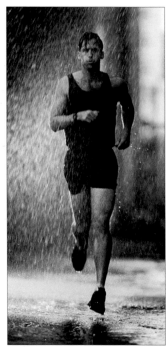

Above: In the gym, many of the machines have heart-rate monitors built into the mechanism.

training, then you may be overtraining. Your body is telling you that it needs to rest – and you should listen to it.

Using your heart-rate monitor regularly in training sessions outdoors is a useful measure of how the weather conditions are affecting your performance. For example, if you are out on your normal cycle route and it is wet and windy, and you are cycling or running directly against the direction of the wind, you may find that you cover the ground slower. Your heart-rate monitor, however, tells you that you are working at the same intensity – if not higher – as you would if there were no wind. This shows that the wind is probably the limiting factor on your time. So, rather than overexerting yourself to beat your previous best time, and in the process increasing your risk of injury, use the heart-rate monitor to keep yourself in the correct zone. If you have not been exercising regularly or you are an athlete

returning from illness, consider using a heart-rate monitor to monitor your heart rate while exercising, that way you won't overdo your first few sessions on the way back to fitness. Avoid letting your heart rate go above 75 per cent of its maximum.

Above: Adverse weather conditions, such as rain or snow, can affect your heart rate.

Below: Cycling against a headwind slows you down and makes you work harder. This causes an increase in the heart rate.

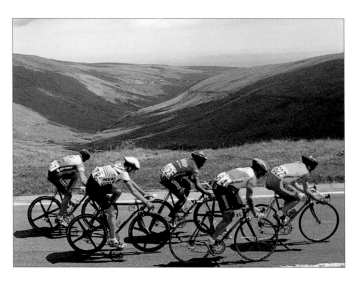

Breathing Technique

There is an art to breathing correctly and getting the most out of each breath.
Good breathing technique will help lower blood pressure, purify the blood, increase
metabolism, improve digestion, promote rapid recovery after exercise and help you to relax.

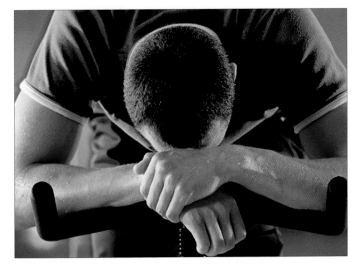

Take a look at a gym full of people exercising and the chances are that you will notice most people resorting to shallow, fast breaths, because they are using only the top part of their chest to breathe. This type of breathing is inefficient and ineffective. Excessive panting is a waste of energy and does not deliver enough oxygen to your lungs. This rapid, shallow breathing may trigger what is known as a 'flight-or-flight' response: your heart rate increases as the heart pumps faster to use what little oxygen it has been given. This increases the stress on your body, which leads, in turn, to poor physical performance and increases the recovery time needed after your training session. Your brain is tricked into thinking you are exercising at high intensity when, in fact, if you were breathing correctly, you would be aware that it is not high intensity at all. Using only the top of the lungs with this type of short, shallow, chest breathing does not make use of the bottom half of your lungs, where

the most efficient exchange of oxygen takes place. It is important to exhale fully before you take in another breath or you simply won't have enough room for the new oxygen to come in.

Above: After strenuous exercise, you will feel less stressed and your recovery will be much quicker if you have been breathing correctly.

Shallow breathing

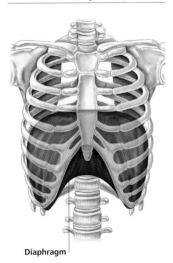

Diaphragm

Breathing exercises

During the week, try to regularly make time for some simple breathing exercises. Remember to keep your posture as upright as possible: relax your shoulders but keep your chest up and make sure your ears, shoulders and hips are all in line to maintain good posture.

If you add these two breathing exercises to your training plan twice a week, you will see the benefits within a few weeks.

Left: When breathing hard during exercise make sure you use the bottom half of the lungs to get maximum oxygen supply to your muscles. The most efficient exchange of oxygen takes place in the bottom half of the lungs. The diaphragm is shaped rather like a parachute.

Emptying your lungs

Breathing out correctly can be likened to emptying your garbage bin to make room for more. You need to empty the whole bin before you start filling it up again. Likewise, you need to empty your lungs completely before you take in another breath.

During any type of exercise, once you have completely breathed out, avoid holding your breath. If you do not breathe in again, you take the risk of depriving the body of oxygen and a dangerous rise in blood pressure. Also, if you are not breathing properly, your performance would be unsatisfactory and you may feel unwell.

After training, slow, deep breathing and slow exhalation can help to relax the body.

Abdominal or diaphragmatic breathing

Practise this technique when you are resting and relaxed, then start to incorporate the technique into your workout sessions. You will soon be able to increase the intensity level of your training session and sustain it at a higher level for longer.

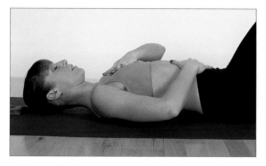

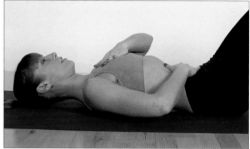

1 *Place one hand on your stomach and the other hand on your chest. As you breathe in, look at your hands. The hand on your stomach should be moving more than the hand on your chest. When this happens, you know you are making good use of the space at the bottom of your lungs.*

2 *Next, take a deep breath in through your nose and out slowly through your mouth. When you think you have breathed out fully, contract your stomach muscles to help empty your lungs completely. Breathing out should take twice as long as breathing in. Repeat this technique for 3 to 4 minutes at a time.*

Bellows breathing

Athletes often use this technique at the start of a competition because, by making the muscles involved in heavy breathing ready for action, it conditions the body to overcome the shock of a sudden demand for more oxygen. This method of breathing can help to combat fatigue, as it releases energizing chemicals to your brain.

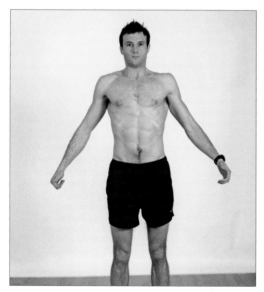

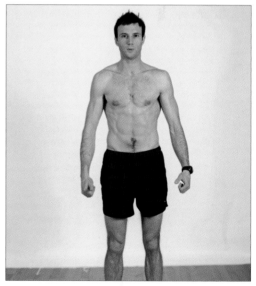

1 *Sit in a chair the first time you attempt bellows breathing because it can cause hyperventilation, and in some cases people may pass out. When you are confident that you can use the technique safely, do it standing up, with your arms out to your side.*

2 *Breathe in fast through your nose and mouth, then breathe out fast through your mouth, using your abdominal muscles to empty your lungs completely. Try bellows breathing for 10 seconds, then increase by 5 seconds each time you practise the exercise.*

Levels of Intensity

Doing the same 30 minutes of cardiovascular exercise every day will not continue to give you the results you need. To prevent your body from getting used to any one style of exercise – and so making it ineffective – you need to vary your intensity levels.

To achieve dramatic results through cardiovascular training, you need to learn more about your training and apply levels of intensity to your training routine. Heart rate is perhaps the best measure of intensity because it indicates how hard your body is working. To get the best results from your exercise routine, follow the four levels of intensity.

Level 1: Steady, long-duration training

This lasts for at least 1 hour. Your heart rate should be between 40 and 60 per cent of maximum and you should be able to hold a normal conversation without effort or panting. If you are new to exercise, this is the level at which you will spend most of your time for the first few weeks. It is the least demanding, but it will start to promote an efficient cardiovascular system. If you are unfit, there is no point in trying to go above

Below: Level 1 is simply walking steadily for about one hour, while still being able to drink and eat.

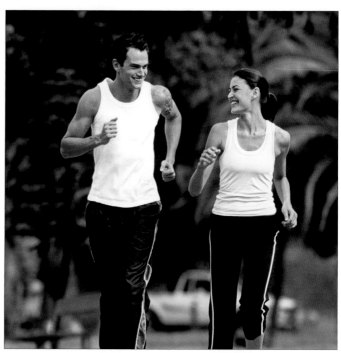

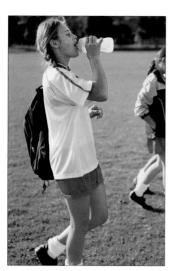

this level quickly, because you will tire too early to get a beneficial session. Walking fast for 40 minutes is far more beneficial than running for 5 minutes and being too tired to go any farther. Top athletes use this level of intensity to begin their warm-ups.

Level 2: Medium-intensity training

You should use this for 15 to 60 minutes of cardiovascular training. Your heart rate should be between 60 and 75 per cent of maximum – a rate at which you can only hold a conversation in short sentences. This level is great for weight loss and improving aerobic capacity without the risk of injury, but you have to make a conscious effort to stay at this level. (Aerobic capacity is the

Above: At Level 2, the pace is faster but still allows joggers to be able to speak comfortably.

highest amount of oxygen consumed during maximal exercise in activities that use the large muscle groups in the legs, or in the arms and legs combined.)

Fat burning myth
It is a myth that to burn fat you need to keep your heart rate low and keep going for a long period of time. In fact, the best way to lose fat is to adjust your intensity to challenge your body by making the exercise much harder, which in turn will burn more calories.

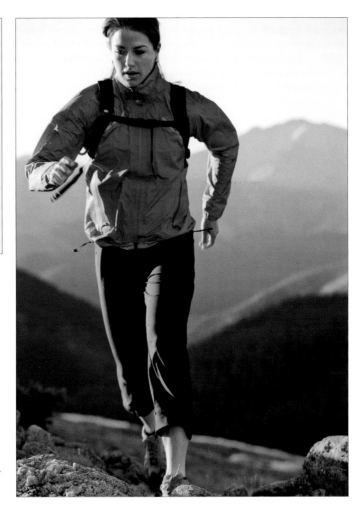

Pyramid of intensity

Imagine a pyramid where the base of the pyramid is Level 1. As you start to go up the pyramid, your level of intensity increases until you are training at Level 4, at the top. The base of the pyramid is wider indicating the amount of time you need to spend at this level of intensity to make your body efficient at coping with the demands of your exercise. If the pyramid has a narrow base, it will be more likely to topple over when you are at the top. This theory applies directly to your training. If you try to train at a high-intensity level without building a good base, you will be prone to injuries and overtraining.

Level 3: High-intensity training

This should last from 1 to 10 minutes, although trained athletes can continue at this level for longer due to their high aerobic capacity. Your heart rate should be between 75 and 90 per cent of maximum. You should only be able to give one-word answers during this type of training as you will be fully focused on breathing in as much oxygen as possible. Athletes often use this level of training in the form of intervals. For

Right: At Level 3, the going gets tougher, with the person running so hard that they start to get out of breath.

Below: The maximum level is Level 4, in which the runner pushes as hard as possible for a short sustained effort.

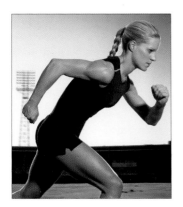

example, 10 minutes at Level 2, then 2 minutes at Level 3, then 2 minutes at Level 2, followed by 4 minutes at Level 3. This is often called Aerobic Interval Training. It is important to vary the duration of the intervals to achieve the best results. This is hard to begin with, but your body will adjust and be able to recover quickly between the intervals. This is the fastest way to develop muscle and increase your fat metabolism.

Level 4: Maximum-intensity training

This should last between 10 seconds and 2 minutes. This level is 90 per cent and above of maximum heart rate.

You will not be able to talk comfortably and you will feel out of breath from start to finish. As with Level 3, this level is used for interval training. For example, after 10 minutes' warm-up, walk for 1 minute, sprint as fast as possible for 30 seconds, then walk for 1 minute and, finally, sprint again for 30 seconds.

Sports people who play in positions that require the maximum amount of speed over short distances should adopt this type of intensity training. Do not, however, attempt to start this extreme type of training unless you have already been doing some reasonably intense training for some time.

Climate and Performance

Temperature, altitude, wind and humidity can all have significant effects on the body's ability to perform. It is absolutely essential that you understand these factors before attempting to train or compete in conditions that could have very serious adverse effects on your body.

One of the biggest factors that can affect your performance when training or competing in sports events is the prevailing temperature.

Your core body temperature is regulated at 37°C/98.6°F. If your body temperature changes by even just a few degrees above or below this level, you will become extremely unwell. Our natural reaction to combat overheating is to sweat. This creates a layer of water on the skin that helps to cool the body. Conversely, if we are too cold, we shiver, which increases muscle activity and in the process generates heat. We can, of course, also help to regulate our temperature by adding or removing layers of clothing.

Extreme heat

Exercising in the heat can be just as dangerous as exercising in low temperatures – and you should never attempt it without a full understanding of all the factors involved and being properly prepared. As soon as the air temperature rises above 32°C/89.6°F, you are entering the danger zone of heat cramps, heat exhaustion or even heatstroke. Heat cramps are similar to muscle cramps, and are caused by exertion and insufficient salts. Heat exhaustion is caused by a lack of the bodily fluids that would normally help cool you down. The signs of heat exhaustion are excessive sweating, pale skin, faster pulse and breathing rates, general weakness, nausea and vomiting. Heatstroke occurs when there is an increase in core body temperature due to a lack of fluids, or when the heat is so extreme that it overpowers your body's cooling mechanism. Too much water is lost via sweating and the volume of blood decreases so that there is less blood flow between the muscles and skin and less cooling, so that the body overheats. The

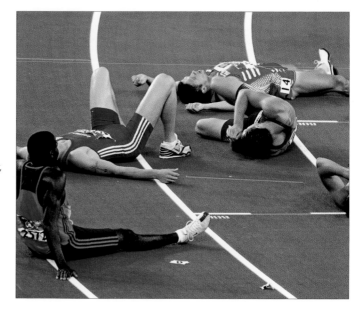

signs of heatstroke are the same as heat exhaustion, with possibly the additional symptom of dilated pupils. Heatstroke can be fatal. To avoid overheating, make sure you do not exercise in extreme temperatures, and avoid dangerous dehydration by drinking plenty of fluids before, during and after exercising. The amount you drink will depend on how hard you are exercising, your weight and the prevailing air temperature.

Wind

Weather conditions such as wind will either help or hinder your performance. For example, if you cycle with the wind

Above: Athletes at the Athens 2004 Olympics lie on the track suffering from heat exhaustion.

behind you, it will help you to go faster. If the wind is blowing toward you, it will slow you down. You should take this into consideration when you are trying to train at certain levels of intensity – there is no point in trying to beat a personal best time if you are cycling or running into a headwind.

Wind will take away the warm air close to your body and replace it with cooler air, lowering your body temperature in the process. The wind

Exercise and high temperatures	
Temperature – °C/°F	**Type of heat injury**
32–40/89.6–104	Heat cramps
40–54/104–129.2	Heat cramps, heat exhaustion, possibility of heatstroke
54/129.2+	Heatstroke very likely

chill factor is a scale that shows the equivalent temperature given to a particular wind speed. In hot conditions, wind will interfere with your body's natural cooling mechanism by drying the layer of sweat on your body that would normally cool you down.

Humidity

The ratio of water in the air at a particular temperature to the total quantity of moisture that could be carried in that air is defined as humidity. It is expressed as a percentage. If the level of humidity is high (30 per cent and above), you will sweat more, but the sweat cannot evaporate, hampering the body's ability to cool itself. This will lead to dehydration and the same problems associated with exercising in hot temperatures. To help overcome high humidity, drink fluids containing essential salts and minerals to keep your body functioning as normally as possible.

Below: When exercising in very cold weather, it is important to keep moving around and to wear adequate clothing.

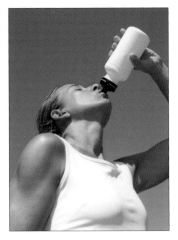

Above: In hot or humid conditions, drink plenty of liquids before, during and after your exercise programme.

Altitude

As altitude increases, atmospheric pressure drops and there is a decrease in the amount of oxygen available. Your maximal aerobic ability is reduced by

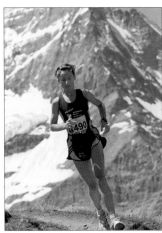

Above: If you run in the mountains, where there is an increase in altitude, you will need a few days to adapt.

1 per cent for every 91m/300ft above 1,372m/4,500ft. To exercise at high altitude, your body will have to go through short- and long-term adaptive changes. At first, you will experience a more rapid breathing rate and increased blood flow when exercising, and you will find yourself tiring very quickly. You may get acute mountain sickness, feelings of nausea, headaches, insomnia, dizziness and muscle weakness.

However, in just one or two days, your body will have adapted. Your resting heart rate will increase, as will your cardiac output (blood flow), in order to compensate for the lack of oxygen. After three to four weeks, your blood haemoglobin level will increase – every drop of blood that supplies the muscle will deliver an increased amount of oxygen. (Haemoglobin is a protein in the blood that contains iron and transports oxygen from the lungs to the rest of the body.)

If you live at high altitude for some time, your body will naturally adapt to the atmospheric conditions by producing more of the myoglobin, mitochondria and metabolic enzymes used for aerobic energy transfer.

However, you can also expect to lose muscle mass and body fat, which may affect your performance.

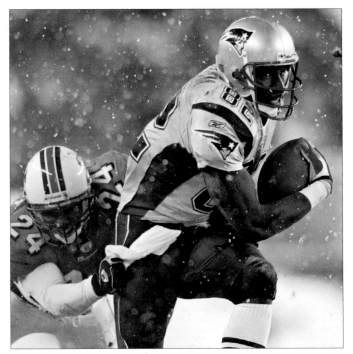

Walking

It's tempting to think that there's nothing to walking beyond putting one foot in front of the other and setting off. True, it is a very accessible form of exercise. However, getting the best from it calls for the right technique, pace, clothing and footwear – and a schedule.

Walking has many benefits. It's free, it's an independent mode of transport and environmentally friendly. It is also a great way to get fit before progressing to harder forms of exercise, such as running or preparing yourself for a bigger goal such as a marathon. Walking at a brisk pace will burn between 300 and 400 calories per hour and because walking has only one-third as much impact as running, it is an ideal form of exercise for people who suffer from bone-degenerating diseases such as osteoporosis.

Technique

Try to focus on a different aspect of your technique each time you walk. It is important to keep your head still with your chin parallel to the ground to eliminate using unnecessary energy. Stand tall when you walk, keep your abdominals and buttocks tensed to keep your spine in a good neutral position, and bend your elbows at 90 degrees. To make your walking workout even more demanding, carry dumbbells or

Below: Listening to the radio or music through headphones will keep you company while you are walking.

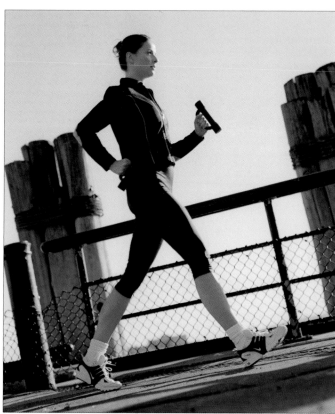

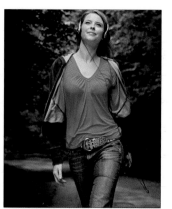

Above: Carrying dumbbells while walking very briskly gives you a much more vigorous workout.

hand weights. The key to walking more efficiently is to increase your stride rate and maintain flexibility in the hips. Your foot should strike the ground with your heel first, before rolling forward on to your toes.

What to wear

It is essential to have the right clothes and footwear for walking exercise. Make sure that you are properly fitted

Walking speed

The following chart will give you a guide to your walking speed. The next time you are walking for an exercise session, try counting the number of strides you take in 1 minute.

Steps per minute	kph	mph
70	3.2	2
90	4	2.5
105	4.8	3
120	5.6	3.5
140	6.4	4

for your walking shoes. There should be a certain amount of comfort to begin with, but be aware that shoes will get more comfortable as the material softens and you wear them in. Therefore, you should buy shoes that are a half to a whole size too large so that you have room for your feet to expand when they get hot. If you are going to walk on the side of the road or on smooth walking tracks, you can wear normal running shoes. However, if you are going off-road, you will need a shoe with ankle support to protect your ankles from turning over on rough terrain. You should also wear several layers of clothing so that you can adjust them as necessary.

Below: Correct clothing and footwear suitable for the weather conditions and terrain are essential.

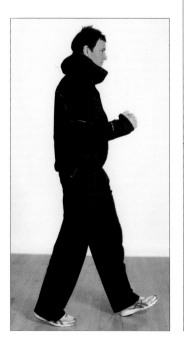

Walking exercises

Follow this six-week walking programme for four days a week, to improve your fitness. Although fast walking has less impact than running, equip yourself with comfortable walking shoes, and wear layers of clothing that you can peel off if you become overheated. The total walking time each week should increase week by week as you progressively get fitter and faster. If you are serious about stepping up your fitness, consider other aspects such as flexibility, core stability, strength and nutrition to get the desired results. After just six weeks of working through these exercises, you should be able to walk across hilly terrain for 60 minutes without stopping. Your recovery should be good enough for you to continue without taking any rests. To avoid dehydration, make sure you take fluids with you if you are out walking for more than 45 minutes.

Time	Intensity/environment
Week 1	
20 minutes	flat terrain
30 minutes	flat terrain, alternating 1 minute fast, 2 minutes slow
30 minutes	hilly terrain
20 minutes	flat or hilly terrain, with hand weights or a backpack

Weekly total: 1 hr 40 minutes

Week 2	
25 minutes,	flat terrain
30 minutes	flat terrain, alternating 2 minutes fast, 2 minutes slow
35 minutes	hilly terrain
20 minutes	flat or hilly terrain, with hand weights or a backpack

Weekly total: 1 hr 50 minutes

Week 3	
25 minutes	flat terrain
30 minutes	flat terrain, alternating 2 minutes fast, 2 minutes slow
40 minutes	hilly terrain
20 minutes	flat or hilly terrain, with hand weights or a backpack

Weekly total: 1 hr 55 minutes

Week 4	
30 minutes	flat terrain
35 minutes	flat terrain, alternating 2 minutes fast, 1 minute slow
40 minutes	hilly terrain
20 minutes	flat or hilly terrain, with hand weights or a backpack

Weekly total: 2 hrs 5 minutes

Week 5	
35 minutes	flat terrain
40 minutes	flat terrain, alternating 2 minutes fast, 1 minute slow
50 minutes	hilly terrain
25 minutes	flat or hilly terrain, with hand weights or a backpack

Weekly total: 2 hrs 30 minutes

Week 6	
35 minutes	flat terrain
40 minutes	flat terrain, alternating 2 minutes fast, 1 minute slow
60 minutes	hilly terrain
25 minutes	flat or hilly terrain, with hand weights or a backpack

Weekly total: 2 hrs 40 minutes

Cross-trainer

The cross-trainer is a highly effective, all-over body exercise that uses a large number of muscles. It offers a great alternative to running and is an excellent way to exercise for people who suffer from back and joint problems.

The cross-trainer is a low-impact alternative that works the same muscles that you use when running, but without the same physical impact of pounding the floor. The action of pushing and pulling with the arms simulates the action of cross-country skiing and hill-walking with poles. It also gives you great upper-body tone. If you are looking to do an all-over body weight-training session, the cross-trainer will provide you with a great warm-up.

Technique

Before you begin exercising on the cross-trainer, check to see if you are in the right position. If your feet are too far apart, your stride may force you to overstretch, which could cause an injury. Adjust the step length until you feel comfortable. Keep your posture upright

Below: Unlike running, the cross-trainer works all the major muscle groups in the body.

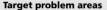

> **Target problem areas**
>
> Change the emphasis of your workout according to the body parts that you want to work hardest. For example, if you want to work your arms, then relax your legs and just let them follow as you drive the machine with your arms. Conversely, relax the arms so you can work the legs.

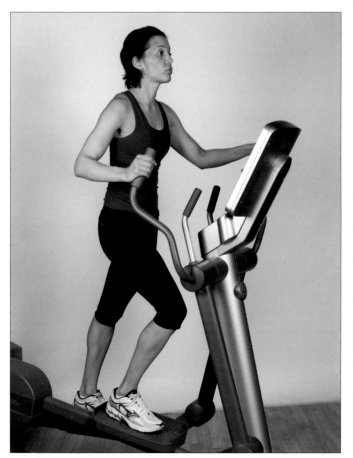

– your back should be straight, your shoulders back, chin up and your core muscles, especially abdominals, switched on to work hard. Try not to let your arms do too much of the work. Instead, really use your legs to drive the machine forward. When your leg drives the foot plate back, ensure that the back of your leg is fully extended to have maximum effect on the muscles at the back of your leg.

Avoid wearing training shoes that have too much grip. Your feet need to be able to move slightly in the shoes to find their natural position as you push down on the footplates.

To make the best use of your legs, resist bending forward when you start to feel fatigued. Bending forward will force your lower back to provide the power to drive the machine, and it will quickly tire. If this happens for long periods of time, you may be at risk of a lower-back overuse injury.

> **Warning**
>
> If you suffer from hip and lower back problems, do not at first spend too much time on the cross-trainer. Start with a maximum of around 10 minutes and gradually build it up, by around 3 to 5 minutes every session, until you are comfortable exercising for about 30 minutes.

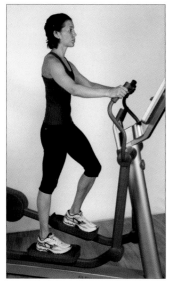

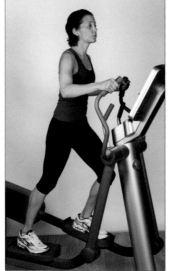

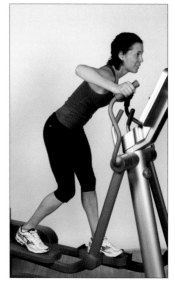

Above: This position is too far back on the cross-trainer to have any significant effect on the muscles.

Above: The ideal position is a straight back, shoulders back and chin up. Let your legs do all the work.

Above: Leaning too far forward will cause strain on the arms and the back and neck will feel uncomfortable.

Getting started

Each cross-trainer will have different resistance or gradient settings. You should adjust these settings depending on your fitness level and weight. Your level should be adjusted depending on the type of training session that you want to do: long and steady to train your endurance; or fast, powerful intervals to increase your aerobic threshold. Rhythm is the key. You should feel as if you are keeping up with the machine or, ideally, you should stay slightly ahead of the machine, rather than losing rhythm and feeling as if you are struggling. To set your training levels, follow the principles relating to levels of intensity set out earlier in the book.

Post injury

If you are recovering from a running injury, use the cross-trainer to do similar training, but without the same physical impact on your joints and muscles, especially after Achilles tendon, feet, knee, pelvic and lower-back injuries.

Cross-trainer exercises

Include the following training sessions in your weekly programme to get the most out of this type of cardiovascular exercise. Check that you are in the correct position on the cross-trainer. Before you begin any of the sessions, make sure you do at least 5 minutes' warm-up at Level 1 intensity, including some stretches for the lower back, quadriceps, hamstrings and calves.

	Fitness level	Distance/time	Intensity
Session 1: aerobic endurance	Below average:	20 minutes	L2 continuous
	Average:	40 minutes	L2 continuous
	Above average:	60 minutes	L2 continuous
Session 2: improved fitness and aerobic capacity	Below average:	4 x 3 minutes	L3 with 3 minutes L1 easy between efforts
	Average:	5 x 4 minutes	L3 with 3 minutes L1 easy between efforts
	Above average:	6 x 4 minutes	L3–L4 with 3 minutes L1 easy between efforts
Session 3: a new level of fitness, and anaerobic workout	Below average:	20 minutes	L2 with 20-second sprints L4 every 4 minutes
	Average:	40 minutes	L2 with 30-second sprints L4 every 3 minutes
	Above average:	60 minutes	L2 with 30-second sprints L4 every 3 minutes

Rowing

Few cardiovascular exercises use the upper body to the same extent that rowing does. Rowing burns 600–1,000 calories per hour, making it one of the most effective exercises for burning calories and losing weight.

As well as giving you an excellent cardiovascular workout, rowing also exercises all the major muscles.

Technique

Hold the handle in front of you, arms straight and in line with the rowing chain. Your body should be curled up toward the front of the machine like a coiled spring. Initiate the pull by driving your legs as if you are doing a leg press. Take your arms with you as you straighten your legs. As your legs straighten, pull the handle in toward your lower chest and abdomen. Pause for 1 second – the recovery phase – then straighten your arms and bring your legs back to the coil position. Take your time in the recovery phase. Check your stroke rate, which will change depending on whether you are doing speed-work intervals or long-distance endurance. Aim for 25–35 strokes per minute. Your breathing needs to be correct, because the large number of muscles used in rowing demand a lot of oxygen. Breathe in as you recover into the coil, and out as you explode back in the pull.

Muscles exercised during rowing

Most of the muscles in your body are used for rowing; the picture below shows the major muscles working. Rowing regularly is a good cardiovascular exercise that is ideal for strengthening your shoulder, arm, abdomen and back muscles.

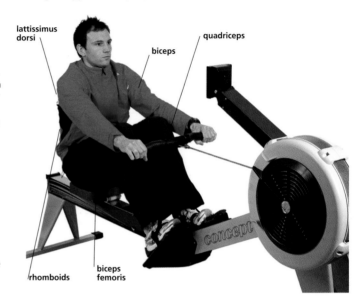

lattissimus dorsi

biceps

quadriceps

rhomboids

biceps femoris

Rowing exercises

Include the following training sessions in your weekly programme to get the most from this cardiovascular exercise. Before any of the sessions, make sure you do at least 5 minutes' warm-up at Level 1 intensity, and because rowing strengthens all the main muscles, it is best to warm them up first with some stretches for the lower back, quadriceps, hamstrings and calves.

	Fitness level	Distance/time	Intensity
Session 1: time trials to help monitor your fitness	Below average:	1km/0.6 miles	L2–L3
	Average:	2km/1.2 miles	L2–L3
	Above average:	2km/1.2 miles	L2–L3
Session 2: improving fitness level and aerobic capacity	Below average:	4 x 200m/219yd	intervals with 60 seconds' rest between each one L3
	Average:	8 x 200m/219yd	intervals with 45 seconds' rest between each one L3
	Above average:	16 x 200m/219yd	intervals with 30 seconds' rest between each one L3
Session 3: improving rowing efficiency and burning calories for weight loss and maintenance	Below average:	2km/1.2 miles	long-distance, steady row L2
	Average:	5km/3.1 miles	long-distance row L2
	Above average:	1km/0.6 miles	long-distance row L2

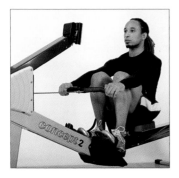

Above: Before starting your rowing exercises, the body is set in a coiled spring position.

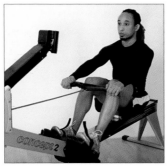

Above: Drive the machine back with the legs, pulling the arms back with you as you begin to straighten your legs.

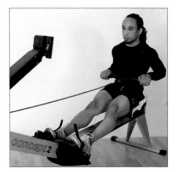

Above: As the legs are extended, pull your arms toward your lower chest and abdomen.

There are a number of technique faults that you should look out for and correct in order to prevent injury and make your rowing more energy-efficient.

Common faults
• Leaning forward as you go into the coil position: keep the back straight and bend your legs more in the coil position so that you don't have to lean forward to get a long stroke.
• Bent arms in the pull phase: correct bent arms by using your legs more. Your legs are approximately five times stronger than your arms, so keep your arms straight until your legs are almost straight, and your legs will do most of the work.
• Leaning back too much at the end of the stroke: leaning back will give you a

Below: Leaning too far forward means that you have to expend far more energy to drive back.

longer pull but can cause lower back injuries. Try to keep your back as upright as possible until you have the core strength to allow you to lean back slightly.
• Grip too tight: a tight grip is fine for short, fast-interval sessions because you get a chance to put the handle down and relax between efforts. However, for longer distances, such as those over 1km/1,094yd, you need to keep your grip relaxed in order to prevent your forearms from getting too tight and cramping. If you are rowing long distances, try changing the position of your thumb. Instead of wrapping it under the handle, rest it on top to use different hand muscles.

Below: Wait for the legs to be fully extended before pulling the arms in toward your chest.

Getting started
If you are using the rowing machine for the first time, start with the below-average fitness sessions (*see* Rowing exercises). After six weeks, move up to the average fitness sessions. Wait at least another six weeks before you attempt the above-average fitness stage. Before you do any of these sessions, start with a 500m/547yd warm-up at Level 1, followed by back, arm and leg stretches.

Set your target
Professional rowers are able to row 2km/1.2 miles in less than 6 minutes. If you are starting out, 8 minutes is a good target to try to achieve for this distance.

Below: Leaning back too much at the end of the stroke can cause injury to your lower back.

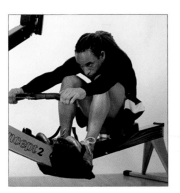

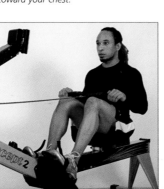

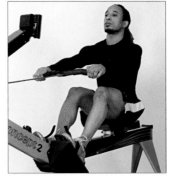

Swimming

For many people, swimming is simply an enjoyable bit of splashing about at the pool or the seaside. Beyond that, though, it can improve your cardiovascular fitness as well as muscular strength without any impact, because it is non-weight bearing.

There are a number of different swimming strokes you can use, which use different muscles. Try to use a combination of strokes to ensure that all your muscles are worked.

Freestyle

Front crawl is usually now referred to as freestyle. The arms are mainly used to get the forward motion, with the legs producing only 10 per cent of the forward energy. However, your legs do play a vital role in keeping your body balanced and in preventing excess drag. Keep your hand slightly cupped as it enters the water and reaches forward

Muscles used in swimming

These are the main muscles used in swimming. Each stroke will place different demands and movement patterns on the muscles. Using these muscles in conjunction with correct technique will improve your swimming.

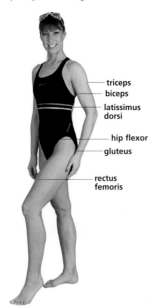

- triceps
- biceps
- latissimus dorsi
- hip flexor
- gluteus
- rectus femoris

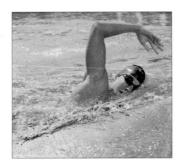

Above: Take a breath as your arm and head come out of the water and before your hand re-enters the water.

and outward to catch the water. Sweep your hand outward and press the water laterally to your body, then sweep your hand in toward your hips. To finish the stroke, press the water down toward your hips, extending your arm as much as possible. On recovery to the next stroke, your elbow leaves the water first. You then reach forward, keeping your elbow high so that you don't slap the water as your hand re-enters it. Keep kicking with your legs at all times.
Tip At mid-stroke, slightly dropping the shoulder of your arm under the water will promote a better stroke and help the opposite arm to recover.

Butterfly

The butterfly is one of the hardest to perfect. The timing of the arm pull and leg kick is essential for a continuous efficient stroke. Your fingers should enter the water first, just as your legs finish their big kick. At this point, your arms should begin to bend as they press laterally, and the small leg kick begins. You then turn your hands and press them toward your body as the small leg kick finishes. You finish the stroke by pushing your hands toward your feet with straight arms, followed by the

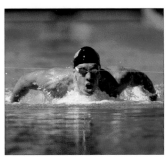

Above: For the butterfly, as you reach forward for the next stroke, your upper body comes up out of the water.

quick exit of the hands from the water and the start of the big leg kick as your arms recover and reach forward to re-enter the water.
Tip Arch your lower back as you do the big kick so that you can help to get your upper body reaching forward for the next stroke.

Backstroke

Your legs are vital in the backstroke and should be kicking all the time below the surface of the water for maximum efficiency. Your little finger

Below: In the backstroke, the arms supply forward movement. One arm is in recovery while the other is in the water.

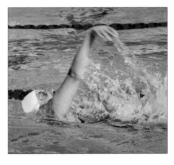

Swimming exercises

If you include the following three sessions as part of your main set of exercises, you will get fitter and faster in the water. Keep a diary of your times and comments to help monitor your improved performance. For the cool-down after you have done the main set of three sessions, choose any stroke you prefer and carry out at least 100m/109yd of easy swimming, focusing on breathing and trying to remain relaxed.

	Fitness level	**Distance/time**	**Intensity**
Session 1: time trials to help monitor your fitness	Below average:	10 minutes' continuous	go as far as you can L2–L3
	Average:	800m/875yd continuous	L2–L3 and note the time
	Above average:	1,500m/1,640yd continuous	L2–L3 and note the time
Session 2: improved fitness level and aerobic capacity	Below average:	8 x 25m/27yd intervals	with 60 seconds' rest between each one L3–L4
	Average:	10 x 50m/55yd intervals	with 30 seconds' recovery between each one L3–L4
	Above average:	10 x 100m/109yd intervals	with 30 seconds' recovery between each one L3–L4
Session 3: improved endurance	Below average:	20 minutes	L2
	Average:	40 minutes	L2
	Above average:	90 minutes	L2

should enter the water first, then your whole arm, with hand cupped to catch the water. Flex your elbow and press the water laterally, then downward, until your hand is just about level with your chest. To finish the stroke, press your hand down toward your feet, keeping it close to your body. When your arm is fully straightened, start the recovery by taking your thumb out of the water first and rotating your shoulder joint, allowing your little finger to enter the water first on re-entry.
Tip Keep your head as flat as possible, with eyes looking up to the ceiling, to minimize drag in the water.

Below: An efficient breathing technique is crucial for a good performance in strokes such as the butterfly.

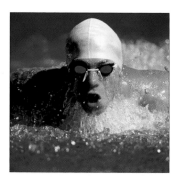

Breaststroke

For an effective breaststroke, it is essential to get the timing of your legs and arms right in order to cover the maximum distance with the least amount of effort. Start by pushing your arms out in front of you to create a forward glide as your legs kick back. Cup the water and press your hands against the water laterally, arms slightly bent, then sweep your hands in toward your chest and start the upward leg movement in preparation for the kick. To complete the stroke, thrust your hands forward to the straight-arm position as the leg kick starts.

Breathing

When you are swimming, breathing correctly takes practice. You should decide which method of breathing works best for you: trickle breathing or explosive breathing. Trickle breathing involves slowly breathing out when your head is down in the water, and then taking a breath in on the recovery as your head comes out of the water. Explosive breathing requires you to hold your breath while your head is in the water, then quickly breathing out and back in as you lift your head out of the water in the recovery.

Warning

Breaststroke can be bad for you if you have a weak lower back, hips or knees, as it involves a strong kicking action in an awkward position.

Getting started

A good swim session should be structured as follows: a good warm-up, main set and cool-down. Doing the technique drills before the main set will remind you what the correct technique should feel like. Before you start, warm-up with 5 minutes of easy swimming.

Below: Good aerodynamic technique is essential to cut through the water in backstroke.

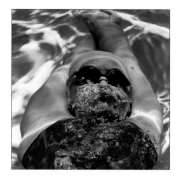

Boxercise

Tense, stressful day at the office? Boxercise is just what you need to work it out of your system. And you don't have to get into the ring to enjoy the benefits of this popular sport. Many sports centres now run boxing-based exercise classes.

Boxercise is a sport that will improve your endurance, speed, power and core stability. It will also strengthen and tone your arms, legs and abdominals. The satisfaction of landing a correct punch will help to alleviate the stress induced by a long day pounding a keyboard or sitting through yet another meeting. It is also a great way to burn up to 500 calories per hour, so it's time to get the gloves on.

Technique

To get the correct stance, stand with your feet just over shoulder-width apart, with one foot slightly in front of the

Muscles used in boxing

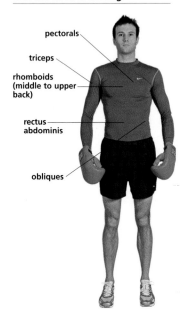

pectorals
triceps
rhomboids
(middle to upper
back)
rectus
abdominis
obliques

The muscles illustrated represent those that are mainly used in boxercise. Some muscles will be used to make the punch while other muscles stabilize the rest of the body making the punch even more powerful.

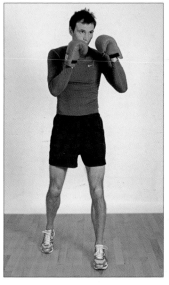

Above: The correct stance when you are ready to attack is feet balanced, with hands raised to protect the face.

other. If you are right-handed, place your right foot slightly behind the line of the left foot, and vice versa if you are left-handed. If you are right-handed, your left hand should be in front. If you are left-handed, your right hand should be in front.

Getting started

Warm up with 5 to 10 minutes of cardiovascular exercise, such as running or rowing, and some light stretches and core exercises to prepare your muscles. You will need a pair of boxing gloves for yourself and pads for your training partner. To avoid injuries, your partner should, ideally, be someone of a similar size to you.

Begin by learning the three different punches – jab, hook and uppercut. Once you have mastered these, slowly build

> **High intensity**
> The level of intensity for boxing is high. Expect to be in Level 3 and 4 for the actual movements of the workout. Between punching combinations, try to take some deep breaths and lower the intensity to Level 2 so that you can recover sufficiently to get enough oxygen to cope with the demands of the next set of combinations.

up combinations to try to make it an exciting workout. Next, you can add some leg exercises, such as squats, lunges and side lunges as you do the boxing combinations to raise the heart rate further and make your legs work harder.

It is important to remember that this is not a contest to see who can hit the hardest. It is, instead, a good way to increase your heart rate to improve your fitness levels and burn calories. To get the most from your muscles, focus on mastering the technique, then you can go on to add speed and power.

Below: When sparring, always hit across at your partner's opposite hand.

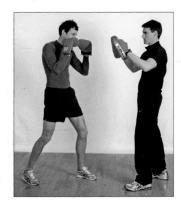

Jab

Though not a particularly hard punch, the jab can be made more powerful by stepping into the punch with a short forward step. To maintain a high heart rate, use the jab more frequently than any other punch.

Watchpoint It is important to control your breathing, especially with long combinations of punches. Experiment to find the best breathing method for you. Try breathing out as you land every third punch, and in before the fourth punch.

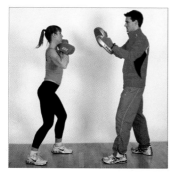

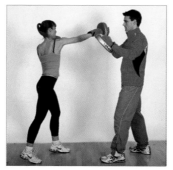

1 *Stand with your feet shoulder-width apart, holding both hands up in front of your face to act as a guard. Your training partner holds the pads out in front of him, at your eye height, his arms slightly bent to absorb the punch.*

2 *With your right arm almost fully extended, throw a quick punch, straight and forward, to make contact with your partner's right pad. Your hand should finish in a horizontal position, the back of your hand facing upward.*

Hook

Aim to get a good follow through with this punch. Use your abdominal muscles to produce a powerful rotation of the body to add extra weight to the punch, and keep them tight to control the follow-through. If your follow-through is too big, you will risk overstretching other muscles, which can cause lower-back problems.

Watchpoint To help prevent wrist injuries, keep your wrists, elbows and shoulders in line at the same height for the jab and the hook punches.

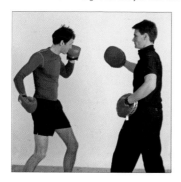

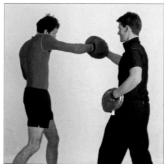

1 *Hold a hand up in front of your face to act as a guard. Your training partner holds the pads out to the side with his palms (face of the pad) facing in toward each other.*

2 *Take your right arm back round to the side of your body and then throw it back around in a semicircle to hit your partner's right pad, with your knuckles pointing forward.*

Uppercut

This is a powerful punch. Due to starting in a lower squatting position, you will use more muscle mass and momentum, so your partner should expect a big impact. Hit upward hard to raise your partner's hand.

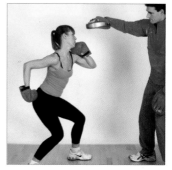

1 *Hold a hand up in front of your face to act as a guard. Squat down slightly by bending both knees. Your training partner stands close to you with the face of the pads facing the floor. Keep your balance throughout the movement.*

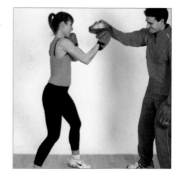

2 *From a bent-arm position, straighten your arms as you straighten your legs, and throw the punch up toward your partner's right pad. Make contact with your knuckles facing away from you.*

Combination punches

Experiment with different combinations of punches. For example, try two jabs with the left hand and then a hook with the right. Having mastered that, try four jabs then a squat, four hooks, a lunge, four uppercuts and a side lunge.

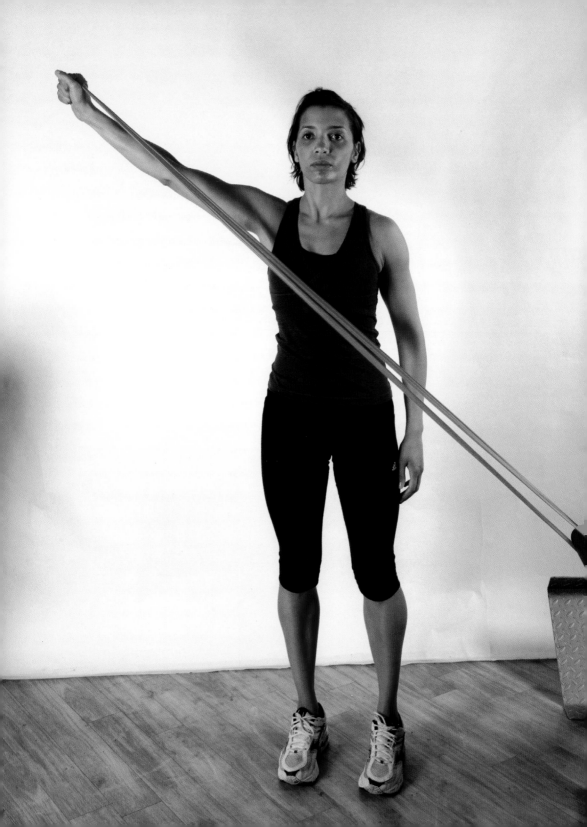

RESISTANCE TRAINING

The benefits of resistance training include weight loss, a faster-acting metabolism and improved body shape. It is particularly good for people who struggle with sustained cardiovascular training. This chapter outlines the muscles involved, and the exercises and techniques that work them effectively and safely. Before you begin, familiarize yourself completely with the exercises and the equipment. To challenge your body and make training fun, make sure to include a variety of exercises in your resistance-training plan.

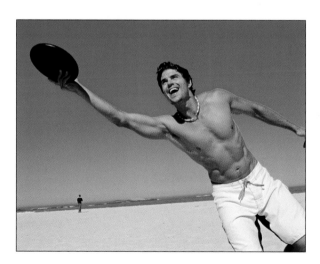

Above: Alternate your time in the gym with fun exercise in the open air.
Left: Correct resistance training will build your strength for different forms of exercise.

Benefits and Principles of Resistance Training

After the age of 30, your metabolic rate starts to decrease every year. Resistance training involves applying resistance to a movement that will not only increase your metabolic rate, but also give you greater strength and more energy.

Resistance training will build muscle and can even reverse the inevitable decline in your metabolic rate. The afterburn (calories expended after exercise) of resistance training will burn far more calories than the afterburn of a cardiovascular session. Knowing that you are still burning calories when you are sitting at your desk, several hours after your training session, is a real bonus.

Resistance training and health
You can build and tone over 600 of your muscles using resistance training; it will help reduce the risk of injury, especially lower back injury, by promoting good balance, co-ordination and posture.

Sports that involve contact, such as rugby or American football, will take their toll on your body. The correct resistance training, however, will give you the strength you need to withstand the impact of the tackle or of falling to the ground. Endurance sports such as running require your muscles to

Below: Press-ups are one of the oldest resistance exercises, but they are still just as effective as ever.

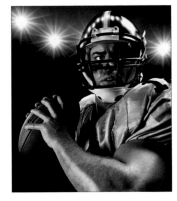

Above: For any sports involving impact, such as American football, resistance training is essential to build muscle.

contract over and over again for long periods of time; resistance training will help give your muscles the strength they need to prevent overuse injuries. Changing your body shape through resistance training will give you improved self-esteem and will motivate you to keep up your training. There are also medical benefits to resistance

training. It will strengthen your bones and reduce the risk of bone degenerating disease such as osteoporosis. Resistance training will also help to lower your blood pressure, lower your resting heart rate, decrease the risk of diabetes, decrease the chance of certain cancers and promote an increase in high-density lipid (HDL) cholesterol, or good cholesterol.

Technique
Start by only using weights that are up to 75 per cent of your One Repetition Maximum (ORM). Each set should consist of at least 12 repetitions and at the end of each set you should feel as if you could do two more repetitions. Do no more than three sets of each exercise to avoid overtraining a muscle

Increase metabolic rate
Having muscle means having more living tissue that is available to burn calories; just in the same way a car with a big engine will burn more fuel than a car with a small engine.

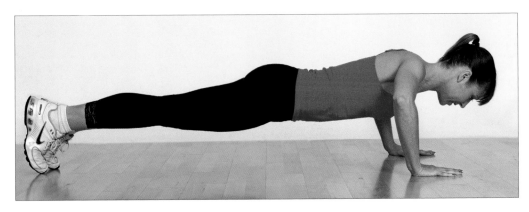

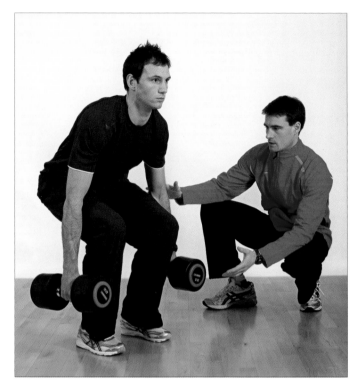

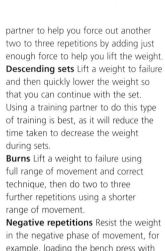

partner to help you force out another two to three repetitions by adding just enough force to help you lift the weight.

Descending sets Lift a weight to failure and then quickly lower the weight so that you can continue with the set. Using a training partner to do this type of training is best, as it will reduce the time taken to decrease the weight during sets.

Burns Lift a weight to failure using full range of movement and correct technique, then do two to three further repetitions using a shorter range of movement.

Negative repetitions Resist the weight in the negative phase of movement, for example, loading the bench press with 100kg/220lb when your ORM is only 80kg/176lb and then resisting the bar as it lowers down to your chest. You may require a training partner to do this, as you will be using a weight that is greater than your ORM. If you don't have a training partner use safety catches to prevent injury.

Below: Cable machines are a very versatile training aid.

Above: Get your trainer or training partner to check your technique while you are exercising.

group. To avoid muscle imbalances and promote good co-ordination, rotate your routine so that you use all your body parts in the week's training. Do not move on to other resistance training methods until you have completed six weeks of basic weight-training. Try to find a training plan that fits in with your goals.

Supersets These will help you to increase the intensity of your workout by decreasing the rest between exercises. This technique involves two exercises with just 5 seconds' rest between each exercise, followed by a 60–90 second rest at the end of a set before repeating.

Exercise opposing muscle groups, such as chest and back, hamstrings and quadriceps or triceps and biceps. This type of supersetting is great if you want to have an express workout

or want to maintain a high heart rate to get cardiovascular benefits and to lose weight.

Pre-exhaustion supersets You may find that when you are working muscles in your upper body, your smaller muscles fatigue before you have worked the bigger muscles; for example, your triceps fatigue before you can work your pectorals hard enough. To combat this employ pre-exhaustion supersets using minimal rest. For example, to work the pectorals superset cable flies and bench presses. Only allow 5 seconds between each exercise so that the pectorals don't get a chance to recover.

Cheating repetitions Lift a weight to failure and then 'cheat' for a further two to three reps. For example, do a set of bicep curls to the point where you can't do another rep using the correct form and then try to do a further cheating rep swinging your upper body to help curl the weights up.

Forced repetitions Lift a weight to failure and then get your training

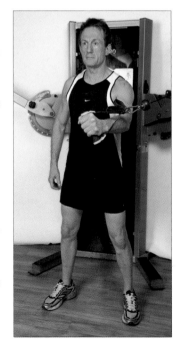

The Muscular System

Many people want to increase their muscle size. However, before you can even begin to think about effective training to achieve that goal, you need to understand how each of your muscles works to enable you to isolate the muscles you want to use.

Muscles are made up of bundles of fibres which are held in place by protective sheaths called fascia. The fibres are then subdivided into myofibrils. They contract when chemically stimulated by the nervous system and extend when the stimulation stops. Weight-training makes muscles grow by increasing the size of the myofibrils, which in turn increases the volume of blood flow to the muscle, the number of nerves that stimulate the muscle and the amount of connective tissue within the muscle cells. Myofibrils are divided again into bundles of myofilaments which are made up from chains of sarcomeres. As you reach the point of fatigue during resistance training, you will get small tears (microtears) in the myofilaments.

Below: The leaner you are, the easier it is to see the muscles you are working during resistance exercise.

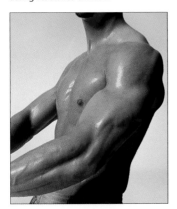

During recovery after exercise your body will repair these small tears by giving the fibres nutrients which will also make these small fibres grow in size. The more exercise you do and the harder the intensity becomes, other

adaptations occur in the muscles. Muscles are able to store more glycogen which will enable the muscles to work even harder in the next workout. This also helps the muscles to slightly increase in size. As you lift a weight and

The muscles of the body

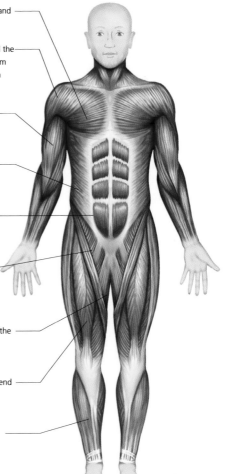

Pectorals these are used to push and pull the arms across the body.

Deltoids these are used to control the movement of the arms, taking them above the head, out to the side, in front and behind.

Biceps these are used to bend the arms at the elbow to bring the hands up toward you.

Obliques these are used to bend to the side and to control the twisting of the upper body.

Rectus abdominis these are used to bend the top half of the body forward.

Hip flexors these are used to lift the upper legs forward and upward.

Adductors these are used to pull the legs inward, toward the body.

Quadriceps these are used to extend and straighten the upper legs.

Tibialis anterior these are used to pull your feet upward, toward your shins.

Visualization
Think about what is going on inside your muscles to help you focus on keeping perfect technique throughout your training session.

cause tension in a muscle, more blood is transferred to that muscle, giving the muscle more oxygen and nutrients to provide energy for hard work.

The muscular nervous system

As you lift a weight and put your muscles under tension your nervous system sends a signal to the sheaths protecting the muscle fibres. This results in the muscle fibres contracting and the weight being lifted. It is important to use good technique in all your resistance training from the start, otherwise your

nervous system will adopt an incorrect sequence of movement, which long-term could lead to you sustaining an injury – and you won't get the desired results from your training. However, if your training is done correctly your nervous system will become even more efficient at telling your muscles when to work. Muscle recruitment is the key to getting stronger.

Right: The more toned you are, the more motivated you will feel about your workouts.

The muscles of the body

Neck muscles (semispinalis capitis muscle) these are used to move the head in a semi-circle from side to side, forward and backward.

Trapezius these are used to lift the shoulders upward and backward.

Rhomboids these are used for pulling movements; they help protect the spine.

Triceps these are used to push and to fully extend the arms.

Latissimus dorsi these are used to pull the arms into the body when there is resistance.

Abductors these are used to pull the legs outward, away from the body.

Gluteus maximus provide strength in powerful movements that involve most of the body. They maintain a connection between the legs and upper body.

Biceps femoris (hamstrings) these are used to bend the legs at the knees and lift them behind.

Gastrocnemius these are used to extend the feet when the legs are straight.

Soleus these are used to extend the feet when the legs are bent at the knee.

Muscular contractions

There are three types of muscular contractions:

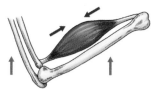

Concentric contraction

The arrows show a decrease in joint angle and muscle shortening. An example of this would be shortening your bicep muscle to bring your hand up toward you.

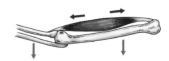

Eccentric contraction

The arrows show an increase in joint angle and muscle lengthening. An example of this would be lengthening of your bicep muscle as it lowers under resistance.

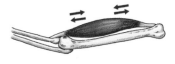

Isometric contraction

The arrows show no change in joint angle and muscle length under constant tension. An example of this would be tensing the abdominal muscles to stay in a fixed plank position.

Muscle Types

Now you know what the muscles of the body are called and where to find them. However, before you head straight to the gym, it is also important that you know what type of muscle you need to help you to achieve your goals.

Your body is made up of more than 250 million muscle fibres. Some muscle fibres consist of a high number of motor units per muscle fibre, such as muscles in the eye, which control small, precise movements. Other muscles, such as the quadriceps, need fewer motor units per muscle fibre, as they control bigger movements.

There are essentially two types of muscle fibre: Type I and Type II. Your genetic make-up does, to some extent, determine your muscle fibre type, but with the correct training and nutrition, you can change the percentage of each type. For endurance sports such as running and cycling, resistance training will give the muscles the strength they need.

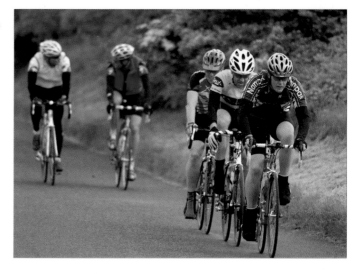

Type I

These are also known as slow-twitch muscle fibres. They are red in colour as a result of their high myoglobin (a protein

Below: Long-distance marathon runners require Type I muscle fibres so they can sustain an effort for a long time.

Above: Cyclists who ride for long distances need Type I muscle fibres so they can keep going for long periods.

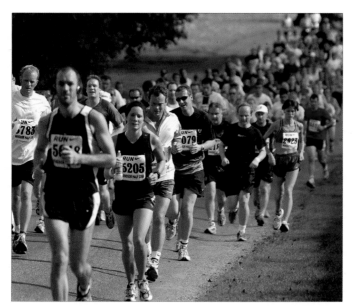

found in heart and skeletal muscles) content and have a high concentration of mitochondria (the 'power plant' of our cells, which use oxygen fat and sugar to release stored energy). A person with this type of muscle fibre is best at long-distance events such as Ironman triathlons or cross-country skiing. People with slow-twitch muscle fibre are likely to be smaller and have an ability to keep going for long periods of time. Type I muscle fibres contract more slowly than Type II muscle fibres, so people with this type of muscle are less good at movements such as throwing a ball fast or throwing a hard, fast punch.

Type II

These are also known as fast-twitch muscle fibres. They are white in colour due to a low myoglobin content and have a low concentration of mitochondria. People with this type

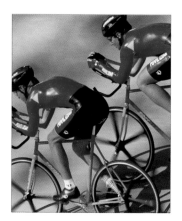

Which type of muscle fibre does your sport require?

This table shows the ratio of Type I muscle fibres to Type II muscle fibres that different athletes are likely to have, and also their VO2 max (ml/kg/min) as an indicator of the level of aerobic capacity they are likely to need for their sport.

Type of activity	Ratio of Type I to Type II	VO2 max ml/kg/min
Cyclist	60–40	60–75
Swimmer	55–45	55–65
Elite distance runner	80–20	70–80
American footballer	40–60	45–55
Ice hockey player	40–60	50–60
Cross-country skier	85–15	75–85
Rower	75–25	50–65
Sprinter	35–65	50–60

Above: Track cyclists need a higher percentage of Type II muscle fibres to pedal faster for short distances.

of muscle fibre are good at shorter athletic events because the muscle fibres contract faster. Power lifters and sprinters need a greater percentage of this type of muscle fibre. People with Type II muscle fibre appear bigger and have a larger amount of muscle mass. Type II muscle fibres can be split further into two subdivisions: IIa and IIb.

Type IIa is similar to a Type I muscle fibre in that it has adapted from being a Type II fibre to be able to assist in endurance events, such as cross-country skiing and marathon running. It is still able to contract fast but also has a well-developed capacity for both aerobic (the body's use of oxygen to generate energy) and anaerobic (without oxygen) energy transfer. This fibre type is more dependent than the others on a ready supply of oxygen.

Type IIb has the ability to work totally anaerobically, or without oxygen, and this athlete is capable of fast contractions using only anaerobic energy transfer.

Training the muscle types

It is possible to train muscle fibre to be of better use to you. For example, if you are a marathon runner, the more long-distance running you do, the better trained your Type I muscle fibre becomes. It is harder to train Type II muscle fibre.

Experiment with low-repetition weight-training on or close to your personal best, or sprint training with short recoveries.

One of the most effective ways of recruiting the fast-twitch muscle fibres is plyometrics training, because it activates the stretch-reflex mechanism of the muscle with an eccentric contraction. Plyometrics uses the acceleration and deceleration of body weight and includes exercises such as jumping and bouncing to enhance neuromuscular co-ordination of muscular movement.

In some sports it is hard to set training plans. For example, tennis requires lots of aerobic training to produce slow-twitch muscle fibres to give the player the endurance to last the entire match. However, this

steady cardiovascular training can interfere with the demand for high power output (fast-twitch muscle fibres) in the actual tennis strokes. Boxing is the same – being able to move around the ring constantly requires lots of endurance training and use of slow-twitch muscle fibres but the ability to give powerful punches means training your fast-twitch muscle fibres.

You should plan out your training sessions carefully, always being clear in your mind which type of muscle you want to train in each session.

Below: Sprinters require a higher percentage of Type II muscle fibres, which contract faster.

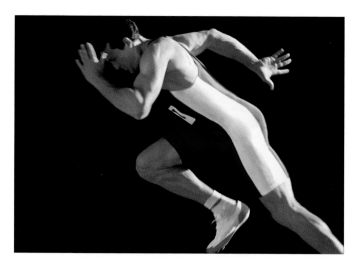

Resistance Training Safety

Every weight room in every gym should have on display a set of rules and regulations pertaining to safety. Make sure that you are fully aware of these rules and don't deviate from them. If you can't see one, ask a member of staff to point you in the right direction.

It is important that you always use the correct technique in all of your workout sessions. Do not copy the bad habits of other gym users who may be taking short cuts to make the training easier. Poor technique is a waste of time and effort because you will not be exercising the right muscles. Good technique, on the other hand, will help to prevent injuries, enabling you to train regularly and achieve your goals sooner. Use lighter weights than you think you might be capable of to start with in order to get your muscles used to the correct movements. Always make sure that you breathe in the correct way; holding your breath during a repetition will cause your blood pressure to rise and, in extreme cases, you could even pass out.

Training partner

If possible, train with another person. Your training partner can monitor and comment on your technique, and help you with heavier weights. If your partner is going to spot for you, make sure that you are both aware of what signal you will give when you are struggling. Your training partner will also need to know

Below: Your trainer or training partner can check your position to ensure that you are exercising safely.

where to stand if he is going to spot for you. For example, in a seated dumbbell shoulder press, he needs to stand behind you and give support to your elbows to help you press the dumbbells up when you are struggling. In an Olympic bar bench press, your partner should stand behind your head, with both hands moving up and down close to the bar, ready to take the bar at any moment; or to help with the press when you start to struggle on the last few repetitions.

Equipment

Wear the correct clothing so that your body temperature does not go down after the warm-up. Have all the equipment you will need for the next few sets ready so that you are not waiting to go from one piece of equipment to the other. This way, you will stay in the right training zone, physically and mentally. Be safe when you are using the equipment – always use collars on the end of barbells and make sure racks have safety catches if you are training on your own. Put the equipment away after you have used it to avoid people tripping up – dumbbells rolling around on the floor are a safety hazard, and safety catches not fully engaged may cause severe injury. Always look to see what condition the equipment is in. Common problems include: dumbbells not screwed together correctly; bench press safety stoppers missing or not aligned correctly; loose foot supports; fraying cables; broken or loose seat supports; loose cable attachments; and slippery floors.

Warm-up

During resistance training, most injuries are caused by an inadequate warm-up and by attempting to lift weights that are too heavy. Warming up lubricates the tissues between the joints and

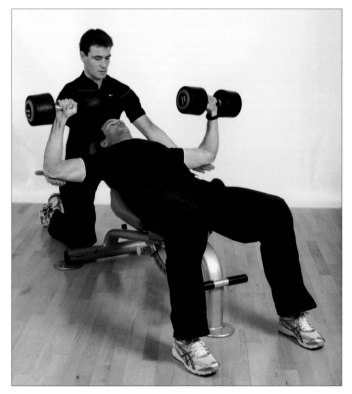

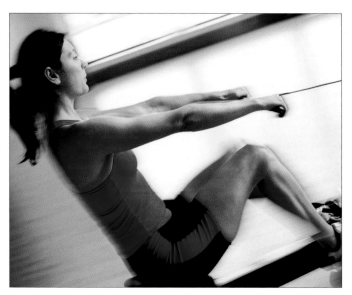

Above: Using a rowing machine is a good way to prepare your body before doing resistance training.

increases the oxygenated blood supply to the muscles you want to work. It is essential to warm up correctly in order to prepare your muscles and joints for action in your exercise session. Wear a

Below: Shoulder press movements are a good way to warm up the upper body before training.

number of layers in the gym to help maintain your body's temperature after the warm-up. You may need three to four layers in cold gyms or winter months. A good warm-up is an indispensable part of your routine for safe training and should never be skipped – even if it means that you have to cut your weight-lifting exercises short.

Below: To prepare for a session in which you will use your legs, stretch the quadriceps beforehand.

Warm-up procedure

Start with a light aerobic exercise such as jogging, cycling or rowing, depending on the body parts that you intend to use in the session. For example, do rowing if you are going to do a heavy session on the back muscles, or cycling if you are going to do a leg weights session.

Exercise for 5 minutes, then build the intensity for a further 5 minutes until your heart rate is up and you start to sweat and you begin to feel slightly short of breath.

For the next stage of the warm-up, simulate the movements you are going to be doing in the workout. For example, do three sets of ten squats if you are planning a leg exercising session, or three sets of ten shoulder presses with no weights if you are planning a shoulder workout.

Follow these exercises with some light stretches on the muscles you want to use, for example a quadriceps stretch for a leg workout and a cross-body shoulder stretch for a shoulder session. Hold each for 30 seconds at a time.

To finish the warm-up, use light weights and high repetitions on the first exercise that you want to do. Do one set of at least 20 repetitions before you move on to heavy weights.

Below: Stretch the shoulders to warm up the upper body in preparation for resistance training.

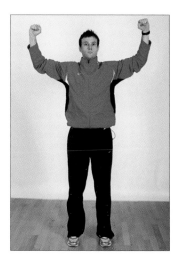

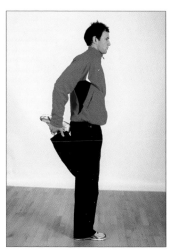

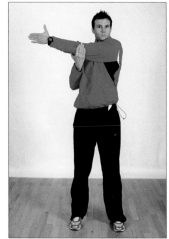

Leg Exercises for Beginners

There are more than 200 muscles in the lower half of the body, so it is no surprise that there are a great number of different leg exercises. To build up your leg muscles safely and effectively, start with these beginners' exercises.

Your legs are five times stronger than your arms because they have to support the body. To get real results from training your legs, you must be prepared to work hard. Take 2 to 3 seconds for each movement. Breathe in at the start of the movement and out as you return to the start position.

Static squat

Muscles used Quadriceps – rectus femoris, vastus lateralis, vastus intermedius

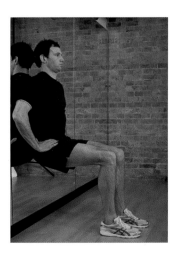

Squat with your back flat against the wall, feet in front of you, knees directly above your ankles, and thighs parallel to the floor. Hold for 60 seconds. When 60 seconds gets easy, make it harder by holding dumbbells.

Beginners' leg exercises	
Exercise	**Sets and repetitions**
Leg press	5 x 8–12
Dumbbell squat	5 x 8–12
Static squat	5 x 20-second holds

Dumbbell squat

Muscles used Quadriceps – rectus femoris, vastus lateralis, vastus intermedius; gluteus medius and maximus

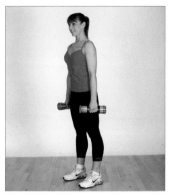

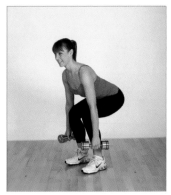

1 *Stand with your feet shoulder-width apart. Hold a dumbbell in each hand, with your palms facing inward.*

2 *Bend your knees until your thighs are almost parallel to the floor. Pause for a second, then push back up.*

Barbell front squat

Muscles used Quadriceps – rectus femoris, vastus lateralis, vastus intermedius; gluteus medius and maximus

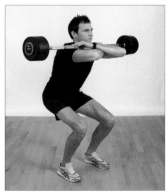

1 *With a barbell across your shoulders (front), squat as for a dumbbell squat.*

Wide-leg power squat

Muscles used Quadriceps – vastus medialis, rectus femoris, vastus lateralis and intermedius; gluteus medius and maximus; abductor magnus

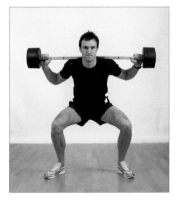

1 *With a barbell across your shoulders (back), squat with your toes at 45 degrees.*

Machine hack squats

Muscles used Quadriceps – vastus medialis, vastus lateralis, rectus femoris

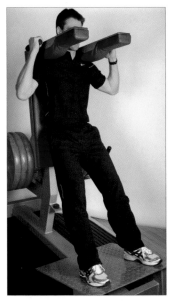

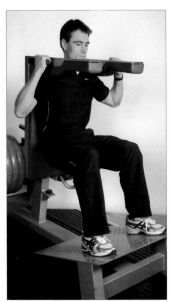

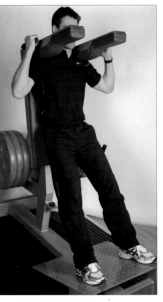

1 *Make sure that your back, shoulders, neck and head are fully supported. Place your feet shoulder-width apart in front of you.*

2 *Release the weight with the handle and squat down, keeping your back flat. With your feet shoulder-width apart, your knees won't go forward of your feet.*

3 *Once your thighs are parallel with the floor, pause for one second, then push the weight back up by straightening your legs.*

Leg press

Muscles used Quadriceps – vastus medialis, rectus femoris, vastus lateralis, vastus intermedius; gluteus maximus; biceps femoris – short head, long head

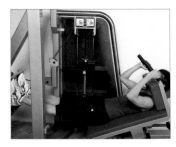

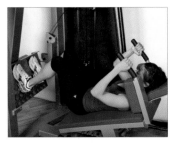

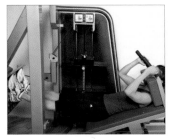

1 *Lie on the machine with your back resting against the back support. Place your feet hip-width apart against the foot support. Focus on tensing the abdominals so that you feel the burn more in that area. Push your weight through the heels to make the quadriceps work harder.*

2 *Carefully release the handle and slowly bend your legs, allowing the weight to come back toward you, until your legs are bent at 90 degrees at the knee. Push firmly down through the heels to get the quadricep muscles working really hard. Try to keep the head and neck relaxed, without any tension.*

3 *Pause for one second and then push the weight back away from you by extending your legs and pressing through your heels. To work your quadriceps, place your feet farther back on the foot plate. To work the hamstrings and gluteus maximus, place your feet farther up the plate.*

Leg Exercises: General

The following exercises use the majority of the leg muscles; they simulate the same muscular movements that you make when you are running, walking or cycling. For athletes wishing to excel, these exercises should play a significant part in your training routine.

You don't have to be a highly competitive athlete to benefit from these exercises. These are also the exercises to do if you simply want to have firm buttocks. The human body – like many large, powerful animals – needs large gluteus muscles (buttocks) to provide power and speed. You don't actually need your gluteus muscles when you are just walking, but as soon as the intensity of the exercise increases, for example when you walk uphill or run, you need them to help extend your hip and keep an upright torso.

The exercises described here will help to train your gluteus muscles and work them in conjunction with your trunk and other lower-body muscles, which will improve your physical performance in your chosen sport.

Many people have weak gluteus muscles because of their sedentary lifestyle. They sit on these muscles but never use them. By putting one foot in front of the other, these exercises simulate everyday sporting movements, especially as they require balance that forces your smaller muscles to act as stabilizers and work in tandem with your core muscles. If the stabilizers around your trunk and lower-body muscles are inactive, you will be prone to injury as the intensity of your exercise increases.

For each exercise, take 2 to 3 seconds for each direction of the movement. Breathe in at the start of the movement, then breathe out as you return to the start position.

Exercises to build powerful buttocks	
Exercise	**Sets and repetitions**
Step-up	5 x 8–10
Bench drop lunge	5 x 8–10
Side lunge	5 x 8–10
Side step-up	5 x 8–10

Step-up

Muscles used Quadriceps – vastus medialis, rectus femoris, vastus lateralis, vastus intermedius; gluteus medius and maximus

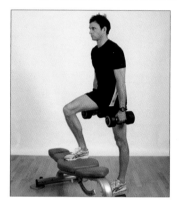 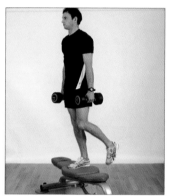

1 With a dumbbell in each hand, place one foot on the aerobics step (or bench). The slower you carry this out, the harder you work the quadriceps.

2 Step up to your full height. Hold the opposite foot in the air to work your leg harder. Pause for 1 second then slowly step back down.

Side step-up

Muscles used Quadriceps – rectus femoris, vastus lateralis, vastus intermedius, vastus medialis; adductor – longus, magnus; gluteus medius and maximus

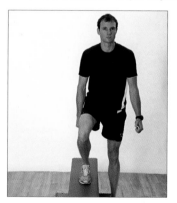 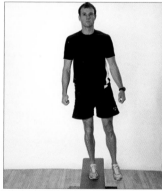

1 Stand side-on to a bench (or aerobics step), with your arms by your side. Place the near foot on the bench.

2 Step up to your full height, pause, then slowly lower yourself back down, using your quadriceps to control the fall.

Static lunge

Muscles used Quadriceps – rectus femoris, vastus lateralis, vastus intermedius, vastus medialis; gluteus maximus

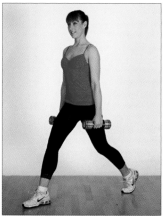

1 *Stand with one foot in front of the other, roughly 60cm/2ft apart, with both feet facing forward, and your body weight suported evenly between your feet. Your back heel will be raised off the floor. Hold a dumbbell in each hand. Keep your hips level, your back straight and your shoulders back.*

Bench drop lunge

Muscles used Quadriceps – rectus femoris, vastus lateralis, vastus intermedius, vastus medialis; gluteus maximus

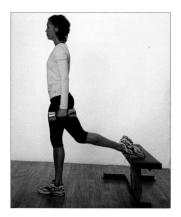

1 *Standing with your back to a bench, with a dumbbell in each hand and your feet roughly 60cm/2ft apart, place one foot up on the bench behind you, with the top of the foot downward.*

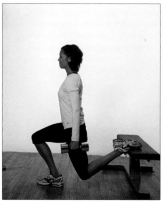

2 *Slowly lower yourself by bending both legs until your front leg thigh is parallel with the floor. Try to get your back knee as low as possible for the best stretch. Pause for 1 second, then push back up.*

Side lunge

Muscles used Quadriceps – rectus femoris, vastus lateralis, vastus intermedius, vastus medialis; gluteus maximus and medius; adductor – longus, magnus; gracilis; pectineus

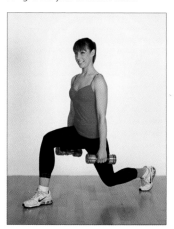

2 *Slowly lower yourself by bending both legs until the thigh of your front leg is parallel with the floor. Pause for 1 second, then slowly push back up to the start position. Keep your chest out to help isolate the legs during the lunge.*

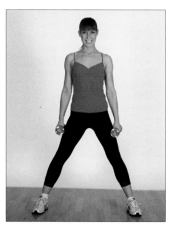

1 *Stand with your feet wide apart and your back straight. Keep your arms straight, your hands just touching the tops of your thighs. Hold a dumbbell in each hand. Keep your abdominals tensed all the time.*

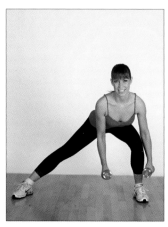

2 *Lunge sideways, shifting your weight behind the bent leg, tensing the abdominals to support the lower back. With the thigh of the lunging leg parallel to the floor, pause for 1 second, extend the leg, then push yourself back to the start position.*

Leg Exercises: Thigh Muscles

There are three sets of strong muscles in your thigh: quadriceps at the front, hamstrings at the back and adductor muscles on the inside. All of these have to work hard when you work out, and you can fully expect to feel like your legs are on fire following these exercises.

Whenever you start to accelerate with a longer stride or to lunge to one side, you are using your inner and outer thigh muscles. These muscles, which are known as the adductors and abductors, help to stabilize your body. For example, if you run and you have lots of lateral movement in the hips, it may cause a snaking effect in your spine, which can lead to back pain. In any case, you want to transfer all your power into going forward, not sideways. When riding a bike, you want all your leg power to go down through the chain to give you more forward speed. When hitting a golf ball, you want good hip stability to allow you to rotate and strike it with as much power and speed as possible.

The following exercises work a number of inner and outer thigh muscles together. There is no time for them to relax – when one is working, the other is acting as a stabilizer. While training these muscles, always contract your core muscles to help isolate the inner and outer thigh muscles you want to work. Be careful when starting your adductor and abductor routine. Begin with a light weight and work up. Don't ignore pain when training these muscles, as you could injure yourself.

For each exercise, take 2 to 3 seconds for each direction of the movement. Breathe in at the beginning of the movement, and breathe out as you return to the start position.

Exercise plan for abductor/ adductor strength and toning	
Exercise	**Sets and repetitions**
Lunge	3 x 20
Side lunge	3 x 20
Cable abduction	3 x 20
Cable adduction	3 x 20
Machine abduction	3 x 20
Machine adduction	3 x 20

Cable hip abduction

Muscle used Gluteus medius

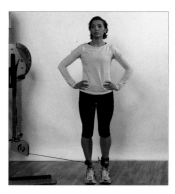 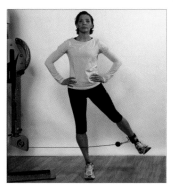

1 *Stand side-on to the cable machine with feet hip-width apart. Attach an ankle strap to the outside leg. Keep the emphasis on the sides of the buttocks throughout the movement.*

2 *Slowly raise the outside leg as far out to the side as possible. Pause for a second, then slowly lower it back down. Doing the exercise slowly ensures that the gluteus is working hard.*

Cable adduction

Muscles used Adductor – longus, magnus; pectineus; gracilis

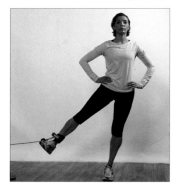 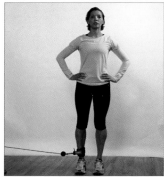

1 *Stand on one leg side-on to the cable machine. The other leg is raised in the air, attached to the cable by an ankle strap. Keep your upper body as still and upright as possible by tensing the abdominals.*

2 *Adduct the attached leg until the legs are together. Pause then lower the weight by taking your leg back out to the start. Start with a weight that is lighter than you think you can manage and then work your way upward.*

Machine abduction

Muscles used Gluteus – medius
and maximus

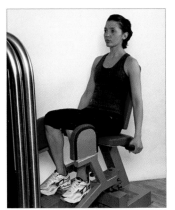

1 *Place your legs against the leg pads.
Hold on to the handles to keep yourself
firmly positioned in the seat. If you
change the angle of your upper
torso by adjusting the back pad
angle you can focus the exercise on
different muscles.*

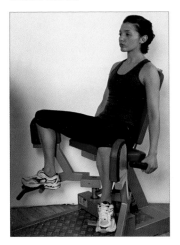

2 *The more vertical the back pad, the
more your gluteus maximus will work,
and the more angled the back pad, the
greater the emphasis on the gluteus
medius. Tense your gluteus and spread
the legs as far apart as comfortable.
Pause for 2 seconds, then slowly bring
your legs back together, while resisting
the weight.*

Machine adduction

Muscles used Adductor muscles – brevis, longus, magnus;
pectineus

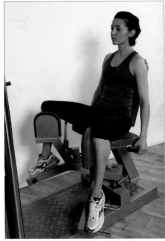

1 *Place your legs into the leg pads and
tense your core muscles to keep your
torso motionless. Hold the handles to
keep yourself in the seat while you do
the exercise. Take this exercise slowly
to begin with.*

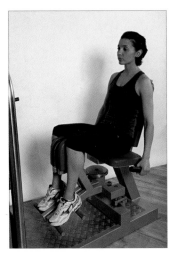

2 *Push in your legs until they meet. Pause
for 2 seconds, then slowly allow them to
be pulled back out, still tensing your
muscles to create resistance. If you have
never worked these muscles before, it will
take some time to build them up.*

Elastic abduction

Muscles used Gluteus – medius, maximus

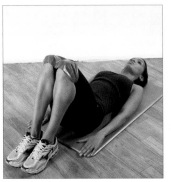

1 *Lie on your back with the legs bent up
at 90 degrees and your feet flat on the
floor in front of you. Place an elastic
strip around your knees and tie it in
a secure knot. Tense your abdominals
so that you can keep your back flat
on the floor.*

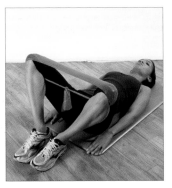

2 *In this exercise, to make your buttocks
work even harder, do a hip raise before
you move your legs apart. Tense the
gluteus muscles and spread the knees as
far apart as possible. Pause for 2 seconds,
then slowly return to the start position,
keeping the abdominals tense.*

Leg Exercises: Calf Muscles

Every time you step forward, you use your calf muscles. For faster activities, such as running and sprinting, strong calf muscles are essential. They maintain your forward motion and provide good strength and stability for the other muscles in your legs.

People often skip calf-strengthening exercises because they think they are dull. This is a mistake – you will not perform at your best with weak calves. Also, you will be prone to injury, particularly Achilles' injuries. Bodybuilders often say they can't be bothered with training their calves because they believe they can't build them up. The main reason for this is that calf muscles are small and it takes a lot of patience to see the gradual improvements in size and definition through the appropriate training. If this is the case for you, take time in your workout and make your calves a priority – even try putting calf exercises at the start of your workout for a few weeks.

Training the calf muscles

There are three muscles that flex and extend the foot to make up the calves. These are: the tibialis anticus, which runs down the front of the shin and contracts to flex the toes toward the knee; the gastrocnemius, a long, wide muscle that connects the bottom part of your upper leg to your heel (it flexes to extend your toes when your leg is straight and contracts to flex all of the muscles in the back of the leg); and the soleus, a shorter muscle that connects to the upper part of the shin and the heel, and works mainly when the leg is already bent at 90 degrees.

If you have been training your calves and seeing no improvement, try changing your routine. To get a better training effect, change the repetition range each time you train them. One day, do 6–10 reps with a heavier weight and, on another day, do 20–30 reps on a lighter weight. Try holding the weight for 3 seconds at the top of each peak contraction to make the calf muscles work even harder. But don't overtrain them and leave at least a day's rest between calf

sessions – otherwise your progress will come to a halt. Also, be careful not to train the calf muscles first if you also want to include bigger leg-muscle exercises in your routine. You need your calf muscles to be fresh if they are to provide enough support and stability when your bigger muscles are working.

Always stretch your calves to prevent them becoming tight and affecting the Achilles' tendon. If you do suffer from tight calves, do some regular stretching and have them massaged before this leads to injury. Stretching the calves can actually make them

bigger and give them a more ripped look. For each of these exercises, take 2 to 3 seconds to carry out each direction of the movement. Breathe in at the start of the movement, then breathe out as you slowly return to the start position.

Exercise plan for stronger calf muscles	
Exercise	**Sets and repetitions**
Double-leg calf raise	3 x 20
Calf press	3 x 20
Seated single-leg calf raise	3 x 20

Double-leg calf raise

Muscles used Triceps surae – gastrocnemius medial head, gastrocnemius lateral head, soleus

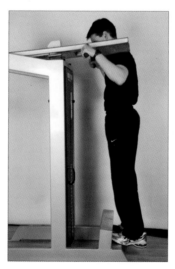 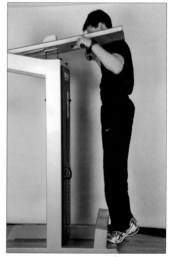

1 Stand on the edge of a step on the balls of your feet. Hold on to the handles for balance. Tense your core muscles and the tops of your legs to keep your body in a straight line. Lower your heels below the line of the step.

2 Pause for a second, tense your calf muscles as much as possible and raise your heels as high as you can above the step. Pause for 2 seconds in this position, then lower yourself back down to the start position.

Calf press

Muscles used Triceps surae – gastrocnemius medial head, gastrocnemius lateral head, soleus

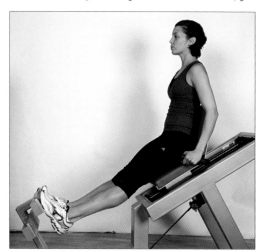 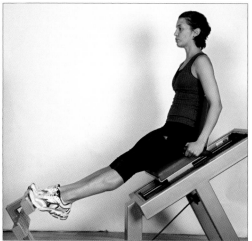

1 *Sit in the calf-press machine, with the back straight and head in line. Hold the handles and place the balls of your feet up against the edge of the leg press plate. To put emphasis on the calf muscles, keep the whole leg as straight as possible and tense your core muscles to keep your back flat.*

2 *Keeping your calf muscles tense, press the plate away from you. Pause for 2 seconds, then slowly relax your calves. Repeat the exercise six to ten times. To make this exercise more demanding and to make sure you have equal strength in both legs, try using one leg only.*

Seated single-leg calf press

Muscles used Triceps surae – gastrocnemius medial head, gastrocnemius lateral head, soleus

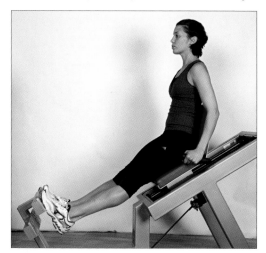 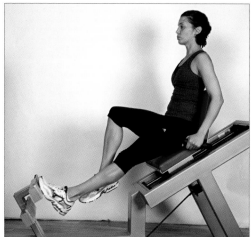

1 *Sit in the calf-press machine, with the back straight. Hold the handles and place the balls of your feet up against the edge of the leg press plate. Straighten your legs and tense your core muscles to keep your back flat.*

2 *Take one leg off the plate, straighten the other, tense your core muscles and your calf muscle, and press the plate away from you. Pause for 2 seconds and slowly relax your calf. If you can do 50 repetitions, you have good calf strength.*

Chest Exercises: Bench Press

The chest muscles are large muscles that cover the upper section of your ribs called the pectorals. They help to drag the upper arm forward via a tendon extending from the side of the upper arm bone to the pectoral muscle.

Bench pressing is the most common chest exercise and is a good exercise for building a bigger chest. There are several variations of the bench press that will help to tone and shape your pectorals. Bench press exercises, however, will only help build the lower and outer edges of the pectoral muscles.

To get the inner and upper parts of your chest working well, and give you good symmetry, you will need to do other exercises.

Top bodybuilders believe bench presses are the key to developing a strong, well-developed chest. There is no doubt that they do bring out the size in the chest and so it is no surprise that they are often referred to as the 'meat and drink' of all upper-body exercises.

Don't try to take the bar too low when doing the bench press or else other muscles will have to work, not just your chest muscles in isolation. Taking your elbows just past the line of your body is enough. As you press the weight back to the top, try to keep your chest as big as possible and force your pectorals to contract as much as possible.

Changing the angle of the position you are pressing from will help to work different parts of the chest. Putting the bench into an incline position will isolate the top part of the chest. It will also make the front of your shoulders work hard to create a strong connection between your chest and shoulders. Putting the bench into a decline bench position will work the lower

part of your chest and your upper-back muscles, forcing a good connection between the chest and back muscles. If the bench press is going to be the biggest upper-body exercise in your routine, do it first, so that all your stabilizing muscles are fresh and can help support your chest muscles. Make sure it has been at least 48 hours since you last trained your triceps, because they can tire fast when you are doing bench presses.

For each exercise take 2 to 3 seconds for each direction of the movement. Breathe in at the beginning of the movement, and breathe out as you return to the start position.

Bench press exercises for bigger chest muscles	
Exercise	**Sets and repetitions**
Incline press	5 x 6–8
Decline press	5 x 6–8
Bench press	5 x 6–8
Incline press	3 x 20+ less than 60 seconds' rest between sets
Decline press	3 x 20+ less than 60 seconds' rest between sets
Bench press	3 x 20+ less than 60 seconds' rest between sets

Bench press

Muscles used Pectorals major; anterior deltoid; triceps brachii – medial head and long head

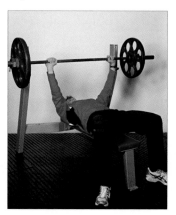 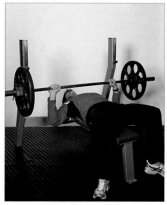

1 Lie on a bench with the head back and the feet on the floor. Grip the bar in both hands and hold it above you, in line with the middle of the chest. Grip it with your hands slightly wider than shoulder-width apart, palms facing outward. Keep the bar in line with your chest and not your shoulders or you might cause yourself an injury.

2 With straight arms, lower the bar down to your chest, bending your elbows to the side. Keep lowering until your elbows are at 90 degrees. Pause for 1 second, then raise the bar to the start position, keeping your abdominals tense. The bar should come down low enough to work your chest, and as you press it back up, push your chest out to make it work harder.

<table>
<tr><td>

Narrow grip bench press

Narrow grip bench press is a variation of the bench press. This involves holding the bar with your hands no more than 15cm/6in apart; this will work the inner pectorals and triceps.

</td></tr>
</table>

Incline press

Muscles used Pectorals major; anterior deltoid; triceps brachii – medial head and long head

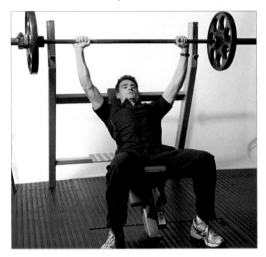 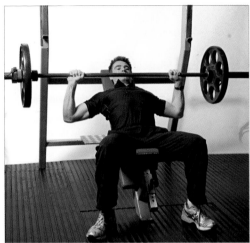

1 *Adjust the bench to a 45-degree incline. Lie on it and grip the bar, your palms facing your feet. Keep your feet flat on the floor. Hold the bar vertically above the top half of your chest. Rest your head on the bench and keep your back flat.*

2 *Lower the bar, taking your elbows out to the side until they are at 90 degrees. Pause for a second, then raise the bar to the start position. Tense your abdominals throughout the movement to help maintain a flat back.*

Decline press

Muscles used Pectorals major; triceps brachii – medial head, long head

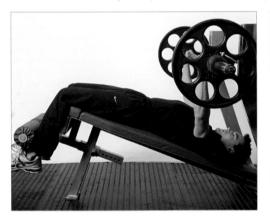 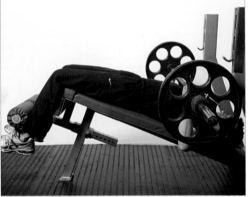

1 *Adjust the bench to a 30-degree maximum decline. Lie on it with your legs hooked over the end to prevent sliding. Grip the bar with your palms facing toward your feet, your hands slightly wider apart than shoulder width. Hold the bar vertically above the lower half of your chest. Rest your head on the bench. This exercise is good for outlining the bottom of the chest. Keep the bar in line with the bottom of the chest and don't allow the shoulders to take over.*

2 *Gripping the bar firmly, lower it toward your chest, taking your elbows out to the side until they are at 90 degrees. Pause for 1 second, then raise the bar to the start position. Tense your abdominals throughout the movement to help maintain a flat back. Try to prevent your shoulders from rising up, which has the effect of tensing your neck muscles. In this way you will be able to place greater emphasis on your chest muscles.*

Chest Exercises: Dumbbell Presses

Dumbbell chest press exercises are similar to bench presses using the same muscles. However, you can go lower with dumbbells because there is no bar directly in front of the chest, thus providing a longer range of movement and a more intense workout for your chest.

The movement involved in dumbbell presses also enables the weight to progress from straight above the chest and out to the sides, making it a more effective exercise to develop the entire set of pectoral muscles.

Many bodybuilders believe they get faster results when they use dumbbells. Because dumbbells have to be balanced to carry out chest press exercises, this involves having to recruit all your stabilizing muscles so that you can control the movement of the dumbbells. As a result, your stabilizing muscles will develop better.

Always have a training partner with you when you are doing heavy dumbbell presses, as you can never tell when you may suddenly weaken, especially as one

arm might prove to be stronger than the other. (The dumbbells will reveal if one side of your body is weaker than the other.) Avoid big increases in weights to prevent injury and always be in control of the movement.

For each chest exercise, take 2 to 3 seconds for each direction of the movement. Don't forget your breathing: breathe in at the beginning of the movement and breathe out as you return to the start position.

Chest building session for beginners

Try doing supersets: pair up two exercises and switch from one exercise to the other with only 5–10 seconds' rest between sets. To get a really good workout, try doing the sets and repetitions twice weekly.

Exercise	Sets and repetitions
Bench press	3 x 8–12
Dumbbell chest press	3 x 8–12
Incline bench press	3 x 8–12
Decline dumbbell press	3 x 8–12

Dumbbell chest press

Muscles used Pectoralis major; triceps brachii; anterior deltoid

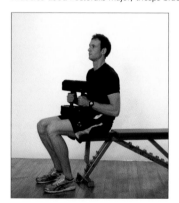 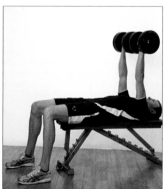 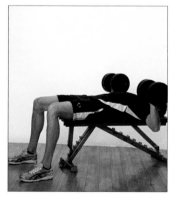

1 Sit on the end of the bench with your feet firmly on the floor in front of you. Hold a dumbbell in each hand, resting on top of your thighs, palms facing toward each other. Keep the dumbbells in line with the middle of the chest. Slowly lie back, taking the dumbbells with you. Tense your abdominals to maintain a flat back.

2 Hold the dumbbells with straight arms above your chest, your palms facing your feet. Keep your feet on the floor, on the bench or in the air, with your legs at 90 degrees. Relax your head and rest it on the bench. Work the chest harder by pushing it out on the return phase. If you need to, rest in between chest presses.

3 Lower the weights, taking your elbows out to the side until they are at 90 degrees. To prevent injury, and isolate the chest and triceps, don't let your elbows go lower than 90 degrees. Raise the dumbbells to the position in step 2. The forearms should always be perpendicular to the ground. Continue with your planned repetitions.

Incline dumbbell chest press

Muscles used Pectoralis major; triceps brachii – long head, medial head; anterior deltoid

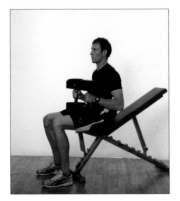

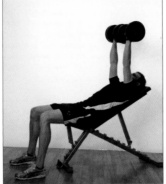

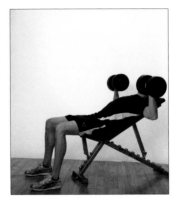

1 *Adjust the bench to a 20- to 60-degree incline. Sit on the end of the bench with your feet on the floor. Hold a dumbbell in each hand, resting on your thighs, your palms facing toward each other. Tense your abdominals throughout the movement to help keep your back flat.*

2 *Lie back, placing your head on the bench, and hold the dumbbells with straight arms above the top half of your chest, with your palms facing your feet. The raising movement here should be slightly rounded as if you are hugging a tree. Your back should be flat against the bench.*

3 *Lower the dumbbells, taking your elbows out to the side, keeping your forearms perpendicular to the ground, until your elbows are at 90 degrees. Pause for 1 second, then raise the dumbbells to the position in step 2. Keep them in line with the upper half of the chest for emphasis on the pectorals.*

Decline dumbbell chest press

Muscles used Pectoralis major; triceps brachii – long head, medial head

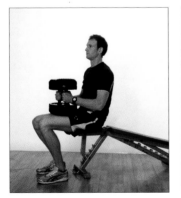

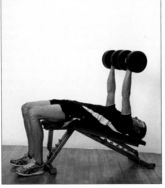

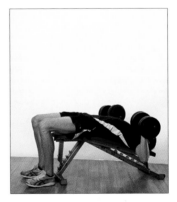

1 *Adjust the bench until it is at a 20- to 60-degree decline. Sit on the end of the bench with your feet placed firmly on the floor. Hold a dumbbell in each hand, resting on the top of your thighs, your palms facing toward each other. Lower yourself down slowly into the decline to give you an opportunity to work your abdominals.*

2 *Hold the dumbbells with straight arms above the lower half of your chest, with your palms facing your feet. Place the head against the bench and hook your legs over the end of the bench, or keep your legs straddling the bench, so that the feet are on the floor. Slowly raise the dumbbells upward above the upper chest so that the arms are straight.*

3 *Lower the dumbbells, taking the elbows out to the sides. Keep your forearms perpendicular to the ground, until your elbows are bent at 90 degrees. Pause for 1 second, then raise the dumbbells to the position in step 2. At the end of the movement, for more emphasis, squeeze the bottom of your pectorals up and together.*

Chest Exercises:
Body Weight-training

There are a variety of chest exercises you can perform using just your body weight. The principal advantage is that you can retain the firm chest you developed in the gym even when you are on holiday or travelling on business.

It is possible to work your chest muscles without going to the gym, and simple press-ups are very effective. Press-ups from different angles work different parts of the pectoral muscles and

can be incorporated into outdoor workouts using park benches. To work the stabilizing muscles surrounding your chest harder, use fit balls and medicine balls.

For each exercise, take 2 to 3 seconds for each direction of the movement. Breathe in at the start of the movement and out as you return to the start position.

Press-up

Muscles used Pectoralis major; anterior deltoid; triceps brachii – medial head, long head

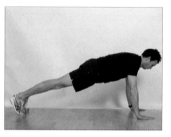

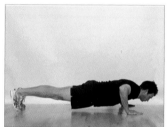

1 *Place your hands on the floor, just over shoulder-width apart, your feet behind you, hip-width apart, elbows in line with your chest. Tense your core muscles and keep your head in line with your spine.*

2 *Keeping your abdominals tight, lower yourself toward the floor, taking your elbows out to the side until your chest is one fist from the floor. Pause for a second, then return to the start position.*

Decline press-up

Muscles used Pectoralis major; triceps brachii – medial head and long head

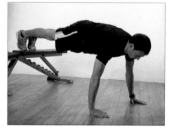

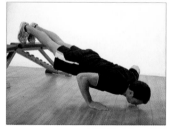

1 *Place your hands on the floor, just over shoulder-width apart, core muscles tense, feet behind you on the bench, hip-width apart, elbows in line with your chest. Keep your head in line with your spine.*

2 *Lower yourself toward the floor, taking your elbows out to the side until your chest is one fist from the floor. Pause for a second, then return to the start position.*

Incline press-up

Muscles used Pectoralis major; anterior deltoid; triceps brachii – medial, long head

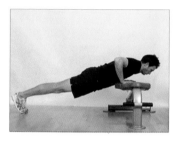

This is a simple variation on the standard press-up. The start position is exactly the same except that you place your hands on an aerobic step instead of on the floor. Then lower yourself toward the step, taking your elbows to the side. Pause for 1 second, then return to the start position. To make sure that your chest does the work, don't push back behind you, and keep your chest up above the bench. Keep the core muscles tensed to hold the straight body position throughout the movement.

Knee press-up

If you haven't done press-ups before, don't press up completely from your arms, start by doing them balancing on your knees. Gradually increase the angle at the back of your knees as you get stronger and can support yourself fully on your arms. This method is recommended for women.

Fit ball press-up

Muscles used Pectoralis major; anterior deltoid; triceps brachii; serratus anterior; abdominals; gluteus

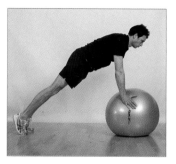

1 *Place your hands on the fit ball. Keep your arms straight, your feet behind you, hip-width apart, and your head in line with your spine. Tense your core muscles to keep your body straight. Turn your hands outward at 45 degrees to avoid wrist injuries.*

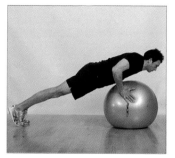

2 *Slowly lower your weight, taking your elbows out to the side until they are bent at 90 degrees. Pause for 1 second, then return to the start. Take extra care, or avoid this exercise if you have weak wrists.*

Chest exercises with little equipment

Exercise	Sets and repetitions
Double-hand medicine ball press-up	3 x 10
Single-hand medicine ball press-up	3 x 10
Decline press-up	3 x 10
Press-up	3 x max
Incline press-up	3 x max

Single-hand medicine ball press-up

Muscles used Pectoralis major; triceps brachii; abdominals

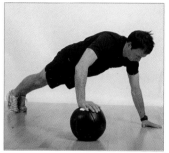

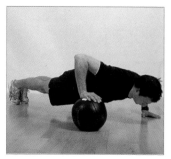

1 *Place one hand on the ball and one hand on the floor, just wider than shoulder-width apart. Your wrist should be in the middle of the top of the ball to prevent wrist injuries. Support your weight on straight arms, your feet out behind you, hip-width apart. Keep your elbows in line with your chest. Use your core muscles to maintain this position. Your head should remain in line with your spine throughout the movement.*

2 *Keeping the core muscles switched on to maintain good balance and posture, slowly lower your body weight, taking your elbows out to the side until they are at 90 degrees. Pause for 1 second before returning to the start position. Keep your abdominal muscles tight throughout the movement to maintain a straight body. As you get stronger, transfer more weight onto the side with the medicine ball so your muscles work harder and improve your stability.*

Double-hand medicine ball press-up

Muscles used Pectoralis major; triceps brachii – medial, long and lateral heads

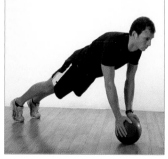

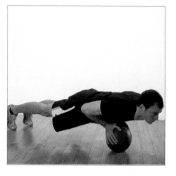

1 *Place both hands on the ball. Support your weight on straight arms, and keep your feet out behind you, hip-width apart, with the toes on the floor and the heels raised. Keep your elbows in line with your chest. Switch on your core muscles to maintain good balance and posture. Your head should remain in line with your spine throughout the movement.*

2 *Keeping your core muscles tense, slowly lower yourself, taking your elbows out to the side until they are at 90 degrees. The angle of the elbows changes the emphasis of the exercise. The closer your elbows are to your ribs the more the triceps will work, the farther away, the harder the chest muscles will work. Pause for 1 second before returning to the start position.*

Back Exercises: The Lats

Your back is one of the strongest areas of your body but one that is often neglected by gym users. This may be because it is difficult to see the back muscles, which makes it harder to monitor them, and therefore to stay motivated to train them.

The following exercises work the large muscles called latissimus dorsi, which are situated on the widest part of the upper back. For each exercise, take 2 to 3 seconds for each direction of the movement. Breathe out at the beginning of the movement, and breathe in as you return to the start position. Try using forced repetitions, when you have done as many reps as possible. Get your training partner to help you do two to three more reps.

Exercises to build stronger back muscles

The back muscles are large, so it takes hard work to train them.

Exercise	Sets and repetitions
Overhand chin-up	5 x max
Lat pull-down, wide grip	3 x 12
Lat pull-down, underhand grip	3 x 12

Lat pull-down, underhand grip

Muscles used Latissimus dorsi; teres major; biceps brachii; brachialis

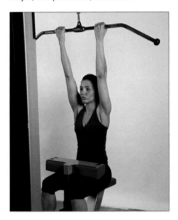

1 Sit on the bench, with your feet shoulder-width apart, between you and the machine. Hold the bar with a close underhand grip. Lean back slightly and keep your head in line with the spine.

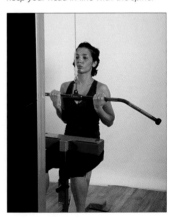

2 Pull the bar toward the bottom of your chest, chest out, elbows out to the side and behind you. When the bar is close to your chest, pause for a second, then slowly return to the start position.

Lat pull-down, wide grip

Muscles used Latissimus dorsi; teres major; biceps brachii; brachialis

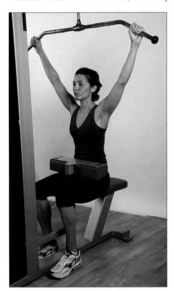 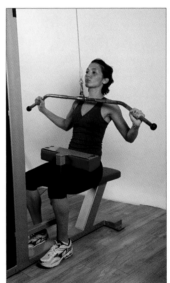

1 Hold the bar using a wide overhand grip. Sit on a seat, bench, fit ball or floor. Place your feet on the floor between you and the machine, shoulder-width apart. Lean back slightly and keep your head in line with your spine. Keep your body fixed in one position with your abdominals tensed.

2 Pull the bar toward the bottom of your chest, your elbows going out to the side and behind you. When the bar is close to the chest, pause for 1 second, then slowly return to the start position. Push your chest out as the bar is pulled in. Focus on using your lat muscles and don't let your shoulders rise up in the movement.

Overhand chin-up, wide grip

Muscles used Latissimus dorsi; teres major; rhomboid – minor, major; biceps brachii; brachialis

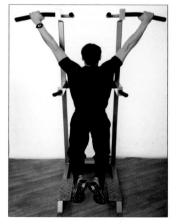

1 Grip the outside of the chin-up bar with an overhand grip so that your palms are facing away from you. Hang from the bar with straight arms and tense core muscles. Keep your head facing forward and in line with your spine. Your legs should be hanging straight under you in line with your body.

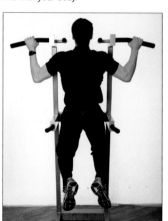

2 Slowly pull your body weight up, with your elbows going out to the sides until your chin is over the top of the bar. Pause for 1 second, then return to the start position. Keep the core muscles tensed at all times, and let your arms go almost straight between repetitions.

Rope pull-down

Muscles used Latissimus dorsi; teres major; biceps brachii; brachialis

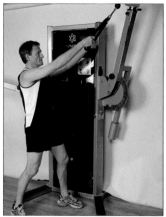

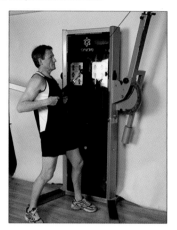

1 Hold the rope using a wide overhand grip. Place your feet on the floor, shoulder-width apart, between you and the machine. Lean back slightly and keep your head in line with your spine. Don't let the weight drag you forward and round your shoulders.

2 Pull the rope toward the bottom of your chest, chest out and elbows to the side and behind you. Push your hips slightly forward and tense your core muscles to emphasize your lats. When the rope is close to your chest, pause for a second, then slowly return to the start.

Straight arm cable pull-down

Muscles used Latissimus dorsi; teres major; triceps brachii – long head

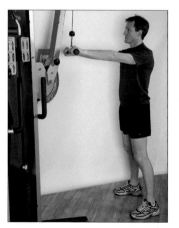

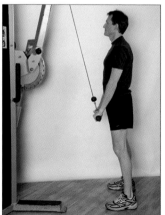

1 Face the cable machine with feet shoulder-width apart. Hold the bar in front of you at eye level, with straight arms. Tense the core muscles during the exercise. Keep your head in line with your spine during the movement.

2 Pull the bar down to below the waist. Keep the grip relaxed so the back, abdominals and triceps work harder. Pause for 1 second, then return to the start. Push the chest out and keep the head facing forward throughout.

Back Exercises: Back Muscles

For these exercises, you will need you to recruit your core muscles more than ever, as they form a strong connection between the upper and lower body. If you want to build body mass and pure lifting strength, these are the right exercises for you.

The following exercises work all the back muscles. They may be of particular use to you for lifting heavy weights and in contact sports such as rugby and American football. These exercises are exhausting, as you use a massive amount of muscle. So, practise getting your breathing right to ensure you are getting enough oxygen to your muscles, especially as you are trying to tense the core muscles as much as possible throughout the movements.

Make sure that you do at least 10 minutes' cardiovascular exercise and some stretching before you start these exercises, to get good blood flow to the muscles and avoid injury. Practise without any weight to get the correct technique before adding weights.

For each exercise, take 2 to 3 seconds for each direction of the movement. Breathe out at the beginning of the movement, and in as you return to the start position.

Exercises to build mass for your back	
Exercise	**Sets and repetitions**
Olympic bar deadlift	3 x 8–10
Single-arm dumbbell row	3 x 8–10
Bent-over barbell row	3 x 8–10
Underarm barbell row	3 x 8–10
Seated cable row	3 x 8–10

Olympic bar deadlift

Muscles used Trapezius; rhomboid major; latissimus dorsi; gluteus maximus; semitendinosus; semimembranosus; biceps femoris – long head and short head; vastus lateralis, medialis; rectus abdominis

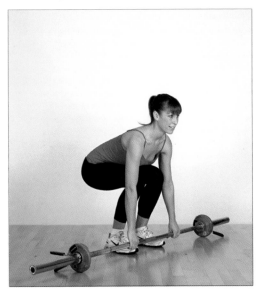
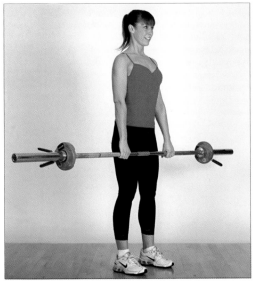

1 *Stand with your feet shoulder-width apart. Bend your knees until your thighs are nearly parallel with the floor, the upper body leaning forward, bending at the hip. Arch your lower back slightly and tense your core muscles as much as possible. They must remain tight throughout this exercise in order to prevent your back from becoming rounded. A rounded back could result in severe spinal disc problems. Look straight ahead, keeping your head in line with the spine.*

2 *Grip the Olympic bar with an overhand grip, with palms facing backward. The hands should be shoulder-width apart, arms straight. Pull the weight up by straightening your legs, with the bar passing close to your shins and over the knees in a smooth, continuous movement. Straighten your upper body until you are completely upright. Pause for 1 second, then slowly reverse the movement back to the start position.*

Bent-over barbell row

Muscles used Latissimus dorsi; teres major; rhomboid major; trapezius; posterior deltoid; biceps brachii; brachialis; brachioradialis

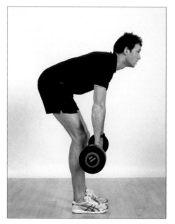

1 Grip the bar with an overhand grip, hands just wider than shoulder-width apart. Bend your hips at just 90 degrees. With your feet shoulder-width apart, legs straight and core muscles tensed, push your hips back and arch your lower back slightly to maintain good body position. The bar should hang, from straight arms, perpendicular to the ground.

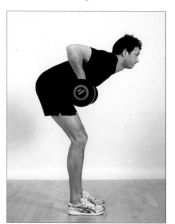

2 Pull the bar toward your chest, with your elbows going out to the sides until the bar is against your chest. Pause for 1 second, then lower the weight back to the start position.

Bench barbell row

Muscles used Latissimus dorsi; teres major; rhomboid major; trapezius; posterior deltoid; biceps brachii; brachialis; brachioradialis

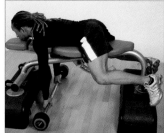

Lie face down on the bench with your abdominals tensed to provide a stable base. Grip the bar using an overhand grip just over shoulder-width apart. Pull the bar up toward you with the elbows passing your ribs at the sides. Once at the top pause for a second and then slowly lower the bar back down. Keep arms straight to work the back muscles through a range of movement.

Bent-over T-bar row

Muscles used Posterior deltoid; teres – minor, major; trapezius; infraspinatus; rhomboid; latissimus dorsi; erector spinae; brachialis; brachioradialis

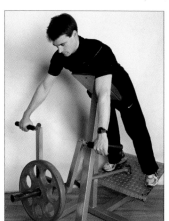

1 Stand with your legs either side of the T-bar, shoulder-width apart. Grip the bar with an overhand grip, slightly bend your knees and bend your upper body at the hips, keeping your torso very still.

Underarm barbell row

Muscles used Latissimus dorsi; teres major; rhomboid major; trapezius; posterior deltoid; biceps brachii; brachialis; brachioradialis

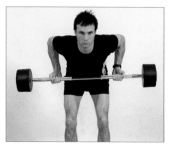

The start position is the same as for the bent-over barbell row (left), except you grip the bar with an underhand grip, hands just wider than shoulder-width apart. Bend the hips at 90 degrees. With your feet shoulder-width apart, legs straight and core muscles tensed, push the hips back and arch your lower back slightly to maintain good body position. The bar hangs perpendicular to the ground.

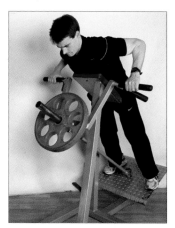

2 Pull the bar in toward your body, with your elbows bending out to the side, behind the line of your body. Once the bar is close to your ribs, pause for a second, then return to the start position.

Shoulder Exercises: General

Many people want wider shoulders. Although you can't increase the actual bone size of the shoulder, you can, with the right exercises, increase your shoulder muscle, which will make your shoulders appear much broader.

For most people, changing the width and depth of their shoulders makes them appear different and can have a dramatic effect on their body shape. Wider shoulders make it much easier to give your torso a great V-shape. Hanging clothes on wide shoulders can make you look more athletic and slimmer.

There are a number of shoulder exercises that you can use to build the depth and increase the width of your shoulder muscles.

To build strong shoulders, you need to use three types of movement: pressing, pulling and raising. It can take a long time to develop really strong shoulders because there are a number of different muscles surrounding a complex joint, and these are not necessarily muscles you use in everyday life.

Your deltoid is the primary muscle in your shoulder and is split into three parts: the anterior deltoid, medial deltoid and posterior deltoid. Depending on the movement you are performing, one part of the deltoid will work more than the others. In most movements, however, two parts of the deltoid will work together, or even all three parts. Make sure that you use the correct weight and warm up sufficiently in order not to damage the smaller muscles in the shoulder (rotator cuff).

When you start training your shoulders, it is important that you use basic pressing exercises to make your shoulder muscle active before moving on to exercises better suited for isolating the different areas of the shoulder. Otherwise, you might injure yourself.

Make sure your lower back is well supported during any pressing movements. As soon as you feel your body starting to twist while trying to do shoulder exercises, your shoulders are fatigued and you should rest. For every exercise, take 2 to 3 seconds for each direction of the movement. Breathe out at the beginning of the movement and in as you return to the start position.

Exercises to build stronger shoulders for beginners	
Exercise	**Sets and repetitions**
Olympic bar front shoulder press	3 x 12
Dumbbell shoulder press	3 x 12
Alternate dumbbell shoulder press	3 x 20

Olympic bar front shoulder press

Muscles used Deltoid – middle, anterior, posterior; triceps brachii – medial head, lateral head and long head

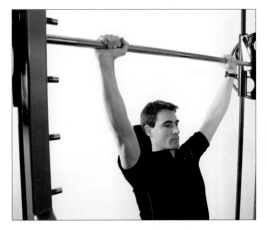 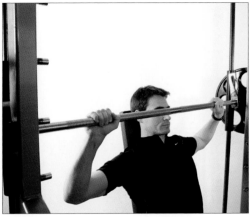

1 *Sit on the bench with your back pushed against the pad and put your feet out in front of you, shoulder-width apart, for support. If possible, put your feet up against a wall or dumbbell rack to help keep your back flat. Grip the bar firmly with both hands using an overhand grip. Always have someone there to spot for you for this exercise.*

2 *Lift the bar from the rack up above your head and hold it in a straight-arm position. Slowly lower the bar down, with the elbows going out to the sides, until the bar is in front of your head at eye level. Pause for 1 second, then press the bar back up to the start position. Take care, the shoulders can fatigue, so that you struggle to get the bar back on the rack.*

Dumbbell shoulder press

Muscles used Deltoid – middle, anterior, posterior; triceps brachii

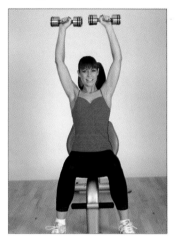

1 *Sit on the bench with your feet in front of you, shoulder-width apart, to make a firm base. Slowly lift the weights up above your shoulders until they are straight up above head height, out to the sides. Try not to let your neck tense, and keep your shoulders working equally.*

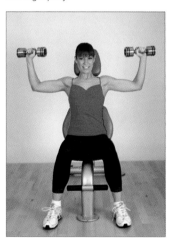

2 *Slowly lower the weights, with your elbows going out to the sides to 90 degrees, the weights level with your ears. Pause for 1 second, then press the weights back up to the start position.*

Alternate shoulder press

Muscles used Deltoid – middle, anterior, posterior; triceps brachii – medial head, lateral head and long head

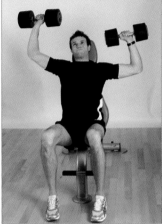

1 *Sit on the bench, feet out in front of you or pressed up against a wall or dumbbell rack, at least shoulder-width apart, to make a firm base. Keep your core muscles tight throughout the movement. With one arm, lift one weight above your shoulders until it is straight up above head height, out to the side. Move slowly, without jerking, so you don't damage any muscles.*

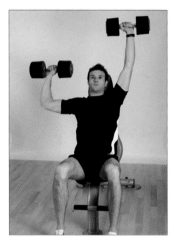

2 *Slowly lower the weight, with your elbow going out to the side, until it is at 90 degrees and the dumbbell is level with your ears. Pause for 1 second, then press the weight back up to the start position. Repeat with the other side. Wait for one arm to complete the press before you start to press the dumbbell up with the other arm.*

Body weight shoulder press

Muscles used Deltoid – middle, anterior, posterior; pectoralis major; triceps brachii – medial head, lateral head, long head

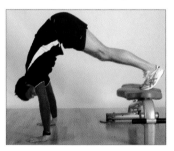

1 *Assume the decline press-up position with your feet up behind you on a bench. Pike at the hips and bring your hands back closer toward you, palms flat on the floor. Avoid this exercise if you have weak wrists.*

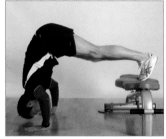

2 *Lower yourself down by bending your elbows until your head is almost touching the floor. Try not to let your back arch. Pause for 1 second, before pressing back up to the position in step 1.*

Shoulder Exercises: Rotational Strength

The following exercises will work the shoulder muscles as well as some of the muscles surrounding them. The range of movement involved will make your core and stabilizing muscles work harder, giving you the benefits of good rotational strength.

Most sports require some rotation at the shoulder joint. Throwing movements use all the muscles in the deltoid and make you over-dominant in one arm, which can lead to muscle imbalances and injury. So it is important that you work both shoulder muscles equally. In these rotational movements, many shoulder muscles have to work together. The rotator cuff, often the site of shoulder injuries, is the main stabilizer during any shoulder movement to keep the ball of the upper arm central. If it is not centred, this can put abnormal stress on the surrounding tissue, making tendonitis, rotator cuff tears and shoulder impingement likely.

As you get older, the tendons in the rotator cuff lose elasticity, making injury more likely. With age, too, comes a gradual decline in the muscle bulk that surrounds the shoulder. The following exercises will help to counteract the effect of aging, allowing you to continue with your chosen sport for longer.

The rotator cuff is made up of three parts: the supraspinatus, located at the top of the shoulder, which adducts the shoulder (raises the upper arm and moves it away from the body); the subscapularis, at the front of the shoulder, which internally rotates the shoulder; and the infraspinatus and teres, at the back of the shoulder, which externally rotates it. The following exercises work all three.

Generally, take 2 to 3 seconds for each direction of the movement. Breathe out at the beginning of the movement, and in as you return to the start position.

Variation: single-arm cable shoulder press

Muscles used Deltoid – middle, anterior, posterior; triceps brachii – medial head, lateral head and long head

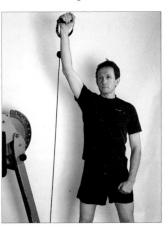

Start by holding one handle of the cable shoulder press above your head until your arm is straight. Pause for 1 second then slowly lower the weight back to the start. Repeat with the other arm.

Cable shoulder press

Muscles used Deltoid – middle, anterior, posterior; triceps brachii – medial head, lateral head and long head

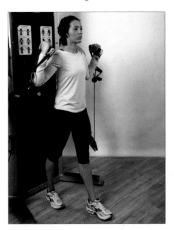

1 *Stand with your feet shoulder-width apart, one foot in front of the other and hold the handles at shoulder height.*

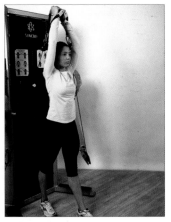

2 *Press the handles above your head until your arms are straight. Pause for a second, then slowly lower the weight back down.*

Exercises to build rotational strength of shoulders

Try some forced sets on the final exercise by getting your partner to help you with the lat two reps after you have already fatigued.

Exercise	Sets and repetitions
Arnie shoulder press	3 x 12
Cable shoulder press	3 x 12
Single-arm shoulder press	3 x 12
Olympic bar front shoulder press	3 x 8–12

Seated reverse dumbbell shoulder press, with rotation

Muscles used Deltoid – middle, anterior, posterior; pectoralis major; triceps brachii – medial head, lateral head and long head

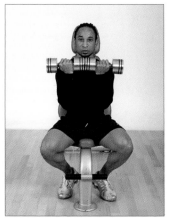

1 *Sit on the bench, with core muscles tense. Bring the dumbbells up in front of your shoulders, palms facing you and your elbows as close together as possible.*

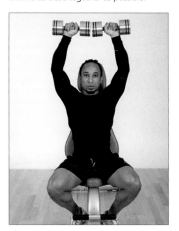

2 *Press the dumbbells upward, palms facing you and elbows as close together as possible. As the dumbbells reach eye level, start to rotate them so that they have rotated through 180 degrees by the time they reach the straight-arm position above your head. Pause at the top, then slowly lower the weights, rotating back to the start position.*

Arnold shoulder press

Muscles used Deltoid – middle, anterior, posterior; pectoralis major; triceps brachii – medial head, lateral head and long head; biceps brachii; brachialis; brachioradialis

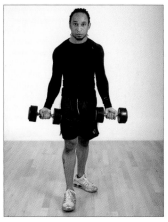

1 *Use a lighter weight than you think you need to keep the emphasis on the deltoids. Stand with the feet shoulder-width apart. Hold one dumbbell in each hand, your arms by your sides, your hands just below hip level.*

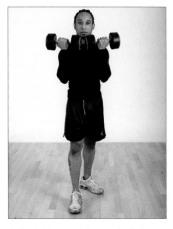

2 *Slowly bicep-curl the dumbbells by bending the elbow until the dumbbells are at shoulder height, with your elbows squeezed into your ribs. Keep your head and back straight and avoid arching the back.*

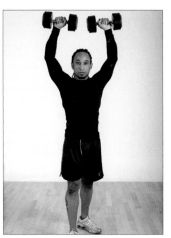

3 *Keeping your palms facing toward you and your elbows close together, press the dumbbells up to eye level before rotating them through 180 degrees to complete the press-up above your head. At the top, pause for a second before slowly lowering the dumbbells, and gradually rotating them through 180 degrees.*

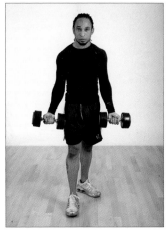

4 *As you complete the 180-degree rotation on the way back down, reverse-curl the dumbbells to the start position. For this exercise, take 4 to 5 seconds in each direction. Don't let the back arch during this exercise. Keep your abdominals tensed throughout the entire movement. If you feel your upper torso twisting, stop immediately.*

Shoulder Exercises: The Anterior Deltoids

The exercises here train the front of the shoulders (anterior deltoids), with little strength coming from other parts of your deltoids. These muscles give you toned shoulders and are essential for exercises, especially those involving pressing big weights above the chest.

The anterior deltoid muscles are involved in stabilizing the muscles during chest presses and are heavily involved when a chest exercise is done on an incline. The high usage of this muscle makes it susceptible to injury. It is a mistake to try to work these muscles using shoulder exercises in the same routine as chest presses or even on the day after. You must try to avoid overtraining the anterior deltoids, so have a day's rest between exercises that involve using them.

All these exercises involve raising movements, so there will be no real help from your triceps. People often choose to work the anterior deltoids harder than other parts of the deltoids because it is easy to see the muscle in the mirror. But this often leads to muscle imbalances and can make the anterior deltoids over-dominant in the movement of the shoulder press exercises, causing the weight to be dragged forward. Your posture will also be affected in that your shoulders will be dragged forward, creating a more rounded upper back. Make sure you balance this out by using the other parts of the deltoid. If you

have poor posture, you need to pay more attention to exercising the medial and posterior deltoid in your workouts. It is worth considering omitting specific exercises for these muscles from your routine, because they will be worked with the chest press exercises anyway.

When planning your routine, make sure that you use each arm equally to prevent one getting stronger than the other. To help isolate the muscle, try

sitting down for some of the exercises in order to prevent your body getting into too much of a swinging motion. You may need to use a lighter weight than you think you need so that you will be able to activate the muscle correctly.

For each exercise, take 2 to 3 seconds for each direction of the movement. Breathe out at the beginning of the movement, and in as you return to the start position.

Single-arm dumbbell frontal raise

Muscles used Deltoids – middle, anterior, posterior; pectoralis major

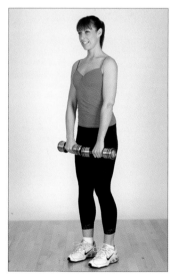

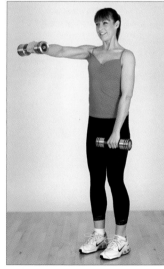

1 *Stand with your head up but relaxed, and your feet shoulder-width apart so that you feel stable and balanced. Take hold of a dumbbell in each hand and hold them close together in front of your thighs, with your arms hanging straight down and the palms facing behind you.*

2 *Pull one arm forward, keeping it straight, until it is in front of you at eye level. Try not to let momentum take over. Pause for 1 second, then slowly lower the weight back to the starting position. Repeat with the other arm. Only lift the weight once the other arm has returned to the start position.*

Exercises to build powerful shoulders

Superset each exercise with the one below, with only five to ten seconds' rest between sets.

Exercise	Sets and repetitions
Olympic bar shoulder press	3 x 8–12
Arnie shoulder press	3 x 8–12
Upright dumbbell row	3 x 8–12
Upright cable row	3 x 8–12
Single-arm dumbbell frontal raise	3 x 8–12
Cable frontal raise	3 x 8–10

Cable frontal raise

Muscles used Deltoids – middle, anterior, posterior; pectoralis major

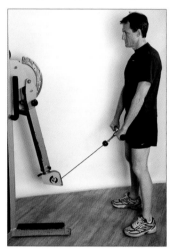

1 Stand with your feet shoulder-width apart, 60cm/2ft from the cable machine. Hold the bar with an overhand grip, with hands just less than shoulder-width apart. Focus on the front of your shoulders. Don't let your back arch.

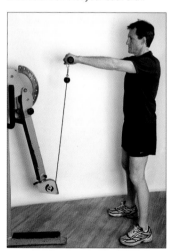

2 Beginning with arms straight down in front of the body, pull the bar up, with your arms straight out in front of you, until it is at eye level. Keep the neck relaxed. Pause for 1 second, then slowly lower it back down to the start position.

Single-arm cable frontal raise

Muscles used Deltoids – middle, anterior, posterior; pectoralis major

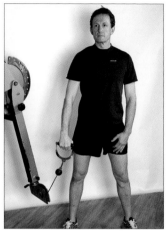
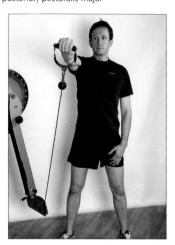

1 Stand with your feet shoulder-width apart, side-on on to the cable machine. Using one hand, hold the bar with an overhand grip, with the palm facing backward. Stay in a position that is square-on to the machine. Focus on the front of the shoulder that is doing the exercise.

2 Keeping your arm straight out in front of you, pull the cable up until it is at eye level. Pause for 1 second, then, without jerking, slowly lower it back down to the start position. Keep the shoulders level and don't let your back arch. Don't hold your breath; keep breathing throughout.

Bench frontal raise

Muscles used Deltoids – middle, anterior, posterior; pectoralis major; rectus abdominis

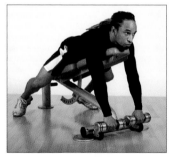
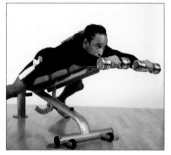

1 Lie face down on a 30-degree incline bench with your arms straight down in front of you just above floor height. Place the balls of your feet on the floor behind you, and out to the sides of the bench. Hold a dumbbell in each hand. Check that the dumbbells are the right weight for you.

2 Lift the dumbbells up in front of you with straight arms, keeping the arms as close to each other as possible. Do not allow your lower back to arch. Once your hands are up to almost shoulder level, pause for 1 second, then slowly lower the weights back down to the start position.

Shoulder Exercises: Stability

The exercises given here use raising movements to place emphasis on the posterior deltoid and middle deltoid muscles – the muscles that provide much-needed stability for a range of movements involved in many sports.

If you want wider, toned shoulders, include the following exercises in your routine. If you have poor posture, use these exercises to prevent rounded shoulders. The exercises will pull your shoulders back and force your back muscles to work in conjunction with your shoulders. They will also help improve your posture. There are many stabilizers in the shoulders, one of which, the scapular (shoulder blade), helps the rotator cuff to stabilize the shoulder joint while in motion. The scapular must be stable – if not, the pressure on it caused by lifting heavy weights may cause injury to the rotator cuff.

These exercises will give you strength with the full range of movement and help to stabilize your shoulder at the same time. Concentrate especially on not using your lower back to help lift the weights. If you are suffering from shoulder injuries, consult your physician before you do these shoulder exercises. While they will help with shoulder stability, your shoulder needs to be sufficiently stable in the first place before you attempt them.

Unless stated otherwise, for each exercise, take 2 to 3 seconds for each direction of the movement. Breathe out at the beginning of the movement, and in as you return to the start position.

Exercises to give wider, toned shoulders	
Exercise	**Sets and repetitions**
Reverse dumbbell shoulder press	3 x 12
Single-arm dumbbell frontal raise	3 x 20
Upright dumbbell row	3 x 12
Bent-over cable lateral raise	3 x 12
Windmill	3 x 12
Single-arm dumbbell lateral raise	3 x 12

Bent-over cable lateral raise

Muscles used Deltoids – middle, anterior, posterior; teres minor; rhomboid; trapezius

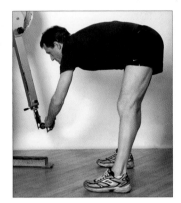 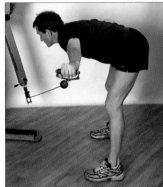

1 *Stand between the two arms of the cable machine, with feet just over shoulder-width apart. Take hold of the handle so that your arm is across your body. Bend the upper body at the hips so that your back is parallel to the floor.*

2 *Pull the handle back across your body with a straight arm until it is out to the side, level with your body like the wing of an airplane. Pause for 1 second, then slowly lower the weight back to the start position.*

Bent-over dumbbell lateral raise

Muscles used Deltoids – middle, anterior, posterior; teres minor; rhomboid; trapezius

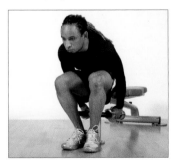 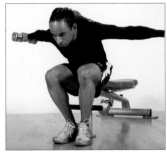

1 *Sit on the end of a bench with your feet on the floor and legs bent at 90 degrees. Lean forward so that your chest is almost resting on your knees. Hold a dumbbell in each hand.*

2 *Pull the dumbbells out to the sides in an arc, arms almost straight, until the weights are level with the line of your shoulders. Pause for a second, then slowly lower your arms back to the start position.*

Windmill

Muscles used Deltoids – middle, anterior, posterior; rhomboid; trapezius

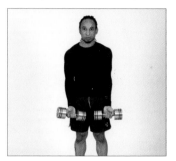

1 *Stand with your feet shoulder-width apart, arms straight, a dumbbell in each hand in front of you.*

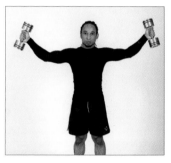

2 *Take your arms out to the side until they are at shoulder level. Pause in this position for 1 second.*

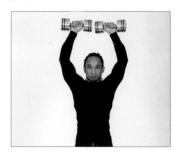

3 *Continue the movement until the weights are above your head. Once they are above your head, slowly lower them back to shoulder level as in step 2, pause for a second, then continue to lower them back to the start position. For this exercise, take 3 to 4 seconds for each direction of the movement.*

Dumbbell lateral raise

Muscles used Deltoids – middle, anterior, posterior

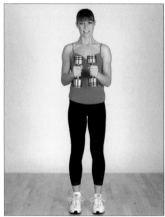
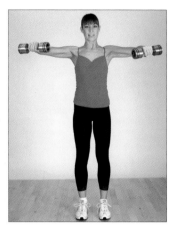

1 *Stand with your feet shoulder-width apart, looking straight ahead, keeping your neck straight. Hold one dumbbell in each hand, with your palms facing toward each other and your elbows tucked in tight against your ribs.*

2 *Keeping your elbows at the same angle, take your arms out to the sides until your upper arm, elbow, forearm and wrist are all level with your shoulders. Pause for a second, then slowly lower back to the start position.*

Single-arm dumbbell lateral raise

Muscles used Deltoids – middle, anterior, posterior

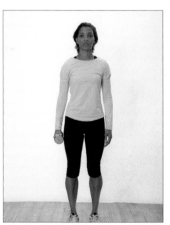
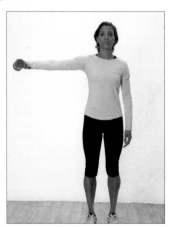

1 *Stand with feet shoulder-width apart, hold a dumbbell in one hand by your side. Let the other hand hang straight and loose by your side to hip level. Tense the core muscles to stop movement and to isolate the deltoid muscle.*

2 *Lift your arm to the side, keeping it straight, until your wrist, forearm and elbow are level with your shoulder. Pause for 1 second, then slowly lower the weight back down to the start position. Repeat with the other arm.*

Biceps Exercises: Powerful Arms

Your biceps make up only 30–40 per cent of your upper arm – the triceps account for most of it – but biceps exercises are probably the most popular upper-body weight-training exercise because, quite simply, many people believe that big biceps look good.

There are two muscle groups in the front of your upper arm. The largest group is the biceps brachii and the smallest is the brachialis. This small area of the body requires a variety of different exercises. It is important to change your bicep routine regularly to get the most from each session. Many gym users use bad technique to lift the heaviest weights they can. The following exercises will ensure that you stick to the correct technique to put the emphasis on your biceps.

For each exercise take 2 to 3 seconds for each direction of the movement. Breathe out at the beginning of the movement, and in as you return to the start position.

Standing barbell bicep curl, wide grip

Muscles used Biceps brachii – long head, short head; brachialis

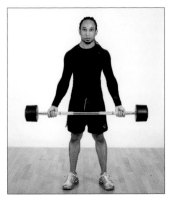 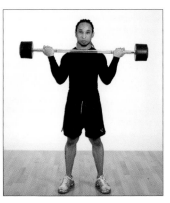

1 Stand with your feet shoulder-width apart so that you feel well balanced and stable. Grip the barbell close to the thighs, with an underhand grip so that your palms are facing forward, your arms straight and your hands just over shoulder-width apart. To prevent any part of your body other than the biceps from working, keep the upper torso still by tensing your core muscles.

2 Keep your elbows at your sides, locked in to your ribs, and curl the bar up to the shoulders. Prevent your elbows from moving forward and backward: imagine a pin going through your elbow into your ribs; rotate on this axis. Stand side-on to a mirror and glance at it in the middle of each set to check your elbow is in the right place. Pause for 1 second, then slowly return to the start position.

Reverse dumbbell bicep curl

Muscles used Brachioradialis; biceps brachii – long head, short head; brachialis; extensor carpi; radialis – longus, brevis; extensor digitorum; extensor digiti minimi; extensor carpi ulnaris

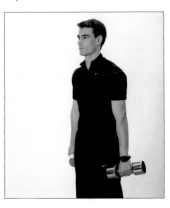

1 Stand with feet shoulder-width apart. With an overhand grip, hold a dumbbell in each hand, close to your thighs.

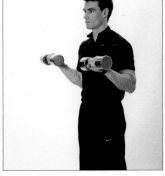

2 Keeping your elbows locked in to the ribs, curl the dumbbells up to your shoulders. Pause for 1 second, then slowly return to the start position.

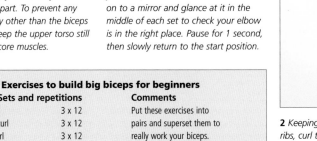

Exercises to build big biceps for beginners		
Exercise	**Sets and repetitions**	**Comments**
Barbell bicep curl	3 x 12	Put these exercises into
Dumbbell bicep curl	3 x 12	pairs and superset them to
Concentration curl	3 x 12	really work your biceps.
Hammer curl	3 x 12	

Standing dumbbell bicep curl

Muscles used Biceps brachii – long head, short head; brachialis

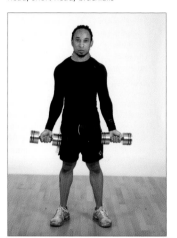

1 Stand, feet shoulder-width apart, a dumbbell in each hand, close to your thighs, using an underhand grip. To prevent your forearms from overworking, don't grip the dumbbells too tightly.

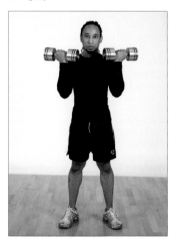

2 Keeping your elbows locked in to your ribs, curl the dumbbells up to your shoulders. Pause for a second, then slowly return to the start position. Keep your palms facing in the same direction. Don't let the weight of the dumbbell twist them, especially on the way back down.

Dumbbell hammer curl

Muscles used Brachioradials; biceps brachii – long head, short head; brachialis

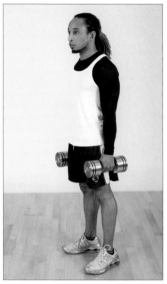

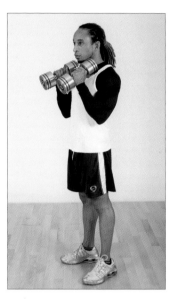

1 Stand with your feet shoulder-width apart, your elbows tucked into your ribs. With an underhand grip, hold one dumbbell in each hand, close to your thighs. Concentrate on the arms doing the work.

2 Keep the elbows close to the ribs. Curl the weights up to the shoulders, turning the angle of the forearms by 90 degrees. At the top of the curl, pull the elbows back, pause for a second, then return to the start position.

Concentration curl

Muscles used Biceps brachii – long head, short head; brachialis

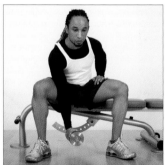

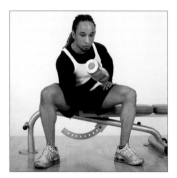

1 Sitting on a bench, take hold of the dumbbell and rest your elbow against your inner thigh. The palm of your hand should be facing away from you. Try to focus on isolating your bicep.

2 Keeping your elbow firmly up against your inner thigh, curl the dumbbell up to your shoulder. Use control to get a good burn. Pause for a second, then lower it down to the start position.

Biceps Exercises: Strong Lower Arms

Most upper-body exercises will help to work your lower arms but you should also regularly use specific lower-arm exercises. Changing the angle of the wrist when doing biceps curls will make the different parts of the bicep work more effectively.

Forearms need to be strong to give you the support to do other exercises, especially when you need to grip hard and pull weights to work the back muscles.

There are three types of forearm muscle structure and function: forearm supinator, a large muscle on the outer part of the forearm, which can be trained with reverse curls and hammer curls; forearm flexor, a small muscle on the inside of the forearm used to close your fist, which can be trained with barbell wrist curls; and forearm extensors, small muscles on the outside of the forearm, which straighten the fingers after your hand has been clenched, and bring your wrist back toward the arms.

There is virtually no sport which doesn't require strong lower arms. You can adapt your resistance exercises to your chosen sport. If you want stronger arms and wrists for mountain biking do more reps and less sets for greater endurance. Hovering with your fingers over the brakes and hands wrapped around the bars for hour after hour will take its toll if you don't do enough of these exercises. Even if a boxer's lower arms and wrists are heavily wrapped, the muscles must still be able to stand up to the impact and maintain stability to keep throwing punches.

Breathe out when you begin each exercise; then breathe in as you return to the start position.

Exercises to tone and strengthen lower arms	
Exercise	**Sets and repetitions**
Cable bicep curl	3 x 12
Single-arm cable bicep curl	3 x 8
Lying-down cable bicep curl	3 x 12
Wrist curl	3 x 15–20
Reverse wrist curl	3 x 15–20
Hammer wrist curl	3 x 15–20

Cable bicep curl

Muscles used Biceps brachii; brachialis

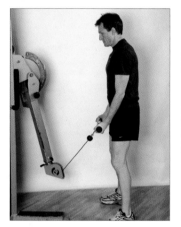 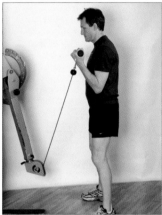

1 *Stand up straight, arms straight down in front of you, core muscles tense, feet shoulder-width apart, 30cm/1ft from the machine. Grip the bar using an underhand grip, so that the bar rests against the tops of your legs.*

2 *Curl the bar up to the shoulders keeping your elbows tucked into your ribs and your feet shoulder-width apart. Pause for 1 second at the top and then slowly return the bar to the start position.*

Lying-down cable bicep curl

Muscles used Biceps brachii; brachialis

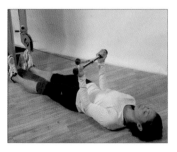 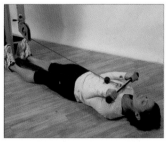

1 *Lie down flat on your back, with your feet close to the cable machine. Hold the bar attached to the cable with an underhand grip, with your hands shoulder-width apart.*

2 *Place the bar down by the front of your legs and curl it up toward your shoulders, keeping your elbows tucked against your ribs. Pause for 1 second then slowly lower it back down.*

Single-arm cable bicep curl

Muscles used Biceps brachii; brachialis

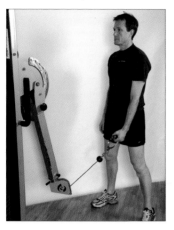

1 *Stand with your feet shoulder-width apart, 30cm/1ft from the cable machine. Grip the bar, with one hand, using an underhand grip, so that it rests against the top of your thigh. Keep your other hand close in by your other thigh. Stand up straight with your core muscles tense. Try to keep the rest of your torso as still as possible.*

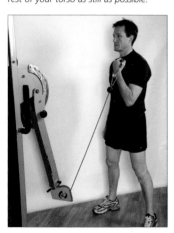

2 *Curl the bar up to the shoulder, keeping your elbow tucked in to your ribs. Focus on getting a good full range of movement. Pause for 1 second at the top, then, keeping the core muscles tense, slowly return the bar to the start position. Repeat the same movement on the other side.*

Wrist curl

Muscles used Flexors – carpi ulnaris, digitorum, carpi radialis; palmaris longus

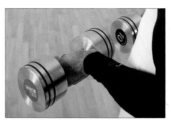
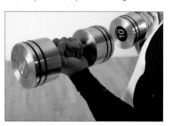

1 *Stand or sit with a barbell in each hand, using an underhand grip, hands shoulder-width apart, elbows at 90 degrees.*

2 *With forearms out in front of you, to isolate the forearm and wrist muscles, curl the weight up as far as possible. Pause for 2 seconds.*

Reverse wrist curl

Muscles used Extensors – carpi radialis longus, carpi radialis brevis, carpi ulnaris, indicis, digitorum

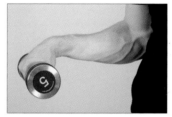
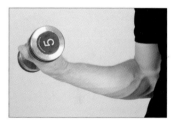

1 *Stand or sit with a dumbbell in one hand, using an overhand grip, elbow bent at 90 degrees to help isolate the forearm and wrist.*

2 *Curl the weight up as far as possible, using just the wrist and forearm muscles, and pause for 2 seconds. Repeat with the other arm.*

Hammer wrist curl

Muscles used Extensors – carpi radialis longus, carpi radialis brevis, carpi ulnaris, digitorum

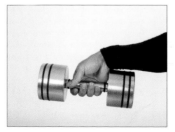
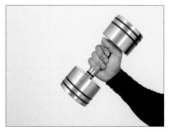

1 *Stand or sit holding the dumbbell in a hammer position, then gradually allow the weight to tilt your wrist away from you.*

2 *Keep the forearm and arm still and use the muscles in the wrist to tilt the dumbbell back up toward you. Pause for a second then lower to the start position.*

Triceps Exercises

All upper-body resistance training that involves pressing movements will also involve the triceps. If you want to build bigger upper arms or press heavier weights, triceps exercises need to be part of your regular routine.

There are three parts to the triceps muscle: the medial head, lateral head and long head. These muscles are positioned at the back of your upper arm and are responsible for extending your upper arm. Always do your chest or shoulder exercises first before training your triceps. If you have a good session on the triceps, and then try to press weights to work your chest or shoulders, you will not achieve very much. Your triceps will be fatigued long before your chest or shoulders have had a good workout. Compared to the chest or shoulder muscles, the triceps are small muscles, so be strict in your technique to ensure that you are working your triceps only and not other larger muscles.

You need to work hard to get bulging triceps. Remember that roughly 70 per cent of your upper arm mass is made up of the triceps. Once you are strong enough, try to include one or two triceps exercises that involve using your body weight as these are often some of the most effective, and can be of most use to you in everyday life and for your sport.

Remember good technique; if your technique is poor you will be recruiting other muscles such as your chest and shoulders, which will not develop the triceps. For each exercise, take 2 to 3 seconds for each direction of the movement. Breathe out at the beginning of the movement, and breathe in as you return to the start position.

Exercises to build bigger triceps	
Exercise	**Sets and repetitions**
Triceps dip	5 x max
Triceps bench dip	5 x max
Cable push-down	3 x 8–10
Reverse cable push-down	3 x 10
Overhead cable triceps extension	3 x 10

Triceps bench dip

Muscles used Triceps brachii – long head, lateral head, medial head; anconeus

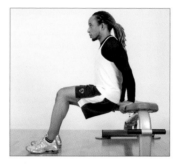 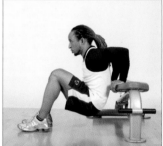

1 Grip the edge of the bench, with the back of your hands facing forward at your sides, arms fully extended to suspend your body weight. Keep your feet flat on the floor in front of you.

2 Lower your body toward the floor, bending your elbows behind you, at 90 degrees. Pause for 1 second, then return to the start position. As you get stronger, take feet farther away from you.

Triceps dip

Muscles used Triceps brachii – long head, lateral head and medial head; anconeus; pectoralis major

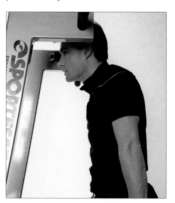 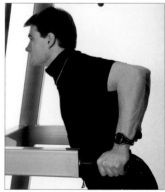

1 Grip the handles of the machine, with an overhand grip, your legs hanging under you. Keep your elbows tucked in to isolate your triceps. Fully extend your arms to suspend your body weight from the machine.

2 Lower your body toward the floor, bending your elbows behind you at 90 degrees. If your elbows are wide apart, you will work the pectorals. Pause for a second, then push yourself back up to the start position.

Cable push-down

Muscles used Triceps brachii – long head, lateral head and medial head

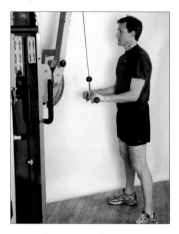

1 Use a lighter weight than you think you need to isolate and work the triceps. Grip the bar with an overhand grip, with hands just less than shoulder-width apart, and your arms bent at 90 degrees. Tuck your elbows in against your ribs. Don't let your shoulders rise up.

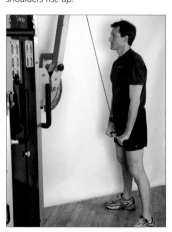

2 Fully extend your arms, keeping the elbows locked in to your ribs, until your hands are down in front of your legs. Pause for 1 second, then slowly bend your arms, allowing the bar to raise. Open your grip at the bottom of the movement when your arms are in full extension to work your triceps harder.

Reverse cable push-down

Muscles used Triceps brachii – long head, lateral head and medial head; anconeus; extensors – carpi radialis brevis, digitorum, carpi ulnaris and carpi radialis longus

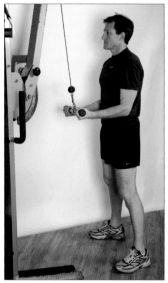

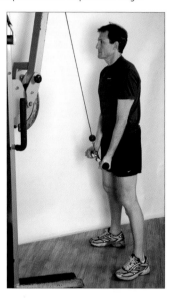

1 Grip the bar with an underhand grip, with your hands just less than shoulder-width apart, and arms bent at 90 degrees. Tuck your elbows in closely against your ribs throughout the whole movement.

2 Fully extend your arms until your hands are down in front of your legs. Pause for 1 second, then slowly bend your arms, allowing the bar to raise. Pause for longer at full extension to get a good burn on the triceps.

Overhead cable triceps extensions

Muscles used Triceps brachii – long head, lateral head and medial head

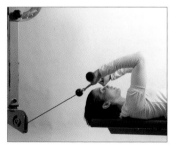

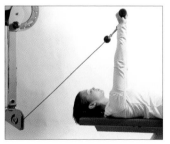

1 Lie on the bench and grip the bar from behind your head with an overhand grip. Pull it forward so that your arms are bent at 90 degrees and the bar is roughly in line with the front of your head. Your elbows should be facing forward and in a fixed position.

2 Bring the bar forward in front of you by fully extending your arms, keeping your elbows as close together as possible. Pause for 1 second on full extension and then bend at the elbow to allow the bar to return to the start position.

Specific triceps exercises

Many bodybuilders in the past have not used specific triceps exercises and have managed to get away with it because the triceps are involved in so many other exercises, especially chest presses and shoulder presses. Now, however, most bodybuilders do exercises specifically to isolate the triceps and give them that ripped look. The danger is that the triceps can easily be overtrained, especially as they are much smaller than other pressing muscles such as the chest and shoulders. So, avoid making the mistake of thinking that your triceps need to be trained more than your biceps because they make up a bigger percentage of the overall size of your arm when so many exercises work the triceps anyway.

The triceps are a three-headed muscle complex that originates in the shoulder and attaches to the forearm after passing over the top of the elbow. Their function is to straighten your arm from a bent position. They can be worked by moving your arm in an arc in front of you until it is straight down by your side, and also function during pressing movements above the chest or the shoulders.

For really ripped triceps, focus on isolation exercises and spend time on cables, which provide continuous tension throughout the entire movement. It is important to feel the muscle you are isolating, yet many people cheat on triceps exercises by allowing their elbows to move back and forth, making their shoulders and back do the work instead of their triceps. You may need to use a lighter weight than you think you need to achieve proper isolation of the muscle.

For each exercise, take 2 to 3 seconds for each direction of the movement. Breathe out at the beginning of the movement; breathe in as you return to the start position.

Exercises to isolate triceps	
Exercise	**Sets and repetitions**
Triceps press-up	5 x max
Overhead triceps extension	3 x 8–10
Lying-down triceps extension	3 x 8–10
Single-arm cable triceps push-down	3 x 8–10

Single-arm cable triceps push-down

Muscles used Triceps brachii – long head, lateral head and medial head; anconeus

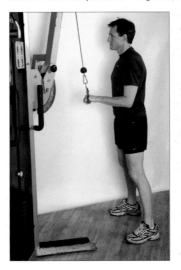
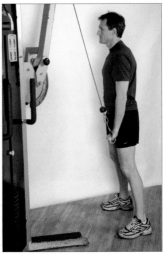

1 *Hold the cable handle in one arm using an overhand grip, with your arm bent at 90 degrees and forearms out in front of you. Keep your elbows close to your ribs. Your other arm should rest at your side. Don't let your shoulders rise up in the movement – keep them level and don't let your body twist to help with the movement.*

2 *Fully extend your arm in a downward direction until your arms are straight and the handle is by your side. Pause for 1 second then slowly allow the arm to bend back up to the starting position at 90 degrees. Hold the full extension for more than 1 second if you want to get even better recruitment of all the tricep muscles.*

Triceps press-up

Muscles used Triceps brachii – long head, lateral head and medial head; anconeus

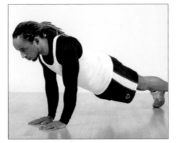
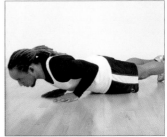

1 *Assume the standard press-up position, with hands on the floor, just less than shoulder-width apart, and fingers facing forward. Hold your body up with straight arms. The toes should touch the floor with heels raised.*

2 *Bend your arms to lower your body, keeping your elbows tucked in close to your ribs. Once the elbows are at 90 degrees pause for 1 second, then press back up extending the arms. This isolates the triceps by using your own body weight.*

Overhead triceps extension

Muscles used Triceps brachii – long head, lateral head and medial head

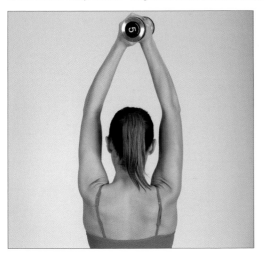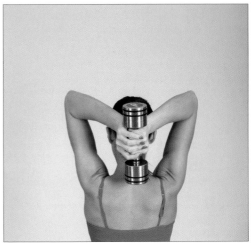

1 *Hold a dumbbell, with an interlocking grip. Slowly take the dumbbell over the top of your head, fully extending your arms. Hold the dumbbell in this position for a few seconds then go on to do step 2. Don't forget to co-ordinate your breathing with the movement and ensure that you are standing in a comfortable position and well balanced.*

2 *Slowly lower the dumbbell behind your head until your arms are bent at 90 degrees. Keep your elbows as close together as possible. Once your elbows go out to the side, you are at the lowest point your flexibility will allow you to go or the weight is too heavy. Pause for 1 second, then push the dumbbell back up above your head by fully extending your arms.*

Lying-down triceps extension

Muscles used Triceps brachii – long head, lateral head and medial head; anconeus

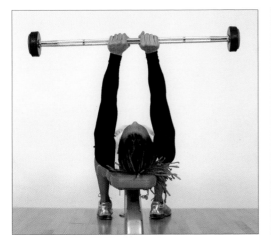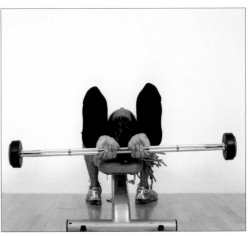

1 *Lie on your back on a flat bench so that your back, shoulders, neck and head are supported. Hold a barbell with an overhand grip, hands no more than shoulder-width apart, up above your shoulders, straight arms, elbows facing forward.*

2 *Keeping your back flat and your feet on the floor, slowly lower the barbell toward your face until your arms are bent at 90 degrees. Pause for 1 second then extend the arm back to the starting position.*

Abdominal Exercises: General

The abdominals are possibly the most important muscles to train in your body. The following exercises, along with the correct techniques to use, provide an effective workout for the full range of abdominal muscles that you need to exercise.

The abdominals, which cover a large area of the mid-section of your body, enable your torso to bend forward and sideways, and to twist. Before you start lifting heavy weights, you need sufficient abdominal training to prevent lower-back injuries. To benefit fully from your training, change the exercises regularly.

These exercises mainly work the rectus abdominis, a large, flat muscle covering the entire front of the abdomen between the lower ribcage and the hips. It contracts to flex your body at the waist and tenses as soon as you start to bring your shoulders and head forward. Sit-ups and leg-raising exercises work the rectus abdominus throughout the entire movement.

For each exercise, take 2 to 3 seconds for each direction of the movement. Breathe out at the beginning of the movement, and breathe in as you return to the start position.

Below: Rectus abdominis, external and internal obliques and the transverse abdominis are the abdominal muscles that support the trunk and hold the organs in place.

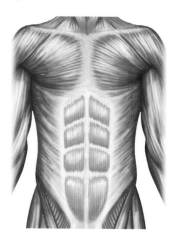

Sit-up

Muscles used Rectus abdominis; obliques – external and internal

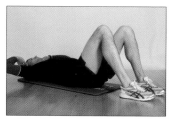

1 *Lie on your back and bend your knees to 90 degrees and place your feet flat on the floor. Put your hands behind your head and elbows back out to the sides.*

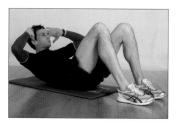

2 *Tense your abdominals and raise your head, shoulders and upper back off the floor. Pause for 1 second, then lower yourself back down. Keep the abdominals tense throughout.*

Sit-up technique
• Keep your feet on the ground or get your training partner to hold them on the floor. Or, put dumbbells on top of your feet.
• If your neck is weak, tuck your chin in to your chest so it does not move during the exercise.
• Keep your elbows back out to the sides to make the exercise harder.
• You do not need to sit-up – if your abdominals are working, a small movement is enough.

Sit-up with Russian twist

Muscles used Rectus abdominis; obliques – external and internal.

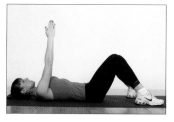

1 *Lie on your back and bend your knees to 90 degrees and place your feet flat on the floor, with your arms up vertically in front of your chest.*

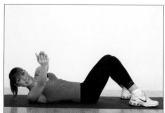

2 *Tense your abdominals and raise your head, shoulders and upper back off the floor. As you sit up, twist your upper body to one side, pause for 1 second, then twist back to straight before slowly returning to the start position. Keep your elbows back out to the sides so that your abdominals will be made to work harder during the movement.*

Exercises to build abdominals for beginners

Exercise	Sets and repetitions
Sit-up	3 x 10
crunch	3 x 10
Sit-up with Russian twist	3 x 10
Reverse crunch with alternate legs bent	3 x 20

Crunch

Muscles used Rectus abdominis; obliques – external and internal

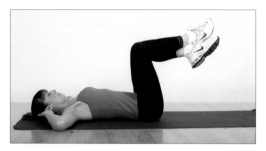

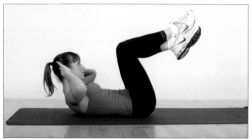

1 Lie on your back and bend your knees to 90 degrees, lifting the feet off the floor. Put your hands behind your head and your elbows back out to the sides. Tense your abdominals.

2 Crunch your knees in and raise your head, shoulders and upper back off the floor. At the top of the crunch pause for 2 seconds, then return to the start position, abdominals still tense.

Reverse crunch with bent legs

Muscles used Rectus abdominis; external oblique; tensor fascia lata

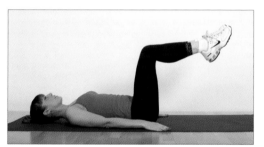

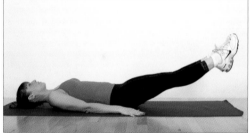

1 Lie on your back. Keeping your abdominals tense, pull your legs in toward your abdomen until they are bent at 90 degrees.

2 Lower your legs until they are almost parallel to the floor, pause for a second, then return to the start position.

Reverse crunch with alternate legs bent

Muscles used Rectus abdominis; external oblique; tensor fascia lata

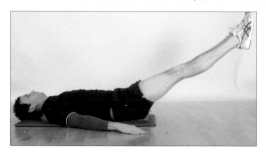

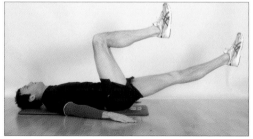

1 For the starting position, lie on your back and raise your legs, keeping your abdominals tense. Place your hands, palms facing down, flat on the floor, out to your sides in line with your hips.

2 Pull one leg in toward your abdomen until the lower part is almost parallel to the floor. Pause for 1 second, then return to the start. Repeat with the other leg. In this way, both sides of your abdominals are working equally.

Abdominal Exercises: The Sides

The following exercises will make you use the sides of your abdominals. To bend to the side and rotate your torso in relation to your hips, you use your oblique muscles, which are made up of the internal obliques, transverse obliques and external obliques.

When you are performing these exercises, stay focused on your abs and be careful to avoid any lateral movement in the hips, because this takes the emphasis away from the abdominal muscles.

If you find it hard to avoid the movement in the hips, try sitting with your legs either side of a bench.

This will prevent your hips moving. Or, you can sit on a fit ball and try to keep the ball as still as possible when you bend to the sides.

For each of these exercises, take 2 to 3 seconds for each direction of the movement. Breathe out at the beginning of the movement, and breathe in as you return to the start position.

Exercises to build side abdominals	
Exercise	**Sets and repetitions**
Side crunch	3 x 20–30
Oblique crunch	3 x 20–30
Dumbbell side bend	3 x 20–30
High cable side bend	3 x 20–30

One-leg crossed crunch

Muscles used Rectus abdominis; external oblique

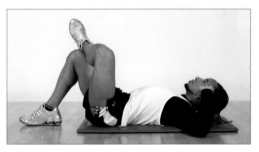

1 Lie on your back, with your arms out to the sides, your fingers touching the sides of your head. Cross your left leg over your right leg so that your left ankle rests on your right knee. Keep the movement slow, and focus on the abdominals.

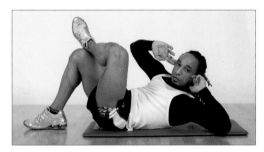

2 Tense your abdominals and crunch up toward your knees. At the top of the crunch, twist to one side so that you are facing your left knee. Pause for a second, then slowly lower back down. Repeat the movement with the left leg crossed over the right leg. To put emphasis on the obliques, keep the elbows back and hands relaxed. Look the way you are turning to help the rotation.

Side crunch

Muscles used Rectus abdominis; obliques – external and internal

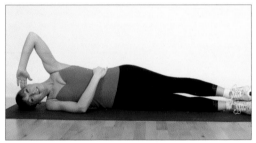

1 Lie on your right side, with your legs slightly bent, your left hand behind your head, and your right arm tucked across your body. Stay as side-on as possible to make the crunch more effective.

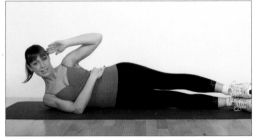

2 Tense your abdominals, keep your feet firmly together and crunch up sideways as far as you can go. Keep your left hand slightly behind your head and your right arm tucked across your body throughout. Turn over and repeat the movement with the opposite side. As long as the obliques are working, the range of movement can be small to begin with.

Dumbbell side bend

Muscles used Rectus abdominis; obliques – external and internal

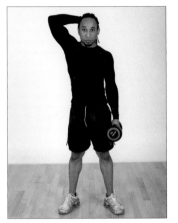

1 *Stand with your legs shoulder-width apart and your right hand behind your head. Hold a dumbbell in your left hand, down at your side.*

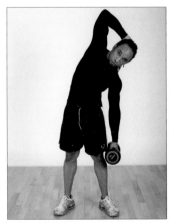

2 *Keeping your abdominals tense and staying side-on, bend at the hips to lower down to the side that holds the dumbbell. Once the dumbbell is level with your knee, pause for 1 second, then raise your body back up to the start position. Repeat with the other side. As you stretch down, you will be lengthening your abdominals, and on the way back up, you will be contracting them to make them work harder.*

High cable side bend

Muscles used Rectus abdominis; obliques – external and internal

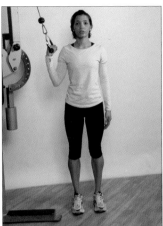

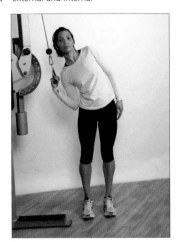

1 *Stand side-on to the cable machine, feet shoulder-width apart. Take hold of the pulley with one hand and hold it at shoulder height, with your arm bent. Let your other hand hang by your side. Keep the arm holding the cable as still as possible to ensure that it is only the abdominals that are doing the work.*

2 *Tense your abdominals and crunch down to the side. Try holding the position at the bottom of the bend for longer to really isolate the correct muscles. Pause at the bottom for 1 second, then slowly come back up to the start position. Repeat the movement on the other side.*

Oblique crunch

Muscles used Rectus abdominis; obliques – external and internal

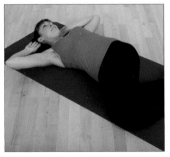

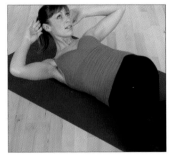

1 *Lie on your back with your legs bent and over to the left side, your feet placed firmly together. Try to keep your shoulders on the floor and your legs as far over to one side as possible. Place your hands behind your head with your elbows out to the side, with your fingers, fully extended, touching the sides of your head.*

2 *Tense your abdominals and crunch up, keeping your upper body as square-on as possible. Pause for a second at the top of the crunch and then, keeping your abdominals tense, slowly return to the start position. To make the abdominals work harder, tense them equally on the way back to the start as you did on the way up. Repeat on the other side.*

Abdominal Exercises: Rotational

It is important to use abdominal exercises that simulate the types of movements you need to do in everyday life and for your sport. The following exercises involve rotational exercises. Virtually every sporting activity calls for good rotational strength.

You should always maintain your abdominal muscles in tension throughout any exercise. If you can practise this in your strength workouts, you will start to use these muscles without having to make any conscious effort to do so. Get in touch with your abdominal muscles mentally – you need to learn how to recruit them and how to isolate the different abdominal muscles with various exercises.

When you train your abdominals, you should feel a burn and as you train harder, the burn should intensify. As your abdominal muscles get stronger, you will feel the burn even more as they work that bit harder. Your abdominals should feel pumped up after a workout, just like any other body part you have been training.

Be careful not to attempt too many repetitions. If your abdominal muscles get tired, you will start to use your lower back, which can lead to back injuries and overdevelopment of the lower-back muscles. To avoid using your lower back, always keep your abdominals tensed as you return to the start position in any abdominal exercise. The negative phase of the movement can make a massive difference in your abdominal development.

For each of these exercises, take 2 to 3 seconds for each direction of the movement. Breathe out at the beginning of the movement; breathe in as you return to the start position.

Excercises to tone and build rotational strength	
Exercise	**Sets and repetitions**
Hanging leg raise with a twist	3 x 10–20
Broomstick twist	3 x 30–40
Kneeling cable rotation	3 x 30–40
Alternating leg crunch	3 x 20–30

Alternating leg crunch

Muscles used Rectus abdominis; obliques – external and internal; tensor fascia lata; quadriceps

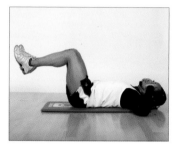
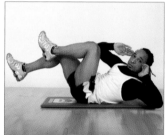

1 *Lie on your back, with your arms out to the sides, your fingers touching the sides of your head. Raise both legs up in the air at 90 degrees so that your calves are parallel to the floor. Keep your feet firmly together. Ensure that the movement is slow and under control to make your abdominals do all the work.*

2 *Straighten your right leg and crunch up with a twist, bringing your right elbow toward your left knee. When your elbow touches your knee, pause for 2 seconds, then return to the start position. Repeat with the other side. To make this exercise harder, try performing it on a slight incline.*

Leg criss-cross

Muscles used Rectus abdominis; obliques – external and internal; tensor fascia lata; quadriceps

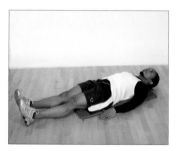
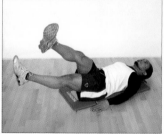

1 *Lie on your back with your legs on the floor stretched straight out in front of you. Put your hands by your sides, with your palms flat on the floor, for added stability. Press your back flat against the floor throughout the movement.*

2 *Lift your legs into the air and criss-cross them, alternating right over left and left over right. Keep your hands by your sides. To check that your lower abdominals are working, put your fingers under your lower back. You will feel it pushing against your fingers.*

Kneeling cable rotation

Muscles used Rectus abdominis; obliques – external and internal

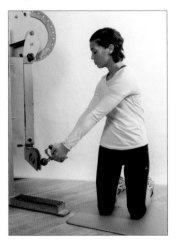

1 Kneel on the floor, side-on to one side of the cable machine. Keeping your arms straight and together in a V shape and your lower body straight from the abdomen down, grip the handle firmly with both hands.

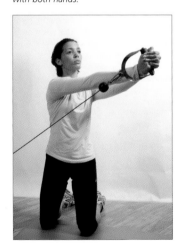

2 Tense your abdominals and rotate at the waist, taking your arms from one side to the other in a semicircular movement. When you have rotated through 180 degrees, pause for 1 second, then return – again through a semicircular movement – to the start position.

Machine trunk rotation

Muscles used Rectus abdominis; obliques – external and internal

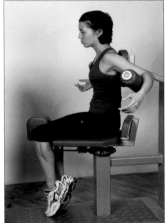

1 Sit on the machine and wrap your arms around the supports to keep yourself facing forward. Emphasize the abdominals throughout the movement.

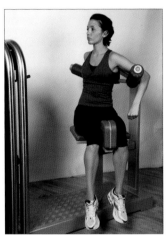

2 Tense your core muscles and rotate from one side to the other, keeping the movement smooth. Try not to move the hips and shoulders too much.

Broomstick twist

Muscles used Rectus abdominis; obliques – external and internal

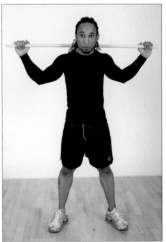

1 Stand with your feet shoulder-width apart so that you feel well balanced. Hold a broomstick or similar lightweight pole behind your head, across the back of your shoulders.

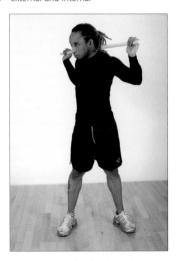

2 Keeping your feet firmly shoulder-width apart, rotate your upper body from one side to the other, keeping your hips as still as possible so that you can put more emphasis on the obliques.

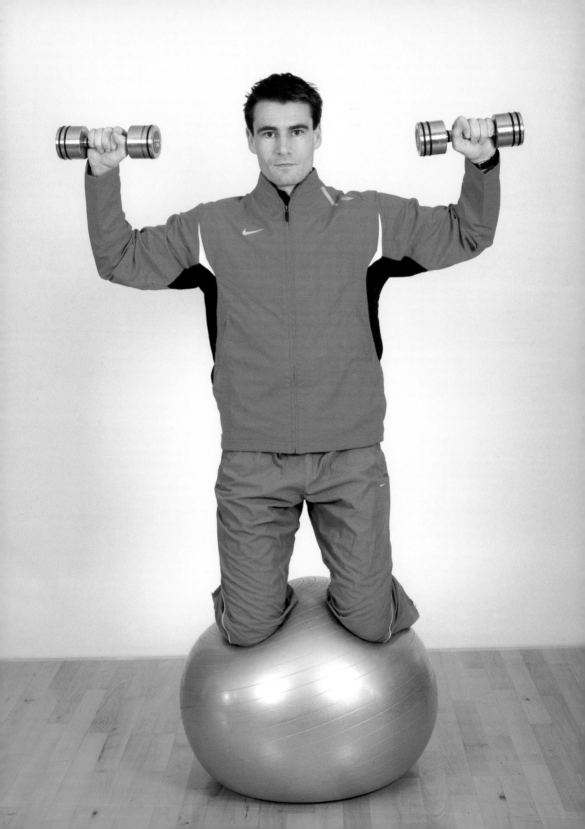

FLEXIBILITY AND CORE STABILITY

Pre-exercise and post-exercise stretches are essential to avoid exercise-related injuries – it is important to include a variety of flexibility exercises in your routine. Core stability is the strength of the muscles that hold the spine and pelvis in place. Without core strength and flexibility, you will be prone to injury and poor performance.

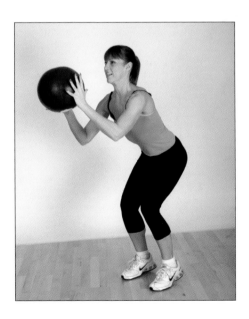

Above: Maintaining a firm position to catch a medicine ball requires good core strength.
Left: Kneeling on a fit ball while holding weights demonstrates balance and stability, owing to core strength.

The Importance of Flexibility

Flexibility training is one of the most frequently ignored and least understood areas of most fitness routines. You should, however, treat it with all the seriousness and commitment that you would accord any other part of your training routine.

There are a number of reasons why flexibility is essential. If, to give one example, your calf muscles are tight before you start a 10km/6.2-mile race or training session, then you are far more likely to suffer from cramps and muscle tears. If you play contact sports, such as American football or rugby, and you go hard into a tackle, your neck may be vulnerable if you don't have a good range of movement – a stiff neck will put the muscles and tendons under significant pressure.

If you are a swimmer with limited mobility around the shoulder joint, the result will be poor technique, a weak performance and likelihood of injury.

Stretching to remain flexible is not a new concept for your body. Everyone is born with great flexibility but as we get older we become less and less flexible due to lack of activity, sitting for long periods of time, and injuries from everyday life and sport. Everyone needs to be flexible.

What is flexibility?
You may often hear the word 'flexibility' used in relation to fitness training, but what is it? It is the range of mobility around a joint and the muscles that surround it. Flexibility training should: reduce the risk of injury; create a good range of movement (especially as a

muscle reaches its outer limits of movement); improve the movement around a joint; reduce muscular ache; increase co-ordination; increase blood flow circulation; break down scar tissue from general and overuse injuries; and equip the body to cope with the demands of a specific type of training or sport.

Sit and reach
The most commonly used test of flexibility is the sit and reach test. Thanks to the ample amount of research that has been carried out on the subject, it is fairly easy to compare yourself with other people. As a test, it illustrates the level of flexibility in your hamstrings and lower back. Studies show that there is direct correlation between flexibility in the hamstrings and the lower back, with muscular pain in the lower back, gait limitation and the risk of falling in older adults. (American College of Sports Medicine 1998.)

Use a sit and reach test box or simply make your own using a box and a solid ruler. Place the soles of your feet up

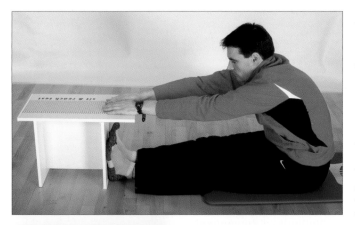

Left: The sit and reach test assesses the flexibility of the back and the hamstrings, at the back of the thigh.

Below left: To keep muscle flexibility during your training, stop now and again to do some stretches.

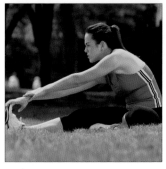

Sit and reach test
This simple test is a reliable measure of the flexibility of the hamstrings and the lower back.

	Male	Female
Very poor	−20cm/−7¾in	−15cm/−6in
Poor	−19 to 9cm/−7½ to 3½in	−14 to 8cm/−5½ to 3in
Fair	−8 to 1cm/−3 to ⅓in	−7 to 0cm/−2¾ to 0in
Average	0 to 5cm/0 to 2in	1 to 10cm/⅓ to 4in
Good	6 to 16cm/2⅓ to 6¼in	11 to 20cm/4⅓ to 7¾in
Excellent	17 to 27cm/6⅔ to 10½in	21 to 30cm/8¼ to 12in
Superior	27cm+/10½in+	30cm+/12in+

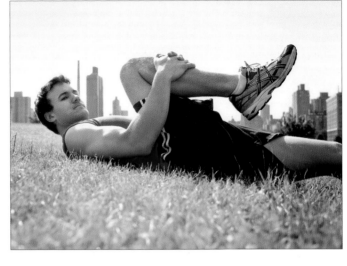

against the box and then, with your arms out in front of you and your legs straight, slowly reach forward along the ruler. After three attempts at stretching forward, you should be at your farthest point. The point where your fingers touch the ruler or box is your score (if you don't make it beyond your toes, you receive a negative score). The ruler should read zero where the soles of your feet are in contact with the box. Compare your score with the data in the box to see how flexible you are. Be aware that warm-up will make a massive difference to your flexibility, so always use the same warm-up before you do the test. About 5 minutes of cardiovascular exercise would be suitable.

When to stretch

You should try to stretch before and after every training session or competition. Before you begin any activity, warm up

Below: After you have completed your training programme, do some stretches to aid recovery.

first with some cardiovascular exercise to promote blood flow and heat in the muscles. For example, if you intend going for a 10km/6-mile run, do 5 minutes' fast walking. Follow this with 5 minutes of stretches, paying particular attention to your hamstrings, quadriceps and calf muscles. After the run, do static stretches in your cool-down. If you are intending to lift heavy weights, do 5 minutes' easy warm-up on the

Below: Stretching is beneficial to everyone, whatever their level of fitness or their age.

Above: When you begin any major training, always include stretches in your warm-up.

rowing machine before you do dynamic or proprioceptive muscular facilitation stretches (PMF stretching), paying particular attention to the muscle regions you may use. For example, before a chest weights session, stretch the pectorals, triceps and lower back. After the weights session, do static stretches to help lengthen the muscles back to full movement and decrease the risk of injury.

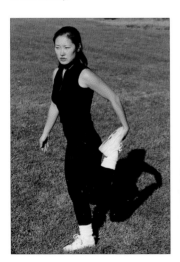

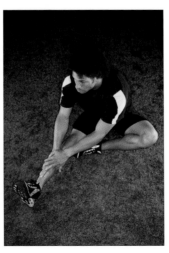

Types of Flexibility

The different types of stretching that should be included in you training programme are static active stretching, static passive stretching, ballistic stretching, isometric stretching and proprioceptive muscular facilitation.

Everyone wants to achieve greater flexibility in the shortest time possible, with minimum pain and risk, so that they can get on with their fitness training programme. The good news is that you can – and you don't need to get yourself into bizarre contortions as if you were auditioning for the circus in order to do so.

There are a number of different types of stretches that are suitable for inclusion in your training programme. First, though, you need to understand how the following types of stretches can help you, when it is appropriate to do them, and what exactly is meant by terms such as 'static active stretching', 'static passive stretching', 'dynamic stretching', 'ballistic stretching', 'isometric stretching' and 'proprioceptive muscular facilitation stretching' (PMF stretching).

When deciding which technique to use, think about the range of movement you are trying to achieve, and always use a variety of stretches to improve your flexibility. It is important to remember that stretching should not be painful. Simply getting into the correct stretching position and starting to feel the tension in the right muscle is enough. Some types of stretching are more aggressive than others, for example dynamic stretching or ballistic stretching. Before you do any of these types of stretches, make sure you warm up for at least 10–15 minutes in order to get adequate blood flow and heat in the muscles.

When not to stretch?

In some situations it may be best not to do any stretches. If you feel any discomfort in the muscle from an injury, leave the injury for at least 48 hours and consult a physician to determine whether it is safe to begin stretching the muscle. Avoid stretching areas that are suffering from muscular and ligament strains or areas of recent fractures. If you are at all unsure, get expert advice.

Static active stretching

This is a method of stretching muscles with minimal movement. An example would be placing one leg on a step and holding it there for 30 seconds. This is the best form of stretching for a cool-down after your training to help re-align the muscles and promote good blood flow. This type of stretch uses the opposing muscles to hold the stretch.

Static passive stretching

This stretch will increase the range of movement of a muscle. Unlike static active stretching, you will need to use an external force to stretch the muscle. Static passive stretching is best used after training or competition to realign the muscle fibres. It is often used for the rehabilitation of torn muscles.

> **Build in flexibility**
> To get the most out of exercise, it is important to get an understanding of which stretches and types of flexibility are going to be good for you.
> Flexibility is as necessary as any other training. Without a good programme of flexibility exercises, you will be more prone to injury. Injuries mean less training, or even no training as a result. So there are no excuses – make flexibility a vital part of your fitness training programme.

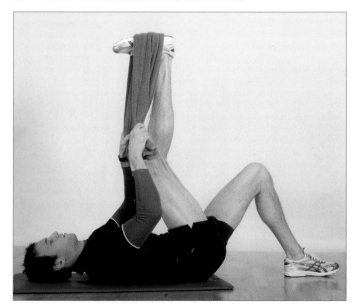

Hold a towel around your foot to pull it up by stretching your hamstrings. Hold the stretch for 20 to 30 seconds.

Dynamic stretching

This is a good way to warm up – but not after injury, as it could cause further damage. It uses training movements, such as lunges and squats, to warm up and stretch the muscles you will use in the activity. Your body's movement and momentum create the stretch. Ensure that your heart rate has been elevated for at least 10 minutes for sufficient blood flow and heat in the muscles.

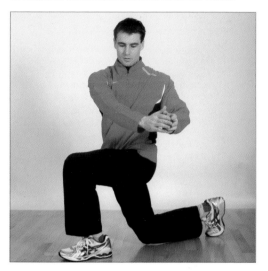

This lunge with rotation has some momentum to get a good dynamic stretch. Maintaining your balance while stretching is important.

Proprioceptive muscular facilitation (PMF) stretching

This is commonly used in sports that require a larger range of movement, such as ballet and gymnastics. It involves a muscle being stretched by a partner. It is perhaps one of the most advanced forms of stretching and can often promote the best results. When contracting the muscles being stretched, do so for only 5 to 6 seconds, then stretch again for 10 seconds.

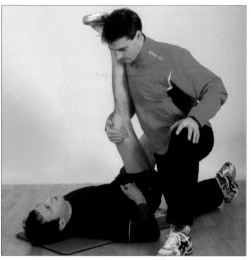

Have your training partner stretch your hamstrings until they reach stretching point. Resist by contracting your hamstrings to try to force your partner's arm back.

Isometric stretching

This uses the contraction of the muscle to stretch muscle fibres that are not being stretched in a normal passive stretch. Following the stretch, allow the quadriceps to contract for 3 to 5 seconds to wake up any fibres that are not being stretched. This creates a greater stretch response in the muscle fibres. When a muscle is contracted during exercise, not all the fibres are contracting; some are at rest. When a muscle is being stretched, some muscle fibres are elongated and some are not. During an isometric contraction, the muscle fibres will be pulled from both ends by the contracting muscles, so the resting fibres are stretched.

Lie on your front and have your training partner bend your leg up behind you to stretch your quadriceps muscles.

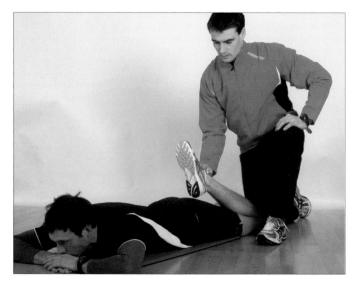

Importance of Core Stability

The term 'core stability' is used to describe the muscles of the trunk that hold and control the position and movement of the lumbar spine and pelvis. Because these muscles are rarely used in everyday life, they require special attention.

Thousands of years ago people had to be physically active to survive; our ancestors were hunters and gatherers who were constantly on the move, lifting materials to build shelters, tracking down animals for food and felling trees for fires. Today, we miss out on these everyday activities. In the past, we would regularly have used all the muscles that control the position and dynamic movements of the lumbar spine

and pelvis. Now, many people live a sedentary lifestyle and have little or no core stability.

You need your core muscles to be strong and active all the time for everyday movements. For example, if you are about to lift something heavy from the floor, your core muscles will have to tense before the rest of your body exerts itself to pick the item up in order to keep a brace-like position to

> **Working together**
> It's not just a case of getting your core muscles to work; they need to work in conjunction with your other muscles and recruit in the correct order to help all your muscles to be effective in establishing core stability in your body.

hold your spine and pelvis in place to assist the lifting movement. If your core muscles are not tensed, your spine and pelvis will not have the strength to maintain their correct position, leaving you prone to injury. Common problems related to poor core stability include lower back pain, rounded shoulders and back, and poor posture. With the appropriate core stability exercises, you will be able to recruit the correct core muscles to support your body effectively; the pressure on your back will dramatically reduce and your posture will improve.

Core stability is also important for optimum performance in many sports. You may have strong legs and shoulders but if your core stability is poor, the middle of your body may twist under pressure in a rugby scrum or tackle, for

Below: Sitting at a desk all day may result in your core muscles becoming even weaker.

The core stability muscles

The major muscles in the trunk that provide you with good core stability are:

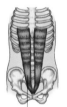

rectus abdominis

Above: This muscle helps you to sit up.

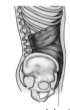

transversus abdominis

Above: This muscle pulls you in and helps you exhale.

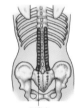

multifidus

Above: Controls movement of the spine in any direction.

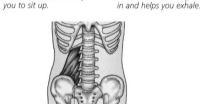

quadratus lumborum

Above: Controls lateral movement of spine.

iliopsoas

Above: Flexes the tops of the legs and hips.

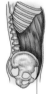

external oblique

Above: Controls lateral and rotational movements.

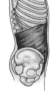

internal oblique

Above: This muscle controls lateral movement of the trunk.

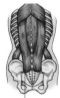

erector spinae

Above: This muscle supports you bending forward.

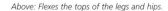
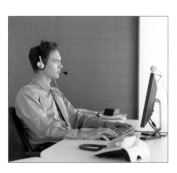

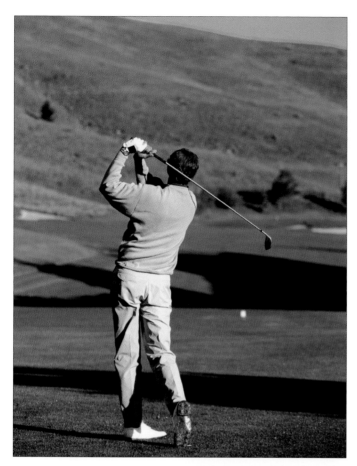

Above: An effective golf swing requires a good level of core stability to control the movement.

use in giving you good core stability, and, most people use poor technique when they do sit-ups and crunches.

Avoiding injury

If you are looking to build strength in your upper and lower body using weights, it is important to have strong core stability to avoid injury. Adding core exercises twice a week to your training programme will give you greater stability and power, and help you to avoid injury. Once your core muscles are switched on and recruiting properly you will feel them working. When you do a chest press tense the core muscles also. The muscles you are targeting in the legs or arms work harder and feel more isolated. Using the core muscles during other exercises will make them stronger and more effective.

Below: In combat sports such as rugby, strong core muscles are essential to avoid sustaining injuries.

example. Likewise, if your torso muscles are weak, your golf swing will suffer: you will not be able to transfer as much power from your body to the ball, and your lack of control in your back swing and follow-through will leave you off balance and at risk of injury.

People often make the mistake of thinking that simply doing lots of sit-ups and crunches will provide them with good core stability – and it's not true. It doesn't matter how many sit-ups and crunches you do, they will only help you to firm up your muscles to make it look like you have a toned, flat stomach. These exercises are, in fact, of very little

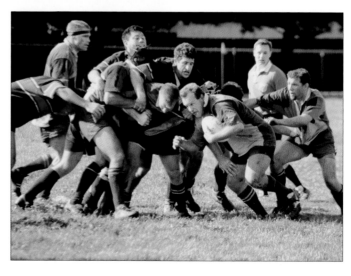

Measuring Core Stability

It is difficult to measure core stability and muscle recruitment outside a laboratory environment. However, there are some basic tests that will reveal whether your core stability is working efficiently enough to support you.

Core strength is so important that if the results of the tests below show that there is any weakness in your core stability, you should take time to work on all aspects of it. The tests not only reveal how much strength you have in your muscles, but also the recruitment pattern of the muscles connected to the core. If your core is weak, these muscles may not be recruiting effectively in the right order.

It is important to consider which core muscles are most important for your sport, and in some cases this means designing a test that is relevant to you. A good physiotherapist or expert in biomechanics should be able to tell you which parts of your body are the most important and which movements

Poor core strength

You may find you get cramp in your feet during these exercises – this is a sign of poor core strength, as your body has to compensate by using other muscles to keep your balance. If this happens to you, stop for a few minutes and try to relax your other muscles.

require help from your core-stability muscles. For example, in your golf swing, you need to have strong core muscles to prevent lateral movement at the hips. Doing a single-leg squat or lunge and watching the lateral movement at the hip closely will help you to see how strong your core is at maintaining the solid position required.

Film yourself from all angles doing the tests so that you can see for yourself where your core stability weaknesses are. Repeat these tests every six weeks to monitor your progress.

Below: You will be more prone to injury if you do not maintain core stability while you are training. A strong core is vital for effective exercising.

Ignore at your peril

Many people, including elite athletes, don't bother with core stability exercises, as it is difficult to measure the results. But core stability and correct muscular recruitment will relate directly to all sporting and exercise activities, so measure it, train it and monitor it.

Single-leg stand

Check your core stability with this simple test: Stand still for at least 30 seconds, without putting your arms out for balance. If you can't do this, your core muscles are not working well. In this exercise, all the core muscles are used.

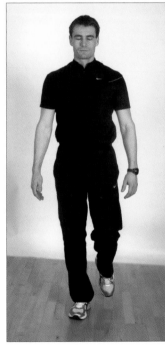

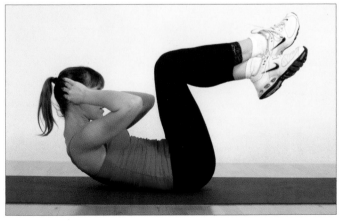

Stand on one leg with your arms by your sides. Shut your eyes and stand still for as long as possible. As soon as you shut your eyes, you should feel your core muscles tightening – they help to hold you still, just like the guy ropes of a tent. Keep your feet as relaxed as possible to put more emphasis on the core stability muscles, thus making them work harder. Restrict movement in the hips when changing from one leg to the other.

Single-leg squat

Do this exercise in front of a mirror to assess which parts of your body are weak. All of the core-stability muscles are used in this exercise.

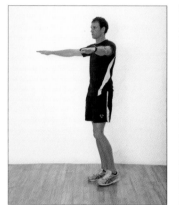

1 *Stand up straight on both legs with your arms out in front of you. Balance well so the head is still (a sign of weak core stability is the head moving from side to side).*

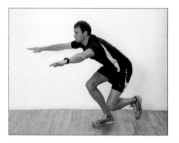

2 *Squat until the thigh of your squatting leg is almost parallel to the ground. Pause for 2 seconds, then slowly stand up.*

Check your core stability

Look out for the signs of weak core stability: head moving from side to side; hips dropping down and not staying level (also indicative of weak gluteus muscles); leg crossing behind your squatting leg during the squat (also indicative of weak buttock muscles); knee wobbling from side to side (indicative of weakness higher up in core muscles); and trunk constantly moving.

The lunge

In this exercise, the signs of a weak core are the same as those for the single-leg squat. Include lunges with leans and lunges with rotation in your exercise plan to make your core muscles strong enough to support your body in your chosen sporting activity. The lunge uses all the core-stability muscles.

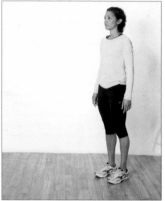

1 *Stand up straight on both legs, with your feet hip-width apart and your arms hanging straight by your side. Try to keep the head and neck totally relaxed before you start the lunge.*

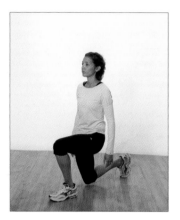

2 *Take a forward stride and lower your body weight by bending both legs, keeping your back as upright as possible. Try to avoid any lateral forward or backward movement during the lunge.*

Plank hand changes

Keep your core muscles switched on through this exercise. All of the core muscles are recruited for this exercise.

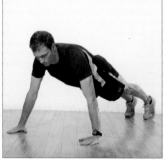

1 *Adopt the standard press-up position, with your legs wide apart and hands with palms flat on the floor, so that you can keep your hips still and progressively move your feet closer together to assess how much your core stability is improving. Focus on the hips and don't move them sideways or rotate them.*

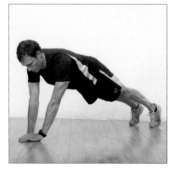

2 *Slowly raise one hand off the floor and place it on top of your other hand. Feel and watch out for any lateral, upward and downward movement of the hips. Your core is working well when there is little trunk movement during the exercise. Lateral movement and/or rotation in the centre of the body will make you prone to injury.*

Basic Core Exercises

It is vital to begin with these basic core exercises in order for your core muscles to recruit correctly. If you jump to more advanced exercises, your core muscles will not benefit, and you will be prone to injury.

In addition to beginning with these exercises so that you can get your muscles recruiting correctly, you should also regularly revert back to using them to check whether you are doing the basics correctly.

If possible, you should also work with a training partner who can observe your exercising and give you some guidance on whether your core muscles are working properly. Where possible, try placing your hands on the core muscles you are supposed to be working during the exercise to see if they are held in tension or not.

For each exercise, take 2 to 3 seconds for each direction of the movement. Breathe out at the beginning of the movement, continue breathing through the hold, and breathe in as you return to the start position.

Think before you tense

It is easy to do core-stability exercises without knowing which muscles you are trying to engage. Take your time to think clearly about which parts of the body are giving you the stability for each exercise, and be patient, focusing intently on that part of the body. If you are in a position that requires you to hold the core muscles tight, then keep your body as still as possible.

Many people think they have mastered an exercise and quickly move on to more advanced core work when, in fact, they only keep their balance by wobbling from side to side, waving their arms around or holding on to a wall. If you are really struggling to feel your core muscles, especially your abdominal muscles, then try feeling them when you are coughing. The tension that you feel around your abdominal area as you are coughing is caused by the core muscles tensing.

Plank (prone bridging)

Muscles used Rectus abdominis; transversus abdominis; internal obliques

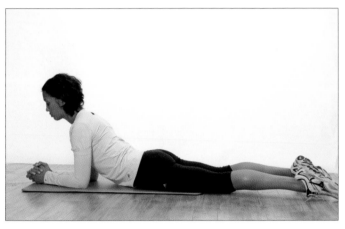

1 *Lie on your front with your legs out straight behind you and your hands clasped together in front of you, with your forearms flat on the floor. Keep your spine in neutral all the time and don't let your back arch.*

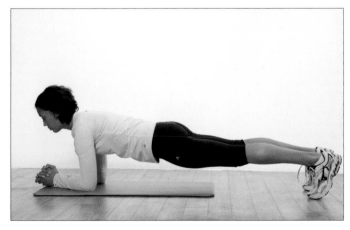

2 *Raise your hips so that only your forearms and toes are resting on the floor. Hold this position for as long as possible by tensing your core muscles. Push your chest out and keep your shoulders back to make the exercise harder. You should aim to hold the plank for as long as you possibly can. Begin by holding the position for 20 seconds, adding 5 seconds each time, until you can stay in this position for at least 1 minute.*

Plank to single-leg raise

Muscles used Rectus abdominis; transversus abdominis; internal obliques

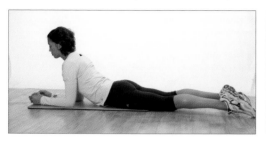

1 Lie on your front with your legs out straight behind you and your hands clasped together in front of you, with your forearms flat on the floor. Keep your spine in neutral and tense your core muscles.

2 Raise your hips, keeping your forearms and toes on the floor, then lift one leg off the ground, keeping it straight out behind you. Hold for up to 30 seconds. Repeat the exercise with the other leg.

Side plank raises (lateral bridging)

Muscles used Obliques – internal and external; transversus abdominis

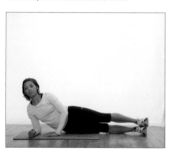

1 Lie on your side, with the legs out straight, a forearm flat on the floor, with the hand in a loose fist position, the other hand palm down on the floor, and one foot resting on top of the other.

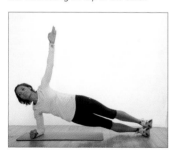

2 Raise your hips, keeping one forearm on the floor and your feet together. Raise the other arm straight up in the air. Hold so your body is in a straight line.

Gluteal bridge

Muscles used Rectus abdominis; gluteus maximus; erector spinae

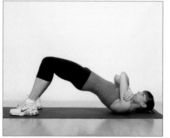

Lie on your back on a mat, with the legs bent at 90 degrees. Tense your core muscles, especially the gluteus muscles, and raise your hips until your body is level in one line, from your knees to your shoulders. Begin by holding the position for 10–20 seconds, gradually building up to a 1-minute hold.

Tips for core exercises
Start by keeping your body as still as possible, then begin tensing your core muscles. Try pushing through your heels to put more emphasis on the gluteus and less stress on your knees. Focus on tensing your buttocks. Keep your hands and elbows off the ground to make your core muscles work harder. Breathe out to begin and in when you return to the start.

Single-leg stand

Muscles used All the core muscles are used for this exercise.

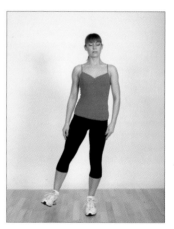

Stand on one leg, with your eyes closed and both arms hanging by your sides. Try to keep your body still and as relaxed as possible, then tense your core muscles to maintain your balance. Hold your position for 10–20 seconds, gradually building up to a 1-minute hold. Keep your spine in neutral throughout the movement and focus on working the obliques. After you have completed a 1-minute hold, try holding the position for as long as possible, tensing your core muscles all the time.

Intermediate Core Exercises

As your core-stability muscles get stronger, you can start to introduce exercises – of the kind given here – that involve making a strong connection between your core muscles and the muscles of your limbs.

When you start using your limbs to press and pull weights, it is important to be able to keep your spine and pelvis in their natural positions in order to make your core-stability muscles stronger for everyday activities and sporting movements.

Remember that you are only as strong as your core-stability muscles. Without strengthening the core, you will not increase your physical power and will always be more prone to injury.

Taking your limbs away from the centre of your body will act as a lever to make your core muscles work even harder. Exercises that involve rotation will force some core muscles to keep your body still, with other core muscles working to allow parts of your body to rotate, but in a controlled way. If you don't take time to get this correct, other muscles – mainly in the lower back – will be forced to do the work, which will not give you the core strength that you are looking for.

For each exercise, take 2 to 3 seconds for each direction of the movement. Breathe out at the beginning of the movement, and breathe in as you return to the start position.

For the following intermediate core exercises, start with three sets of five repetitions and build up gradually over the weeks until you are doing five sets of ten repetitions.

Rest-day exercise

For you to get the maximum benefit from your core exercises, they need to be given your full attention and energy. At the intermediate stage you should try to plan two core-stability workouts a week. You need to do these sessions separately from your normal cardiovascular or strength-training sessions. Try fitting them in on the days that you would normally rest.

Plank leg kick

Muscles used Rectus abdominis; transversus abdominis; internal obliques; gluteus maximus; tensor fascia lata

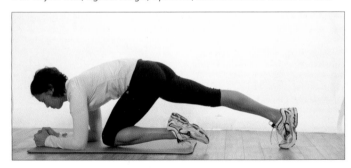

1 *Lie on your front, legs out straight, hips raised, with forearms and toes on the floor.*

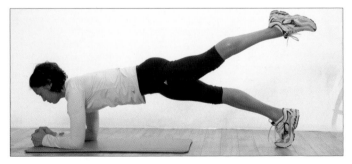

2 *Raise one foot, bend your knee and bring it in toward your chest until your thigh is perpendicular to the ground.*

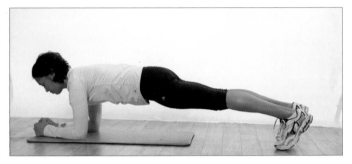

3 *Kick the leg back out, slowly but forcefully, until it is straight out behind you. Hold for 5 seconds, then bring the knee in. Repeat with the other leg.*

Hip-raise, single-leg changeovers

Muscles used Rectus abdominis; gluteus maximus; erector spinae

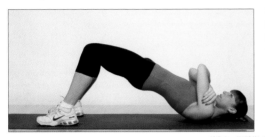

1 *Adopt the gluteal bridge position. Tense your core muscles, especially the gluteus muscles. Raise your hips until your body is in one line from your shoulders to the knees.*

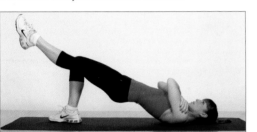

2 *Slowly raise one leg until it is in line with the rest of your body. Hold this position for 5 seconds then change legs, keeping your hips off the floor and your body in line.*

Superman

Muscles used Erector spinae; gluteus maximus; rectus abdominis

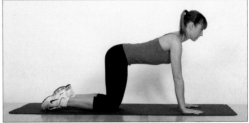

1 *Start with your hands and knees on the floor, and your belly button pulled in toward your spine to keep your core muscles tense.*

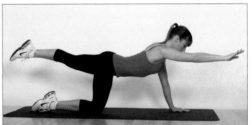

2 *Raise your right leg off the floor, straighten it behind you, lift and straighten your left arm in front of you. Hold for 5 seconds, return to the start position and repeat with the opposite limbs.*

Cable wood chops, high to low

Muscles used Rectus abdominis; obliques – internal and external

Work the core muscles

Try to visualize a poker going through the top of your head and down the length of your spine. If you imagine turning on this 'axis', you will find that the exercise is more effective.

Use a weight that is lighter than you think you need to start with. Use a mirror to check your technique, to help you eliminate any lateral hip movement.

With rotational exercises, your hips will try to move. To create a strong core, keep the hips still; get the core muscles to work.

This is a great exercise for golfers as it involves the same muscles used for the golf swing.

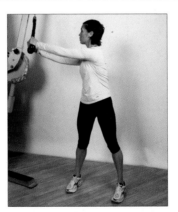

1 *Stand side-on to the cable machine, with your feet just over hip-width apart. Turn toward the machine by twisting upward from just above the hips, and grip the rope in both hands.*

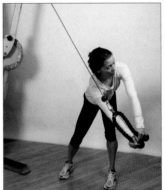

2 *Slowly rotate your upper body, keeping your arms straight out in front, until the handle is level with your opposite knee. Pause for a second, then slowly rotate back to the start position.*

Advanced Core Exercises

When you get to an advanced stage of your core-stability training, you can start to involve dynamic exercises that will simulate the movements you might use in your sport. These exercises make it hard to balance, so that your core muscles have to work hard.

Most people believe that you are either naturally blessed with having good balance or not, when in fact it really comes down to your core muscles giving you enough stability to achieve really good balance.

Most sporting movements call for good balance to cope with changes in direction and transferring weight and stress from one limb to another. Some of the following exercises use weights to make the exercise harder and to help build core muscles. If you want to move your limbs with strong, rapid movements, you will need to have very strong core stability with great balance.

For each exercise, take 2 to 3 seconds for each direction of the movement. Breathe out at the beginning of the movement, continue breathing through the hold, and breathe in as you return to the start position.

For all of these exercises, begin with three sets of repetitions each side of the body, gradually building up to five sets of ten repetitions each side.

> **Exercise to stay injury-free**
> When you have reached the advanced stage, just build the exercises into your normal training programme. Do them between cardiovascular exercises and resistance exercises to help keep your core muscles switched on through all of your movements. It will also help you avoid injuries in training and make the core muscles focus and become recruited to support your limbs as they start to fatigue.

Two-point superman

Muscles used Erector spinae; gluteus maximus; rectus abdominis

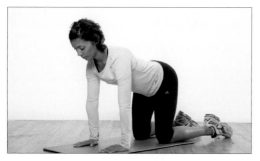

1 Start on all fours on a mat, with both hands and knees on the floor, hands palm down. Try to prevent your lower back from arching.

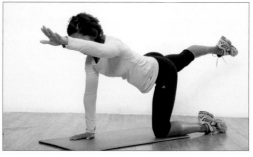

2 Raise and straighten your right leg out behind you. At the same time, raise and straighten your left arm in front of you. Pull your belly button in toward your spine.

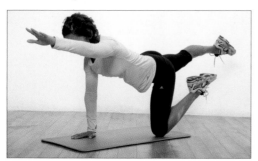

3 To make this a two-point superman, lift the foot of your supporting leg off the floor to work your core muscles harder.

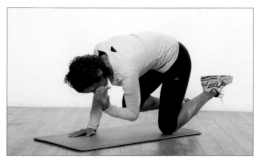

4 Hold for 5 seconds, then bring your right leg and left arm in until the knee and elbow touch. Repeat on the other side.

Press-up plank to side waves

Muscles used Rectus abdominis; obliques – internal and external; pectoralis major

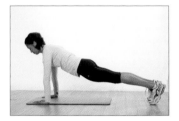

1 *Start in a standard press-up position.*

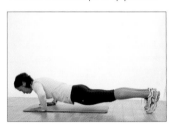

2 *Lower your body toward the floor by bending your elbows out to the sides.*

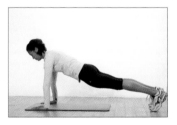

3 *With elbows bent at 90 degrees, hold for 2 seconds then push back up.*

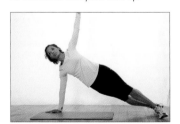

4 *Take one arm out to the side and twist your body until you are side-on to the floor in a side plank position. Think of your trunk as a brace and don't let your hips drop in the rotation. Let your feet rotate over on to their sides.*

Single-leg cable wood chops, high to low

Muscles used Erector spinae; gluteus – maximus, medius; rectus abdominis

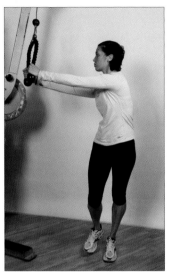

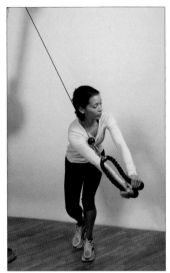

1 *Stand on one leg, with the other foot raised just slightly off the floor, side-on to the cable machine. Turn your upper torso slowly toward the machine and grip the rope with both hands. Try doing this exercise sitting on a fit ball, with only one foot on the floor.*

2 *Slowly rotate your upper body, keeping your arms straight out in front of you until the handle is level with your opposite knee. Pause for a second, then slowly rotate back to the start position. Keep your hips facing forward to put greater emphasis on the core muscles.*

Superman row

Muscles used Erector spinae; rectus abdominis; obliques; latissimus dorsi

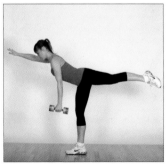

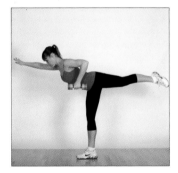

1 *Stand on one leg and hold your other leg straight out behind you, and your opposite arm straight out in front of you. Hold a dumbbell in the other hand at knee height. Keep your back parallel to the floor.*

2 *Pull the dumbbell up to your ribs, taking your elbow past your ribs and back behind the line of your body. Avoid twisting your trunk as you pull the weight up. Pause for 1 second, then return to the start position.*

Fit Ball Core Exercises

The fit ball is an effective piece of equipment for improving core stability, because it forces your body to stimulate more neuromuscular pathways, which in turn activate a larger number of muscle fibres in the core.

The fit ball was first introduced in the 1980s as a way of improving posture and rehabilitation for injuries. But because the fit ball helped to achieve great results in increased core stability among top athletes, it has become a great tool for people of all abilities.

Being round, a fit ball is an unstable surface to work on, unlike a conventional flat bench in the gym. As a result, core-stability muscles have to stay switched on throughout any movement when you are on the fit ball if you want to stay on the ball. Just sitting on a ball holding your body upright requires the majority of your core-stability muscles to work. The ball also allows you to get a greater range of movement for exercises that you would usually do on the floor. For example, with gluteal bridges, you can lower your hips to the ground before tensing them to come back up.

By using a fit ball, your body awareness and balance will improve, which is a bonus for any sporting activity. Do not try using these exercises until you have completed the intermediate stage of your core-stability training.

Building connections
Replace some of your regular gym exercises with fit ball exercises to build the connection between your core and limbs. For example, when training your legs, include some single-leg fit ball squats; for a chest session, include fit ball press-ups; and for a shoulder workout, include some fit ball shoulder presses. Many of the exercises used in the gym can be replicated using the fit ball; this will make them significantly harder and ensure that you are using your core muscles correctly. Many world-class athletes have stated that using a fit ball made a big difference to their performance.

Fit ball hip raises, feet on ball

Muscles used Gluteus maximus and medius; rectus abdominis; obliques – internal and external; biceps femoris

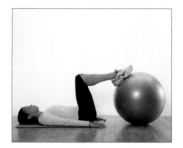 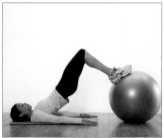

1 *Lie on your back on a gym mat on the floor, with your feet on the top of the fit ball and your hands flat on the floor, palms down. Tense your core muscles, especially your buttocks. Keep the ball as still as possible.*

2 *Raise your hips until your body is in one line from your shoulders to your knees. Try to maintain your balance throughout. Hold this position for 5 seconds, then slowly return to the start position.*

Single-leg fit ball squat

Muscles used Rectus abdominis; gluteus medius; quadriceps

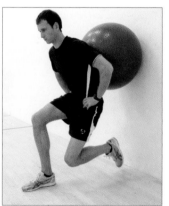 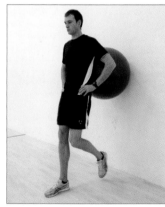

1 *With the fit ball between your lower back and a wall, slowly squat in front of a mirror, pushing your weight through your heels, until your heel is almost parallel to the floor.*

2 *Pause for 2 seconds, check that your hips are staying in line, then gradually extend your legs until you are standing fully upright. Tense your buttocks as your legs straighten.*

Fit ball plank

Muscles used Rectus abdominis; transversus abdominis; internal obliques

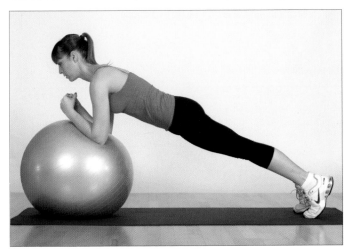

Adopt a plank position with your elbows and forearms resting on the ball and your feet out behind you, resting on your toes. Hold this position for as long as possible by tensing your core muscles. Keep your spine in neutral all the time and don't let your back arch. If your back does start to arch, stop the exercise immediately; it will have a negative effect by teaching your body to do the exercise using the wrong muscles. Aim to hold the plank for as long as possible. Begin by holding the position for 20 seconds, building up to a 1-minute hold for three sets.

Fit ball side roll

Muscles used Obliques; gluteus medius; rectus abdominis; tensor fascia lata

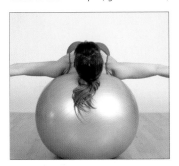

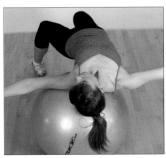

1 Rest the fit ball under your shoulders and neck. Keep your knees bent at 90 degrees and your feet flat on the floor. Tense your core muscles to keep your hips up in line with your knees and shoulders. Look down toward your feet to help you balance at first. Focus on working your obliques and gluteus medius.

2 Roll your upper body over to one side of the fit ball until you reach the point where you start to lose your balance. Pause for 2 seconds, then slowly return to the start position. Start with your feet wide apart and gradually bring them closer together as you get better at the exercise. Start with three sets of five repetitions to each side.

Fit ball shoulder press

Begin with three sets of five repetitions, then build up to five sets of ten repetitions.

Muscles used Rectus abdominis; gluteus – maximus and medius; deltoid

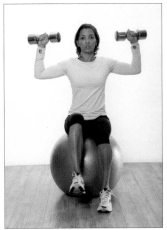

1 Holding dumbells in each hand, sit on the fit ball, raise one foot off the floor and lift the dumbbells up to ear level. Have a training partner close to you throughout this exercise to help you get used to balancing on the ball.

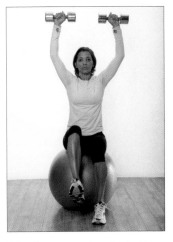

2 Keeping your core tensed, raise the dumbbells up above your head, pause for 2 seconds, then slowly return to the start position.

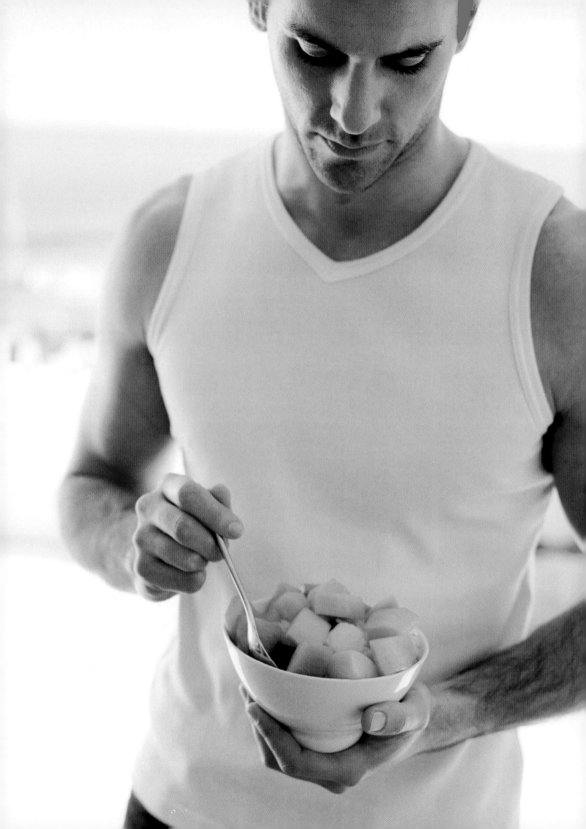

NUTRITION

To get the most from your fitness training, you need to focus on nutrition as much as exercise. No matter how hard you train, if you eat the wrong food at the wrong time, you will hinder your progress and may also experience fatigue, illness and injury. This chapter reveals the reality behind quick-fix diets and explains why you should simply eat healthily. The key is to know which foods are good for you, when to eat them and their effect on your performance. Equipped with this knowledge you can adopt a healthy eating plan to suit your lifestyle and help achieve your exercise goals.

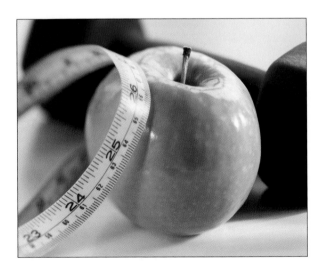

Above: The tape measure will reveal whether you are eating an appropriate diet.
Left: Enjoy getting fit and healthy with exercise and nutritious food.

Eating Healthily

With so much conflicting advice on how to eat healthily, it can be difficult knowing which foods are best and the correct time to eat them, especially when you are exercising hard. But it doesn't have to be such a problem.

A regular exercise routine throws up many questions about diet. Should you eat a diet rich in carbohydrates or go for the high protein option? Should you have separate protein days and carbohydrate days? Should you focus on eating foods labelled low fat? Is it best to have three meals a day or several smaller meals? If you are exercising hard, what and when should you eat? Which diet will work for you?

Diet confusion

Before changing your eating habits, consider what our ancestors ate 10,000 years ago. After all, the human body has not changed in all that time, and neither have our dietary requirements. We are designed to be hunter-gatherers, not to live sedentary lifestyles, consuming convenience foods rich in sugar, saturated fats and salt. Despite the lack of healthcare, our ancestors had relatively good health – chronic diseases, such as obesity, diabetes, liver disease and heart disease were far less prevalent than they are today. There are still areas of the world where people live as our ancestors did 10,000 years ago.

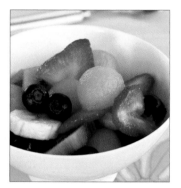

Above: Fruits tend to be low in calories and fat and provide fibre and vitamins as well as natural sugars.

These people do not suffer from high cholesterol, high blood pressure and insulin problems. Instead, they have a low percentage of body fat and very efficient cardiovascular systems.

A natural diet

Hunter-gatherers had to think of food as fuel. They ate what they were naturally meant to eat. In the modern developed

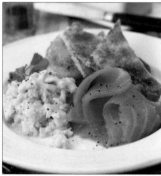

Above: Fish, such as smoked salmon with scrambled eggs, makes a tasty and delicious start to the day.

world, people choose foods that satisfy their tastebuds without considering how it will affect their daily performance, whether it's running for the bus or concentrating in the office. Far too many modern-day city dwellers do not eat a natural diet, as dictated by our genes. Instead, the supermarkets tell us what we should eat, even though 75 per cent of the food available in those packed aisles would not have been available 200 years ago. For example, adverts extol the virtues of cereal as a breakfast food, but cereals were only introduced at the time of the agricultural revolution.

Below: Apples and carrots make a great, low-calorie snack when you are hungry. And they are full of vitamins and fibre.

Below: Don't rely on fast food; take your own healthy lunch of nuts, seeds, dried fruit and canned fish.

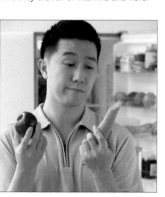

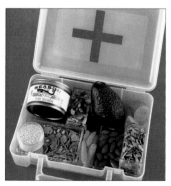

Slowly does it

Don't alter your eating habits all at once; it is important to remember that you should make any changes to your diet gradually so that your body can adjust and get used to the healthier foods. Don't expect to see spectacular results such as weight loss overnight. The first thing you should notice, though, if you are making the right changes to your diet is an increase in your energy levels.

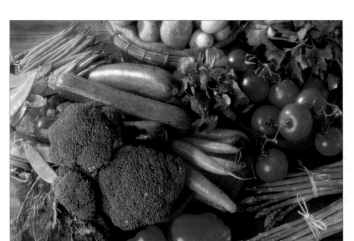

Above: Fresh vegetables supply vitamins and minerals. It is important to eat a good variety to get vitamins A and C.

Many types of cereals are of little nutritional value. Eating fresh fish and fruit for the first meal of the day is a much healthier option than a bowl of cornflakes.

What's on your plate?
Because we are not eating a diet to which we are naturally suited, we are suffering from a wide range of health problems. Just as you need to use the correct fuel in your car, your body needs the correct food to function properly, and to avoid being damaged. So, take time to study foods and find out where the food you eat comes from. Are the meats, fruit and vegetables on your plate organically or agrochemically produced? Wherever possible, it is better to eat organic food for a number of reasons:
• Organic foods contain higher levels of essential vitamins and minerals.
• It tastes better, especially fruit and vegetables, which take a longer

time to grow and contain a lower proportion of water than the equivalent agrochemical produce.
• Only 32 of the 290 food additives used in food production are used in organic food. Many food additives have been linked with health problems.
• Organic foods have not been genetically modified.
• There are no drugs in organic foods.
• Organic foods contain none of the many chemicals used to make agrochemical foods grow faster.
• Producers of organic foods undergo regular inspection to ensure high standards are maintained.
• Organic food production does not contribute to the pollution and degradation of the environment.
• Animal welfare is a priority for organic producers. Animals reared humanely and fed the appropriate diet in free-range environments means better, more nutritious food – which, in turn, means a healthier you.

The bonfire theory
Your body's metabolism works in exactly the same way as a bonfire. But which type? Essentially, there are two types to choose from:
The log bonfire is fed with logs every two to three hours. It takes time to light this fire, but once lit, it burns with intense heat for a long time.
The twig bonfire is easy to light, but soon goes out and emits very little heat.

Eat little and often
If you leave a gap of more than three to four hours between eating, your metabolism will slow down, just like the bonfire that goes out if it is not fed every two to three hours.

If you fuel your body with foods high in sugar, your metabolism will be very sluggish and your body will only be able to perform when you keep taking more sugar. In this scenario, your metabolism is just like the twig bonfire. Your body never burns fat because it is constantly being provided with top-ups of sugar to keep it going.

However, fuelling your body with the correct fats, proteins and natural, slow-releasing carbohydrates will keep your metabolism high and enable your body to use fat as a good energy source – just like the log bonfire. If you can follow this theory for most of your everyday meals, you will be on the way to becoming a healthier person, and you will soon experience an increase in energy levels and improved body shape.

Below: The bonfire analogy is that, fed with nourishing food every few hours, the body will keep going for a long time.

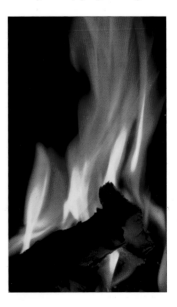

Quality not quantity
You should concentrate on the type of calories that you eat and timing when you eat, rather than focus on the number of calories consumed.

Carbohydrates, Proteins and Fats

These are the three pillars of diet that keep the human body fit, functioning and healthy – as long as they are in correct proportion and balance. All too often, unfortunately, that's not the case. It's time to redress the balance.

A balanced diet consists of three main essential food groups: carbohydrates, protein and fats.

Carbohydrates

There are two types of carbohydrates: simple carbohydrates and complex carbohydrates, also known as sugars and starches. Simple carbohydrates are higher in refined sugars, contain empty calories (non-nutritious) and can cause food cravings and upset your energy levels. Complex carbohydrates are also high in sugars but take longer to digest and absorb and keep blood sugar levels stable.

Good carbs, bad carbs For athletes, a carbohydrate-rich diet is essential for constant energy. For those living a sedentary lifestyle, carbohydrates are less essential. Common foods high in carbohydrate are pasta, bread, potatoes, rice, fruit, vegetables, jams and honey. Carbohydrates account for more than 50 per cent of our daily food intake in

> **Cholesterol and heart disease**
> Found in every cell in the body, cholesterol is an essential lipid for good health. However it is present as two different types of lipoproteins: low-density lipoproteins and high-density lipoproteins. Low-density lipoproteins are the bad guys. They cause surplus fat to build up on the walls of the arteries that supply the heart and brain. High-density lipoproteins are good cholesterols – they are essential for a healthy immune system and for controlling weight.

the developed world, while for our ancestors, they made up less than 35 per cent. We simply eat too much carbohydrate. You can be forgiven for assuming that all carbohydrates are good for you – because some of them are. But take time to work out which ones are, and which are not. For example, most breakfast cereals contain around

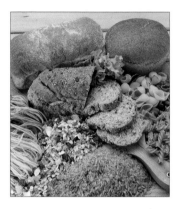

Above: When it is made from whole grains, bread supplies us with fibre, essential fatty acids and some protein.

70g/2.5oz carbohydrate per 100g/3.5oz. Cereal, however, has little nutritional value and will affect your metabolism because the rate of sugar release is too rapid. It can also contain anti-nutrients, which actually stop you absorbing proper nutrients that are vital for digestion and the immune system. Oats, however, are a good source of protein and help to reduce low-density lipid (LDL) cholesterol; the so-called 'bad' cholesterol.

Fruit and vegetables are sources of good carbohydrates. They have a slower rate of energy release and also provide more fibre in your diet. Ultimately, it is not a matter of how much you eat, but what you eat. If you are unsure which carbohydrates are good for you, then choose fruit and vegetables, preferably those that have been grown organically, as they are much more nutritious and tasty.

Proteins

Essential amino acids from proteins help to repair muscle. Fish, poultry, meat, eggs, milk and cheese are examples of protein-rich foods. In the US and most western countries, protein provides only

Food pyramid

The food pyramid suggests how our daily diet should be divided, for optimum nutrition, depending on your age, sex and physical activity.

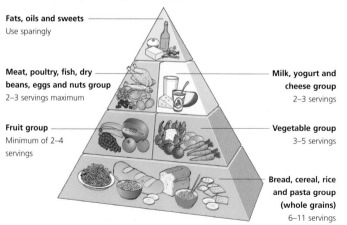

Fats, oils and sweets
Use sparingly

Meat, poultry, fish, dry beans, eggs and nuts group
2–3 servings maximum

Milk, yogurt and cheese group
2–3 servings

Fruit group
Minimum of 2–4 servings

Vegetable group
3–5 servings

Bread, cereal, rice and pasta group (whole grains)
6–11 servings

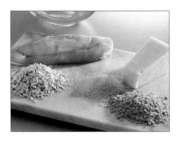

Above: Chicken, cheese, lentils, couscous and oats contain protein, which provides energy and nutrients.

15 per cent of daily food intake. We should be consuming closer to 30–40 per cent. Protein provides useful energy that helps to burn calories and promote weight loss. Without protein, your muscles cannot be fed with the correct nutrients for repair and growth. Some foods contain more protein than others, and those with a higher protein content often contain less fat. For example, the calorie content of two slices of skinless turkey breast contains 3g/0.1oz fat, 0g/0oz carbohydrate, 11g/0.4oz protein, 75 calories, 32 milligrams cholesterol and 1g/0.04oz saturated fat. By comparison, a fried egg contains 7g/0.3oz fat, 1g/0.04oz carbohydrate, 6g/0.2oz protein, 90 calories, 211 milligrams cholesterol and 1.9g/0.07oz saturated fat.

Whereas, today, we mainly get our protein from animals, 10,000 years ago, we obtained it from pulses, nuts and seeds, and animals. Our current over-reliance on animal protein is responsible for the high LDL (bad) cholesterol levels in developed countries. So, take time to compare the labels on the foods that you buy to make sure that the meat and fish you eat is high in protein, and not high in saturated fats.

Fats

The majority of people, particularly overweight people, eat too much fat. Though essential for energy, fat takes a lot longer to break down than carbohydrate. Fat provides energy for long periods of exercise but the exercise intensity has to be lower so that there is a good supply of oxygen available for the fat to burn. Examples of foods high in fats are cheese, butter, oil and some meat. Per gram or ounce, fat provides twice as many calories as carbohydrates and proteins. The World Health Organization recommends that 25–30 per cent of daily calories should come from fat, but most of the population in the developed world get 40–50 per cent of their daily energy from fat.

Saturated and unsaturated fats The problem is not necessarily the amount of fat that you eat but the type of fat. Saturated fats clog arteries and cause poor health, such as heart disease, obesity and cancer. Foods containing saturated fats include meat, eggs, dairy products and foodstuffs containing these ingredients, such as cakes and chocolate, pastries and pies.

Regulating fat intake
- Eat lean meat and cut off visible fat. Choose poultry, where the fat is in the skin and is easy to remove, over red meat.
- Eat oily fish containing polyunsaturated fats (see below)
- Choose low-fat varieties of dairy products and limit the use of butter and spreads.
- For cooking, only use oils that contain lower levels of saturated fat and which also contain monounsaturated and polyunsaturated fats, which help reduce your LDL (bad) cholesterol.
- Eat chocolate, cake and biscuits only on rare occasions.

Unsaturated fats are better for you. They promote high-density lipid (HDL) or good cholesterol and reduce the risk of illness. Oily fish – for example salmon, herring, mackerel, fresh tuna (not canned), anchovies, sardines, kippers and whitebait, among others – are rich in beneficial omega 3 polyunsaturated fat, which can help protect against heart disease. Vegetables oils like sesame, olive, sunflower, corn, soya bean, walnut and canola are sources of monounsaturated and polyunsaturated fats.

Below: Oily fish, such as sardines, mackerel and anchovies are a good source of essential oils. Two to four portions a week are recommended.

Oily fish – recommended weekly portions

The Food Standards Agency (UK) recommends the following portions, according to age and gender:

Age group/gender	Weekly portion
Girls under 16	Up to 2 portions (280g/10oz)
Boys under 16	Up to 4 portions (560g/20oz)
Women over 16	Up to 4 portions (560g/20oz)
Women who are pregnant, who might be pregnant or breastfeeding	Up to 4 portions (560g/20oz)
Men over 16	Up to 4 portions (560g/20oz)

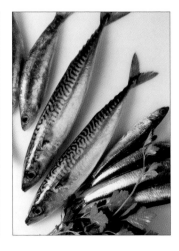

Healthy Eating for Vegetarians

A vegetarian diet can be healthier than a meat-based diet, but it's not just a question of cutting out meat. It takes knowledge and adequate preparation for a meat-free diet to include enough protein, vitamins and minerals for you to stay fit and healthy.

Many people believe that eating a vegetarian diet will help them to lose weight and this can be true, but zero animal fat does not necessarily equate to a low-fat diet. In fact, since vegetarians rely on foods such as eggs, cheese and other dairy products for protein, they can easily consume as much fat as a meat-eater.

A healthy vegetarian diet calls for a finely balanced, closely monitored diet. Adequate protein must be consumed for growth and maintenance of the muscles and for wound healing – otherwise the metabolism will decline, which can result in weight increase. Proteins are also a source of energy.

Below: Vegetarians can select foods such as nuts, grains and seeds to ensure they get sufficient essential nutrients, such as protein.

Protein intake

A vegetarian diet can be deficient in protein. To combat this, make sure that you include eggs and dairy products in your diet. This will also increase the availability of minerals such as calcium, phosphorous and especially vitamin B12, which is otherwise difficult to obtain.

However, dairy intake must also be regulated to prevent weight gain. If you are exercising hard, careful planning is vital to make sure that you can keep up with the demands of your training plan.

What to eat

To achieve a good balance of nutrients and amino acids from a vegetarian diet, you should include a wide variety of foods in your diet. A combination of

RDAs of protein

The following table shows recommended daily amounts (RDAs) of protein. The UK's Department of Health advises vegetarians and vegans to multiply the figure for their age group and gender by a factor of 1.1, because protein from plant sources is harder to digest than other sources.

Boys/girls	RDA
0–12 months	12.5g/0.4oz
1–3 years	14.5g/0.5oz
4–10 years	19.7g/0.7oz
Girls	
11–14 years	41.2g/1.5oz
15–18 years	45g/1.6oz
Boys	
11–14 years	42.1g/1.5oz
15–18 years	55.2g/1.9oz
Women	
19–50	45g/1.58oz
50 +	46.5g/1.6oz
In pregnancy	extra 6g/day
Breastfeeding 0–6 month	extra 11g/day
6 months +	extra 8g/day
Men	
19–50	55.5g/1.9oz
50 +	46.5g/1.6oz

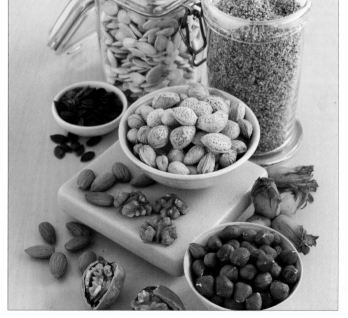

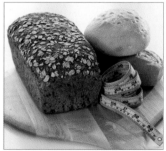

Below: Bread is a carbohydrate, and while it is beneficial, it is not enough to sustain a healthy diet.

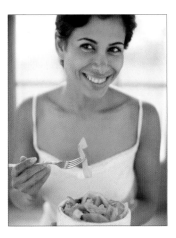

Above: You can't look and feel fit and healthy unless you plan a nutritious diet that includes vegetables and fruits.

foods is vital, as different foods contain different nutrients: grains are rich in sulphur but lack lysine, an essential amino acid, whereas beans, peas and lentils are high in lysine but lack sulphur.

Pros and cons of a veggie diet

Most vegetarian diets are high in carbohydrates, fibre, fruit and vegetables. Health problems such as heart disease, increased blood pressure

Below: Some fats are needed in the diet, but saturated fats such as butter, cheese and ice cream should be eaten sparingly.

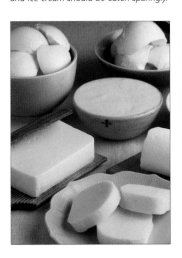

Foods for vegetarians and vegans	

Commonly available foods that provide the most protein in a vegan diet are:

Pulses – peas, beans, lentils and soya products
Grains – wheat, oats, rice, barley, buckwheat, millet, pasta and bread
Nuts – brazil nuts, hazelnuts, almonds and cashew nuts
Seeds – sunflower, pumpkin and sesame
Eggs – hen's eggs
Dairy foods – milk, cheese and yogurt

Foods that provide 10g/0.4oz of protein, eaten in the following amounts:

Eggs	1 whole egg
Low-fat cheese	30g/1.1oz
Low-fat milk	300ml/½ pint/1¼ cups
Low-fat yogurt	300ml/½ pint/1¼ cups
Soya flour	24g/0.8oz
Peanuts	39g/1.4oz
Pumpkin seeds	41g/1.5oz
Almonds	47g/1.7oz
Brazil nuts	50g/1.8oz
Sesame seeds	55g/1.9oz
Hazelnuts	71g/2.5oz
Wholemeal (whole-wheat) bread	95g/3.4oz
Lentils	114g/4oz
Chickpeas	119g/4.2oz
Kidney beans	119g/4.2oz
Wholemeal (whole-wheat) spaghetti	213g/7.5oz
Brown rice	385g/13.6oz

---

and obesity may be reduced due to the low cholesterol and high antioxidant content of a vegetarian diet. However, the lack of low-fat protein can lead to a deficiency in vitamins B6 and B12, and calcium so vegetarians must include quantities of low-fat dairy products,

cereals, nuts and seeds, particularly in the winter months, to ensure that they receive all the necessary nutrients.

Below: Beans and lentils are a source of protein for vegetarians; nuts and rice also contain small amounts of protein.

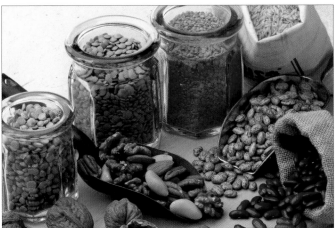

Fluid Intake

Your body is 70 per cent water and you should do your best to keep it that way during exercise, so fluid intake is vital. Fluid loss will depend on the intensity of your exercise, the duration, temperature, humidity and your fitness level.

Muscles produce heat, which makes you sweat. This, in turn, provides a layer of moisture on the skin that helps to keep the core temperature down. Your body's temperature has to remain between 37°C/98.6°F and 38°C/100.4°F for it to function properly. For every 1 litre/ 2 pints of sweat that evaporates, you lose 600kcal of heat energy. A depletion of body fluids is called dehydration.

Below: Dehydration is one of the main causes for poor sporting performance. Your body is 70 per cent water and needs hydration during sporting activities.

It is important to know how to avoid becoming dehydrated, and to recognize the symptoms if you become dehydrated. One simple test is to weigh yourself before and after exercise. Typically, you will lose 1 litre/2 pints of fluid per hour and around 2 litres/4 pints per hour when the temperature and humidity are high.

A 2 per cent weight loss will mean a 20 per cent decrease in performance; lose 4 per cent and you may have nausea, vomiting and diarrhoea; 5 per cent and your brain will start to shut down; 7 per cent and you hallucinate; 10 per cent and heatstroke sets in.

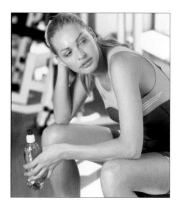

Above: Always carry water with you so you can keep well hydrated at all times in training at the gym.

Exercise and hydration

To avoid dehydration, drink plenty of fluids before, during and after exercise. Drink 400–600ml/13–20fl oz of fluid in the two hours before exercise. It may be fairly easy to drink on a bike, but it is much harder to drink during activities such as running, so make sure that you have plenty of fluid in your system before you start exercising. It is not possible to take in extra fluid and store it. Above a certain level, your body will pass it as urine. Include some carbohydrates in a drink, such as simple sugars: 1g/0.04oz of carbohydrate for every 1kg/2.2lb of body weight, or 14g/0.5oz per 18kg/40lb will help to sustain energy levels.

To maintain the exercise intensity level during exercise, you must replace 80 per cent of your fluid loss during exercise.

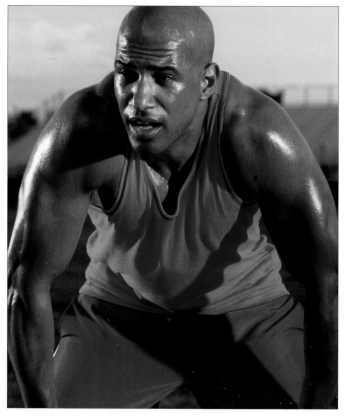

Dehydration test
Check the colour of your urine – the darker the urine, the more dehydrated you have become.

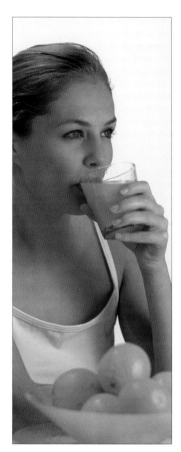

Above: Staying hydrated means you will need to calculate how much fluid to drink, how often and what your fluids should contain.

Try to drink before you feel thirsty. Aim to drink 400–1,000ml/13–34fl oz per hour. If you leave it too long, you may end up feeling sick and bloated. Drink plain water if exercise lasts up to 1 hour. For longer exercise sessions, use sports drinks that contain hypotonic or isotonic solutions, which will help with water absorption; and glucose polymers, which will allow you to absorb a greater quantity of carbohydrate to keep your energy levels high.

The following is a guide to which drinks are best according to the exercise you are doing:

• Isotonic: Use for middle- or long-distance running events and team sports. It provides glucose, the body's preferred source of energy. For a concentration of 6–10 per cent, for example, try Lucozade Sport, 515g/18oz, and High Five; or mix 200ml/6.7fl oz orange squash, 1 litre/2 pints water and 1g/0.04oz salt.

• Hypotonic: Use for car racing and horse-racing. It quickly replaces fluid loss but contains no carbohydrate; mix 100ml/3.4fl oz orange squash, 1 litre/2 pints water and 1g/0.04oz salt.

• Hypertonic: Use to top up carbohydrate during long-distance events. It is suitable when energy is required for long periods, can be taken on the move and is easy to digest; mix 400ml/13.5fl oz orange squash, 1 litre/2 pints water and 1g/0.04oz salt.

After exercise To enable a fast, efficient recovery, slowly drink 1.5 litres/3 pints of fluid for every 1kg/2.2lb of weight loss. Between exercise sessions, drink 1 litre/2 pints for every 1,000kcal of energy expenditure.

Overhydration

It is possible to overhydrate if you drink too much. This leads to circulatory problems and dizziness as the blood becomes too diluted, or even seizures or coma if overhydration occurs quickly. If you suspect that you are overhydrated, stop drinking and consume something salty, as your sodium levels will probably have become dangerously low.

Caffeine

Your performance can be improved by caffeine; it helps your body to use fatty acids instead of glycogen, which will enable you to exercise at a high intensity for longer. But more than 300mg of caffeine can be detrimental to your health, as it may cause dehydration (a cup of coffee typically contains 50–100mg of caffeine). Increase your water intake to counteract the dehydrating effect of caffeine.

Alcohol

There are very few benefits to drinking alcohol. It may be useful in social situations – even then, in moderation only – but beyond that, there's little to recommend it. It will affect your reaction time and co-ordination, and you will experience a decline in your speed, power and strength. It will hinder your body's ability to regulate temperature and can lead to blood-sugar level problems and dehydration. The empty calories in alcohol will also lead to weight gain. If you do choose to drink alcohol, make sure that you also drink plenty of water to dilute its effects and reduce the risk of dehydration.

Below: Drinking tea and coffee will make you even more dehydrated. It is best to stick to water or juice.

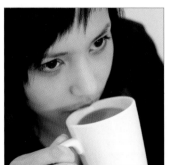

Below: Lack of fluid can make you prone to headaches, lower your energy levels and make you feel unwell.

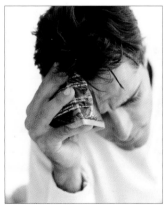

Vitamins and Minerals

The importance of vitamins and minerals is well known, but where do they come from and what are they for? The information below highlights some of the most important vitamins and minerals, their uses and where to find them.

Vitamins are essential for your body to function properly. Vitamins fall into two categories: fat-soluble and water-soluble. Fat-soluble vitamins are found in animal fats and other fatty foods. These vitamins are stored in the body for long periods of time. They are available when you need them, so you do not have to eat fatty foods every day.

Water-soluble vitamins can be found in a wide variety of foods. Unlike fat-soluble vitamins, these are not stored in the body, so you need to make sure that you have an adequate amount of them in your daily diet. Don't take too many vitamins especially vitamins A, D, E and K as the body finds it harder to get rid of the excess in the urine. To get the most from your food, steam it or eat it raw. Baking, grilling and frying all lower the vitamin content of food. Be aware that as fruit and vegetables age they lose their vitamin content, so try to eat fruit and vegetables that are as fresh as possible. Frozen vegetables from the supermarket, in which the vitamin content has been preserved, are often better than fresh.

Trace elements

Compared with vitamins and minerals, far smaller amounts of trace elements are required for optimum health, proper growth and development. With today's modern diet and cooking methods, there is concern that the body is not getting an adequate supply of trace elements.

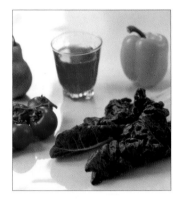

Above: Discover what vitamins are present in your vegetables so that you can design a balanced diet.

It is possible to take supplements but the correct dosage is difficult to work out because different foods and diets have varying concentrations of trace elements, and their rate of absorption also differs. It is better to consume trace elements as part of your daily diet.

Below: Citrus fruits such as oranges and lemons are rich in vitamin C, which is essential in the diet for healthy skin, joints, bones and the immune system.

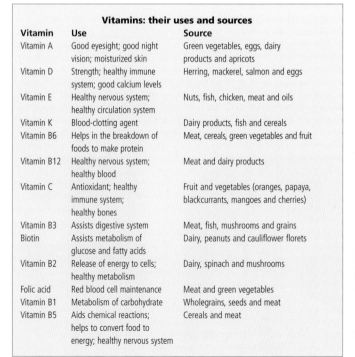

Vitamins: their uses and sources		
Vitamin	**Use**	**Source**
Vitamin A	Good eyesight; good night vision; moisturized skin	Green vegetables, eggs, dairy products and apricots
Vitamin D	Strength; healthy immune system; good calcium levels	Herring, mackerel, salmon and eggs
Vitamin E	Healthy nervous system; healthy circulation system	Nuts, fish, chicken, meat and oils
Vitamin K	Blood-clotting agent	Dairy products, fish and cereals
Vitamin B6	Helps in the breakdown of foods to make protein	Meat, cereals, green vegetables and fruit
Vitamin B12	Healthy nervous system; healthy blood	Meat and dairy products
Vitamin C	Antioxidant; healthy immune system; healthy bones	Fruit and vegetables (oranges, papaya, blackcurrants, mangoes and cherries)
Vitamin B3	Assists digestive system	Meat, fish, mushrooms and grains
Biotin	Assists metabolism of glucose and fatty acids	Dairy, peanuts and cauliflower florets
Vitamin B2	Release of energy to cells; healthy metabolism	Dairy, spinach and mushrooms
Folic acid	Red blood cell maintenance	Meat and green vegetables
Vitamin B1	Metabolism of carbohydrate	Wholegrains, seeds and meat
Vitamin B5	Aids chemical reactions; helps to convert food to energy; healthy nervous system	Cereals and meat

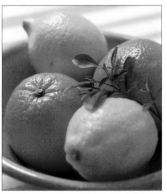

Essential minerals and trace elements

Daily consumption of the following minerals and trace elements is essential in order for your body to function efficiently. They help the body turn the food you eat into energy and maintain a healthy body. Deficiencies in vitamins and minerals lead to illness.

Mineral	Use	Source	Daily amounts
Sodium	Healthy water balance	Cereals, bread and dairy	6g/0.2oz
Magnesium	Structure of bone and tendons	Wholegrains, cereals, fruit, cocoa and seeds	Men 300mg; Women 270mg
Iron	Maintains red blood cells; oxygen in blood	Meat, raisins and kidney beans	Men 8.7mg; Women 14.8mg
Calcium	Strong bones and teeth; helps convert food to energy; healthy muscular nervous system	Dairy, sardines, broccoli and dark green vegetables	700mg
Potassium	Healthy muscular nervous system; maintains fluid balance	Nuts, fruit, broccoli, mushrooms and seeds	3,500mg
Phosphorus	Strong bones and teeth; helps convert food to energy; healthy muscular nervous system	Dairy, chicken, eggs and nuts	550mg

Trace element	Use	Source	Daily amounts
Selenium	Antioxidant; aids metabolism	Fish, eggs, meat and cereals	200mcg
Manganese	Bone structure; aids metabolism	Bread, nuts, cereals, vegetables, soya beans and chickpeas are good sources	5mg
Molybdenum	Metabolism of proteins	Nuts, wholegrains	500mcg
Zinc	Healthy skin; immune system	Meat, fish and dairy	15mg
Iodine	Healthy nervous system; cell maintenance	Fish (haddock, mackerel, herring, trout and salmon are good sources), salt and vegetables	75mcg
Chromium	Regulates blood-sugar levels	Dairy, wholegrains and meat	200mcg
Fluoride	Teeth and bones	Fish	3mg

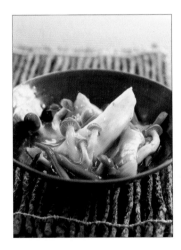

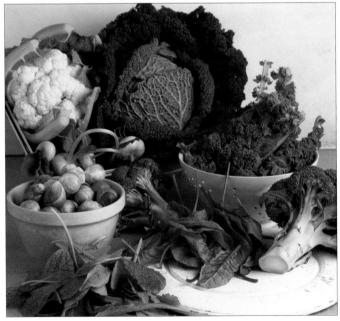

Above: Steaming vegetables seals in the flavour and retains taste and food value.

Right: You will need a variety of vegetables to get all the essential minerals and vitamins you need.

Glycaemic Index

Using the GI system, carbohydrate foods are divided into three categories – low, medium and high – according to the speed with which they raise the body's blood-sugar levels compared with pure glucose.

Carbohydrates with a high glycaemic index (GI) release sugar fast, and are far more likely to cause you to put on weight and therefore slow your athletic performance. The reason for this is a complex glucose–insulin reaction that takes place in your body when you eat. Your body needs to produce glucose from food in order to survive. This production can be rapid or slow, depending on the GI of the food consumed. High GI foods lead to the rapid production of blood glucose,

which in turn has a feedback response that can lead to the body releasing high levels of insulin in an attempt to deal with high glucose levels in the blood. This will then turn the glucose into fat, causing weight gain and, over time – if

left unchecked – obesity and type II diabetes, which are currently reaching epidemic proportions in developed societies, among young children and adults. There is evidence, however, that some people who eat a lot of high GI

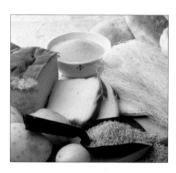

Above: Some foods affect your blood sugar more than others; using the GI system will help you choose carefully.

Below: People with type II diabetes need to test for blood sugar regularly. Understanding the glycaemic index will help you deal with diabetes.

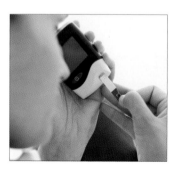

High, medium and low GI foods

Breakfast
High GI: most refined cereals with added sugar
Medium GI: porridge and fruit muesli
Low GI: oat meal, rolled oats, natural muesli and rice bran

Breads
High GI: white, French bread, bagel and black rye bread
Medium GI: pitta bread, wholemeal (whole-wheat), wholemeal roll and fruit bread
Low GI: soy bread, sourdough rye, wholegrain and pumpernickel

Dairy
High GI: ice cream and cheesecake
Medium GI: fruit yogurts
Low GI: full-fat (whole) milk, semi-skimmed (low-fat) milk, skimmed milk and natural yogurt

Vegetables
High GI: parsnips, pumpkin, turnips, swedes (rutabagas), carrots, squashes and pumpkins
Medium GI: beetroots (beets), corn on the cob, kidney beans, pinto beans, dried green peas and carrots
Low GI: peas, corn, broccoli, cauliflower florets, onions, peppers, tomatoes, cabbages, mushrooms, lettuces, aubergines (eggplant), courgettes (zucchini), sprouts, cucumbers, green beans, rocket (arugula), spinach, asparagus, artichokes, kale, radishes and celery sticks

Fruit
High GI: watermelons, dates, bananas, raisins, dried apricots, dried peaches, dried apples, pineapples and cantaloupe melon, canned fruits in syrup
Medium GI: papayas, mangoes, blueberries, sultanas (golden raisins), figs, pears, grapes, orange juice, apple juice, grapefruit juice and fruit cocktail
Low GI: prunes, peaches, pears, grapefruits, apples, kiwi fruits, cherries, plums, apricots, raspberries, strawberries, blueberries, blackberries and avocados

Staples
High GI: white rice, mashed potato and French fries
Medium GI: gnocchi, basmati rice, cornmeal, couscous, baked potato, wild rice, buckwheat, barley, noodles and new potatoes
Low GI: wholemeal (whole-wheat) spaghetti, quinoa and egg noodles

Snacks
High GI: rice cakes, biscuits (cookies), doughnuts, cakes, pretzels, jelly babies and wine gums (fruit candy), jam, French fries, potato crisps (chips)
Medium GI: muffins, oatmeal cookies, muesli bars and chocolate bars
Low GI: cashew nuts, peanuts, mixed nuts and raisins, carrot cake, seeds, hummus and peanut butter

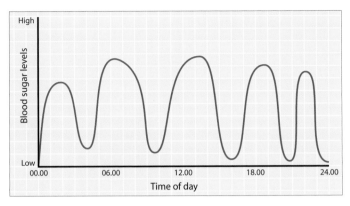

Above: High GI foods can cause sharp increases and falls in blood sugar through the day, as this chart shows.

foods – in Asia and Peru, for example – do not suffer high levels of obesity or diabetes. This is because they also eat a lot of fresh fruit and vegetables, which counteract the effect of the high GI foods. Mixing high and low GI foods produces moderate GI values.

Foods with a low GI have little effect on your body's blood-sugar level because it takes the body a long time to

Below: To keep sugar levels balanced, mix high GI foods with those which have a lower GI.

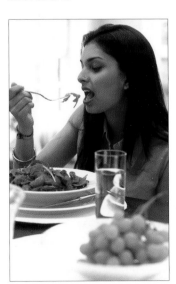

metabolize them. Foods with a high GI, however, cause an immediate increase in blood-sugar levels.

Advantages of a low GI diet

Eating low GI foods will help you to lose weight, reduce the risk of certain cancers, increase the amount of fibre in your diet, decrease the chances of developing type II diabetes and coronary heart disease, boost your immune system, and increase your stamina and energy levels. There are no disadvantages to eating low GI foods.

Below: Before a competition, eat the right mix of high and low GI foods for optimum performance.

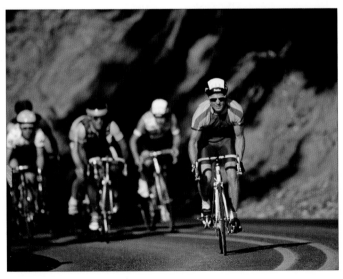

Surprisingly high

You may be surprised to find that some of your favourite foods are high GI. To help balance your body's blood-sugar levels, and to give you energy for the whole day, you should avoid or cut down on these foods. Following the principles of the GI will help you to lose weight, improve your sporting performance and aid recovery after exercise.

Athletes

Ultra-marathon runners and Ironman triathletes who take part in events lasting more than two hours, have become increasingly aware of the importance of the GI value of foods taken before and after competition. In preparation for training or events, athletes need to consume low GI foods in order to release energy slowly. During their training or event, athletes should try to balance high and low GI foods to maintain their energy levels on an even keel.

Mix high and low

If you still feel the need to include some high GI foods in your diet, make sure you counteract the effect of the high GI food by also eating lots of foods that have a low GI.

Eating to Lose Weight

Fad diets are everywhere and promise miraculous results. In truth, however, beyond healthy book sales and magazine circulation figures, they do little good. Long-term weight loss involves a realistic plan that encompasses lifestyle, diet and exercise.

No single diet, whether it is low fat, reduced calorie or low carbohydrate, will help you to maintain your new size once you have lost the initial weight. One of the first things all of these diets do is lower your normal calorie intake. This will cause you to lose weight, but much of this weight loss will be muscle, which you need to retain, because it is living tissue that helps you to maintain a high metabolism and keep you trim. If you want to lose weight, and keep it off, you need to change your lifestyle and eating habits. Another important factor is to understand the relationship between what you eat and what you look like. Also regular exercise will help you in your goal.

Here are 16 steps that will help you to lose weight:

1 Portion control This is one of the fastest ways to lose weight. If you use a smaller plate, and don't pile food up, you will soon find that your stomach starts to shrink and that you feel full

Below: When you are trying to lose weight, choose ingredients for your meal that are fresh and healthy.

after eating less food. Aim to eat 80 per cent of what you think you need at each meal.

2 Eat slowly Chew each mouthful at least 20 times before you swallow it. Taking longer to eat your food will send a signal to your brain to register that your stomach is full. While you are chewing, put your knife and fork down to create a slight pause between mouthfuls. Again, this will enable you to feel full before you have time to have a second plateful.

3 Leave leftovers Only eat the food on your plate if you really need it. There is no shame in not finishing a meal, especially if you are out in a restaurant and you have been presented with a larger portion than you wanted.

4 Less fat Eat less fatty food. In particular, avoid eating fat from foods that have been processed. Also, cook with less fat to avoid adding extra fat to your meal.

5 More fruit and vegetables A low-calorie way to feel full is to eat lots of fruit and vegetables. Eating more of these foods will also help to increase the fibre in your diet, which will help

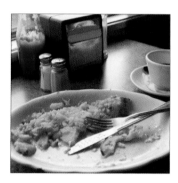

Above: Don't feel you always have to finish everything on your plate – stop eating when you are satisfied.

to lower your cholesterol level. Aim for at least five portions of fruit and vegetables each day.

6 Read the label Be wary of foods that are labelled 'low fat'. They may be low in saturated fats but the likelihood is that they are high in sugar, which will

Below: Eat foods that are not processed and are as natural as possible so you know what is in them.

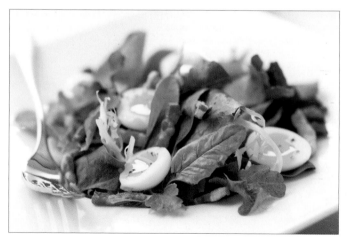

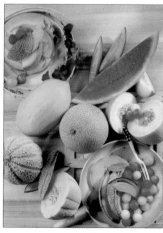

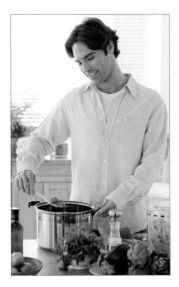

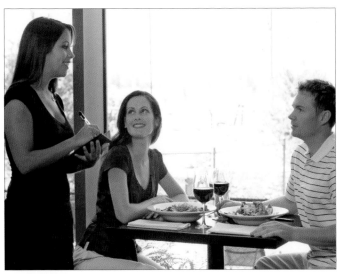

Above: Above: If you need to lose weight, select low-fat foods, such as fruits and vegetables, and control the portion size.

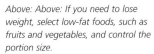

Above: If you are trying to lose weight, and you eat in a restaurant, ask about the ingredients and how the food is cooked so you can make the right choice.

have the effect of raising your blood sugar, then your insulin levels and make you deposit fat.

7 Low GI Eat low GI foods to prevent your body becoming insulin-resistant (a pre-diabetic state in which normal amounts of insulin are no longer sufficient to produce a normal insulin response from fat, muscle and liver cells). Eating low GI foods will keep your blood-sugar levels constant and enable you to feel good and crave healthy foods.

8 Be prepared When travelling, take with you food such as nuts and fruits, so that you don't have to rely on what is on offer at the service station or garage and be tempted to buy chocolate.

9 Little and often Eat small meals regularly to make sure that your metabolism is working all the time. Don't let yourself go hungry, because your body will then go into 'famine mode' and start to store all the calories, thinking it won't be fed again for a while.

10 Drink more water You might often think that you are hungry when, in fact, you are just thirsty. Avoid excessive

calories from other beverages such as fizzy drinks and alcohol. Aim for eight 200ml/6.7-fl oz glasses per day.

11 Avoid sugary snacks You may think that just one sugary snack a day won't do much harm when you count the small number of calories in it. However, the knock-on effect on your energy levels, and the associated problems with insulin levels, should not be underestimated.

12 Ask about what you are eating If you are eating out, find out what the ingredients of a dish are, and don't be embarrassed to ask the chef to omit a sauce, dressing or gravy, if necessary.

13 Get active No matter how healthily you eat, if you don't do any activity, you will not be able to burn off calories. You need to be burning off more calories in a day than you consume in order to lose weight.

14 Slowly does it Don't rush it – aim to lose weight at a sensible speed. A loss of 0.5–1kg/1.1–2.2lb per week is sustainable, and will give your body a chance to adjust to the changes it is going through.

15 Obstacles Note down anything that gets in the way of losing weight, then work out ways that you can get around these obstacles.

16 Downfalls List the foods that made you put on weight in the first place. You need to understand which foods are bad for you in order to make yourself avoid them altogether by not buying them or, at least, cut down on the amount you eat.

Below: Sugary snacks such as chocolate will be detrimental to weight loss; instead, opt for fruit or nuts.

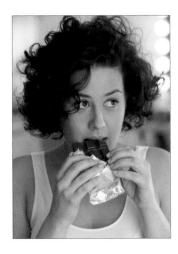

Eating to Gain Muscle

Some people think that hour after hour at the gym is all they need to build muscle. You can train all day long, but if you don't put the right fuel into your body, your muscles will fail to recover after exercising and simply will not grow.

To gain muscle, you need to adopt a diet that is rich in carbohydrate and protein, with some fat. Choose low GI foods over high GI ones and consider including a dietary supplement.

Small and frequent meals will help to increase metabolism, burn more fat and give you better muscle definition – great definition will make your muscles look bigger, even if they aren't. Eat little and often; every three to four hours to avoid going into a catabolic state, in which your body starts to eat muscle to get energy, resulting in more fat and less muscle.

A balanced diet

Each meal should consist of 40 per cent carbohydrate, 40 per cent protein and 20 per cent fat. You need protein to build muscle and carbohydrates to give you the energy to turn protein into muscle. Fats are also important, as every cell in the body has fat in it and hormones are made from fats. Choose unsaturated fats – good sources are fish oils, peanut butter and olive oil.

Testosterone is the most important hormone as far as muscle growth is concerned. A low-fat diet leads to low

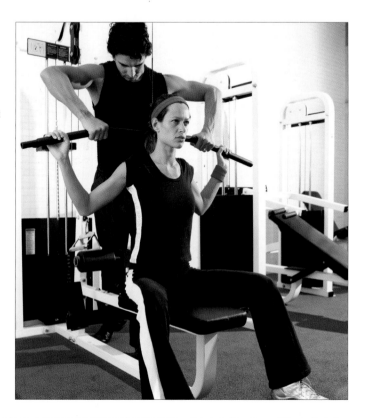

Above: Putting in a sustained effort at each session in the gym will pay off over time as you get fitter.

Left: Protein, such as a lean steak, is an essential nutrient for repairing and building muscles.

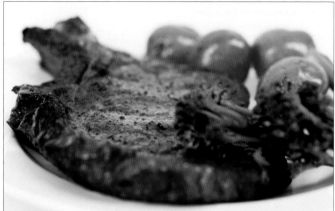

Measure fat

You should aim to gain around 250g/0.5lb of muscle per week. If you gain any more than that, you will be in danger of putting on fat instead of muscle. In addition to using the scales, measure your body fat on a regular basis.

levels of testosterone, and therefore no muscle growth. Every tissue in the body is made from protein, so it is very important to maintain a high-protein diet, especially if you need to repair damaged tissue after exercise.

Protein levels

For basic training of up to an hour a day, you need to consume 2.5g/0.08oz of protein per 1kg/2.2lb of body weight. If you aim to train hard and gain muscle, you will need to increase this to 3–4g/0.10–0.14oz of protein per 1kg/2lb of body weight, or approximately 57–85g/2–3oz per 18kg/40lb.

There is no point in eating more than 4g/0.14oz of protein per 1kg/2.2lb of body weight, or approximately 3oz per 40lb, as your body cannot utilize more than this quantity of protein.

Low GI and high fibre

Eat low GI foods for a sustained slow, but constant release of energy, and to maximize recovery of your muscles. Always include fibre in your diet. Five to ten servings of fruit and vegetables a day will help to keep your digestive system working efficiently, which is especially important if you are eating extra protein. Fibre will slow down the digestion of the protein giving your body more time to absorb the amino acids.

Below: Peanut butter provides essential fats and protein for building muscles and a long steady release of energy.

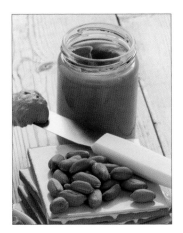

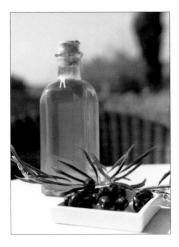

Above: Avoid saturated fats; choose healthy oils instead, such as olive oil or various types of nut oils.

Food supplements

Creatine supplementation will help to increase muscle mass. It is possible to gain up to 3 per cent muscle mass in one week, if you consume 7g/0.25oz of creatine a day. Creatine works by dragging water into the cells, which then stimulate protein synthesis.

There are some side effects – water retention, cramping, kidney and muscle damage and dehydration. The best form of creatine is creatine monohydrate, which is readily available and easy for the body to utilize.

People with fewer fast-twitch muscle fibres may struggle to get the maximum benefit from taking creatine. If you are a long-distance athlete looking to put on weight, use creatine after meals containing carbohydrates, as the increase in the insulin level after the meal can help with the uptake of creatine into the muscle cells. Drink plenty of water after taking creatine to compensate for its dehydrating effect.

Meal-replacement drinks If you lead a busy lifestyle, it can be hard to prepare meals with enough calories and nutritional value. A meal-replacement drink (MRP) will take care of that. Most MRP drinks contain essential amino acids and creatine

Calorie count

If you are attempting to put on muscle, try increasing your carbohydrate consumption to 50 per cent and your fat consumption to 25 per cent, while decreasing your protein consumption to 25 per cent. This will mean that instead of consuming 12 calories per 500g/1.1lb of body weight, which is an average amount, you will double your calories and consume 24 calories per 500g/1.1lb of body weight. Extra calories are essential if you want to put on more muscle, especially if you are burning off more energy because you have recently stepped up your physical training.

and glutamine to aid recovery and promote muscle growth. They typically contain 40g/1.4oz of protein and 60g/2oz of carbohydrates.

Exercise and rest

To prevent calories from being burnt, avoid cardiovascular exercise and ensure you do appropriate weight-training. Use free weights to work throughout the entire movement and provide good stability. Rest is very important. If your body has maximum recovery after a workout, it will also have maximum potential for growth.

Below: Adding protein and fruit shakes to your diet will ensure that you get a supply of high-quality protein.

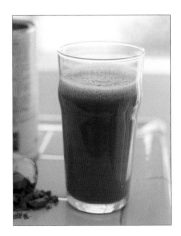

Index

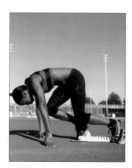

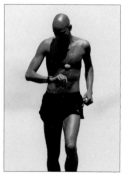

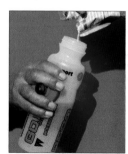

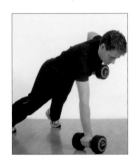
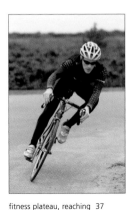

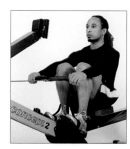
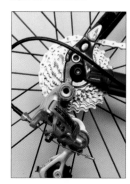

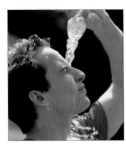

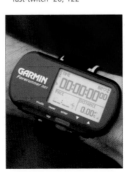

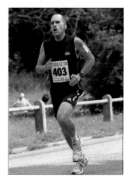

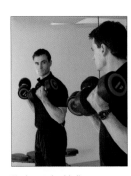
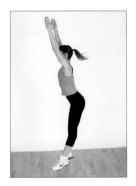

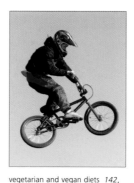

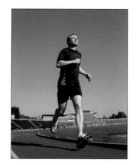

Acknowledgements

Picture Credits

l=left, r=right, t=top, b=bottom, bl=bottom left, br=bottom right, c=centre, tr=top right.

2:09 events: 86, 114b, 158t, 165tl, 171br.

Alamy: 21b, 230, 369bl, 372bl, 372br, 375bl, 407tr, 408b.

Andy Jones: 212t, 256t, 261tl, 263t, 264b, 268, 279c, 322, 324br.

Banayote Photography: 95b.

The Boston Marathon: 88b.

Peter Bull illustration: 26, 27, 39, 70, 71, 72, 73, 75.

MHFS 10k for Men: 108b.

Corbis: 10, 16, 17t, 17b, 21t, 47tl, 47tr, 58, 82t, 87, 90t, 90b, 93t, 96t, 97t, 97b, 111t, 119, 126t, 128, 129t, 130t, 130b, 132t, 132b, 133, 136, 137b, 140t, 141b, 141tr, 142b, 152t, 156b, 164b, 167b, 170t, 170b, 182, 183br, 194, 188, 190, 191, 192l, 201t, 201bl, 202t, 206 (both), 207b, 207tl, 208r, 214b, 214tc, 216, 217, 234tr, 242 (all), 243 (both), 244, 246t, 247bl, 247br, 249 (both), 251tc, 259br, 264tr, 267tr, 277b, 278t, 281tl, 309tl, 309bl, 309br, 315tr, 315b, 340br, 342, 343bl, 344br, 355tr, 355bl, 370 (both), 372t, 373bl, 374tr, 376bl, 378tr, 379tl, 379tc, 379bl, 406, 407b, 408t, 415bl, 424bl, 470bl, 471tr, 471bc, 491br, 494tr, 500tr, 502t, 503tc.

Peter Drake: 237 (all).

The Flora London Marathon: 96b.

Fotolibra: 233tr, 235t, 240 (both), 241t, 245tr, 245bl, 245br, 306, 307 (all).

Geoff Waugh: 204, 205 (all), 218t, 221bl, 232l, 282, 283, 284 (both), 285 (both), 286 (both), 287 (all), 288 (both), 289 (both), 290 (all), 291 (all), 292 (both), 293 (all), 294 (both), 295 (all), 296 (all), 297 (all), 298, 299 (all), 300 (both), 301 (all), 302 (all), 303 (all), 304 (both), 305 (all), 308, 309tr, 310 (both), 311 (all), 312 (both), 313 (all), 316, 346, 347, 348, 349 (all), 350 (both), 351 (all), 352 (both), 353 (all), 354 (all), 355bl, 361tr.

Getty Images: 93b, 94t, 95t, 127, 135br, 135bl, 135t, 137t, 181t, 234b, 245tl, 248t, 278bl, 367, 368tr, 368bl, 369, 371tl, 371b, 373cl, 373r, 374, 377bl, 377bc, 377br, 381br, 382 (both), 385cr, 385bl, 386 (all), 394, 395, 397tc, 397tr, 397b, 398t, 399b, 401tr, 402t, 404 (both), 405 (both), 414tl, 414tr, 414br, 415br, 419, 420t, 422l, 423tr, 425 (both), 468, 474br, 476bl, 486, 487, 488tc, 488bl, 488bc, 489br, 492br, 493tl, 494bl, 495bc, 495br, 498bl, 500bl, 500br, 501tr, 501br, 502bl, 503br.

Pete Hartley: 85t, 177t.

iStockphoto: 38br, 53t, 57t, 55br, 78t, 79t, 80b, 122bl, 148bl, 150b, 165tr, 208l, 209l, 232r, 236bl, 236br, 238tr, 238tl, 241b, 246b, 250t, 261br, 378bl, 407tl.

Mike King: 18bl, 18br, 20b, 22bl, 22bc, 23, 28l, 28tc, 28tr, 29t (3 pics), 29bl, 29bc, 32t, 34b, 35bl, 35br, 37tr, 44, 46t, 48br, 48bl, 49b, 50b, 51t, 55t, 55b, 56b, 57bl, 60b, 62t, 72tl, 72tr, 76b, 77tl, 77tr, 82bl, 84b, 85b, 107b, 109br, 118, 120 (all), 121 (all), 131 (all), 152br, 170t, 174b, 175tr, 179br, 180tr, 201br.

Philip O'Connor: 13, 14, 15, 19t, 20b, 24t, 25br, 30 (all), 31 (all), 32b, 34t, 35tl, 35tr, 36, 37tl, 37tr, 38l, 40(all), 41 (all), 42, 43, 45t, 45b, 46b, 49tr, 50t, 51b, 52t, 52b, 53b, 56t, 59, 62b, 68, 71tr, 73br, 74, 76t, 88t, 89t, 91b, 98, 102, 103t, 107t, 108, 112t, 113bl, 113br, 114t, 116br, 117t, 122t, 122bc, 122br, 123(all), 124 (all), 125 (all), 134, 138, 143t, 148t, 149b, 152bl, 153, 154br, 156t, 160t, 160b, 162, 164, 165b, 168t, 168b, 169, 171 (all), 173bl, 173bc, 173br, 174t, 175tc, 175tl (x2), 176b, 177, 180b, 181b, 184, 185, 192t, 193 (both), 194, 195 (all), 196 (all), 197 (all), 198 (both), 199tl, 199c, 199r, 200 (both), 202b, 203t, 203c, 203br, 210 (both), 211 (all), 212bl, 212bc, 214tr, 215 (both), 218bl, 218br, 219 (all), 220 (all), 221tl, 221tc, 221tr, 221c, 222 (both), 223 (all), 224 (all), 225 (all), 226 (all), 227 (all), 228 (all), 229 (all), 233t, 233c, 233b, 238b, 251tl, 252, 253, 254, 255, 2560b, 257 (both), 258, 259tl, 259tc, 259tr, 259bl, 262t, 265t, 265c, 266t, 267tl, 268b, 269tl, 170b, 171 (all), 272 (both), 273, 279b, 319, 320 (both), 321tr, 321bl, 321br, 322bl, 323 (all), 324tl, 325 (both), 326 (both), 327 (all), 328, 329 (all), 330, 331 (all), 332 (both), 333 (both), 334t, 334bl, 335 (all), 356, 357 (all), 358, 359 (all), 360 (all), 361 (all), 362, 363, 364-5, 366, 368tl, 375t, 377t, 380 (both), 381tl, 381tr, 381bl, 383 (all), 384, 385tl, 385tr, 387 (both), 388 (all), 389 (all), 390 (both), 391 (all), 392 (both), 393 (all), 396, 398bl, 399t, 400 (all), 401tl, 401b, 403 (all), 409, 410, 411 (all), 412, 413 (all), 414bl, 416 (all), 417 (all), 618, 420b, 421 (both), 426, 427bl, 427bc, 427br, 428–467, 470cl, 472, 473 (all), 476cr, 477 (all), 478–485.

Offside: 218, 274, 275, 276, 277t, 280 (both), 281tr, 281b, 334br, 338 (both), 339 (all), 340 tl, 340tr, 340bl, 341 (all), 243tl, 243t, 344tr, 344bl, 345 (both).

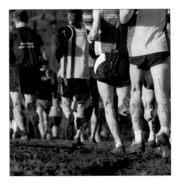

Photolibrary: 235b.

Photoshot: 239, 247c, 314, 315tl, 376tl, 379tr, 501tl.

Race for the Cure: 89b, 92t.

Runner's World Magazine: 18t, 19b, 22t, 28br, 29br, 49tl, 54, 63tl, 63tr, 84t, 91t, 92b, 99, 100, 101, 103b, 104t, 105, 110, 111br, 140b, 112b, 117b, 139, 149t, 155t, 162b, 163, 166, 167t, 167bl, 167br, 171t, 171bl, 173t, 175b, 176t, 178b, 179t, 179bl, 180tl, 183bl.

Superstock: 203bl, 209tr, 209b, 236t, 248t, 250b, 321tl, 427tl

Triathlon magazine: 336 (both), 337 (all).

Wheelbase: 199b, 207tc, 207t, 231, 266bl.

The author and publishers would like to thank the following individuals for their valuable contributions to this book and the companies who kindly supplied their expertise, picture research, equipment, clothing and locations for photography:

Keith Anderson, Rupert Elkington-Cole, Margaret and Scott Dick, Mike Gratton, Suzi Hall, Steven Seaton, Steve Smythe, Brooks, Karen, Sarah, Helen, her family, and the staff of *Runner's World* magazine (UK), Endura, Evans Cycles, Greenwich Leisure Ltd (GLL) Hawkes BMX Club, Triathlon magazine, Zyro

Models: Tyler Bowcombe, Emily Crompton, Elise Dick, Dan Duguid, Michael Egbor, Jo Freeman, Christophe Fromont, Chanelle Garnett, Suzi Hall (www.innovatefitness.com), Elizabeth Hufton, Sharon Knight, Mark Leary, Catherine Lee, Cressida Lorenz, Freddie Lorenz, David McCombes, Sophie Meer, Amber Milligan, Andrew Milligan, Jay Milligan, Philip Mosley, Jamie Newall, George Pagliero, Russ Peake, Edward Pickering, Rebecca Rideout, Jessica Rideout, Oliver Stafford.

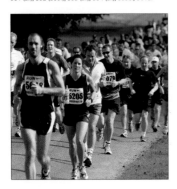

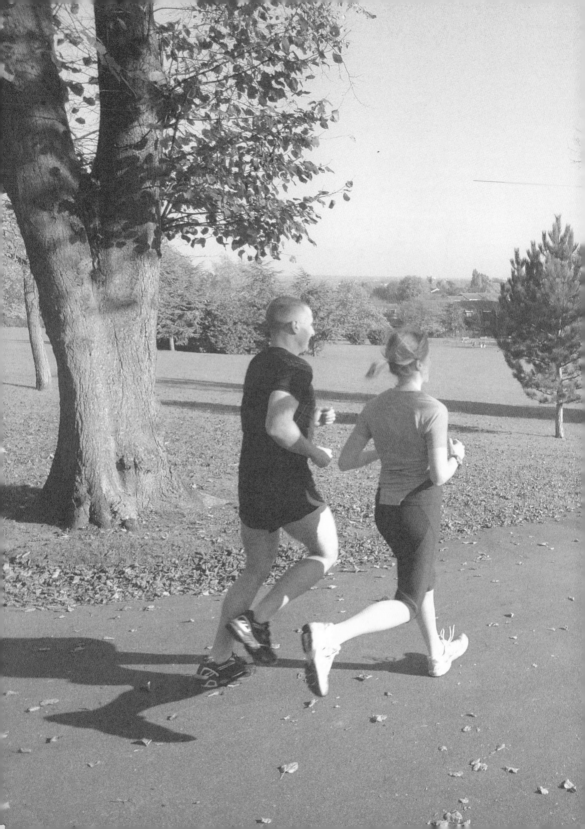